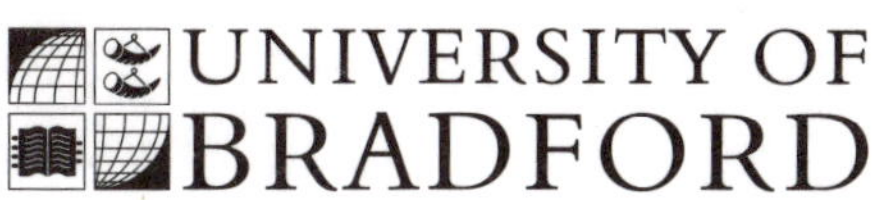

COMPUTER APPLICATIONS IN PHARMACEUTICAL RESEARCH AND DEVELOPMENT

WILEY SERIES IN DRUG DISCOVERY AND DEVELOPMENT

Binghe Wang, Series Editor

Computer Applications in Pharmaceutical Research and Development
Edited by Sean Ekins

COMPUTER APPLICATIONS IN PHARMACEUTICAL RESEARCH AND DEVELOPMENT

SEAN EKINS, M.SC., PH.D., D.SC.

WILEY-INTERSCIENCE
A JOHN WILEY & SONS, INC., PUBLICATION

Published by John Wiley & Sons, Inc., Hoboken, New Jersey
Published simultaneously in Canada

For general information on our other products and services or for technical support, please contact our Customer Care Department within the United States at (800) 762-2974, outside the United States at (317) 572-3993 or fax (317) 572-4002.

Wiley also publishes its books in a variety of electronic formats. Some content that appears in print may not be available in electronic formats. For more information about Wiley products, visit our web site at www.wiley.com.

Library of Congress Cataloging-in-Publication Data:

Computer applications in pharmaceutical research and development / [edited by] Sean Ekins.
p. ; cm.—(Wiley series in drug discovery and development)
Includes bibliographical references and index.
ISBN-13: 978-0-471-73779-7 (cloth)
ISBN-10: 0-471-73779-8 (cloth)
1. Pharmacy—Data processing. 2. Pharmacology—Data processing. 3. Pharmaceutical industry—Data processing. I. Ekins, Sean. II. Series.
[DNLM: 1. Drug Industry. 2. Medical Informatics. 3. Drug Approval—methods. 4. Drug Evaluation—methods. 5. Drug Evaluation, Preclinical—methods.
QV 26.5 C7374 2006]
RS122.2.C66 2006
615'.10285—dc22

2005033608

Printed in the United States of America
10 9 8 7 6 5 4 3 2 1

For Rosalynd

Failures are not something to be avoided. You want them to happen as quickly as you can so you can make progress rapidly
—Gordon Moore

CONTENTS

PREFACE

In less than a generation we have seen the impressive impact of computer science on many fields, which has changed not only the ways in which we communicate in business but also the processes in industry from product manufacturing to sales and marketing. Computing has had a wide influence by implementation of predictions based on statistics, mathematics, and risk assessment algorithms. These predictions or simulations represent a way to rapidly make decisions, prototype, innovate, and, importantly, learn quickly from failure. The computer is really just a facilitator using software and a user interface to lower the threshold of entry for individuals to benefit from complex fields such as mathematics, statistics, physics, biology, chemistry, and engineering. Without necessarily having to be an expert in these fields the user can take advantage of the software for the desired goal whether in the simulation of a process or for visualization and interpretation of results from analytical hardware.

Within the pharmaceutical industry we have progressed from the point where computers in the laboratory were rarely present or used beyond spreadsheet calculations. Now computers are ubiquitous in pharmaceutical research and development laboratories, and nearly everyone has at least one used in some way to aid in his or her role. It should come as no surprise that the development of hardware and software over the last 30 years has expanded the scope of computer use to virtually all stages of pharmaceutical research and development (data analysis, data capture, monitoring and decision making). Although there are many excellent books published that are focused on in-depth discussions of computer-aided drug design, bioinformatics, or other related individual topics, none has addressed this broader utilization of computers in pharmaceutical research and development in as comprehensive or integrated manner as attempted here. This presents the editor of such a volume with some decisions of what to include in a book of this nature when trying to show the broadest applications of computers to pharmaceutical research and development. It is not possible to exhaustively discuss all computer applications in this area; hence there was an attempt to select topics that may have a more immediate impact and relevance to improving the research and development process and that may influence the present and future generations of scientists. There are attendant historical, regulatory, and ethical considerations of using computers and software in this industry, and these should be considered equally alongside their applications. I have not solicited contributions that address the role of computers in manufacturing, packaging, finance, communication, and administration, areas that are common to other industries and perhaps represent the content of a future volume. The book is therefore divided into broad sections, although there are certainly overlaps as some chapters could be considered to belong in more than one section.

The intended audience for this book is comprised of students, managers, scientists, and those responsible for applying computers in any of the areas related to pharmaceutical research and development. It is my desire that pharmaceutical executives will also see the wide-ranging benefits of computers as their influence and impact is often not given its due place, probably because there is always a human interface that presents the computer-generated output. I hope this book shows the benefits for a more holistic approach to using computers rather than the frequently observed narrowly defined vertical areas of applications fragmented on a departmental or functional basis. This book therefore describes the history, present, future applications, and consequences of computers in pharmaceutical research and development with many examples of where computers have impacted on processes or enabled the capture, calculation, or visualization of data that has ultimately contributed to drugs reaching the market. Readers are encouraged to see this broader picture of using computers in pharmaceutical research and development and to consider how they can be further integrated into the paradigms of the future. The whole is certainly greater than the sum of the parts.

I hope that readers who have not used computers in their pharmaceutical research and development roles will also feel inspired by the ideas and results presented in the chapters and want to learn more, which may result in them using some if not many of the approaches. It is also my hope that the vision of this book will be realized by computers being directly associated with the continued success of the pharmaceutical, biotechnology, and associated industries, to ultimately speed the delivery of therapeutics to the waiting patients. I sincerely believe you will enjoy reading and learning about the broad applications of computers to this industry, as I have done during the editing process. This is just a beginning of imagining them as a continuum.

ACKNOWLEDGMENTS

I am sincerely grateful to Dr. Binghe Wang for inviting me to write a book on a topic of my choosing; without his initiation this book might have just remained an idea. I am appreciative of the editorial assistance, overall advice, and patience provided by Jonathan Rose at John Wiley & Sons during the last year. My anonymous proposal reviewers are thanked for their considerable encouragement and suggestions, which helped expand the scope of the book beyond my initial outline. Dr. Jean-Pierre Wery kindly provided valuable suggestions for contributing authors early on, along with the many other scientists contacted who responded by providing ideas for additional authors. As an editor I am entirely dependent on the many authors who have contributed their valuable time and effort to provide chapters for this book, given only a brief title and an overview at the start. I thank them sincerely for making this book possible and for sharing their enthusiasm and expertise with a wider audience as well as bearing up with my communications through the year. I would also like to acknowledge Rebecca J. Williams for kindly providing artwork for the cover image.

My interest in computational approaches applied to the pharmaceutical industry was encouraged nearly a decade ago while at Lilly Research Laboratories by Dr. Steven A. Wrighton, Mr. James H. Wikel, and Dr. Patrick J. Murphy. The generous collaborations with colleagues in both industry and academia since are also acknowledged, and several of these collaborators are contributors to this book. Two books, *The Logic of Failure* by Dietrich Dorner and *Serious Play* by Michael Schrage, were introductions to the global uses of computer simulation 5 years ago, which sowed the seed for considering all the areas where computers and their simulation possibilities could be applied in pharmaceutical research and development. I hope this book builds on the work of the pioneers in the many fields described in the following chapters, and I take this opportunity to acknowledge their contributions where they are not explicitly recognized.

My family has always provided considerable support, from my first interest in science through university to the present, even though we are now separated by the Atlantic. I dedicate this book to them and to Maggie, whose sustained valuable advice, tolerance of late nights and weekends at the computer, and general encouragement has helped me to see this project through from conception.

Sean Ekins

Jenkintown, Pennsylvania
October 2005

CONTRIBUTORS

Mazen Abdellatif, Hines VA Cooperative Studies Program Coordinating Center (151K), P.O. Box 5000, 5th Ave. and Roosevelt Rd. Bldg. 1, Rm. B240, Hines, IL 60141-5000, USA. (mazen.abdellatif@med.va.gov).

Heather Ahlborn, IBM Business Consulting Services, Pharma and Life Sciences, Armonk, NY 10504, USA. (ahlborn@us.ibm.com).

Konstantin V. Balakin, ChemDiv, Inc. 11558 Sorrento Valley Rd., Ste. 5, San Diego, CA 92121, USA. (kvb@chemdiv.com).

Kenneth Banks, Global Analytical Development, Johnson & Johnson Pharmaceutical Research & Development (J&JPRD), 1000 Route 202, Raritan, NJ 08869, USA.

Benoit Beck, Lilly services SA, European Early Phase Statistics, Mont Saint Guibert, Belgium. (Beck_benoit@lilly.com).

James R. Bosley, Jr., Rosa Pharmaceuticals, Inc., P.O. Box 2700, Cupertino, CA 95015, USA. (jim_bosley@comcast.net).

Bruno Boulanger, Lilly services SA, European Early Phase Statistics, Mont Saint Guibert, Belgium.

Donald B. Boyd, Department of Chemistry, Indiana University-Purdue University at Indianapolis (IUPUI), Indianapolis, IN 46202-3274, USA. (boyd@chem.iupui.edu).

Eric J. Buenz, Complementary and Integrative Medicine Program, Mayo Clinic College of Medicine, 200 First Street SW, Rochester, MN 55905, USA. (buenz.eric@mayo.edu).

Andrew Chadwick, PA Consulting Group, Chamber of Commerce House 2nd floor, 75 Harborne Road, Birmingham, B15 3DH, UK. (andrew.chadwick@paconsulting.com).

Cheng Chang, Division of Pharmaceutics, College of Pharmacy, The Ohio State University, Columbus, OH 43210 (chang.440@osu.edu).

Elizabeth A. Colbourn, Intelligensys Ltd., Belasis Business Centre, Belasis Hall Technology Park, Billingham, Teesside, UK.

Daniel Cronenberger, Novartis Institutes for BioMedical Research, Lichstrasse 35, 4002 Basel, Switzerland.

Nick Davies, Pfizer Limited, Sandwich, Kent, CT13 9NJ, UK. (nicholas.davies@pfizer.com).

John C. Dearden, School of Pharmacy and Chemistry, Liverpool John Moores University, Byrom Street, Liverpool L3 3AF, UK. (j.c.dearden@livjm.ac.uk).

David J. Edwards, Accelrys Inc, 10188 Telesis Court, Suite 100, San Diego, CA 92121, USA. (dje@accelrys.com).

Sean Ekins, 601 Runnymede Ave., Jenkintown, PA 19046. (ekinssean@yahoo.com).

Richard Farris, Health Decisions, Inc. 6350 Quadrangle Drive, Suite 300, Chapel Hill, NC 27517, USA. (rfarris@healthdec.com).

Darren R. Flower, Edward Jenner Institute for Vaccine Research, High Street, Compton, Berkshire, RG20 7NN, UK. (darren.flower@jenner.ac.uk).

Andrea de Gaetano, CNR IASI Laboratorio di Biomatematica UCSC – Largo A. Gemeli, 8-00168 Roma, Italy. (andrea.degaetano@gmx.net).

Valerie J. Gillet, Department of Information Studies, University of Sheffield, Western Bank, Sheffield S10 2TN, UK. (v.gillet@sheffield.ac.uk).

Craig N. Giroux, Institute of Environmental Health Sciences, Wayne State University, 2727 Second Avenue, Room 4000, Detroit, MI 48201, USA. (cgiroux@genetics.wayne.edu).

Renée J. Goldberg Arnold, President and CEO, Arnold Consultancy & Technology, LLC, 1 Penn Plaza, 36th Floor, New York, NY 10119. (rarnold@arnoldllc.com).

Nicolas Grandjean, Novartis Institutes for BioMedical Research, Lichstrasse 35, 4002 Basel, Switzerland.

Robert Harrison, 24IP Law Group, Herzogspitalstrasse 10a, 80331 Munich, Germany. (harrison@24ip.com).

Stuart T. Henderson, IBM Business Consulting Services, Pharma and Life Sciences, Armonk, NY 10504, USA. (sthender@us.ibm.com).

Roderick E. Hubbard, Structural Biology Laboratory, University of York, Heslington, York, YO10 5DD, UK and Vernalis (R&D) Ltd, Granta Park, Abington, Cambridge, CB1 6GB, UK. (rod@ysbl.york.ac.uk, r.hubbard@vernalis.com).

Maggie A. Z. Hupcey, PA Consulting Group, 600 College Road East, Suite 1120, Princeton, NJ 08540, USA. (Maggie.Hupcey@PAConsulting.com).

Michael Jones, Molecular Informatics, Triangle Molecular, 1818 Airport Road, Chapel Hill, NC 27514, USA.

Alex Kiselyov, ChemDiv, Inc. 11558 Sorrento Valley Rd., Ste. 5, San Diego, CA 92121, USA.

Olivier Kreim, Novartis Institutes for BioMedical Research, Lichstrasse 35, 4002 Basel, Switzerland.

Hugo Kubinyi, Donnersbergstrasse 9, D-67256 Weisenheim am Sand, Germany. (kubinyi@t-online.de).

Christophe G. Lambert, Golden Helix Inc., P.O. Box 10633, Bozeman, MT 59719, USA. (lambert@goldenhelix.com).

Jonathan G. Levine, Office of Post-marketing and Statistical Science Immediate Office, Center for Drug Evaluation and Research, Food and Drug Administration; Rockville, MD 20857, USA.

Weiyong Li, Global Analytical Development, Johnson & Johnson Pharmaceutical Research & Development (J&JPRD), 1000 Route 202, Raritan, NJ 08869, USA. (wli1@prdus.jnj.com).

Max M. Marsh, Department of Chemistry, Indiana University-Purdue University at Indianapolis (IUPUI), Indianapolis, IN 46202-3274, USA.

Matthew K. McGowan, Business Management & Administration, Bradley University, Peoria, IL 61625, USA. (mmcgowan@bradley.edu).

Richard J. McGowan, Philosophy and Religion Department, Butler University, Indianapolis, IN 46208, USA. (rmcgowan@butler.edu).

Jonathan Moore, PA Consulting Group, One Memorial Drive, Cambridge, MA 02142, USA.

Alfred Nehme, CambridgeSoft Corporation, 100 Cambridgepark Drive, Cambridge, MA 02140, USA. (anehme@cambridgesoft.com).

Simona Panunzi, CNR IASI Laboration di Biomatematica UCSC – Largo A. Gemeli, 8-00168 Roma, Italy.

Pierre Parisot, Novartis Institutes for BioMedical Research, Lichstrasse 35, 4002 Basel, Switzerland.

Anthony Parsons, 3 Harkness Drive, Canterbury CT2 7RW, UK. (tony@parsonsparaphernalia.com).

Manuel C. Peitsch, Novartis Institutes for BioMedical Research, Lichstrasse 35, 4002 Basel, Switzerland. (Manuel.peitsch@novartis.com).

Robin Purshouse, PA Consulting Group, 19 York Street, Manchester, M23BA, UK.

Martin Romacker, Novartis Institutes for BioMedical Research, Lichstrasse 35, 4002 Basel, Switzerland.

Michael Rosenberg, Health Decisions, Inc. 6350 Quadrangle Drive, Suite 300, Chapel Hill, NC 27517, USA. (mrosenberg@healthdec.com).

Raymond C. Rowe, The PROFITS Group, Institute of Pharmaceutical Innovation, University of Bradford, Bradford, West Yorkshire BD7 1DP, UK. (rowe@intelligensys.co.uk).

Nikolay P. Savchuk, ChemDiv, Inc., 11558 Sorrento Valley Rd., Ste. 5, San Diego, CA 92121, USA.

Robert A. Scoffin, CambridgeSoft Corporation, 8 Signet Court, Swann's Road, Cambridge, CB5 8LA, UK. (rscoffin@cambridgesoft.com).

Richard K. Scott, Walk House, Church Lane, Chatteris, Cambridgeshire, PE16 6JA, UK. (DrRKScott@gmail.com).

Jun Shimada, Columbia Universiy, Department of Chemistry, 3000 Broadway, New York, NY 10032, USA. (js2786@columbia.edu, shimadajun@yahoo.com)

Peter W. Swaan, Department of Pharmaceutical Sciences, University of Maryland, 20 Penn Street, Baltimore, MD 21201, USA. (pswaan@rx.umaryland.edu).

Ana Szarfman, Office of Post-marketing and Statistical Science Immediate Office, Center for Drug Evaluation and Research, Food and Drug Administration, Rockville, MD 20857, USA. (SZARFMAN@cder.fda.gov).

Joseph M. Tonning, Office of Post-marketing and Statistical Science Immediate Office, Center for Drug Evaluation and Research, Food and Drug Administration; Rockville, MD 20857, USA.

Thérèse Vachon, Novartis Institutes for BioMedical Research, Lichstrasse 35, 4002 Basel, Switzerland.

Paolo Vicini, Resource Facility for population kinetics, Room 241 AERL Building, Depatment of Bioengineering, Box 352255, University of Washington, Seattle, WA 98195-2255, USA. (vicini@u.washington.edu).

Sandy Weinberg, Fast Trak Vaccines, GE Healthcare 5348 Greenland Road, Atlanta, GA 30342, USA. (sandy.weinberg@ge.com).

David J. Wild, Indiana University School of Informatics, 1900 E. Tenth Street, Bloomington, IN 47406, USA. (djwild@indiana.edu).

Peter Willett, Department of Information Studies, University of Sheffield, Western Bank, Sheffield S10 2TN, UK. (p.willett@sheffield.ac.uk).

S. Stanley Young, CGStat, L.L.C., 3401 Caldwell Drive, Raleigh, NC 27607, USA. (genetree@bellsouth.net).

Weifan Zheng, Cheminformatics Research Resources, Division of Medicinal Chemistry, School of Pharmacy, University of North Carolina at Chapel Hill, NC 27599-7360, USA. (weifan_zheng@unc.edu).

PART I

COMPUTERS IN PHARMACEUTICAL RESEARCH AND DEVELOPMENT: A GENERAL OVERVIEW

1

HISTORY OF COMPUTERS IN PHARMACEUTICAL RESEARCH AND DEVELOPMENT: A NARRATIVE

DONALD B. BOYD AND MAX M. MARSH

Contents

1.1 INTRODUCTION

Today, computers are so ubiquitous in pharmaceutical research and development that it may be hard to imagine a time when there were no computers to assist the medicinal chemist or biologist. A quarter-century ago, the notion of a computer on the desk of every scientist and company manager was not even contemplated. Now, computers are absolutely essential for generating, managing, and transmitting information. The aim of this chapter is to give a

Computer Applications in Pharmaceutical Research and Development, Edited by Sean Ekins.
ISBN 0-471-73779-8

brief account of the historical development. It is a story of ascendancy and one that continues to unfold.

Owing to the personal interest and experience of the authors, the emphasis in this chapter is on using computers for drug discovery. But the use of computers in laboratory instruments and for analysis of experimental and clinical data is no less important. This chapter is written with young scientists in mind. We feel it is important that the new investigator have an appreciation of how the field evolved to its present circumstance, if for no other reason than to help steer toward a better future for those scientists using or planning to use computers in the pharmaceutical industry.

Computers began to be deployed at pharmaceutical companies as early as the 1940s. These early computers were usually for the payroll and for accounting, not for science. Pharmaceutical scientists did eventually gain access to computers, if not in the company itself, then through contractual agreements with nearby educational institutions or other contractors.

There were several scientific and engineering advances that made possible a computational approach to what had long been exclusively an experimental art and science, namely, discovering a molecule with useful therapeutic potential. One fundamental concept understood by chemists was that chemical structure is related to molecular properties including biological activity. Hence if one could predict properties by calculations, one might be able to predict which structures should be investigated in the laboratory. Another fundamental, well-established concept was that a drug would exert its biological activity by binding to and/or inhibiting some biomolecule in the body. This concept stems from Fischer's famous lock-and-key hypothesis (Schlüssel-Schloss-Prinzip) [1, 2]. Another advance was the development of the theory of quantum mechanics in the 1920s [3]. This theory connected the distribution of electrons in molecules with observable molecular properties. Pioneering research in the 1950s attacked the problem of linking electronic structure and biological activity. A good part of this work was collected in the 1963 book by Bernard and Alberte Pullman of Paris, France, which fired the imagination of what might be possible with calculations on biomolecules [4]. The earliest papers that attempted to mathematically relate chemical structure and biological activity were published in Scotland all the way back in the middle of the nineteenth century [5, 6]. This work and a couple of other papers [7, 8] were forerunners to modern quantitative structure-activity relationships (QSAR) but were not widely known. In 1964, the role of molecular descriptors in describing biological activity was reduced to a simplified mathematical form, and the field of QSAR was propelled toward its modern visage [9, 10]. (A descriptor is any calculated or experimental numerical property related to a compound's chemical structure.) And, of course, there was the engineering development of computers and all that entailed. The early computers were designed for military and accounting applications, but gradually it became apparent that computers would have a vast number of uses.

One of us (MMM) was one of the first people in the pharmaceutical industry to perceive that computer-aided drug design was something that might be practical and worthy of investigation. He pioneered a sustained, industrial research program to use computers in drug design. After retiring from Eli Lilly and Company in 1986, he became a Visiting Research Scientist and later an Adjunct Professor in the Department of Chemistry, Indiana University, Bloomington. Section 1.2 is his personal account of the early steps at Lilly.

1.2 COMPUTATIONAL CHEMISTRY: THE BEGINNINGS AT LILLY

This narrative was first presented at Don Boyd's third annual Central Indiana Computational Chemistry Christmas Luncheon (CICCCL-3) on December 18, 1997. Although it is specific for Eli Lilly and Company, the progress and problems that transpired there were probably not too different from developments at other large, forward-looking, research-based pharmaceutical companies.

> This little story contains mainly my personal recollection about how the computational chemistry project in the Lilly Research Laboratories began. An advantage of living longer than one's contemporaries is that there is no one around among the early participants to contradict my reminiscences. A more comprehensive history of this discipline may be found in the Bolcer and Hermann chapter in *Reviews of Computational Chemistry* [11]. I shall confine this commentary to what I remember about my own involvement.
>
> I began work at Eli Lilly and Company in March 1942 as a laboratory aide in the analytical department. At that time, there was very little sophisticated instrumentation in the laboratory. The most complex calculations were carried out using a slide rule. After military service in World War II and an educational leave of absence to complete my undergraduate studies in chemistry at Indiana University, I returned to the Lilly analytical group in 1947. Slide rules were still much in evidence but were soon augmented with mechanical calculators—usually Monroe or Friden models.
>
> It was not until 1949 that the company actually acquired a stored-program computer; at that time an IBM 704 system was purchased—for about $1 million. In spite of the fact that it was a vacuum tube machine—with considerable concomitant downtime—several business operations were carried out using it. A number of inventories and the payroll were successfully handled. However, no scientific calculations were performed with it. The system was replaced in a few years with an IBM 709—again only for business and financial operations.
>
> In the late 1950s or early 1960s, the first computers to have stored programs of scientific interest were acquired. One of these was an IBM 650; it had a rotating magnetic drum memory consisting of 2000 accessible registers. The programs, the data input, and the output were all in the form of IBM punched cards. A major concern was keeping those card decks intact and in order as they were

moved about from user to machine and back. My recollection is that some statistical calculations by Lilly's research statistics group under Dr. Edgar King were carried out on this machine.

At about the same time, one of the business groups obtained an IBM 610 computer. This device was simpler to use than the 650, and it utilized punched paper tape input, program, and output. The tape was generated on a typewriter. Programs were developed using an essentially algebraic language peculiar to the machine. After the program tape was read in, a tape containing sequentially the data to be processed was fed in. The output tape was carried back to a tape reader linked to a typewriter where the results were ultimately typed out. I used this machine.

My interest at that time revolved around evaluating optical rotary dispersion data [12]. The paired values of optical rotation vs. wavelength were used to fit a function called the Drude equation (later modified to the Moffitt equation for William Moffitt [Harvard University] who developed the theory) [13]. The coefficients of the evaluated equation were shown to be related to a significant ultraviolet absorption band of a protein and to the amount of alpha-helix conformation existing in the solution of it.

Interest in possible applications of computers at the Lilly Research Laboratories began to broaden in the early 1960s. Dr. King (then director of the statistical research group) and I appeared before the Lilly board of directors, submitting a proposal to acquire a computer and ancillary equipment to be devoted primarily to research needs. The estimated cost was a little more than $250,000. In those days, an expenditure of that large an amount required board approval. Today, I suppose a division director or even a department head could sign off on a personal computer with vastly more power than any computer of the 1960s!

The board of directors approved our proposal. The system that was purchased was an IBM 1620 with the necessary card punches and reader plus tape drives. In addition to statistical and some analytical chemistry applications, Dr. Charles Rice (then head of the radiochemistry group) and I initiated Lilly's first computer-based information retrieval system. Through an agreement with the Institute for Scientific Information (ISI, Philadelphia), Lilly was able to receive magnetic tapes containing computer-searchable title information on current scientific journals from ISI every 10 days. Interest profiles of individual Lilly scientists were then used to generate the famous (or infamous!) "hit" cards that were distributed to members of the research staff. The cards contained journal citations to articles matching the recipient scientist's profile. This service continued until the advent of electronic literature alerts in the 1980s.

Stemming from my growing interest in and enthusiasm for the potential use of computed values of atomic and molecular properties in pharmaceutical research, I was able to gain approval for a requisition for a scientist who knew how to use computers to determine molecular properties. The person I hired was Dr. Robert B. Hermann, our first theoretical chemist. It was 1964. He obtained his Ph.D. with Prof. Norman L. Allinger at Wayne State and then did postdoctoral research with Prof. Joseph O. Hirschfelder at Wisconsin and with Prof. Peter Lykos at the Illinois Institute of Technology. When Bob joined us, he brought along a semiempirical molecular orbital program that he had personally written. He planned to use this to estimate molecular properties of drug-type molecules, but Lilly computers were incapable of handling the necessary matrix multiplication steps. This obstacle was overcome by going outside the company. We were able to develop a working agreement with the engineering component of Allison Transmission Division of General Motors to use their IBM 7094 after regular working hours. Since the system was used only by Allison and Lilly, data security was not an issue. However, considerable time was spent transporting punched card decks and printouts between the Lilly Research Laboratories near downtown Indianapolis and the Allison facility in nearby Speedway, Indiana.

Looking back, it is difficult for me to pinpoint the factors leading to my initiation of the molecular modeling and drug design effort at Lilly. Certainly, the developments of Prof. Lou Allinger and his associates (at Wayne State and the University of Georgia) in the 1960s to use calculations to study conformation played an important part [14]. Similarly, the publishing of an EHT program by Prof. Roald Hoffmann (Harvard University) in 1963 was a significant impetus. The introduction of the pi-sigma correlation equation by Prof. Corwin Hansch (Pomona College) in 1964 added another facet of interest. Also that year, Dr. Margaret Dayhoff (a theoretical chemist who became the first prominent woman in what would become the field of bioinformatics and who was at the National Biomedical Research Foundation in Maryland) published a method for arriving at the geometry of a polypeptide or protein via internal coordinates [15]. This methodology also encouraged me to begin thinking about enzyme-inhibitor interactions and the three-dimensional requirements for molecular design.

It was not until 1968, when Don Boyd joined us as the second theoretical chemist in our group, that the computers at Lilly started to reach a level of size, speed, and sophistication to be able to handle some of the computational requirements of our various evaluation and design efforts. Don brought with him Hoffmann's EHT program from Harvard and Cornell. Due to the length of our calculations and due to the other demands on the computer, the best we could obtain was a one-day turnaround.

The preceding years involved not only the Allison agreement (for which we paid a modest fee) but also later ones with Purdue University (West Lafayette, Indiana) and Indiana University, Bloomington computing centers. These latter arrangements involved Control Data Corporation (CDC) systems that were much faster than the IBM 7094. Use of the Purdue computer, which continued after Don joined our group, involved driving to the near north side of Indianapolis where the Purdue extension campus was located. In the basement of their science building was a computer center connected to the CDC 7600 in West Lafayette. Computer card decks of data and the associated program for approximate molecular orbital calculations could be left with the machine operators. With luck, the card decks and computer printouts could be retrieved the next day. Security was more of a problem with the academic facilities because they had a large number of users. The concern was enhanced when—on one occasion—I received, in addition to my own output, the weather forecast data and analysis for the city of Kokomo, Indiana! Even though it was unlikely that anyone could make use of our information except Bob, Don, or myself, it was a relief to research management when we were able to carry out all our computations in-house.

> These reminiscences cover about the first 15 years of the Lilly computational chemistry effort. Considering the strong tradition of lead generation emanating from the organic chemistry group, the idea that molecular modeling could make a significant contribution to drug design was slow to be accepted. Nevertheless, enough research management support was found to spark the small pioneering project and to keep it going in the face of strong skepticism. Regrettably, a considerable amount of my time in this critical period was spent attempting to convince management and the scientific research staff of the logic and significance of these studies. Because we entered the field at a very early stage, a great deal of effort went into the testing, evaluation, and establishment of the limits of application of the various computational methods. This kind of groundwork was not always well understood by the critics of our approach.

In what follows, we review events, trends, hurdles, successes, people, hardware, and software. We attempt to paint a picture of happenings as historically correct as possible but, inevitably, colored by our own experiences and memories. The time line is broken down by decade from the 1960s through the turn of the century. We conclude with some commentary on where the field is headed and lessons learned. For some of the topics mentioned, we could cite hundreds of books [16] and thousands of articles. We hope that the reader will tolerate us citing only a few examples. We apologize to our European and Japanese colleagues for being less familiar with events at their companies than with events in the United States. Before we start, we also apologize sincerely to all the many brilliant scientists who made landmark contributions that we cannot cover in a single chapter.

1.3 GERMINATION: THE 1960s

We can state confidently that in 1960 essentially 100% of the computational chemists were in academia, not industry. Of course, back then they were not called computational chemists, a term not yet invented. They were called theoretical chemists or quantum chemists. The students coming from those academic laboratories constituted the main pool of candidates that industry could hire for their initial ventures into using computers for drug discovery. Another pool of chemists educated using computers were X-ray crystallographers. Some of these young theoreticians and crystallographers were interested in helping solve human health challenges and steered their careers toward pharmaceutical work.

Although a marvel at the time, the workplace of the 1960s looks archaic in hindsight. Computers generally resided in computer centers, where a small army of administrators, engineers, programming consultants, and support people would tend the mainframe computers then in use. The computers were kept in locked, air-conditioned rooms inaccessible to ordinary users. One of the largest computers then in use by theoretical chemists and crystallographers was the IBM 7094. Support staff operated the tape readers, card readers, and printers. The users' room at the computer centers echoed with the clunk-clunk-clunk of card punches that encoded data as little rectangular holes in the so-called IBM cards [see reference 11]. The cards were manufactured in different colors so that users could conveniently differentiate their many card decks. As a by-product, the card punches produced piles of colorful rectangular confetti. There were no Delete or Backspace keys; if any mistake was made in keying in data, the user would need to begin again with a fresh blank card. The abundance of cards and card boxes in the users' room scented the air with a characteristic paper smell. Programs were written in FORTRAN II. Programs used by the chemists usually ranged from half a box to several boxes long. Carrying several boxes of cards to the computer center was good for physical fitness. If a box was dropped or if a card reader mangled some of the cards, the tedious task of restoring the deck and replacing the torn cards ensued. Input decks were generally smaller—consisting of tens of cards—and were sandwiched between JCL (job control language for IBM machines) cards and bound by rubber bands. Computer output usually came in the form of ubiquitous pale green and white striped paper (measuring 11 by 14-7/8 inches per page). Special cardboard covers and long nylon needles were used to hold and organize stacks of printouts.

Mathematical algorithms for common operations such as matrix diagonalization had been written and could be inserted as a subroutine in a larger molecular orbital program, for instance. Programs for chemistry were generally developed by academic groups, with the graduate students doing most or all of the programming. Partly, this was standard practice because the professors at different universities were in competition with each other and wanted a better program than their competitors had access to. (Better means running faster, handling larger matrices, and doing more.) Partly, this situation was standard practice so that the graduate students would learn by doing. Obviously, this situation led to much duplication of effort: the proverbial reinventing the wheel. To improve this situation, Prof. Harrison Shull and colleagues at Indiana University, Bloomington, conceived and sold the concept of having an international repository of software that could be shared. Thus was born in 1962 the Quantum Chemistry Program Exchange (QCPE). Competitive scientists were initially slow to give away programs they worked so hard to write, but gradually the depositions to QCPE increased. We do not have room here to give a full recounting of the history of QCPE [17], but suffice it to say that QCPE proved instrumental in advancing the field of computational chemistry including that at pharmaceutical companies. Back in the 1960s and 1970s, there were no software companies catering to the computational chemistry market, so QCPE was the main resource for the entire community. As the name implies, QCPE was initially used for exchanging subroutines and programs for ab initio and approximate electronic structure calculations. But QCPE evolved to encompass programs for molecular mechanics and a wide range of calculations on molecules. The quarterly *QCPE Newsletter* (later renamed the *QCPE Bulletin*), which was edited by Mr. Richard W. Counts, was for a long time the main vehicle for computational chemists to announce programs and other news of interest. QCPE membership included industrial computational chemists.

Finally in regard to software, we note one program that came from the realm of crystallography. That program was ORTEP (Oak Ridge Thermal Ellipsoid Program), which was the first widely used program for (noninteractive) molecular graphics [18]. Output from the program was inked onto long scrolls of paper run through expensive, flat-bed printers. The ball-and-stick ORTEP drawings were fine for publication, but routine laboratory work was easier with graph paper, ruler, protractor, and pencil to plot the Cartesian coordinates of a molecule the chemist wanted to study. Such handmade drawings quantitated molecular geometry. Experimental bond lengths and bond angles were found in a British compilation [19].

Also to help the chemist think about molecular shape, hand-held molecular models were widely used by experimentalists and theoreticians alike. There were two main types. One was analogous to stick representations in which metal or plastic rods represented bonds between atoms, which were balls or joints that held the rods at specific angles. Metal wire Drieding models were among the most accurate and expensive. The other type was space filling. The expensive CPK (Corey–Pauling–Koltun) models [20, 21] consisted of three-dimensional spherical segments made of plastic that were color-coded by element (white for hydrogen, blue for nitrogen, red for oxygen, etc.). From this convention, came the color molecular graphics we are familiar with today.

In the 1960s, drug discovery was by trial and error. Interesting compounds flowed from two main sources in that period. The smaller pipeline was natural products, such as soil microbes that produced biologically active components or plants with medicinal properties. The dominant pipeline, however, was classic medicinal chemistry. A lead compound would be discovered by biological screening or by reading the patent and scientific literature published by competitors at other pharmaceutical companies. From the lead, the medicinal chemists would use their ingenuity, creativity, and synthetic expertise to construct new compounds. These compounds would be tested by the appropriate in-house pharmacologists, microbiologists, and so forth. Besides the intended biological target, the compounds would often be submitted to a battery of other bioactivity screens being run at the company so that leads for other drug targets could be discovered. The most potent compounds found would become the basis for another round of analog design and synthesis. Thus would evolve in countless iterations a structure-activity relationship (SAR), which in summary would consist of a table of compounds and their activities. In fortuitous circumstances, one of the medicinal chemists would make a compound with sufficient potency that a project team consisting of scientists from drug discovery and drug development would be assembled to oversee further experiments on the compound to learn whether it had the appropriate characteristics to become a pharmaceutical product. The formula for career success was simple: The medicinal chemist who invented or could claim authorship of a project team compound would receive kudos from management.

What happens when a theoretical chemist is thrown into this milieu? Well, initially not much because the only theoretical methods of the 1960s that could treat drug-sized (200–500 Da) molecules were inaccurate and limited. These molecular orbital methods were extended Hückel theory [22, 23] and soon thereafter CNDO/2 (complete-neglect-of-differential-overlap/second parameterization) [24, 25]. Although approximate by today's standards and incapable of giving accurate, energy-minimized ("optimized"), three-dimensional molecular geometries (bond lengths, bond angles, and torsional angles), they were far more appropriate for use than other methods available at the time. One of these other methods was Hartree–Fock [26–29] (also called self-consistent field or nonempirical in the early literature, or ab initio in recent decades). Although Hartree–Fock did fairly well at predicting molecular geometries, the computers of the era limited treatment to molecules not much larger than ethane. Another class of methods such as simple Hückel theory [30–32] and Pariser–Parr–Pople (PPP) theory [33] could treat large molecules but only pi electrons. Hence, they were formally limited to planar molecules, but not many pharmaceuticals are planar.

In addition to the quantum chemistry in use in the 1960s, an independent approach was QSAR, as already alluded to. Here the activity of a compound is assumed to be a linear (or quadratic or higher) function of certain molecular descriptors. One of the commonly used descriptors was the contribution of an atom or a functional group to the lipophilicity of a molecule; this descriptor was designated pi (π). Other famous descriptors included the Hammett sigma (σ) values for aromatic systems and the Taft sigma (σ^*) values for aliphatic systems; both came from physical organic chemistry [34–36]. The sigma values measured the tendency of a substituent to withdraw or donate electron density in relation to the rest of the molecule.

Abbott, Schering-Plough, and Upjohn were among the first companies, besides Lilly, to venture into the area of using computers for attempts at drug discovery. Dow Chemical, which had pharmaceutical interests, also initiated an early effort. Generally, the first steps consisted of either hiring a person with theoretical and computer expertise or allowing one of the company's existing research scientists to turn attention to learning about this new methodology. Much effort was expended by these early pioneers in learning the scope of applicability of the available methods. Attempts to actually design a drug were neither numerous nor particularly successful. This generalization does not imply that there were no successes. There were a few successes in finding correlations and in better understanding what was responsible for biological activity at the molecular level. For example, early work at Lilly revealed the glimmer of a relationship between the calculated electronic structure of the beta-lactam ring of cephalosporins and antibacterial activity. The work was performed in the 1960s but was not published until 1973 [37] because of delays by cautious research management and patent attorneys at the company. (The relationship was elaborated in subsequent years [38, 39], but no new pharmaceutical product resulted [40].)

1.4 GAINING A FOOTHOLD: THE 1970s

Some of the companies that first got into this game dropped out after a few years (but returned later), either for lack of management support or because the technology was not intellectually satisfying to the scientist involved. Other companies, like Lilly, persisted. Lilly's pioneering effort paid off in establishing a base of expertise. Also, quite a few papers were published, almost like in an academic setting. In hindsight, however, Lilly may have gotten in the field too early because the initial efforts were so limited by the science, hardware, and software. First impressions can be lasting. Lilly management of the 1970s thwarted further permanent growth but at least sustained the effort. (It was not until near the end of the 1980s that Lilly resumed growing its computational chemistry group to catch up to the other large pharmaceutical companies.) It was generally recognized that Lilly was a family-oriented company committed to doing what was right in all phases of its business. There was great mutual loyalty between the company and the employees. Other companies such as Merck and Smith Kline and French (using the old name) entered the field a few years later. Unlike Lilly, they hired chemists trained in organic chemistry and computers and with a pedigree traceable back to Prof. E. J. Corey at Harvard and his attempts at computer-aided synthesis planning [41–43].

Regarding hardware of the 1970s, pharmaceutical companies invested money from the sale of their products to buy better and better mainframes. Widely used models included members of the IBM 360 and 370 series. Placing these more powerful machines in-house made it easier and more secure to submit jobs and retrieve output. But output was still in the form of long printouts. Input had advanced to the point where punch cards were no longer needed. So-called dumb terminals, that is, terminals with no local processing capability, could be used to set up input jobs for batch running. For instance, at Lilly an IBM 3278 and a Decwriter II (connected to a DEC-10 computer) were used by the computational chemistry group. The statistics program MINITAB was one of the programs that ran on the interactive Digital Equipment Corporation machine. Card punches were not yet totally obsolete, but received less and less use. The appearance of a typical office for computational chemistry is shown in Figure 1.1.

The spread of technology at pharmaceutical companies also meant that secretaries were given word processors (such as the Wang machines) to use in addition to typewriters, which were still needed for filling out forms. Keyboarding was the domain of the secretaries, the data entry technicians, and the computational chemists. Only a few managers and scientists would type their own memos and articles.

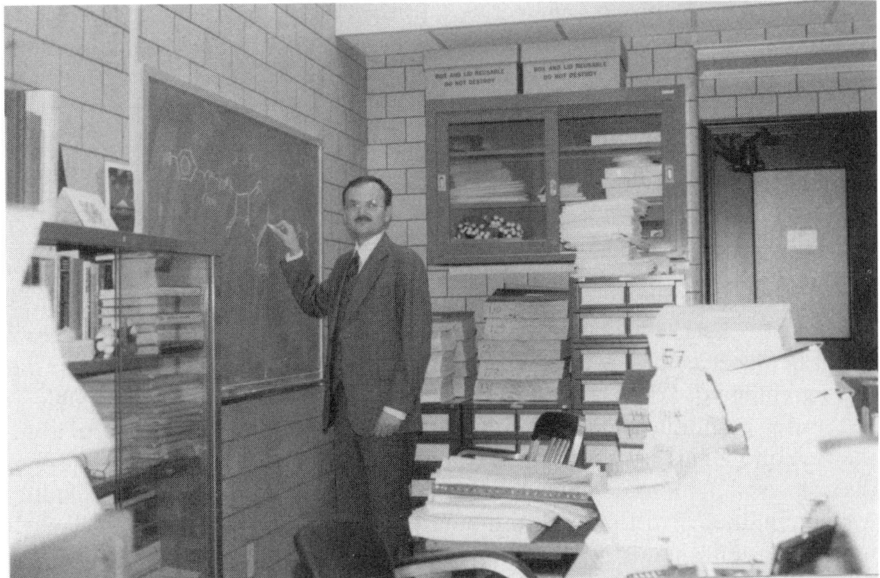

Figure 1.1 Offices used by computational chemists were filled with stacks of printouts and banks of file cabinets with legacy card decks. This photograph was taken in 1982, but the appearance of the environs had not changed much since the mid-1970s.

Software was still written primarily in FORTRAN, now mainly FORTRAN IV. The holdings of QCPE expanded. Among the important acquisitions was Gaussian 70, an ab initio program written by Prof. John A. Pople's group at Carnegie-Mellon University. Pople made the program available in 1973. (He later submitted Gaussian 76 and Gaussian 80 to QCPE, but they were withdrawn when the Gaussian program was commercialized by Pople in 1987.) Nevertheless, ab initio calculations, despite all the élan associated with them, were still not very practical or helpful for pharmaceutically interesting molecules. Semiempirical molecular orbital methods (EHT, CNDO/2, MINDO/3) were the mainstays of quantum chemical applications (MINDO/3 [44] was Prof. Michael J. S. Dewar's third refinement of a modified intermediate neglect-of-differential-overlap method).

The prominent position of quantum mechanics led a coterie of academic theoreticians to think that their approach could solve research problems facing the pharmaceutical industry. These theoreticians, who met annually in Europe and on Sanibel Island in Florida, invented the new subfields of quantum biology [45] and quantum pharmacology [46]. These names may seem curious to the uninitiated. They were not meant to imply that some observable aspect of biology or pharmacology stems from the wave-particle duality seen in the physics of electrons. Rather, the names conveyed to cognoscenti that they were applying their trusty old quantum mechanical methods to compounds discussed by biologists and pharmacologists [47]. However, doing a calculation on a system of pharmacological interest is not the same as designing a drug. For instance, calculating the molecular orbitals of serotonin is a far cry from designing a new serotonin reuptake inhibitor that could become a pharmaceutical product.

Nonetheless, something even more useful came on the software scene in the 1970s. This was Prof. N. L. Allinger's MMI/MMPI program [48, 49] for molecular mechanics. Classic methods for calculating conformational energies date to the 1940s and early 1960s [50, 51]. Copies of Allinger's program could be purchased at a nominal fee from QCPE. Molecular mechanics has the advantage of being much faster than quantum mechanics and capable of generating common organic chemical structures approaching "chemical accuracy" (bond lengths correctly predicted to within about 0.01 Å). Because of the empirical manner in which force fields were derived, molecular mechanics was an anathema to the quantum purists, never mind that Allinger himself used quantum chemistry, too. Molecular mechanics became an important technique in the armamentarium of industrial researchers. Meanwhile, a surprising number of academic theoreticians were slow to notice that the science was transitioning from quantum chemistry to multifaceted computational chemistry [52, 53].

Computational chemists in the pharmaceutical industry also expanded from their academic upbringing by acquiring an interest in force field methods, QSAR, and statistics. Computational chemists with responsibility to work on pharmaceuticals came to appreciate the fact that it was too limiting to confine one's work to just one approach to a problem. To solve research problems in industry, one had to use the best available technique, and this did not mean going to a larger basis set or a higher level of quantum mechanical theory. It meant using molecular mechanics or QSAR or whatever.

Unfortunately, the tension between the computational chemists and the medicinal chemists at pharmaceutical companies did not ease in the 1970s. Medicinal chemists were at the top of the pecking order in corporate research laboratories. This was an industry-wide problem revealed in conversations at scientific meetings where computational chemists from industry (there were not many) could informally exchange their experiences and challenges. (Readers should not get the impression that the tension between theoreticians and experimentalists existed solely in the business world. It also existed in academic chemistry departments.)

The situation was that as medicinal chemists pursued an SAR, calculations by the computational chemists might suggest a structure worthy of synthesis. Maybe the design had the potential of being more active. But the computational chemist was totally dependent on the medicinal chemist to test the hypothesis. Suddenly, the medicinal chemist saw himself going from being the wellspring of design ideas to being a technician who was implementing someone else's idea. Although never intended as a threat to the prestige and hegemony of the organic chemistry hierarchy, proposals from outside that hierarchy were often perceived as such.

Another problem was that on a computer it was easy to change a carbon to a nitrogen or any other element. It was easy to attach a substituent at any position in whatever stereochemistry seemed best for enhancing activity. It was easy to change a six-member ring to a five-member ring or vice versa. Such computer designs were frequently beyond the possibilities of synthetic organic chemistry, or at least beyond the fast-paced chemistry practiced in industry. This situation contributed to the disconnect between the computational chemists and medicinal chemists. What good is a computer design if the molecule is impossible to make?

If the computational chemist needed a less active compound synthesized to establish a computational hypothesis, such as for a pharmacophore, that was totally out of the question. No self-respecting medicinal chemist would want to admit to his management that he purposely spent valuable time making a less active compound. Thus the 1970s remained a period when the relationship between computational chemists and medicinal chemists was still being worked out. Management people, who generally rose from the ranks of medicinal chemists, were often unable to perceive a system for effective use of the input computational approaches might provide. In addition, many managers were not yet convinced that the computational input was worth anything.

The computational chemists at Lilly tackled this problem of a collaboration gap in several ways. One was to keep the communication channels open and constantly explain what was being done, what might be doable, and what was beyond the capabilities of the then-current state of the art. For organic chemists who had never used a computer, it was necessary to gently dispel the notion that one could push a button on a large box with blinking lights and the chemical structure of the next $200 million drug would tumble into the output tray of the machine. (Back in those days, $200 million in annual sales was equivalent to a blockbuster drug.) The limited capability to predict molecular properties accurately was stressed by the computational chemists. Moreover, it was up to the human, not the machine, to use chemical intuition to capitalize on relationships found between calculated physical properties and sought-after biological activities. Also, it was important for the computational chemist to avoid theory and technical jargon when talking with medicinal chemists. The computational chemists, to the best of their ability, had to speak the language of the organic chemists, not vice versa.

In an outreach to the medicinal chemists at Lilly, a one-week workshop was created and taught in the research building where the organic chemists were located. (The computational chemists were initially assigned office space with the analytical chemists and later with the biologists.) The workshop covered the basic and practical aspects of performing calculations on molecules. The input requirements (which included the format of the data fields on the punch cards) were taught for several programs. One program was used to generate Cartesian atomic coordinates. Output from that program was then used as input for the molecular orbital and molecular mechanics programs. Several of the adventurous young Ph.D. organic chemists took the course. The outreach was successful in that it empowered a few medicinal chemists to do their own calculations for testing molecular design ideas. It was a foot in the door. These young medicinal chemists could set an example for the older ones. An analogous strategy was used at some other pharmaceutical companies. For instance, Merck conducted a workshop on synthesis planning for their chemists [54].

Despite these efforts, medicinal chemists were slow to accept what computers were able to provide. Medicinal chemists would bring a research problem to the computational chemists, sometimes out of curiosity about what computing could provide, sometimes as a last resort after a question was irresolvable by any other approach. The question might range from explaining why adding a certain substituent unexpectedly decreased activity in a series of compounds to finding a QSAR for a small set of compounds. If the subsequent calculations were unable to provide a satisfactory answer, there was a tendency among some medicinal chemists to dismiss the whole field. This facet of human nature of scientifically educated people was difficult to fathom. A perspective that was promoted by one of us (DBB) to his colleagues was that computers should be viewed as just another piece of research apparatus. Experiments could be done on a computer just like experiments could be run on a spectrometer or in an autoclave. Sometimes the instrument would give the results the scientist was looking for; other times, the computational experiment would fail. Not every experiment—at the bench or in the computer—works every time. If a reaction failed, a medicinal chemist would not dismiss all of synthetic chemistry. Instead, another synthetic route would be attempted. However, the same patience did not seem to extend to computational experiments.

Finally, in regard to the collaboration gap, the importance of a knowledgeable (and wise) mentor—an advocate—cannot be overstated. For a nascent effort to take root in a business setting, the younger scientist(s) had to be shielded from excessive critiquing by higher management and powerful medicinal chemists.

The computational chemists were able to form collaborations with their fellow physical chemists. Some of the research questions dealt with molecular conformation and spectroscopy. The 1970s were full of small successes such as finding correlations between calculated and experimental properties. Some of these correlations were published. Even something so grand as the de novo design of a pharmaceutical was attempted but was somewhat beyond reach.

Two new computer-based resources were launched in the 1970s. One was the Cambridge Structural Database (CSD) [55], and the other was the Protein

Data Bank (PDB) [56]. Computational chemists recognized that these compilations of 3D molecular structures would prove very useful, especially as more pharmaceutically relevant compounds were deposited. The CSD was supported by subscribers, including pharmaceutical companies. On the other hand, the PDB was supported by American taxpayers.

We have not discussed QSAR very much, but one influential book of the 1970s can be mentioned [57]. Dr. Yvonne Martin began her scientific career as an experimentalist in a pharmaceutical laboratory, but after becoming interested in the potential of QSAR she spent time learning the techniques at the side of Prof. Corwin Hansch and also Prof. Al Leo of Pomona College in California. As mentioned in her book, she encountered initial resistance to a QSAR approach at Abbott Laboratories. Another significant book that was published in the late 1970s was a compilation of substituent constants [58]. These parameters were heavily relied upon in QSAR investigations.

The decade of the 1970s saw the administration in Washington, DC, set the laudatory goal of conquering cancer. Large sums of taxpayer dollars were poured into the National Cancer Institute for redistribution to worthy academic research projects. Naturally, many professors, including those whose work was related to cancer in the most tenuous and remote way, lined up to obtain a grant. The result was that many academic theoretical chemistry papers published in the 1970s included in their introduction rather farfetched claims as to how the quantum chemical calculations being reported were going to be applicable (someday) to the design of anticancer agents. Computational chemists in industry were not touched by this phenomenon because they were supported by the sales efforts of the manufacturers of the pharmaceuticals and were more focused on the real task of aiding drug discovery.

1.5 GROWTH: THE 1980s

If the 1960s were the Dark Ages and the 1970s were the Middle Ages, the 1980s were the Renaissance, the Baroque Period, and the Enlightenment all rolled into one. The decade of the 1980s was when the various approaches of quantum chemistry, molecular mechanics, molecular simulations, QSAR, and molecular graphics coalesced into modern computational chemistry.

In the world of scientific publishing, a seminal event occurred in 1980. Professor Allinger launched his *Journal of Computational Chemistry*. This helped stamp a name on the field. Before the journal began publishing, the field was variously called theoretical chemistry, calculational chemistry, modeling, etc. Interestingly, Allinger first took his proposal to the business managers for publications of the American Chemical Society (ACS). Unfortunately, they rejected the concept. Allinger turned to publisher John Wiley & Sons, which went on to become the premier producer of journals and books in the field. Nearly 25 years passed before the ACS moved to rectify its mistake, and in 2005 it remolded its *Journal of Chemical Information and Computer*

Sciences (JCICS) in an attempt to meet the needs of today's computational chemists. JCICS was becoming the most popular venue for computational chemists to publish work on combinatorial library designs (see Fig. 1.2 and Section 1.6 on the 1990s).

Several exciting technical advances fostered the improved environment for computer use at pharmaceutical companies in the 1980s. The first was a development of the VAX 11/780 computer by Digital Equipment Corporation (DEC) in 1979. The machine was departmental size, that is, the price, dimen-

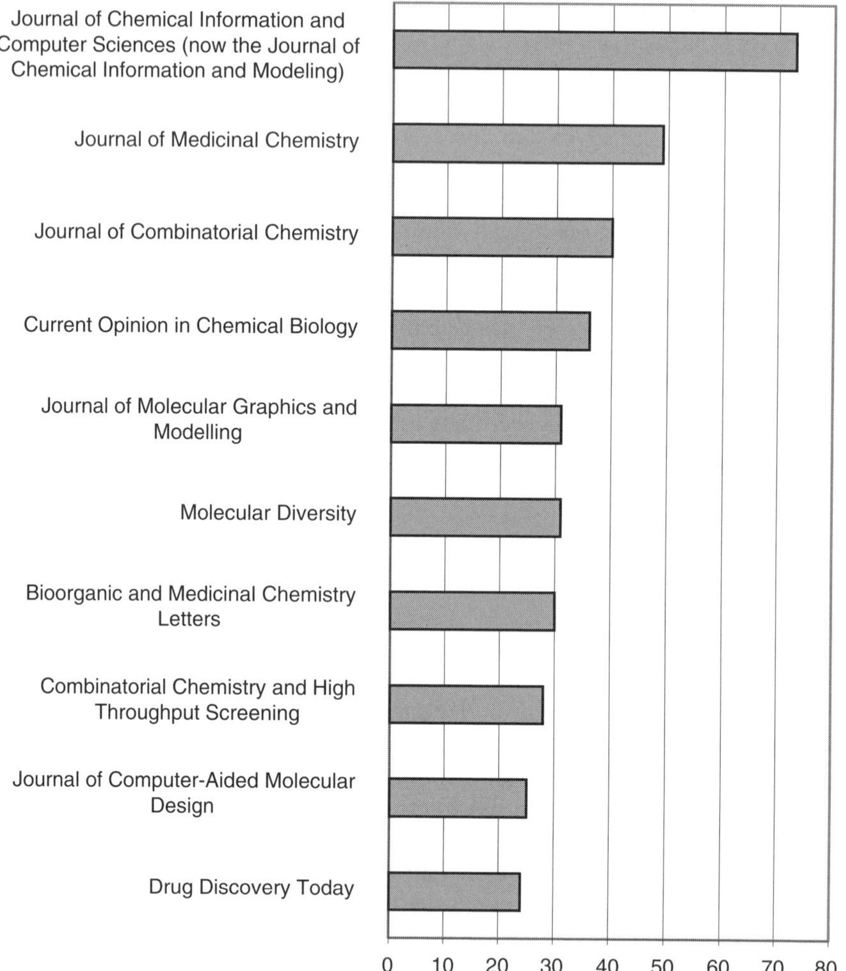

Figure 1.2 Journals that have published the most papers on combinatorial library design. Total number of papers published on this subject according to the Chemical Abstract Service's CAPLUS and MEDLINE databases for all years through 2004 plus three-quarters of 2005.

sions, and easy care of the machine allowed each department or group to have its own superminicomputer. This was a start toward noncentralized control over computing resources. At Lilly, the small-molecule X-ray crystallographers were the first to gain approval for the purchase of a VAX, around 1980. Fortunately, the computational chemists and a few other scientists were allowed to use it, too. The machine was a delight to use and far better than any of the batch job-oriented IBM mainframes of the past. The VAX could be run interactively. Users communicated with the VAX through interactive graphical terminals. The first terminals were monochrome. The first VAX at Lilly was fine for one or two users but would get bogged down, and response times would slow to a crawl if more than five users were logged on simultaneously. Lilly soon started building an ever more powerful cluster of VAXes (also called VAXen in deference to the plural of "ox"). Several other hardware companies that manufactured superminicomputers in the same class as the VAX sprung up. But DEC proved to be a good, relatively long-lasting vendor to deal with, and many pharmaceutical companies acquired VAXes for research. (However, DEC and those other hardware companies no longer exist.)

The pharmaceutical companies certainly noticed the development of the IBM personal computer (PC), but its DOS (disk operating system) made learning to use it difficult. Some scientists bought these machines. The Apple Macintosh appeared on the scene in 1984. With its cute little, lightweight, all-in-one box including monochrome screen, the Mac brought interactive computing to a new standard of user friendliness. Soon after becoming aware of these machines, nearly every medicinal chemist wanted one at work. The machines were great at word processing, graphing, and managing small (laboratory) databases. The early floppy disks formatted for the Macs held only 400 KB, but by 1988 double-sided, double-density disks had a capacity of 1400 KB, which seemed plenty in those days. In contrast to today's huge applications requiring a compact disk for storage, a typical program of the 1980s could be stuffed on one or maybe two floppy disks.

On the software front, three advances changed the minds of the medicinal chemists from being diehard skeptics to almost enthusiastic users. One advance was the development of electronic mail. As the Macs and terminals to the VAX spread to all the chemists in drug discovery and development, the desirability of being connected became obvious. The chemists could communicate with each other and with management and could tap into databases and other computer resources. As electronic traffic increased, research buildings had to be periodically retrofitted with each new generation of cabling to the computers. A side effect of the spread of computer terminals to the desktop of every scientist was that management could cut back on secretarial help for scientists, so they had to do their own keyboarding to write reports and papers.

The second important software advance was ChemDraw, which was released first for the Mac in 1986 [59–62]. This program gave chemists the ability to quickly create two-dimensional chemical diagrams. Every medicinal chemist could appreciate the aesthetics of a neat ChemDraw diagram. The diagrams could be cut and pasted into reports, articles, and patents. The old plastic ring templates for hand drawing chemical diagrams were suddenly unnecessary.

The third software advance also had an aesthetic element. This was the technology of computer graphics, or when 3D structures were displayed on the computer screens, molecular graphics. Whereas a medicinal chemist might have trouble understanding the significance of the highest occupied molecular orbital or the octanol-water partition coefficient of a structure, he or she could readily appreciate the stick, ball-and-stick, tube, and space-filling representations of 3D molecular structures [63–65]. The graphics could be shown in color and, on more sophisticated terminals, in stereo. These images were so stunning that one director of drug discovery at Lilly decreed that terms like "theoretical chemistry," "molecular modeling," and "computational chemistry" were out. The whole field was henceforth to be called "molecular graphics" as far as he was concerned. A picture was something he could understand!

Naturally, with the flood of new computer technology came the need to train the research scientists in its use. Whereas ChemDraw running on a Mac was so easy that medicinal chemists could learn to use it after an hour or less of training, the VAX was a little more formidable. One of the authors (DBB) was involved in preparing and teaching VAX classes offered to the medicinal chemists and process chemists at Lilly.

Computer programs that the computational chemists had been running on the arcane IBM mainframes were ported to the VAXes. This step made the programs more accessible because all the chemists were given VAX accounts. So, although the other programs (e.g., e-mail and ChemDraw) enticed the medicinal chemist to sit down in front of the computer screen, he or she was now more likely to experiment with molecular modeling calculations. (As discussed elsewhere [66], the terms computational chemistry and molecular modeling were used more or less interchangeably at pharmaceutical companies.) Besides the classes and workshops, one-on-one training was offered to help the medicinal chemists run the computational chemistry programs. This was generally fruitful but occasionally led to amusing results such as when one medicinal chemist burst out of his lab to happily announce his discovery that he could obtain a correct-looking 3D structure from MM2 optimization even if he did not bother to attach hydrogens to the carbons. However, he had not bothered to check the bond lengths and bond angles for his molecule.

On a broader front, large and small pharmaceutical companies became aware of the potential for computer-aided drug design. Although pharmaceutical companies were understandably reticent to discuss what compounds they were pursuing, they were quite free in disclosing their computational chemistry infrastructure. For instance, Merck, which had grown its modeling group to be one of the largest in the world, published its system in 1980 [67]. Lilly's infrastructure was described at a national meeting of the American Chemical Society in 1982 [68].

A few years later, a survey was conducted of 48 pharmaceutical and chemical companies that were using computer-aided molecular design methods and were operating in the United States [69]. Between 1975 and 1985, the number of computational chemists employed at these companies increased from less than 30 to about 150, more than doubling every five years. Thus more companies were jumping on the bandwagon, and companies that were already in this area were expanding their efforts. Hiring of computational chemists accelerated through the decade [70]. Aware of the polarization that could exist between theoretical and medicinal chemists, some companies tried to circumvent this problem by hiring organic chemistry Ph.D.s who had spent a year or two doing postdoctoral research in molecular modeling. This trend was so pervasive that by 1985 only about a fifth of the computational chemists working at pharmaceutical companies came from a quantum mechanical background. Students, too, became aware of the fact that if their Ph.D. experience was in quantum chemistry, it would enhance their job prospects if they spent a year or two in some other area such as molecular dynamics simulations of proteins.

The computational chemistry techniques used most frequently were molecular graphics and molecular mechanics. Ab initio programs were in use at 21 of the 48 companies. Over 80% of the companies were using commercially produced software. Two-thirds of the companies were using software sold by Molecular Design Ltd. (MDL). A quarter were using SYBYL from Tripos Associates, and 15% were using the molecular modeling program CHEMGRAF by Chemical Design Ltd.

The following companies had five or more scientists working full-time as computational chemists in 1985: Abbott, DuPont, Lederle (American Cyanamid), Merck, Rohm and Haas, Searle, SmithKline Beecham, and Upjohn. Some of these companies had as many as 12 people working on computer-aided molecular design applications and software development. For the 48 companies, the mean ratio of the number of synthetic chemists to computational chemists was 29:1. This ratio reflects not only what percentage of a company's research effort was computer based, but also the number of synthetic chemists that each computational chemist might serve. Hence, a small ratio indicates more emphasis on computing or a small staff of synthetic chemists. Pharmaceutical companies with low ratios (less than 15:1) included Abbott, Alcon, Allergan, Norwich Eaton (Proctor & Gamble), and Searle. The most common organizational arrangement (at 40% of the 48 companies) was for the computational chemists to be integrated in the same department or division as the synthetic chemists. The other companies tried placing their computational chemists in a physical/analytical group, in a computer science group, or in their own unit.

About three-quarters of the 48 companies were using a VAX 11/780, 785, or 730 as their primary computing platform. The IBM 3033, 3083, 4341, etc. were being used for molecular modeling at about a third of the companies. (The percentages add up to more than 100% because larger companies had several types of machines.) The most commonly used graphics terminal was the Evans and Sutherland PS300 (E&S PS300) (40%), followed by Tektronix, Envison, and Retrographics VT640 at about one-third of the companies each and IMLAC (25%). The most-used brands of plotter in 1985 were the Hewlett-Packard and Versatec.

As cited above, the most widely used graphics terminal in 1985 was the E&S PS300. This machine was popular because of its very high resolution, color, speed, and stereo capabilities. (It is stunning to think that a company so dominant during one decade could totally disappear from the market a decade later. Such are the foibles of computer technology.) At Lilly, the E&S PS300 was set up in a large lighted room with black curtains enshrouding the cubicle with the machine. Lilly scientists were free to use the software running on the machine. In addition, the terminal also served as a showcase of Lilly's research prowess that was displayed to visiting Lilly sales representatives and dignitaries. No doubt a similar situation occurred at other companies.

The 1980s saw an important change in the way software was handled. In the 1970s, most of the programs used by computational chemists were exchanged essentially freely through QCPE, exchanged person to person, or developed in-house. But in the 1980s, many of the most popular programs—and some less popular ones—were commercialized. The number of software vendors mushroomed. For example, Pople's programs for ab initio calculations were withdrawn from QCPE; marketing rights were turned over to a company he helped found, Gaussian Inc. (Pittsburgh, Pennsylvania). This company also took responsibility for continued development of the software. In the molecular modeling arena, Tripos Associates (St. Louis, Missouri) was dominant by the mid-1980s. Their program SYBYL originally came from academic laboratories at Washington University (St. Louis) [71].

In the arena of chemical structure management, MDL (then in Hayward, California) was dominant. This company, which was founded in 1978 by Prof. Todd Wipke and others, marketed a program called MACCS for management of databases of compounds synthesized at or acquired by pharmaceutical companies. The software allowed substructure searching and later similarity searching [72, 73]. The software was vastly better than the manual systems that pharmaceutical companies had been using for recording compounds on file cards that were stored in filing cabinets. Except for some companies such as Upjohn that had their own home-grown software for management of their corporate compounds, many companies bought MACCS and became dependent on it. As happens in a free market where there is little competition, MACCS was very expensive. Few if any academic groups could afford it. A serious competing software product for compound management did not reach the market until 1987, when Daylight Chemical Information Systems was founded. By then, pharmaceutical companies were so wedded to MACCS that there was great inertia against switching their databases to another platform, even if it was cheaper and better suited for some tasks. In 1982, MDL started selling REACCS, a database management system for chemical reactions. Medicinal chemists liked both MACCS and REACCS. The former could be used to check whether a compound had previously been synthesized at a company and how much material was left in inventory. The latter program could be used to retrieve information about synthetic transformations and reaction conditions that had been published in the literature.

Some other momentous advances occurred on the software front. One was the writing of MOPAC, a semiempirical molecular orbital program, by Dr. James J. P. Stewart, a postdoctoral associate in Prof. Michael Dewar's group at the University of Texas at Austin [74–76]. The program was the first widely used program capable of automatically optimizing the geometry of molecules. This was a huge improvement over prior programs that could only perform calculations on fixed geometries. Formerly, a user would have to vary a bond length or a bond angle in increments, doing a separate calculation for each, then fit a parabola to the data points and try to guess where the minimum was. Hence MOPAC made the determination of 3D structures much simpler and more efficient. The program could handle molecules large enough to be of pharmaceutical interest. In the days of the VAX, a geometry optimization could run in two or three weeks. An interruption of a run due to a machine shutdown meant rerunning the calculation from the start. For the most part, however, the VAXes were fairly stable.

MOPAC was initially applicable to any molecule parameterized for Dewar's MINDO/3 or MNDO molecular orbital methods (i.e., common elements of the first and second rows of the periodic table). The optimized geometries were not in perfect agreement with experimental numbers but were better than what could have been obtained by prior molecular orbital programs for large molecules (those beyond the scope of ab initio calculations). Stewart made his program available through QCPE in 1984, and it quickly became (and long remained) the most requested program from QCPE's library of several hundred [77]. Unlike commercialized software, programs from QCPE were attractive because they were distributed as source code and cost very little.

In the arena of molecular mechanics, Prof. Allinger's continued, meticulous refinement of a experimentally based force field for organic compounds was welcomed by chemists interested in molecular modeling at pharmaceutical companies. The MM2 force field [78, 79] gave better results than MMI. To fund his research, Allinger sold distribution rights for the program initially to Molecular Design Ltd. (At the time, MDL also marketed some other molecular modeling programs.)

A program of special interest to the pharmaceutical industry was CLOGP. This program was developed by Prof. Al Leo (Pomona College) in the 1980s [80–82]. It was initially marketed through Daylight Chemical Information Systems (then of New Orleans and California). CLOGP could predict the lipophilicity of organic molecules. The algorithm was based on summing the contribution from each fragment (set of atoms) within a structure. The fragment contributions were parameterized to reproduce experimental octanol-water partition coefficients, log $P_{o/w}$. There was some discussion among scientists about whether octanol was the best organic solvent to mimic biological tissues, but this solvent proved to be the most used. To varying degrees, lipophilicity is related to many molecular properties including molecular volume, molecular surface area, transport through membranes, and binding to receptor surfaces, and hence to many different bioactivities. The calculated log $P_{o/w}$ values were widely used as a descriptor in QSAR studies in both industry and academia.

Yet another program was Dr. Kurt Enslein's TOPKAT [83, 84]. It was sold through his company, Health Designs (Rochester, New York). The software was based on statistics and was trained to predict the toxicity of a molecule from its structural fragments. Hence compounds with fragments such as nitro or nitroso would score poorly, basically confirming what an experienced medicinal chemist already knew. The toxicological end points included carcinogenicity, mutagenicity, teratogenicity, skin and eye irritation, and so forth. Today, pharmaceutical companies routinely try to predict toxicity, metabolism, bioavailability, and other factors that determine whether a highly potent ligand has what it takes to become a medicine. But back in the 1980s, the science was just beginning to be tackled. The main market for the program was probably government laboratories and regulators. Pharmaceutical laboratories were aware of the existence of the program but were leery of using it much. Companies trying to develop drugs were afraid that if the program, which was of unknown reliability for any specific compound, erroneously predicted danger for a structure, it could kill a project even though a multitude of laboratory experiments might give the compound a clean bill of health. There was also the worry about litigious lawyers. A compound could pass all the difficult hurdles of becoming a pharmaceutical, yet some undesirable, unexpected side effect might show up in some small percentage of patients taking it. If lawyers and lay juries, who frequently have trouble understanding science, the relative merits of different experiments, and the benefit-risk ratio associated with any pharmaceutical product, learned that a computer program had once put up a red flag for the compound, the pharmaceutical company could be alleged to be at fault.

We briefly mention one other commercially produced program. That program was SAS, a comprehensive data management and statistics program. The program was used mainly for handling clinical data that was analyzed by the statisticians at each company. Computational chemists also used SAS and other programs when statistical analyses were needed. SAS also had unique capabilities for graphical presentation of multidimensional numerical data [85] (this was in the days before Spotfire).

With the widespread commercialization of molecular modeling software in the 1980s, came both a boon and a bane to the computational chemist and pharmaceutical companies. The boon was that the software vendors sent marketing people to individual companies as well as to scientific meetings. The marketeers would extol the virtues of the programs they were pushing.

Great advances in drug discovery were promised if only the vendor's software systems were put in the hands of the scientists. Impressive demonstrations of molecular graphics, overlaying molecules, and so forth convinced company managers and medicinal chemists that here was the key to increasing research productivity. As a result of this marketing, most pharmaceutical companies purchased the software packages. The bane was that computer-aided drug design (CADD) was oversold, thereby setting up unrealistic expectations of what could be achieved by the software. Also, unrealistic expectations were set for what bench chemists could accomplish with the software. Unless the experimentalists devoted a good deal of time to learning the methods and limitations, the software was best left in the hands of computational chemistry experts.

Also in the 1980s, structure-based drug design (SBDD) underwent a similar cycle. Early proponents oversold what could be achieved through SBDD, thereby causing pharmaceutical companies to reconsider their investments when they discovered that SBDD too was no panacea for filling the drug discovery cornucopia with choice molecules for development. Nevertheless, SBDD was an important advance.

All through the 1970s, computational chemists were often rhetorically quizzed by critics about what if any pharmaceutical product had ever been designed by computer. Industrial computational chemists had a solid number of scientific accomplishments but were basically on the defensive when challenged with this question. Only a few computer-designed structures had ever been synthesized. Only a very tiny percentage of molecules—from any source—ever makes it as far as being a clinical candidate. The stringent criteria set for pharmaceutical products to be used in humans winnowed out almost all molecules. The odds were not good for any computational chemist achieving the ultimate success, a drug derived with the aid of the computer. In fact, many medicinal chemists would toil diligently their whole career and never have one of their compounds selected as a candidate for clinical development.

Another factor was that there were only a few drug targets that had had their 3D structures solved prior to the advancing methods for protein crystallography of the 1980s. One such early protein was dihydrofolate reductase (DHFR), the structures of which became known in the late 1970s [86, 87]. This protein became a favorite target of molecular modeling/drug design efforts in industry and elsewhere in the 1980s. Many resources were expended trying to find better inhibitors than the marketed pharmaceuticals of the antineoplastic methotrexate or the antibacterial trimethoprim. Innumerable papers and lectures sprung from those efforts. Scientists do not like to report negative results, but finally a frank admission came in 1988. A review concluded that none of the computer-based efforts at his company or disclosed by others in the literature had yielded better drugs [88].

Although this first major, widespread effort at SBDD was a disappointment, the situation looked better on the QSAR front. In Japan, Koga employed classic (Hansch-type) QSAR while discovering the antibacterial agent norfloxacin around 1982 [89–91]. Norfloxacin was the first of the third-generation analogs of nalidixic acid to reach the marketplace. This early success may not have received the notice it deserved, perhaps because the field of computer-aided drug design continued to focus heavily on computer graphics, molecular dynamics, X-ray crystallography, and nuclear magnetic resonance spectroscopy [92]. Another factor may have been that medicinal chemists and microbiologists at other pharmaceutical companies capitalized on the discovery of norfloxacin to elaborate even better quinoline antibacterials that eventually dominated the market.

As computers and software improved, SBDD became a more popular approach to drug discovery. One company, Agouron in San Diego, California, set a new paradigm for discovery based on iterations of crystallography and medicinal chemistry. As new compounds were made, some could be cocrystallized with the target protein. The 3D structure of the complex was solved by rapid computer techniques. Observations of how the compounds fit into the receptor suggested ways to improve affinity, leading to another round of synthesis and crystallography. Although considered by its practitioners and most others as an experimental science, protein crystallography (now popularly called structural biology, see also Chapter 12) often employed a step whereby the refraction data were refined in conjunction with constrained molecular dynamics (MD) simulations. Dr. Axel Brünger's program X-PLOR [93] met this important need. The force field in the program had its origin in CHARMM developed by Prof. Martin Karplus's group at Harvard [94]. Pharmaceutical companies that set up protein crystallography groups acquired X-PLOR to run on their computers.

The SBDD approach affected computational chemists positively. The increased number of 3D structures of therapeutically relevant targets opened new opportunities for molecular modeling of the receptor sites. Computational chemists assisted the medicinal chemists in interpreting the fruits of crystallography for design of new ligands.

Molecular dynamics simulations can consume prodigious amounts of computer time. Not only are proteins very large structures, but also the MD results are regarded as better the longer they are run because more of conformational space is assumed to be sampled by the jiggling molecules. Even more demand for computer power appeared necessary when free energy perturbation (FEP) theory appeared on the scene. Some of the brightest luminaries in academic computational chemistry proclaimed that here was a powerful new method for designing drugs [95, 96]. Pharmaceutical companies were influenced by these claims [97]. On the other hand, computational chemists closer to the frontline of working with medicinal chemists generally recognized that whereas FEP was a powerful method for accurately calculating the binding energy between ligands and macromolecular targets, it was too slow for extensive use in actual drug discovery. The molecular modifications that could be simulated with FEP treatment, such as changing one substituent to another, were relatively minor. Because the FEP simulations had to be run so long to obtain good results, it was often possible for a medicinal chemist to synthesize the new modification in less time than it took to do the calculations. Also, for cases in which a synthesis would take longer than the calculations, not many industrial medicinal chemists would rate the modification worth the effort. Researchers in industry are under a great deal of pressure to tackle problems quickly and not spend too much time on them.

The insatiable need for more computing resources in the 1980s sensitized the pharmaceutical companies to the technological advances leading to the manufacture of supercomputers [98]. Some pharmaceutical companies opted for specialized machines such as array processors. By the mid-1980s, for example, several pharmaceutical companies had acquired the Floating Point System (FPS) 164. Other pharmaceutical companies sought to meet their needs by buying time and/or partnerships with one of the state or national supercomputing centers formed in the United States, Europe, and Japan. For instance, in 1988 Lilly partnered with the National Center for Supercomputing Applications (NCSA) in Urbana-Champaign, Illinois. Meanwhile, supercomputer manufacturers such as Cray Research and ETA Systems, both in Minnesota, courted scientists and managers at the pharmaceutical companies.

A phrase occasionally heard in this period was that computations were the “third way” of science. The other two traditional ways to advance science were experiment and theory. The concept behind the new phrase was that computing could be used to develop and test theories and to stimulate ideas for new experiments.

1.6 FRUITION: THE 1990s

The 1990s was a decade of fruition because the computer-based drug discovery work of the 1980s yielded an impressive number of new chemical entities reaching the pharmaceutical marketplace. We elaborate on this statement later in this section, but first we complete the story about supercomputers in the pharmaceutical industry.

Pharmaceutical companies were accustomed to supporting their own research and making large investments in it. In fact, the pharmaceutical industry has long maintained the largest self-supporting research enterprise in the world. However, the price tag on a supercomputer was daunting. To help open the pharmaceutical industry as a market for supercomputers, the chief executive officer (CEO) of Cray Research took the bold step of paying a visit to the CEO of Lilly in Indianapolis. Apparently, Cray’s strategy was to entice a major pharmaceutical company to purchase a supercomputer, and then additional pharmaceutical companies might follow suit in an attempt to keep their research competitive. Lilly was offered a Cray-2 at an irresistible price. Not only did Lilly buy a machine, but other pharmaceutical companies either bought or leased a Cray. Merck, Bristol-Myers Squibb, Marion Merrell Dow (then a large company in Cincinnati, Ohio), Johnson & Johnson, and Bayer were among the companies that chose a Cray. Some of these machines were the older X-MP or the smaller J90 machine, the latter being less expensive to maintain.

After Lilly's purchase of the Cray 2S-2/128, line managers were given the responsibility to make sure the purchase decision had a favorable outcome. This was a welcome opportunity because line management was fully confident that supercomputing would revolutionize research and development [99]. The managers believed that a supercomputer would enable scientists to test more ideas than would be practical with older computers. Management was optimistic that a supercomputer would foster collaborations and information sharing among employees in different disciplines at the company. The managers hoped that both scientific and business uses of the machine would materialize. Ultimately, then, supercomputing would speed the identification of promising new drug candidates. Scientists closer to the task of using the supercomputer saw the machine primarily as a tool for performing longer molecular dynamics simulations and quantum mechanical calculations on large molecules. However, if some other computational technique such as QSAR or data mining was more effective at discovering and optimizing new lead compounds, then the supercomputer might not fulfill the dreams envisioned for it. A VAX cluster remained an essential part of the technology infrastructure best suited for management of the corporate library of compounds (see more about this below).

Lilly organized special workshops to train potential users of the Cray. This pool of potential users included as many willing medicinal chemists and other personnel as possible. In-house computational chemists and other experts were assigned the responsibility of conducting the off-site, week-long workshops. The workshops covered not only how to submit and retrieve jobs but also the general methods of molecular modeling, molecular dynamics, quantum chemistry, and QSAR. The latter, as mentioned, did not require supercomputing resources, except perhaps occasionally to generate quantum mechanical descriptors. Mainly, however, the training had the concomitant benefit of exposing more medicinal chemists, including younger ones, to what could be achieved with the current state of the art of computational chemistry applied to molecular design.

As the role of the computational chemist became more important, attitudes toward them became more accepting. At some large, old pharmaceutical houses, and at many smaller, newer companies, it was normal practice to allow computational chemists to be co-inventors on patents if the computational chemists contributed to a discovery. Other companies, including Lilly, had long had a company-wide policy that computational chemists could not be on patents. The policy was changed at Lilly as the 1990s dawned. Computational chemists were becoming nearly equal partners in the quest to discover drugs.

Lilly's Cray also served as an impressive public relations showcase. The machine was housed in a special, climate-controlled room. One side of the darkened room had a wall of large glass windows treated with polymer-dispersed liquid crystals. The thousands of visitors who came to Lilly each year were escorted into a uniquely designed observation room where an excellent video was shown that explained the supercomputer and how it could be used for drug discovery. The observation room was automatically darkened at the start of the video. At the dramatic finish of the video, the translucent glass wall was turned clear and bright lights were turned on inside the computer room, revealing the Cray-2 and its cooling tower for the heat transfer liquid. The visitors enjoyed the spectacle.

To the disappointment of Lilly's guest relations department, Lilly's Cray-2 was later replaced with a Cray J90, a mundane-looking machine. But the J90 was more economical, especially because it was leased. The supercomputers were almost always busy with molecular dynamics and quantum mechanical calculations [100]. Of the personnel at the company, the computational chemists were the main beneficiaries of supercomputing.

At the same time supercomputers that were creating excitement at a small number of pharmaceutical companies, another hardware development was attracting attention at just about every company interested in designing drugs. Workstations from Silicon Graphics Inc. (SGI) were becoming increasingly popular for molecular research. These high-performance, UNIX-based machines were attractive because of their ability to handle large calculations quickly and because of their high-resolution, interactive computer graphics. Although a supercomputer was fine for CPU-intensive jobs, the workstations were better suited for interactive molecular modeling software being used for drug research. The workstations became so popular that some medicinal chemists wanted them for their offices, not so much for extensive use but rather as a status symbol.

Another pivotal event affecting the hardware situation of the early 1990s merits mention. As already stated, the Apple Macintoshes were well liked by scientists. However, in 1994 Apple lost its lawsuit against Microsoft regarding the similarities of the Windows graphical user interface (GUI) to Apple's desktop design. Also, the price of Windows-based PCs dropped significantly below that of Macs. The tables tilted in favor of PCs. More scientists began to use PCs. At Lilly, and maybe other companies, the chief information officer (a position that did not even exist until computer technology became so critical to corporate success) decreed that the company scientists would have to switch to PCs whether they wanted to or not. The reasons for this were severalfold. The PCs were more economical. With PCs being so cheap, it was likely more people would use them, and hence there was a worry that software for Macs would become less plentiful. Also, the problem of incompatible files would be eliminated if all employees used the same type of computer and software.

On the software front, the early 1990s witnessed a continued trend toward commercially produced programs being used in pharmaceutical companies.

Programs such as SYBYL (Tripos), Insight/Discover (BIOSYM), and Quanta/CHARMm (Polygen, and later Molecular Simulations Inc., and now Accelrys) were popular around the world for molecular modeling and simulations. Some pharmaceutical companies bought licenses to all three of these well-known packages. Use of commercial software freed the in-house computational chemists from the laborious task of code development, documentation, and maintenance, so that they would have more time to work on actual drug design. Another advantage of using commercial software was that the larger vendors would have a help desk that users could telephone for assistance when software problems arose, as they often did. The availability of the help desk meant that the in-house computational chemists would have fewer interruptions from medicinal chemists who were having difficulty getting the software to work. On the other hand, some companies, particularly Merck and Upjohn, preferred to develop software in-house because it was thought to be better than what the vendors could provide.

Increasing use of commercial software for computational chemistry meant a declining role for software from QCPE. QCPE had passed its zenith by about 1992, when it had almost 1900 members and over 600 programs in its catalog. This catalog included about 15 molecular modeling programs written at pharmaceutical companies and contributed for the good of the community of computational chemists. Among the companies contributing software were Merck, DuPont, Lilly, Abbott, and Novartis. When distribution rights for MOPAC were acquired by Fujitsu in 1992, it was a severe blow to QCPE. After a period of decline, the operations of QCPE changed in 1998. Today only a web-based operation continues at Indiana University, Bloomington.

The 1990s was a decade of change for the software vendors also. The California company that started out as BioDesign became Molecular Simulations Inc. (MSI). MSI went on a buying spree starting in 1991. It grew large by acquiring other small software companies competing in the same drug design market, including Polygen, BIOSYM, BioCAD, Oxford Molecular (which had already acquired several other start-ups), and others [101]. Pharmaceutical companies worried about this accretion because it could mean less competition and it could mean that their favorite molecular dynamics (MD) program might no longer be supported in the future. This latter possibility has not come to pass because there has been sufficient loyalty and demand for each MD package to remain on the market.

Researchers from pharmaceutical companies participated in user groups set up by the software vendors. Pharmaceutical companies also bought into consortia created by the software vendors. These consortia, some of which dated back to the 1980s, aimed at developing new software tools or improving existing software. The pharmaceutical companies hoped to get something for their investments. Sometimes the net effect of these investments was that it enabled the software vendors to hire several postdoctoral research associates who worked on things that were of common interest to the investors. Although the pharmaceutical companies received some benefit from the consortia, other needs such as more and better force field parameters remained underserved. Inspired by the slow progress in one force field development consortium, Merck single-handedly undertook the de novo development of a force field they call the Merck Molecular Force Field (MMFF94). This force field, which targeted the modeling of pharmaceutically interesting molecules well, was published [102–108], and several software vendors subsequently incorporated it in their molecular modeling programs. The accolades of fellow computational chemists led to the developer being elected in 1992 to become chairman of one of the Gordon Research Conferences on Computational Chemistry [109].

On the subject of molecular modeling and force fields, a general molecular modeling package was developed in an organic chemistry laboratory at Columbia University in New York City [110]. Perhaps because MacroModel was written with organic chemists in mind, it proved popular with industrial medicinal chemists, among others. The program was designed so that versions of several good force fields could easily be invoked for any energy minimization or molecular simulation.

The 1990s witnessed other exciting technological developments. In 1991, Dr. Jan K. Labanowski, then an employee of the Ohio Supercomputer Center (Columbus, Ohio), launched an electronic bulletin board called the Computational Chemistry List (CCL). Computational chemists rapidly joined because it was an effective forum for informal exchange of information. Computational chemists at pharmaceutical companies were among the 2000 or so members who joined in the 1990s. Often these employees would take the time to answer questions from beginners, helping them learn about the field of computer-aided drug design. The CCL was a place where the relative merits of different methodologies and computers and the pros and cons of various programming languages could be debated, sometimes passionately.

In 1991, MDL came out with a new embodiment of its compound management software called ISIS (Integrated Scientific Information System). Pharmaceutical companies upgraded to the new system, having become so dependent on MDL. In general, managers of information technology at pharmaceutical companies preferred one-stop solutions. On the other hand, computational chemists found Daylight Chemical Information Systems software more useful for developing new research applications.

MACCS and then ISIS gave researchers exceptional new tools for drug discovery when similarity searching came along. Chemical structures were stored in the database as connectivity tables (showing which atoms were connected by bonds). In addition, chemical structures could be stored as a series of on-off flags ("keys") indicating the presence or absence of specific atoms or combinations of atoms and/or bonds. The similarity of compounds could be quantitated by the computer in terms of the percentage of keys that the compounds shared in common. Thus, if a researcher was aware of a lead structure from in-house work or the literature, it was possible to find compounds in the corporate database that were similar and then get these compounds assayed for biological activities. Therefore the technique of data mining became important. Depending on how large the database was, it was fairly easy to find compounds with low levels of activity by this method. Some of these active compounds might have a skeleton different from the lead structure. The new skeleton could form the basis for subsequent lead optimization. As Dr. Yvonne C. Martin (Abbott) has wryly commented in her lectures at scientific meetings, one approach to drug discovery is to find a compound that the target receptor sees as the same as an established ligand but which a patent examiner sees as a different compound (and therefore satisfying the novelty requirement for patentability).

Many or most of the results from data mining in industry went unpublished. More recently, when a few academic researchers gained access to data mining software, the weakly active compounds they found were excitedly published. This difference between industry and academia in handling similar kinds of results is a matter of priorities. In industry, the first priority is to find marketable products and get them out the door. In academia, the priority is to publish (especially in high-impact journals). Contrary to a common misconception, scientists in industry do publish, a point we return to below.

Software use for drug discovery and development can be classified in various ways. One way is technique based. Examples would be programs based on force fields or on statistical fitting (the latter including log P prediction or toxicity prediction). Another way to classify software is according to whether the algorithm can be applied to cases in which the 3D structure of the target receptor is known or not. An example of software useful when the receptor structure is not known is Catalyst [111]. This program, which became available in the early 1990s, tried to produce a 3D model of a pharmacophore based on a small set of compounds with a range of activities against a given target. The pharmacophore model, if determinable, could be used as a query to search databases of 3D structures in an effort to find new potential ligands.

In situations in which the computational chemist had the benefit of the 3D structure of the target receptor, three methodologies came into increased usage. One was docking, that is, letting an algorithm try to fit a ligand structure into a receptor. Docking methodology dates back to the 1980s, but the 1990s saw more crystal structures of pharmaceutically relevant proteins being solved and used for ligand design [112]. A second technique of the 1990s involved designing a computer algorithm to construct a ligand de novo inside a receptor structure. The program would assemble fragments or "grow" a chemical structure such that the electrostatic and steric attributes of the receptor would be complemented by the ligand [113–115]. The third technique of the 1990s was virtual screening [116, 117]. The computer would screen hypothetical ligand structures, not necessarily compounds in bottles, against the 3D structure of a receptor in order to find those most likely to fit and therefore worthy of synthesis and experimentation.

A new approach to drug discovery came to prominence around 1993. The arrival of this approach was heralded with optimism reminiscent of earlier waves of new technologies. The proponents of this innovation—combinatorial chemistry—were organic chemists. The thinking behind combinatorial chemistry seemed to be as follows. The chance of finding a molecule with therapeutic value was extremely low (one in 5000 or one in 10,000 were rough estimates that were often bandied about). Attempts at rational drug design had not significantly improved the odds of finding those rare molecules that could become a pharmaceutical product. Because the low odds could not be beat, make tens of thousands, . . . no, hundreds of thousands, . . . no, millions of compounds! Then, figuratively fire a massive number of these molecular bullets at biological targets and hope that some might stick. New computer-controlled robotic machinery would permit syntheses of all these compounds much more economically than the traditional one-compound-at-a-time process of medicinal chemistry. Likewise, computer-controlled robotic machinery would automate the biological screening and reduce the cost per assay.

Proponents promised that combinatorial chemistry was the way to keep the drug discovery pipeline full. Pharmaceutical companies made massive investments in people and machinery to set up the necessary equipment in the 1990s. Some companies built large refrigerated storage rooms where the libraries of compounds could be stored and retrieved by robots. The computers to run the equipment had to be programmed. This work was done by instrument engineers, although chemists helped set up the systems that controlled the syntheses.

Combinatorial chemistry increased the rate of output of new compounds by three orders of magnitude. Before combi-chem, a typical SAR at a pharmaceutical company might have consisted of fewer than a couple hundred compounds, and a massive effort involving 10–20 medicinal chemistry laboratories might have produced two or three thousand compounds over a number of years. In 1993, with traditional one-compound-at-a-time chemistry it took one organic chemist on average one week to make one compound for biological testing. Some years later, with combi-chem a chemist could easily produce 2000 compounds per week.

With the arrival of combi-chem, computational chemists had a new task in addition to what they had been doing. Computational chemistry was needed so that the combinatorial chemistry was not mindlessly driven by whatever reagents were available in chemical catalogs or from other sources. There were several strategies to library design [118]. The first was to cover as much of "compound space" as possible, that is, to produce a variety of structures to increase the likelihood that one of the compounds would stick to the target. Then after the drug discovery researchers had gained a general idea of what structure(s) would bind to the target receptor, a second strategy would come into play: to design compounds similar to the lead(s). Another need was to assess the value of libraries being offered for sale by various outside intermediaries. Computational chemists could help determine whether these libraries complemented or duplicated a company's existing libraries of compounds and determine the degree of variety in the compounds being offered. How does one describe chemical space and molecular similarity? Computational chemists had already developed the technologies of molecular descriptors and substructure keys, which we mentioned above. With these tools, the computational chemist could discern where structures were situated in multidimensional compound or property space and provide advice to the medicinal chemists.

Along with all the data generated by combi-chem and high-throughput screening (HTS) came the need to manage and analyze the data. Hence, computers and the science of informatics became increasingly vital.

The computational chemist was now more important to drug discovery research than ever before. Hence by 1993–1994, these technological changes possibly helped save the jobs of many computational chemists at a time when pharmaceutical companies in the United States were downsizing, as we now explain. In 1992–1993 an acute political force impinged on the pharmaceutical industry in the United States. That force was the healthcare reform plan proposed by Hillary and Bill Clinton. Readers who are well versed in history of the 1930s will be aware of the economic system handed down from pre-World War II Europe. Under that system, the means of production, that is, industry, remains in private ownership but the prices that the companies can ask for their products are regulated by government. That was the scheme underlying the healthcare reform proposal. Pharmaceutical companies in the United States generally favored any proposal that would increase access to their products but feared this specific proposal because of the great uncertainty it cast over the status quo and future growth prospects. As a result, thousands of pharmaceutical workers—including research scientists—were laid off or encouraged to retire. Rumors swirled around inside each pharmaceutical company about who would be let go and who would retain their jobs. When word came down about the corporate decisions, the computational chemists were generally retained, but the ranks of the older medicinal chemists were thinned. A new generation of managers at pharmaceutical companies now realized that computer-assisted molecular design and library design were critical components of their company's success. One is reminded of the observation of the Nobel laureate physicist Max Planck, "An important scientific innovation rarely makes its way by gradually winning over and converting its opponents. . . . What does happen is that its opponents gradually die out and the growing generation is familiarized with the idea from the beginning."

Nevertheless, the Clintons' healthcare reform scheme had a deleterious effect on the hiring of new computational chemists. The job market for computational chemists in the United States fell from a then record high in 1990 to a depression in 1992–1994 [119]. This happened because pharmaceutical companies were afraid to expand until they were sure that the business climate was once again hospitable for growth. The healthcare reform proposal was defeated in the United States Congress, but it took a year or two before pharmaceutical companies started rebuilding their workforces.

Toward the mid-1990s, a new mode of delivering content came to the fore: the web browser. Information technology (IT) engineers and computational chemists help set up intranets at pharmaceutical companies. This allowed easy distribution of management memos and other information to the employees. In addition, biological screening data could be posted on the intranet so that medicinal chemists could quickly access it electronically. Computational chemists made their applications (programs) web-enabled so that medicinal chemists and others could perform calculations from their desktops.

The hardware situation continued to evolve. Personal computers became ever more powerful in terms of speed and the amount of random access memory (RAM) and hard drive capacity. The price of PCs continued to fall. Clusters of PCs were built. Use of the open-source Linux operating system spread in the 1990s. Distributed processing was developed so a long calculation could be farmed out to separate machines. Massively parallel processing was tried. All these changes meant that the days of the supercomputers were numbered.

Whereas the trend in the 1980s was toward dispersal of computing power to the departments and the individual user, the IT administrators started bringing the PCs under their centralized control in the 1990s. Software to monitor each machine was installed so that what each user did could be tracked. Following the example of other industries, some pharmaceutical companies turned over the technical work of managing their networks of PCs to outside contractors. Gradually, computational chemists and other workers lost control over what could and could not be installed on their office machines. One type of hardware, however, persisted through the 1990s and even to today: the SGI workstations. These UNIX machines became more powerful and remained popular for molecular modeling. Silicon Graphics Inc. acquired the expiring Cray technology, but it did not seem to have much effect on their workstation business.

Traditionally, in pursuit of their structure-activity relationships, medicinal chemists had focused almost exclusively on finding compounds with greater and greater potency. However, these SARs often ended up with compounds that were unsuitable for development as pharmaceutical products. These compounds would be too insoluble in water, or were not orally bioavailable, or were eliminated too quickly or too slowly from mammalian bodies. Pharmacologists and pharmaceutical development scientists for years had tried to preach the need for medicinal chemists to also think about other factors that determined whether a compound could be a medicine. Table 1.1 lists a number of factors that determine whether a potent compound has what it takes to become a drug. Experimentally, it was difficult to quantitate these other factors. Often, the necessary manpower resources would not be allocated to a compound until it had already been selected for project team status.

At the beginning of the 1990s, the factors in Table 1.1 were generally beyond the capability of computational chemistry methods to predict reliably. However, as the decade unfolded, computational chemists and other scientists

TABLE 1.1 What It Takes for a Compound (Ligand) to Become a Pharmaceutical Product

Absorption into the body, i.e., bioavailability
Behavior in humans as anticipated from preliminary testing in animal models, i.e., no untoward species differences
Distribution among the appropriate tissues of the body
Metabolism by the body or organisms living in the body
Ease of production, including, for instance, the existence of environmentally safe routes of isolation or synthesis
Efficacy, i.e., whatever the compound does at its site(s) of action; the net effect is to elicit a desirable therapeutic outcome
Elimination from the body, i.e., excretion
Medical need, which affects marketability
Novelty, which determines patentability
Pharmaceutical "elegance," which encompasses factors related to route of administration (taste, color, mixability with excipients, etc.)
Side effects of the compound and its degradation products are minimal or at least tolerable
Solubility, preferably in water
Stability, so the compound will not degrade before being consumed and can reach its site of action in a bioactive form
Therapeutic ratio, so that the concentration of the compound to elicit its therapeutic effect is much lower than the concentration that would cause untoward effects
Toxic effects of the compound and its degradation products are minimal

created new and better methodologies for selecting compounds with the characteristics necessary to become a drug. In 1997, Lipinski's now famous "Rule of Five" was published [120]. These simple rules were easily encoded in database mining operations at every company, so that compounds with low prospects of becoming an orally active, small-molecule drug (less than 500 MW) could be weeded out by computer.

The computational methods used in the 1980s focused, like medicinal chemistry, on finding compounds with ever-higher affinity between the ligand and its target receptor. That is why in the past we have advocated use of the term computer-aided ligand design (CALD) rather than CADD. However, with increased attention to the factors listed in Table 1.1, the field was finally becoming more literally correct in calling itself CADD.

Another important change started in the mid-1990s. Traditionally, a QSAR determined at a pharmaceutical company might have involved only 5–30 compounds. The size depended on how many compounds the medicinal chemist had synthesized and submitted to testing by the biologists. Sometimes this size data set sufficed to reveal useful trends. Other times, though, the

QSARs were not very robust in terms of predictability. As large libraries of compounds were produced, data sets available for QSAR analysis became larger. With all that consistently produced (although not necessarily perfectly accurate) biological data and a plethora of molecular descriptors, it was possible to find correlations with good predictability. In fact, QSAR proved to be one of the best approaches to providing assistance to the medicinal chemist in the 1990s. Computational chemists were inventive in creating new molecular descriptors. Hundreds have been described in the literature [121–123].

As stated in the opening of this section, the 1990s witnessed the fruition of a number of drug design efforts. Making a new pharmaceutical product available to patients is a long, difficult, and costly enterprise. It takes 10–15 years from the time a compound is discovered in the laboratory until it is approved for physicians to prescribe. Hence, a molecule that reached the pharmacies in the 1990s was probably first synthesized at a pharmaceutical company well back in the 1980s. (Most of today's medicines come from the pharmaceutical industry rather than from government or academic laboratories.) The improved methodologies of computational chemistry that became available in the 1980s would therefore start to show their full impact in the 1990s. (Likewise, the improved experimental and computational methodologies of the 1990s should be bearing fruit now.)

Table 1.2 lists medicines whose discovery was aided in some way by computer-based methods. Those compounds marked "CADD" were pub-

TABLE 1.2 Marketed Pharmaceuticals Whose Discovery Was Aided by Computers

Generic Name	Brand Name	Year Approved in United States	Discovery Assisted by	Activity
Norfloxacin	Noroxin	1983	QSAR	Antibacterial
Losartan	Cozaar	1994	CADD	Antihypertensive
Dorzolamide	Trusopt	1995	CADD/SBDD	Antiglaucoma
Ritonavir	Norvir	1996	CADD	Antiviral
Indinavir	Crixivan	1996	CADD	Antiviral
Donepezil	Aricept	1997	QSAR	Anti-Alzheimer's
Zolmitriptan	Zomig	1997	CADD	Antimigraine
Nelfinavir	Viracept	1997	SBDD	Antiviral
Amprenavir	Agenerase	1999	SBDD	Antiviral
Zanamivir	Relenza	1999	SBDD	Antiviral
Oseltamivir	Tamiflu	1999	SBDD	Antiviral
Lopinavir	Aluviran	2000	SBDD	Antiviral
Imatinib	Gleevec	2001	SBDD	Antineoplastic
Erlotinib	Tarceva	2004	SBDD	Antineoplastic
Ximelagatran	Exanta	2004	SBDD	Anticoagulant

licized in a series of earlier publications [references 124–128; see also references 129 and 130, and Chapter 16 for other discussion]. These examples of CADD successes were gathered in 1997 when one of us (DBB) undertook a survey of the corresponding authors of papers published after 1993 in the prestigious *Journal of Medicinal Chemistry.* Authors were asked whether calculations were crucial to the discovery of any compounds from their laboratory. Of the hundreds of replies, we culled out all cases in which calculations had not led to drug discovery or had been done post hoc on a clinical candidate or pharmaceutical product. We have always felt strongly that the term "computer-aided drug design" should be more than just doing a calculation; it should be providing information or ideas that directly help with the conception of a useful new structure. We retained only those cases where the senior author of a paper (usually a medicinal chemist) vouched that computational chemistry had actually been critically important in the research process that led to the discovery of a compound that had reached the market. As seen in Table 1.2, there were seven compounds meeting this criterion in the period 1994–1997. The computational techniques used to find these seven compounds included QSAR, ab initio molecular orbital calculations, molecular modeling, molecular shape analysis [131], docking, active analog approach [132], molecular mechanics, and SBDD.

More recently, a group in England led by a structural biologist compiled a list of marketed medicines that came from SBDD [133]. These are labeled "SBDD" in Table 1.2. It can be seen that there is only a little overlap between the two compilations (CADD and SBDD). It can also be seen that the number of pharmaceuticals from SBDD is very impressive. Computer-based technologies are clearly making a difference in helping bring new medicines to patients.

Looking at the success stories, we see that it has often been a team of researchers working closely together that led to the success. It took quite a while for other members of the drug discovery research community to appreciate what computational chemistry could provide. There remains room for further improvement in this regard. Computational chemistry is probably most effective when researchers work in an environment where credit is shared [134]. If management adopts a system whereby company scientists are competing with each other, then collaborations are tempered. On the other hand, if all members of an interdisciplinary team of scientists will benefit when the team succeeds, then collaboration increases, synergies can occur, and the team is more likely to succeed. Sometimes it helps to put the computational chemistry techniques in the hands of the medicinal chemists, but it seems that only some of these chemists have the time and inclination to use the techniques to best advantage. Therefore, computational chemistry experts play an important role in maximizing the potential benefits of computer-based technologies.

1.7 EPILOGUE

To close, we distill in Figure 1.3 the essence of what we have described about the history of computing at pharmaceutical companies over the last four decades. We plot the number of papers published (and abstracted by Chemical Abstracts Service) for each year from 1964 through 2004, the most recent

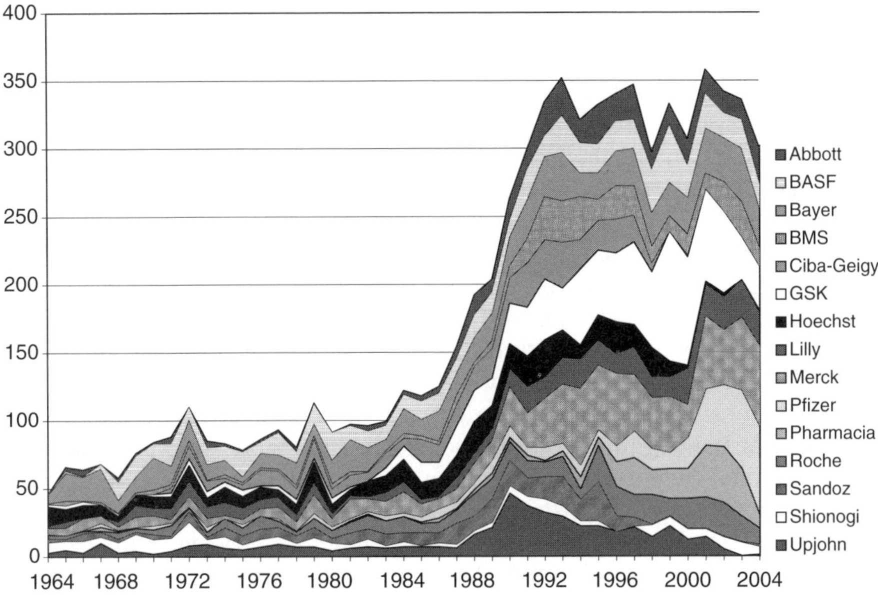

Figure 1.3 Annual number of papers published by researchers at pharmaceutical companies during a 41-year period. The data were obtained by searching the CAPLUS and MEDLINE databases for papers related to "computer or calculation." Then these hits were refined with SciFinder Scholar by searching separately for 48 different company names. Well-known companies from around the world were included. Companies with more than 250 total hits in the period 1964–2004 are included in the plot. The indexing by CAS is such that a search on SmithKline Beecham gave the same number of hits as for GlaxoSmithKline (GSK) but much more than Smith Kline and French. The downward trend of the sum after 2001 can be traced to fewer papers coming from GSK. Initially, we had wanted to structure our SciFinder Scholar search for all papers using terms pertaining to computational chemistry, molecular modeling, computer-aided drug design, quantitative structure-activity relationships, and so forth. However, CAS classifies these terms as overlapping concepts, and so SciFinder Scholar was unable to do the searches as desired. Searching on "computer or calculation" yields many relevant hits but also a small number of papers that are of questionable relevance. This contamination stems from the subjective way abstractors at CAS have indexed articles over the years. The irrelevant papers introduce noise in the data, but hopefully the systematic error is relatively constant over the period covered. CAPLUS covers 1500 journals. See color plate.

complete year. These are papers that were indexed as pertaining to "computer or calculation" and that came from pharmaceutical companies. We can learn several things from Figure 1.3. First, industrial scientists do publish. Second, the figure includes a list of pharmaceutical companies that have done the most publishing of papers pertaining to computers or calculations. There are 15 companies with more than 250 papers each in the 41-year period. Some of these companies ceased publishing simply because they were acquired by other pharmaceutical companies, and hence the affiliation of the authors changed. The companies are headquartered in the United States, Switzerland, Germany, and Japan. Third, the number of publications increased slowly but fairly steadily from 1964 through the mid-1980s. Then, from 1986 through 1992, the annual number of papers grew rapidly. This period is when the superminicomputers, supercomputers, and workstations appeared on the scene. We also learn from Figure 1.3 that since 1994 the sum of the annual number of papers published by the 15 companies has zigzagged around 325 papers per year. Curiously, the recent years show no evidence of an upward trend.

As the twentieth century came to a close, the job market for computational chemists had recovered from the 1992–1994 debacle. In fact, demand for computational chemists leaped to new highs each year in the second half of the 1990s [135]. Most of the new jobs were in industry, and most of these industrial jobs were at pharmaceutical or biopharmaceutical companies. As we noted at the beginning of this chapter, in 1960 there were essentially no computational chemists in industry. But 40 years later, perhaps well over half of all computational chemists were working in pharmaceutical laboratories. The outlook for computational chemistry is therefore very much linked to the health of the pharmaceutical industry itself. Forces that adversely affect pharmaceutical companies will have a negative effect on the scientists who work there as well as at auxiliary companies such as software vendors that develop programs and databases for use in drug discovery and development.

Over the last four decades, we have witnessed waves of new technologies sweep over the pharmaceutical industry. Sometimes these technologies tended to be oversold at the beginning and turned out to not be a panacea to meet the quota of the number of new chemical entities that each company would like to launch each year. Experience has shown that computer technology so pervasive at one point in time can almost disappear 10 years later.

Discovering new medicines is a serious, extremely difficult, and expensive undertaking. Tens of thousands of scientists are employed in this activity. Back in 1980, pharmaceutical and biotechnology companies operating in the United States invested in aggregate about $2000 million in R&D. The sum has steadily increased (although there was the slight pause in 1994 that we mentioned above). By 2003, R&D investments had grown to $34,500 million. In 2004, the total jumped to $38,800 million. The United States pharmaceutical industry invests far more in discovering new and better therapies than the pharmaceutical industry in any other country or any government in the world. Despite the ever-increasing investment in R&D each year, the annual number of new chemical entities (NCEs) approved for marketing in the United States (or elsewhere) has not shown any overall increase in the last 25 years. The number has fluctuated between 60 and 20 NCEs per year and has been around 30 per year recently. This very uncomfortable fact was not widely discussed before the late 1990s [124] but is now well known. A recent analysis of NCE data was able to find some reason for optimism that innovation is bringing to market drugs with substantial advantage over existing treatments [136]. However, deciding whether R&D is becoming more productive depends on how the NCE data are handled. Generally, most people in the field realize that discovery research is not as easy or as productive as they would like.

In an attempt to boost NCE output, executives at pharmaceutical companies have put their researchers under extreme pressure to focus and produce. Since the early 1990s, this pressure has moved in only one direction: up.

During two million years of human evolution, better intelligence at creating and using tools has meant the difference between survival and extinction. In a similar way, those pharmaceutical companies with scientists who are best at creating and using tools will be able to innovate their way to the future. In contrast to the days of the hunter-gatherer cracking stones, today the tools are computers and software, as well as chemistry and biology. With combinatorial chemistry, high-throughput screening, genomics, and structural biology firmly embedded in modern drug discovery efforts, computers are indispensable.

All musical composers work with the same set of notes, but the geniuses put the notes together in an extraordinarily beautiful way. Synthetic chemists all have available to them the same elements. The successful medicinal chemist will combine atoms such that amazing therapeutic effect is achieved with the resulting molecule. The computational chemist's goal should be to help the medicinal chemist by providing information about structural and electronic requirements to enhance activity, namely, information about which regions of compound space are most propitious for exploration.

Fortunately, all the effort that goes into pharmaceutical R&D does benefit society. In nations where modern medicines are available, life expectancy has increased and disability rates among the elderly have declined. Considering all of the things that can go wrong with the human body, many challenges remain for the pharmaceutical researcher. Hopefully, this chapter will inspire some young readers to take up the challenge and join the noble quest to apply science to help find cures to improve people's lives.

ACKNOWLEDGMENTS

We are grateful to Dr. Sean Ekins for the opportunity to participate in this book and for his painstaking editing. We thank our many colleagues over the years for what they taught us or tried to teach us. Some of the historical events reviewed here occurred during the period of our respective tenures as members of the staff at the Lilly Research Laboratories of Eli Lilly and Company. We thank Prof. Norman L. Allinger, Mr. Douglas M. Boyd, Dr. David K. Clawson, Dr. Richard D. Cramer III, Dr. David A. Demeter, Mr. Gregory L. Durst, Dr. Richard W. Harper, Dr. Robert B. Hermann, Dr. Stephen W. Kaldor, Dr. Yvonne C. Martin, Dr. Samuel A. F. Milosevich, and Dr. Terry R. Stouch for aiding us as we wrote this review. Creation of this review was also assisted by the computer resources of SciFinder Scholar, Google, and Wikipedia. No slight is intended for any scientist not mentioned or any publication not cited in this brief history. Our small recitation here should not add to or subtract from the already established achievements of our fellow scientists living or dead.

REFERENCES

1. Fischer E. Einfluß der Konfiguration auf die Wirkung der Enzymen. *Ber Dtsch Chem Ges* 1894;27:2985–93.
2. Silverman RB. *The organic chemistry of drug design and drug action*. San Diego: Academic Press, 1992.
3. Messiah A. *Quantum mechanics*, Vol. I. (Translated from the French by Temmer GM). New York: Wiley, 1966.
4. Pullman B, Pullman A. *Quantum biochemistry*. New York: Interscience Publishers, Wiley, 1963.
5. Crum Brown A, Frazer TR. On the connection between chemical constitution and physiological action. Part I. On the physiological action of the salts of the ammonium bases, derived from strychnia, brucia, thebaia, codeia, morphia, and nicoti. *Trans R Soc Edinburgh* 1869;25:151–203.
6. Crum Brown A, Frazer TR. On the connection between chemical constitution and physiological action. Part II. On the physiological action of the ammonium bases derived from atropia and conia. *Trans R Soc Edinburgh* 1869;25:693–739.
7. Bruice TC, Kharasch N, Winzler RJ. A correlation of thyroxine-like activity and chemical structure. *Arch Biochem Biophys* 1956;62:305–17.
8. Zahradnik R. Correlation of the biological activity of organic compounds by means of the linear free energy relations. *Experimentia* 1962;18:534–6.
9. Hansch C, Fujita T. ρ–σ–π Analysis; method for the correlation of biological activity and chemical structure. *J Am Chem Soc* 1964;86:1616–26.
10. Free SM Jr, Wilson JW. A mathematical contribution to structure-activity studies. *J Med Chem* 1964;7:395–9.
11. Bolcer JD, Hermann RB. The development of computational chemistry in the United States. In: Lipkowitz KB, Boyd DB, editors. *Reviews in computational chemistry*, Vol. 5. New York: VCH, 1994. p. 1–63.
12. Marsh MM. Spectropolarimetric studies on proteins. Bovine plasma albumin and insulin. *J Am Chem Soc* 1962;84:1896–900.
13. Moffitt W. Optical rotatory dispersion of helical polymers. *J Chem Phys* 1956;25:467–78.

14. Allinger N, Allinger J. *Structures of organic molecules*. Englewood Cliffs, NJ: Prentice-Hall, 1965.
15. Dayhoff MO. Computer search for active-site configurations. *J Am Chem Soc* 1964;86:2295–7.
16. Lipkowitz KB, Boyd DB, editors. Books Published on the Topics of Computational Chemistry. In: *Reviews in Computational Chemistry*, Vol. 17. New York: Wiley-VCH, 2001. p. 255–357.
17. Lipkowitz KB, Boyd DB, editors. A tribute to the halcyon days of QCPE. In: *Reviews in Computational Chemistry*, Vol. 15. New York: Wiley-VCH, 2000. p. v–xi.
18. Johnson CK. Drawing crystal structures by computer. *Crystallographic Computing*, Proceedings of the International Summer School held 1969, 1970. p. 227–30.
19. Sutton LE, Jenkin DG, Mitchell AD, Cross LC, editors. *Tables of interatomic distances and configuration in molecules and ions*, Special Publ No. 11. London: The Chemical Society, 1958.
20. Koltun WL. Precision space-filling atomic models. *Biopolymers* 1965;3:665–79.
21. Boyd DB. Space-filling molecular models of four-membered rings. Three-dimensional aspects in the design of penicillin and cephalosporin antibiotics. *J Chem Educ* 1976;53:483–8.
22. Hoffmann R, Lipscomb WN. Theory of polyhedral molecules. I. Physical factorizations of the secular equation. *J Chem Phys* 1962;36:2179–89.
23. Hoffmann, R. An extended Hückel theory. I. Hydrocarbons. *J Chem Phys* 1963;39:1397–412.
24. Pople JA, Segal GA. Approximate self-consistent molecular orbital theory. II. Calculations with complete neglect of differential overlap. *J Chem Phys* 1965;43: S136–49.
25. Pople JA, Beveridge DL. *Approximate molecular orbital theory*. New York: McGraw-Hill, 1970.
26. Hartree, DR. The wave mechanics of an atom with a non-coulomb central field. I. Theory and methods. *Proc Cambridge Phil Soc* 1928;24:89–110.
27. Hartree, DR. The wave mechanics of an atom with a non-coulomb central field. II. Some results and discussion. *Proc Cambridge Phil Soc* 1928;24:111–32.
28. Hartree, DR. Wave mechanics of an atom with a non-coulomb central field. III. Term values and intensities in series in optical spectra. *Proc Cambridge Phil Soc* 1928;24 (Pt. 3):426–37.
29. Fock, V. "Self-consistent field" with interchange for sodium. *Zeitschrift für Physik* 1930;62:795–805.
30. Roberts JD. *Notes on molecular orbital calculations*. New York: Benjamin, 1962.
31. Neely WB. The use of molecular orbital calculations as an aid to correlate the structure and activity of cholinesterase inhibitors. *Mol Pharmacol* 1965;1:137–44.
32. Schnaare RS, Martin AN. Quantum chemistry in drug design. *J Pharmaceut Sci* 1965;54:1707–13.

33. Parr RG. *Quantum theory of molecular electronic structure.* New York: Benjamin, 1963.
34. Hammett LP. *Physical organic chemistry; reaction rates, equilibria, and mechanisms*, 2nd edition. New York: McGraw-Hill, 1970.
35. Taft RW Jr. Linear free-energy relationships from rates of esterification and hydrolysis of aliphatic and ortho-substituted benzoate esters. *J Am Chem Soc* 1952;74:2729–32.
36. Gould ES. *Mechanism and structure in organic chemistry.* New York: Holt Reinhart Winston, 1959.
37. Hermann RB. Structure-activity correlations in the cephalosporin C series using extended Hückel theory and CNDO/2. *J Antibiot* 1973;26:223–7.
38. Boyd DB, Hermann RB, Presti DE, Marsh MM. Electronic structures of cephalosporins and penicillins. 4. Modeling acylation by the beta-lactam ring. *J Med Chem* 1975;18:408–17.
39. Boyd DB, Herron DK, Lunn WHW, Spitzer WA. Parabolic relationships between antibacterial activity of cephalosporins and beta-lactam reactivity predicted from molecular orbital calculations. *J Am Chem Soc* 1980;102:1812–14.
40. Boyd DB. Beta-lactam antibacterial agents: Computational chemistry investigations. In: Greenberg A, Breneman CM, Liebman JF, editors. *The amide linkage: Structural significance in chemistry, biochemistry, and materials science.* New York: Wiley, 2000. p. 337–75.
41. Corey EJ, Wipke WT, Cramer RD III, Howe WJ. Computer-assisted synthetic analysis. Facile man-machine communication of chemical structure by interactive computer graphics. *J Am Chem Soc* 1972;94:421–30.
42. Corey EJ, Wipke WT, Cramer RD III, Howe WJ. Techniques for perception by a computer of synthetically significant structural features in complex molecules. *J Am Chem Soc* 1972;94:431–9.
43. Wipke, WT, Gund P. Congestion. Conformation-dependent measure of steric environment. Derivation and application in stereoselective addition to unsaturated carbon. *J Am Chem Soc* 1974;96:299–301.
44. Bingham RC, Dewar MJS, Lo DH. Ground states of molecules. XXV. MINDO/3. Improved version of the MINDO semiempirical SCF-MO method. *J Am Chem Soc* 1975;97:1285–93.
45. Löwdin PO, editor. Proceedings of the international symposium on quantum biology and quantum pharmacology, Held at Sanibel Island, Florida, January 17–19, 1974. *Int J Quantum Chem, Quantum Biol Symp* No. 1. New York: Wiley, 1974.
46. Richards WG. *Quantum pharmacology.* London, UK: Butterworths, 1977.
47. Olson EC, Christoffersen RE, editors. *Computer-assisted drug design*, Based on a symposium sponsored by the Divisions of Computers in Chemistry and Medicinal Chemistry at the ACS/CSJ Chemical Congress, Honolulu, Hawaii, April 2–6, 1979. ACS Symposium Series 112. Washington, DC: American Chemical Society, 1979.
48. Allinger NL, Miller MA, Van Catledge FA, Hirsch JA. Conformational analysis. LVII. The calculation of the conformational structures of hydrocarbons

by the Westheimer-Hendrickson-Wiberg method. *J Am Chem Soc* 1967;89: 4345–57.

49. Gygax R, Wirz J, Sprague JT, Allinger NL. Electronic structure and photophysical properties of planar conjugated hydrocarbons with a 4n-membered ring. Part III. Conjugative stabilization in an "antiaromatic" system: The conformational mobility of 1,5-bisdehydro[12]annulene. *Helv Chim Acta* 1977;60:2522–9.
50. Westheimer FH, Mayer JE. The theory of the racemization of optically active derivatives of biphenyl. *J Chem Phys* 1946;14:733–8.
51. Hendrickson JB. Molecular geometry. I. Machine computation of the common rings. *J Am Chem Soc* 1961;83:4537–47.
52. Boyd DB, Lipkowitz KB. Molecular mechanics. The method and its underlying philosophy. *J Chem Educ* 1982;59:269–74.
53. Boyd DB, Lipkowitz KB, editors. Preface on the meaning and scope of computational chemistry. In: *Reviews in Computational Chemistry*, Vol. 1. New York: VCH, 1990. p. vii–xii.
54. Gund P, Grabowski EJJ, Smith, GM, Andose JD, Rhodes JB, Wipke WT. In: Olson EC, Christoffersen RE, editors. *Computer-assisted drug design*. ACS Symposium Series 112. Washington, DC: American Chemical Society, 1979. p. 526–51.
55. Allen FH, Bellard S, Brice MD, Cartwright BA, Doubleday A, Higgs H, Hummelink T, Hummelink-Peter BG, Kennard O, Motherwell WDS, Rodgers JR, Watson DG. The Cambridge Crystallographic Data Centre: Computer-based search, retrieval, analysis and display of information. *Acta Crystallogr, Sect B* 1979; B35:2331–9.
56. Bernstein FC, Koetzle TF, Williams GJB, Meyer EF Jr., Brice MD, Rodgers JR, Kennard O, Shimanouchi T, Tasumi M. The Protein Data Bank: A computer-based archival file for macromolecular structures. *J Mol Biol* 1977;112:535–42.
57. Martin YC. *Quantitative drug design. A critical introduction*. New York: Dekker, 1978.
58. Hansch C, Leo A. *Substituent constants for correlation analysis in chemistry and biology*. New York: Wiley, 1979.
59. Corey EJ, Long AK, Rubenstein SD. Computer-assisted analysis in organic synthesis. *Science* 1985;228:408–18.
60. Rubenstein SD. Electronic documents in chemistry, from ChemDraw 1.0 to present. Abstracts of Papers, 228th ACS National Meeting, Philadelphia, PA, August 22–26, 2004. CINF-054.
61. Helson HE. Structure diagram generation. In: Boyd DB, Lipkowitz KB, editors. *Reviews in Computational Chemistry,* Vol. 13. New York: Wiley-VCH, 1999. p. 313–98.
62. Monmaney T. Robert Langridge: His quest to peer into the essence of life no longer seems so strange. *Smithsonian* 2005;36 (8):48.
63. Langridge R. Computer graphics in studies of molecular interactions. *Chem Industry (London)* 1980 (12):475–7.
64. Langridge R, Ferrin TE, Kuntz ID, Connolly ML. Real-time color graphics in studies of molecular interactions. *Science* 1981;211 (4483):661–6.

65. Vinter JG. Molecular graphics for the medicinal chemist. *Chem Britain* 1985;21(1), 32, 33–5, 37–8.
66. Boyd DB. Molecular modeling—Industrial relevance and applications. In: *Ullmann's Encyclopedia of Industrial Chemistry*, 6th edition. Weinheim, Germany: Wiley-VCH, 1998.
67. Gund P, Andose JD, Rhodes JB, Smith GM. Three-dimensional molecular modeling and drug design. *Science* 1980;208 (4451):1425–31.
68. Boyd DB, Marsh MM. Computational chemistry in the design of biologically active molecules at Lilly. Abstracts of 183rd National Meeting of the American Chemical Society, Las Vegas, Nevada, March 28–April 2, 1982.
69. Boyd DB. Profile of computer-assisted molecular design in industry. *Quantum Chemistry Program Exchange (QCPE) Bulletin* 1985;5:85–91.
70. Lipkowitz KB, Boyd DB. Improved job market for computational chemists. In: *Reviews in Computational Chemistry*, Vol. 12. New York: Wiley-VCH, 1998. p. v–xiii.
71. Marshall GR, Barry CD, Bosshard HE, Dammkoehler RA, Dunn DA. The conformational parameter in drug design: The active analog approach. *Computer-assisted drug design*. ACS Symposium Series 112. Washington DC: American Chemical Society, 1979. p. 205–26.
72. Martin YC, Bures MG, Willett P. Searching databases of three-dimensional structures. In: Lipkowitz KB, Boyd DB, editors. *Reviews in Computational Chemistry,* Vol. 1. New York: VCH, 1990. p. 213–63.
73. Grethe G, Moock TE. Similarity searching in REACCS. A new tool for the synthetic chemist. *J Chem Inf Comput Sci* 1990;30:511–20.
74. Dewar MJS, Healy EF, Stewart JJP. Location of transition states in reaction mechanisms. *J Chem Soc, Faraday Transactions 2: Mol Chem Phys* 1984;80:227–33.
75. Stewart JJP. MOPAC: A semiempirical molecular orbital program. *J Computer-Aided Mol Des* 1990;4:1–105.
76. Stewart JJP. Semiempirical molecular orbital methods. In: Lipkowitz KB, Boyd DB, editors, *Reviews in Computational Chemistry*, Vol. 1. New York: VCH, 1990. p. 45–81.
77. Stewart JJP. MOPAC: A semiempirical molecular orbital program. Quantum Chemistry Program Exchange, 1983. Prog. 455.
78. Allinger NL. Conformational analysis. 130. MM2. A hydrocarbon force field utilizing V1 and V2 torsional terms. *J Am Chem Soc* 1977;99:8127–34.
79. Burkert U, Allinger NL. *Molecular mechanics.* ACS Monograph 177. Washington DC: American Chemical Society, 1982.
80. Leo AJ. Some advantages of calculating octanol-water partition coefficients. *J Pharmaceut Sci* 1987;76:166–8.
81. Leo AJ. Hydrophobic parameter: measurement and calculation. *Methods Enzymol* 1991;202:544–91.
82. Leo, AJ. Calculating log P_{oct} from structures. *Chem Rev* 1993;93:1281–306.
83. Enslein, Kurt. Estimation of toxicological endpoints by structure-activity relationships. *Pharmacol Rev* 1984;36 (2, Suppl.):131–5.

84. Enslein, K. An overview of structure-activity relationships as an alternative to testing in animals for carcinogenicity, mutagenicity, dermal and eye irritation, and acute oral toxicity. *Toxicol Industrial Health* 1988;4:479–98.
85. Boyd DB. Application of the hypersurface iterative projection method to bicyclic pyrazolidinone antibacterial agents. *J Med Chem* 1993;36:1443–9.
86. Matthews DA, Alden RA, Bolin JT, Filman DJ, Freer ST, Hamlin R, Hol WG, Kisliuk RL, Pastore EJ, Plante LT, Xuong N, Kraut J. Dihydrofolate reductase from *Lactobacillus casei*. X-ray structure of the enzyme methotrexate-NADPH complex. *J Biol Chem* 1978;253:6946–54.
87. Matthews DA, Alden RA, Freer ST, Nguyen HX, Kraut J. Dihydrofolate reductase from *Lactobacillus casei*. Stereochemistry of NADPH binding. *J Biol Chem* 1979;254:4144–51.
88. Everett AJ. Computing and trial and error in chemotherapeutic research. In: Leeming PR, editor. *Topics in Medicinal Chemistry*, Proceedings of the 4th SCI-RSC Medicinal Chemistry Symposium, Cambridge, UK, Sept. 6–9, 1987. Special Publication 65. London: Royal Society of Chemistry, 1988. p. 314–31.
89. Ito A, Hirai K, Inoue M, Koga H, Suzue S, Irikura T, Mitsuhashi S. In vitro antibacterial activity of AM-715, a new nalidixic acid analog. *Antimicrob Agents Chemother* 1980;17:103–8.
90. Koga H, Itoh A, Murayama S, Suzue S, Irikura T. Structure-activity relationships of antibacterial 6,7- and 7,8-disubstituted 1-alkyl-1,4-dihydro-4-oxoquinoline-3-carboxylic acids. *J Med Chem* 1980;23;1358–63.
91. Koga H. Structure-activity relationships and drug design of pyridonecarboxylic acid type (nalidixic acid type) synthetic antibacterial agents. *Kagaku no Ryoiki, Zokan* 1982;136:177–202.
92. Perun TJ, Propst CL, editors. *Computer-aided drug design: Methods and applications.* New York: Dekker, 1989.
93. Brünger A, Karplus M, Petsko GA. Crystallographic refinement by simulated annealing: application to crambin. *Acta Crystallogr*, Sect A 1989; A45:50–61.
94. Brooks BR, Bruccoleri RE, Olafson BD, States DJ, Swaminathan S, Karplus M. CHARMM: A program for macromolecular energy, minimization, and dynamics calculations. *J Comput Chem* 1983;4:187–217.
95. Kollman, P. Molecular modeling. *Annu Rev Phys Chem* 1987;38:303–16.
96. McCammon, JA. Computer-aided molecular design. *Science* 1987;238(4826): 486–91.
97. Reddy MR, Erion MD, Agarwal A. Free energy calculations: Use and limitations in predicting ligand binding affinities. In: Lipkowitz KB, Boyd DB, editors. *Reviews in Computational Chemistry,* Vol. 16. New York: Wiley-VCH, 2000. p. 217–304.
98. Karin S, Smith NP. *The supercomputer era.* Boston: Harcourt Brace Jovanovich, 1987.
99. Wold JS. Supercomputing network: A key to U.S. competitiveness in industries based on life-sciences excellence. Testimony before the U.S. Senate, Commerce, Science and Transportation Committee Science, Technology and Space Subcommittee. http://www.funet.fi/pub/sci/molbio/historical/biodocs/wold.txt

100. Milosevich SAF, Boyd, DB. Supercomputing and drug discovery research. *Perspect Drug Discovery Design* 1993;1:345–58.

101. Richon AB. A history of computational chemistry. http://www.netsci.org/Science/Compchem/feature17a.html.

102. Halgren TA. The representation of van der Waals (vdW) interactions in molecular mechanics force fields: Potential form, combination rules, and vdW parameters. *J Am Chem Soc* 1992;114:7827–43.

103. Halgren TA. Merck molecular force field. I. Basis, form, scope, parameterization and performance of MMFF94. *J Comput Chem* 1996;17:490–519.

104. Halgren TA. Merck molecular force field. II. MMFF94 van der Waals and electrostatic parameters for intermolecular interactions. *J Comput Chem* 1996;17:520–52.

105. Halgren, T. A. Merck Molecular Force Field. III. Molecular geometrics and vibrational frequencies for MMFF94. *J Comput Chem* 1996, 17:553–86.

106. Halgren TA, Nachbar RB. Merck molecular force field. IV. Conformational energies and geometries. *J Comput Chem* 1996;17:587–615.

107. Halgren TA. Merck molecular force field. V. Extension of MMFF94 using experimental data, additional computational data and empirical rules. *J Comput Chem* 1996;17:616–41.

108. Halgren TA. MMFF VI. MMFF94s option for energy minimization studies. *J Comput Chem* 1999;20:720–29.

109. Boyd DB, Lipkowitz KB, History of the Gordon Research Conferences on Computational Chemistry. In: Lipkowitz KB, Boyd DB, editors. *Reviews in Computational Chemistry*, Vol. 14. New York: Wiley-VCH, 2000. p. 399–439.

110. Mohamadi F, Richards NGJ, Guida WC, Liskamp R, Lipton M, Caufield C, Chang G, Hendrickson T, Still WC. MacroModel—An integrated software system for modeling organic and bioorganic molecules using molecular mechanics. *J Comput Chem* 1990;11:440–67.

111. Sprague PW. Catalyst: A computer aided drug design system specifically designed for medicinal chemists. *Recent Advances in Chemical Information*, Special Publication 100, Royal Society of Chemistry, 1992. p. 107–11.

112. Blaney JM, Dixon JS. A good ligand is hard to find: Automated docking methods. *Perspect Drug Discovery Design* 1993;1:301–19.

113. Boehm H-J. Fragment-based de novo ligand design. *Proceedings of the Alfred Benzon Symposium No. 39*, 1996. p. 402–13.

114. Murcko MA. Recent advances in ligand design methods. In: Lipkowitz KB, Boyd DB, editors. *Reviews in Computational Chemistry,* Vol. 11. New York: Wiley-VCH, 1997. p. 1–66.

115. Clark DE, Murray CW, Li J. Current issues in de novo molecular design. In: Lipkowitz KB, Boyd DB, editors. *Reviews in Computational Chemistry,* Vol. 11. New York: Wiley-VCH, 1997. p. 67–125.

116. Lauri G, Bartlett PA. CAVEAT: A program to facilitate the design of organic molecules. *J Comput-Aided Mol Des* 1994;8:51–66.

117. Walters WP, Stahl MT, Murcko MA. Virtual screening—An overview. *Drug Discovery Today* 1998;3:160–78.

118. Lewis RA, Pickett SD, Clark DE. Computer-aided molecular diversity analysis and combinatorial library design. In: Lipkowitz KB, Boyd DB, editors. *Reviews in Computational Chemistry*, Vol. 16. New York: Wiley, 2000. p. 1–51.

119. Boyd DB, Lipkowitz KB, editors. Trends in the job market for computational chemists. *Reviews in Computational Chemistry*, Vol. 7. New York: VCH, 1996. p. v–xi.

120. Lipinski CA, Lombardo F, Dominy BW, Feeney PJ. Experimental and computational approaches to estimate solubility and permeability in drug discovery and development settings. *Adv Drug Deliv Rev* 1997;23:3–25.

121. Hansch C, Leo A, Hoekman D. *Exploring QSAR: Hydrophobic, electronic, and steric constants.* Washington DC: American Chemical Society, 1995.

122. Todeschini R, Consonni V. *Handbook of molecular descriptors.* Berlin: Wiley-VCH, 2000.

123. Karelson M. *Molecular descriptors in QSAR/QSPR.* New York: Wiley, 2000.

124. Boyd DB. Progress in rational design of therapeutically interesting compounds. In: Liljefors T, Jørgensen FS, Krogsgaard-Larsen P, editors. *Rational molecular design in drug research.* Proceedings of the Alfred Benzon Symposium No. 42. Copenhagen: Munksgaard, 1998. p. 15–23.

125. Boyd DB. Innovation and the rational design of drugs. *CHEMTECH* 1998;28 (5):19–23.

126. Boyd DB. Rational drug design: Controlling the size of the haystack. *Modern Drug Discovery*, November/December 1998. p. 41–8.

127. Boyd DB. Drug design. In: Schleyer PvR, Allinger NL, Clark T, Gasteiger J, Kollman P, Schaefer HF III, editors. *Encyclopedia of computational chemistry*, Vol. 1. Chichester: Wiley, 1998. p. 795–804.

128. Boyd DB. Is rational design good for anything? In: Parrill AL, Reddy MR, editors, *Rational drug design: Novel methodology and practical applications.* ACS Symp Series 719. Washington, DC: American Chemical Society, 1999. p. 346–56.

129. Zurer P. Crixivan. *Chem Eng News*, June 20, 2005. p. 54.

130. Dyason JC, Wilson JC, Von Itzstein M. Sialidases: Targets for rational drug design. In: Bultinck P, De Winter H, Langenaeker W, Tollenaere JP, editors, *Computational medicinal chemistry for drug discovery.* New York: Dekker, 2004.

131. Walters DE, Hopfinger AJ. Case studies of the application of molecular shape analysis to elucidate drug action. *THEOCHEM* 1986 27:317–23.

132. DePriest SA, Mayer D, Naylor CB, Marshall GR. 3D-QSAR of angiotensin-converting enzyme and thermolysin inhibitors: a comparison of CoMFA models based on deduced and experimentally determined active site geometries. *J Am Chem Soc* 1993;115:5372–84.

133. Congreve M, Murray CW, Blundell TL. Structural biology and drug discovery. *Drug Discovery Today* 2005;10:895–907.

134. Boyd DB, Palkowitz AD, Thrasher KJ, Hauser KL, Whitesitt CA, Reel JK, Simon RL, Pfeifer W, Lifer SL, Takeuchi K, Vasudevan V, Kossoy AD, Deeter JB, Steinberg MI, Zimmerman KM, Wiest SA, Marshall WS. Molecular modeling and quantitative structure-activity relationship studies in pursuit of highly

potent substituted octanoamide angiotensin II receptor antagonists. In: Reynolds CH, Holloway MK, Cox HK, editors. *Computer-aided molecular design: Applications in agrochemicals, materials, and pharmaceuticals*, ACS Symp. Series 589, Washington, DC: American Chemical Society, 1995. p. 14–35.

135. Boyd DB, Lipkowitz KB. Examination of the employment environment for computational chemistry. In: Lipkowitz KB, Boyd DB, editors. *Reviews in Computational Chemistry*, Vol. 18. New York: Wiley-VCH, 2002. p. 293–319.

136. Schmid EF, Smith DA. Is declining innovation in the pharmaceutical industry a myth? *Drug Discovery Today* 2005;10:1031–9.

2

COMPUTERS AS DATA ANALYSIS AND DATA MANAGEMENT TOOLS IN PRECLINICAL DEVELOPMENT

WEIYONG LI AND KENNETH BANKS

Contents

Computer Applications in Pharmaceutical Research and Development, Edited by Sean Ekins.
ISBN 0-471-73779-8

2.1 INTRODUCTION

Scientists from many different disciplines participate in pharmaceutical development. Their research areas may be very different, but they all generate scientific data (and text documents), which are the products of development laboratories. Literally, truckloads of data and documents are submitted to the regulatory authorities in support of investigational and marketing authorization filings. For example, even a typical Investigational New Drug (IND) application requires around 50,000 pages of supporting documents. One way or another, every single data point has to go through the acquiring, analyzing, managing, reporting, auditing, and archiving process according to a set of specific rules and regulations. Needless to say, the wide use of computers has tremendously increased efficiency and productivity in pharmaceutical development. On the other hand, it has also created unique problems and challenges for the industry. This overview discusses these topics briefly by focusing on the preclinical development area (also known as the area of Chemical Manufacturing and Control, or CMC). Considering the pervasiveness of computer applications in every scientist's daily activities, special emphases are put on three widely used computer systems:

- CDS—chromatographic data systems
- LIMS—laboratory information management systems
- TIMS—text information management systems

It is probably fair to say that these three computer systems handle the majority of the work in data/document management in the preclinical area, supporting the New Drug Application (NDA) and Marketing Authorization Application (MAA) filings. For each of these three types of systems, there are many vendors who provide various products. The selection of the right product can be complicated, and a mistake made in the process can also be costly. This overview tries to list some of the vendors that are more focused on serving the pharmaceutical industry. The lists are by no means comprehensive. The readers are encouraged to contact the vendors for more in-depth information.

It may also be beneficial to the reader if we define the sources of the scientific data in preclinical development. The following are examples of the development activities that generate the majority of the data:

- Drug substance/drug product purity, potency, and other testing
- Drug substance/drug product stability testing
- Method development, validation, and transfer
- Drug product formulation development
- Drug substance/drug product manufacturing process development, validation, and transfer

- Master production and control record keeping
- Batch production and control record keeping
- Equipment cleaning testing

Another important aspect for discussion is the impact of regulations, specifically the regulation on electronic document management and electronic signatures, 21 CFR Part 11, published by the Food and Drug Administration (FDA) for the first time in 1997 [1] (also see Chapter 26, which covers 21 CFR Part 11 in detail). Since that time the draft rules of Part 11 have been withdrawn and reissued along with various guidance documents [2–3]. Some of the key points of Part 11 are as follows:

- Computer systems must be validated to ensure accuracy, reliability, and consistency with intended performance.
- Computer systems must provide time-stamped audit trails to record actions that create, modify, or delete electronic records.
- Computer system access must be limited to authorized personnel.
- Computer systems should have configurable user capabilities.

Even though Part 11 has not yet been enforced by the FDA, the rules have impacted CDS, LIMS, and TIMS with regard to architectural design and security of these systems.

2.2 CHROMATOGRAPHIC DATA SYSTEMS (CDS)

The importance of CDS is directly related to the roles that chromatography, particularly high-performance liquid chromatography (HPLC) and gas chromatography (GC), play in pharmaceutical analysis. HPLC and GC are the main workhorses in pharmaceutical analysis. In today's pharmaceutical companies, development work cannot be done without HPLC and GC. CDS are also used for several other instrumental analysis technologies such as ion (exchange) chromatography (IC), capillary electrophoresis (CE), and supercritical fluid chromatography (SFC).

2.2.1 The Days Before CDS

In the 1960s and early 1970s, chromatographs were relatively primitive and inefficient. Chromatographers had to use microsyringes for sample injection and stopwatches for measurement of retention times. The chromatograms were collected with a strip chart recorder. Data analysis was also performed manually. Peak areas were obtained by drawing a "best fit" triangle manually for each peak and then using the equation Area = ½Base × Height. At that time, the management of chromatographic data was essentially paper based and very inefficient [4].

However, compared with the traditional analytical methods, the adoption of chromatographic methods represented a significant improvement in pharmaceutical analysis. This was because chromatographic methods had the advantages of method specificity, the ability to separate and detect low-level impurities. Specificity is especially important for methods intended for early-phase drug development when the chemical and physical properties of the active pharmaceutical ingredient (API) are not fully understood and the synthetic processes are not fully developed. Therefore the assurance of safety in clinical trials of an API relies heavily on the ability of analytical methods to detect and quantitate unknown impurities that may pose safety concerns. This task was not easily performed or simply could not be carried out by classic wet chemistry methods. Therefore, slowly, HPLC and GC established their places as the mainstream analytical methods in pharmaceutical analysis.

As chromatographic methods became more and more important in the pharmaceutical industry as well as in other industries, practical needs prompted instrument vendors to come up with more efficient ways for collecting and processing chromatographic data. In the mid-1970s, the integrator was introduced. At first, the integrator worked similarly to a strip chart recorder with the added capabilities of automatically calculating peak area and peak height. Because of limited available memory, chromatograms could not be stored for batch processing. However, new models with increasing capabilities quickly replaced the older ones. The newer models had a battery back-up to maintain integration parameters and larger memory modules to allow the storage of chromatograms for playback and reintegration. At that time, the integrator increased productivity and efficiency in pharmaceutical analysis, which in turn made HPLC and GC even more popular.

2.2.2 The Emergence and Evolution of CDS

For some instrument vendors, the early CDS were developed as proprietary products to help with the sale of instruments. The first generation of CDS systems were based on a working model of multiuser, time-sharing minicomputers. The minicomputers were connected to terminals in the laboratory that the analysts would use. The detector channels of the chromatographs were connected to the data system through a device called the analog-to-digital (A/D) converter, which would convert the analog signals from the detectors into digital signals. In the late 1970s, Hewlett-Packard introduced the HP-3300 series data-acquisition system. Through the A/D converters, the HP system was able to collect chromatographic data from up to 60 detector channels. This represented the beginning of computerized chromatographic data analysis and management [5].

Because the CDS used a dedicated hardware and wiring system, it was relatively expensive to install. It was also difficult to scale up because more minicomputers would be needed with increases in the number of users.

Another drawback of the system was that the performance of the system would degrade as the number of users increased.

The next generation of CDS systems did not appear until the start of the personal computer (PC) revolution in the 1980s. The early PCs commercialized by Apple and IBM were not very reliable or powerful compared with today's PCs. The operating systems were text based and difficult to use. However, it was economically feasible to put them on the desktop in each laboratory, and they were evolving rapidly to become more powerful in terms of hardware and software. By the early 1990s, the PCs were reaching the calculation speed of a minicomputer with a fraction of the cost. A graphics-based operating system also made them more user-friendly.

Taking advantage of the PC revolution, a new generation of CDS appeared on the market that utilized a client/server model. In the new CDS, the client provided the graphical and user interface through a PC and was responsible for some or most of the application processing. The server typically maintained the database and processed requests from the clients to extract data from or update the database. This model was adopted widely in the industry for almost a decade because of its scalability. It also facilitated the activities of data sharing, method transfer, result review and approval, and troubleshooting at different laboratories and locations. It also overcame the problem of scale-up. During this period of time, in parallel with the progress in CDS, chromatography itself was developing rapidly. Instrumentation had adopted modular design so that each functional part became more reliable and serviceable. Progress in microelectronics and machinery made the solvent delivery pump more accurate and reproducible. The accuracy and precision of auto samplers also were significantly improved. Compared with the time when chart recorders or integrators were used, the fully automated HPLC could now be programmed to run for days and nights nonstop. Results could also be accessed and processed remotely. With the help of sophisticated CDS, chromatography finally established its dominance in pharmaceutical analysis.

As instrumental analysis played an increasingly important part in pharmaceutical development, an ever-larger percentage of the data in Good Manufacturing Practice and/or Good Laboratory Practice (GMP/GLP) studies were captured and stored electronically. As CDS became more sophisticated, new functions such as electronic approval became available. However, the legal issues related to electronic signatures needed to be addressed and recognized by the regulatory authorities. To clarify the confusion and provide clear guidelines regarding electronic data, the FDA issued 21 CFR Part 11 rules to address concerns regarding the electronic media of scientific data. With respect to the FDA's expectations, the CDS operated with the client/server model had a significant drawback. In the client/server model, the client must retain parts of the applications. To fulfill the requirements of system qualification, performance verification, and validation, one must validate not only the server, but also each PC used by the client. This created an enormous burden for the customer, which resulted in the adoption of a new operating model of server-based computing.

With server-based computing, the applications are deployed, managed, supported, and executed on a dedicated application server. Server-based computing uses a multiuser operating system and a method for distributing the presentation of an application's interface to a client device. There are no software components installed on the client PC. The client's PC simply acts as the application server's display. CDS using this model significantly reduced the total cost in implementation and maintenance and significantly increased its compliance with regulatory guidelines.

2.2.3 The Modern CDS

Use of server-based computing is only one of the important features of the modern CDS. The other two important features are the use of embedded data structure and direct instrument control. The earlier generations of CDS used a directory file structure, meaning that the raw data and other files such as the instrument method and data processing method were stored at separate locations. There would either be no connections or only partial connections between these files. The most significant drawback of this type of file management was the potential for methods and raw data to be accidentally overwritten. To prevent this from happening, the raw data and result files must be locked. If in some cases the locked data needed to be reprocessed, the system administrator must unlock the files. The embedded relational database has been widely used for LIMS and is a much better file structure. The embedded data structure can be used to manage not only chromatographic data, but also all aspects of the CDS, including system security and user privileges. The embedded data structure maintains all information and changes by date- and time stamping them to prevent accidental overwriting of raw data and method files. It controls versions of all processed result files, acquisition methods, processing methods, and reporting methods to provide full audit trails. All of the metadata (acquisition, process, and reporting methods) related to a specific result are tied together.

Direct instrument control (or the lack of it) was an important issue for the earlier version of CDS. The scheme of connecting the detector channels through A/Ds to CDS worked well in analytical laboratories across the pharmaceutical industry. The scheme provided enough flexibility so that the CDS could collect data from a variety of instruments, including GC, HPLC, IC, SFC, and CE. It was equally important that the CDS could be connected to instruments that were manufactured by different vendors. It was not uncommon to find a variety of instruments from different vendors in a global pharmaceutical research company. The disadvantage of this scheme was that the instrument metadata could not be linked to the result file of each sample analyzed. It could not be guaranteed that the proper instrument parameters were used in sample analysis. Another need came from the increased use of information-rich detectors such as photodiode array detectors and mass spectrometer (MS) detectors. To use these detectors in the GMP/GLP environment, data security had to be ensured. The data from these detectors could not be collected by CDS through A/Ds. This represented an important gap in reaching full compliance of the 21 CFR Part 11 regulations. In addition, the use of A/D inevitably introduced additional noise and nonlinearity. Direct instrument control would avoid these problems. To address these problems, the instrument vendors had to cooperate by providing each other with the source codes of their software. Some progress has been made in this area. A good example is that of the CDS Empower (Waters), which now can directly control HPLC and GC equipment manufactured by Agilent. Table 2.1 lists several of the major CDS vendors and current contact information.

2.2.4 Summary

CDS have certainly served the pharmaceutical industry well by being continuously improved. CDS have helped the pharmaceutical industry to increase efficiency and productivity by automating a large part of pharmaceutical analysis. But CDS still have room for improvement. So far the main focus of CDS has been on providing accurate and reliable data. The current regulatory trend in the pharmaceutical industry is to shift from data-based filings to information-based filings, meaning that the data must be analyzed and converted into information. This implies that enhancements in data searching and trend analysis capabilities will be desirable in the future.

2.3 LABORATORY INFORMATION MANAGEMENT SYSTEMS (LIMS)

Laboratory information management systems, or LIMS represent an integral part of the data management systems used in preclinical development. LIMS

TABLE 2.1 Major CDS Vendors and Their Products

Product	Vendor	URL
Atlas	Thermo Electron Co.	www.thermolabsystems.com
Cerity	Agilent Technologies, Inc.	www.agilent.com
Chromeleon	Dionex Co.	www.dionex.com
Class VP	Shimadzu Scientific Inst.	www.shimadzu.com
Empower	Waters Co	www.waters.com
EZChrom Elite	Scientific Software, Inc	www.scisw.com
Galaxie	Varian Inc.	www.varianinc.com
TotalChrom	Perkin-Elmer, Inc.	www.perkinelmer.com

are needed partly because CDS cannot provide enough data management capability. For example, CDS cannot handle data from nonchromatographic tests.

Another important use of LIMS is for sample management in preclinical development, more specifically in drug substance and drug product stability studies. Stability studies are very labor intensive, and the results have an important impact on regulatory filings. LIMS are designed to automate a large part of these stability studies including sample tracking, sample distribution, work assignment, results capturing, data processing, data review and approval, report generation, and data archiving, retrieving, and sharing.

2.3.1 LIMS Hardware and Architectures

Commercial LIMS appeared on the market in the early 1980s. These operated on then state-of-the-art minicomputers such as the 16-bit Hewlett-Packard 1000 and 32-bit Digital VAX system. By the late 1980s, several DOS-based PC LIMS operating on the primitive PC network were available. By the early 1990s, most LIMS started using commercial relational database technology and client/server systems, which operated on UNIX or the new Windows NT platform. The most advanced LIMS utilize server-based architecture to ensure system security and control.

There are four main types of architectural options when implementing LIMS [6]. The first is the LAN (local area network) installation. In a multiple-site situation and through the standard client/server setup, the application would be hosted separately on a server at each site connected to PC clients. In this setup, the LIMS are installed on both the clients and the server. System administration is required at each facility.

The second type is the WAN (wide area network) installation. In this setup the LIMS take advantage of telecommunication technology to cover a great distance. The setup can also be used to connect disparate LANs together. In this configuration, the LIMS are installed on both the clients and a central server. The third type is the so-called "centrally hosted thin client installation". For this setup, system administration is managed at a corporate center, where the LIMS are hosted and distributed via a WAN or the Internet with a virtual private network (VPN). The last and also the newest type is the ASP (Application Service Provision provider)-hosted installation. In this setup, the LIMS are hosted on a centrally managed server form and maintained by third-party specialists. Users access the LIMS with any Internet-connected PC with a standard Web browser.

2.3.2 Different Types of LIMS

The implementation of LIMS requires a significant amount of investment in capital money and manpower. There are large numbers of established vendors that provide commercial LIMS with a similar range of core functionality, but few of them are dedicated to the pharmaceutical industry because of the market size (Table 2.2). The following discussion is not intended to categorize different types of LIMS; rather, we briefly point out the most obvious characteristics of different LIMS. LIMS may possess certain distinctive features, but their core functionalities may be very similar.

Customer-tailored LIMS—In an implementation of this type of LIMS, the customer purchases a generic product from the vendor. The vendor and customer will work together over a period of time to configure the software to adapt it to meet end user needs. This usually involves extensive programming, which can be performed by the trained end user or dedicated supporting personnel on the customer side. Programming support is usually needed for the entire life of the LIMS to accommodate changes in development projects. The advantage is that the LIMS functions relatively closely to the business practices of the customer and the system can be tailored to fit the needs of the customer's development projects. The disadvantage is that it takes considerable resources to implement and maintain the LIMS.

Preconfigured LIMS—This LIMS does not require extensive customer programming. To meet specific needs of end users, the vendors provide a comprehensive suite of configuration tools. These tools allow end users to add new screens, menus, functions, and reports in a rapid and intuitive manner. The tools also allow the LIMS to be more easily integrated with other business applications such as document processing, spreadsheets, and manufacturing systems.

Specialized LIMS—This type of LIMS is based on the fact that certain laboratories have a range of well-defined processes (e.g., stability testing) that are performed according to a specific set of regulations and by using well-established tests. The tests are done according to industry-wide accepted protocols. Specialized LIMS are tailor-made for certain types of laboratories. Therefore the performance can be optimized for clearly defined work process.

TABLE 2.2 Selected LIMS Vendors Specialized in Pharmaceutical Industry

Product	Vendor	URL
Debra	LabLogic Systems Ltd	www.lablogic.com
Q-DIS/QM	Waters	www.waters.com
QC Client	Agilent	www.agilent.com
WinLIMS	QSI	www.lims-software.com
ACD/SLIMS	Advanced Chemistry Development	www.acdlabs.com
V-LIMS	Advance Technology Corp	www.vetstar.com
VET/HEX	HEX Laboratory Systems	www.hexlab.com
BioLIMS	PE Informatics	www.pebiosystems.com
LabCat	Innovative Programming Assoc.	www.labcat.com

LIMS as rented service—The application service provision provider (ASP) is a means of obtaining access to software applications without the need to acquire expensive licenses and hardware or employ high-cost support resources [7]. The application is hosted on a third-party site with system maintenance, backup, and recovery provided by a third party. Products and services can be rented for a contract period on a fixed cost per user/per month basis. The advantages of obtaining LIMS in this fashion include reduced cost in initial investment and reduced requirement of resources for maintaining the LIMS. The continued security and integrity of the data transferred over the Internet is a major concern for this type of LIMS.

2.3.3 Implementation of LIMS

Because of their complexity, implementing LIMS usually is a traumatic process. Good communication and planning can reduce the level of turmoil caused by LIMS [8].

Planning (defining expectations) is the first step in a lengthy process of acquiring the LIMS. The LIMS vendor and customer have to work very closely at this stage. A series of meetings must be held between the LIMS vendor and potential end users and laboratory supervisors. The business processes and sample flows need to be mapped and documented to prepare for future system configuration. For each type of sample to be tracked by the LIMS, the attributes related to the samples must be defined. Even the data format has to be decided so that it is consistent with existing procedures and practices of the organization. When the expectations are compiled and analyzed, it is important to balance the needs of the end users from different disciplines because they may have different concerns, priorities, and requirements. Mistakes made in the planning stage can be very costly later on over the life span of the LIMS.

The LIMS for GMP/GLP use must be validated [10]. Validation includes design qualification, installation qualification, operational qualification, performance qualification, and final documentation. Each of these steps needs good planning and documentation. The compliance function (QA) of the development organization will need to be involved in reviewing and approving the plan and in the audit of the final report. During validation, the system is tested against normal, boundary value, and invalid data sets. Invalid data should be identified and flagged by the software. Dynamic "stress" tests should also be done with large data sets to verify whether the hardware is adequate. The validation work usually is conducted on a test system that is an exact copy of the production system to protect the data integrity of the production system.

One of the major undertakings during LIMS implementation is user training, which should cover not only the LIMS itself but also the standard operating procedures (SOPs) that govern use, administration, training, and other aspects of the LIMS. The training should be conducted on the test system instead of the production system. The trainers should keep in mind that the LIMS is one of the less user-friendly systems for end users because of its complexity and rigid audit trail setups. Adequate support after training and rollout may have a long-lasting impact on the success of the new LIMS.

2.3.4 Summary

LIMS is a complex system and requires significant capital and manpower investment. Selection of the right LIMS product is a daunting task, and the outcome can have a significant impact on the business.

Compared with CDS, LIMS has more core functionalities in managing laboratory data and other electronic information. It also has much stronger search and reporting capabilities. It is interesting to point out that some LIMS vendors have started to use the term "data mining" in their product introduction brochures. This means that they are aware of a new trend in the pharmaceutical industry, especially in preclinical development, namely, toward a better understanding and control of data in pharmaceutical manufacturing. The FDA has issued a new Guidance on Process Analytical Technologies (PAT), [9] promoting the concepts of "quality by design," "process understanding," and "real-time assurance of quality." These concepts may have a profound impact on how pharmaceutical development is conducted in the future. To put these concepts into practice will mean an explosion in the amount of scientific data, not only through standard testing such as HPLC and GC but also through nonstandard technologies such as near-infrared spectroscopy, Raman spectroscopy, various particle size analysis techniques, etc. More importantly, the data will need to be analyzed with new (e.g., chemometrics) tools to generate process/product information and knowledge. The current LIMS are not designed to handle large amounts of spectral data. We will have to see whether the core functionalities of LIMS can be expanded or totally new information management systems will have to be developed to meet the new challenges.

2.4 TEXT INFORMATION MANAGEMENT SYSTEMS (TIMS)

The name "text information management system" is not as widely used as the name "laboratory information management system." Nevertheless, a text document management system is essential in preclinical development because huge numbers of text documents and other related information such as images, drawings, and photographs are generated in the area. All these documents and information are considered intellectual property and require protection and easy access.

One of the characteristics of the pharmaceutical industry is large quantities of paperwork, particularly in areas where GMP/GLP are strictly enforced. The slogan "documentation, documentation, and documentation . . ." is always in the mind of laboratory scientists.

The scientists in preclinical development spend quite a large percentage of their working time writing compound documents (reports). The report generation, review, approval, filing, and retrieval process can be very inefficient or even bureaucratic in a pharmaceutical company, partly because of the strict regulations. The following scenario could be seen often as recently as the late 1980s: The scientist would prepare his report with one type or another of text and graphic software, often through multiple cut-and-paste procedures to include pictures or images. Then the scientist would make hard copies of the report for review by managers and the department head. After all the corrections were made, the scientist would print out another copy for the QA auditor for auditing (this is only done for the documents used for submission). It could take months before the report was finally ready to be filed in the company record center, where photocopies and microfilms were made and indexing took place. When an end user needed a copy of the report, he would have to make a request to the record center for a hard copy.

When TIMS is used in today's workflow, the scientist can use a report template to facilitate report writing. Some cut-and-paste procedures are still needed to include data and figures. After the draft report is completed, the scientist can send the reviewers an electronic link for the document. The reviewers can review the document and make changes and corrections with the "tracking change" function. When the review is completed, the author can choose to accept the changes or deny them. If auditing is needed, the same process can be used. The finalized document is issued within the TIMS by adding an issue date and signatures, if necessary, and converting into an unalterable PDF file. Future changes made after issuance are captured through version control. End users can also access the issued document electronically and remotely. Comparison of the new process vs. the old one has demonstrated the advantages of TIMS.

2.4.1 Documentation Requirements in Preclinical Development

In preclinical development, the GMP/GLP regulations are enforced not only for scientific data but also for text documents. This section discusses several types of controlled text documents used in preclinical development. Most of these documents are managed by the fully validated TIMS.

Product specification documents and analytical test methods—In preclinical development, these are important documents and they evolve along with the development phases. Drug substances and products for clinical trials are tested based on these documents, and so are the stability samples. It is critical to ensure that the analyst will perform the right tests against the right specifications with the correct version of the test method. Therefore a mechanism must be in place to control these documents. This can be done manually or with TIMS. A manually controlled system would require the analyst to sign out hard copies of the documents from a central location. After the testing is done, the analyst would have to return these controlled documents to the central location. Sometimes mistakes can be made with regard to the correct documents, and this will result in repetition and unnecessary investigation. If TIMS is implemented, the analyst can obtain the documents from the secured database and then the documents should be destroyed after the test is completed.

Standard operating procedures (SOPs)—The SOPs are controlled in a way similar to that of specification documents and analytical methods. It must be ensured that the correct versions of the SOPs are accessed and used by the scientists. After use, the hard copies should be destroyed and disposed of properly. An added requirement is that the SOPs should be accessible during working hours without interruption. Hard copies should be available at a manageable location so that the SOPs are available when the electronic system is down.

Research reports—Research reports such as stability reports, method validation and transfer reports, and pharmaceutical development reports are key documents used for NDA/MAA filings. These documents are strictly version controlled.

Laboratory notebooks—It may be debatable to consider laboratory notebooks as text documents, but they should be mentioned here because of their importance in preclinical development. Laboratory notebooks are used to record experimental procedures, observations, raw data, and other important information. Although laboratory notebooks are rarely used for submission to regulatory agencies directly, they are available for inspection by the authorities in the Preapproval Inspection (PAI) and other GMP/GLP-related inspections. Currently, most of the major pharmaceutical companies still use paper-based laboratory notebooks. Electronic-based notebook systems are being developed and commercialized, which are discussed in Chapter 9.

2.4.2 Current TIMS Products

Various so-called Enterprise Content Management (ECM) systems are commercially available that can meet different end user requirements (Table 2.3). TIMS used in preclinical text document management usually is a simplified version of ECM. At the highest enterprise platform level, ECM vendors include Documentum, FileNet, Interwoven, Stellent, and Vignette. At a lower level, the upper-tier products are provided by Day Software, FatWire, and IBM. For less costly products, there are Ingeniux, PaperThin, RedDot Solutions, and Serena Software. It should also be pointed out that the cost of acquiring and maintaining a fully validated TIMS is much higher than that of a non-GMP/GLP system. Therefore many of the non-GMP/GLP documents in early-phase development are managed with nonvalidated TIMS.

2.4.3 Summary

TIMS has helped the pharmaceutical industry to improve efficiency in managing business-critical text documents. However, it is still a time-consuming

TABLE 2.3 Selected TIMS Vendors and Their Products

Product	Vendor	URL
Documentum Web Publisher	Documentum	www.documentum.com
P8 WCM	FileNet	www.filenet.com
TeamSite	Interwoven	www.interwoven.com
Stellent Content Management Suite	Stellent	www.stellent.com
V7 Content Management Suite	Vignette	www.vignette.com
Communique	Day Software	www.day.com
Content Server	FatWire	www.fatwire.com
Workplace WCM	IBM	www.ibm.com
Mediasurface	Mediasurface	www.mediasurface.com
Ingeniux CMS	Ingeniux	www.ingeniux.com
CommonSpot	PaperThin	www.paperthin.com
RedDot CMS	RedDot Solutions	www.reddot.com
Collage	Serena Software	www.serena.com

process to write, review, audit, approve, and publish text documents for submission. The pharmaceutical industry is working toward making submissions electronically. However, this may take time, and the industry may need many changes in business practices to reach the goal.

REFERENCES

1. FDA. "Code of Federal Regulations, Title 21 Food and Drugs, Part 11 Electronic Records; Electronic Signatures: Final Rule," *Fed Regr* 62 (54), 13429–13466 (20 March 1997).
2. FDA. "Withdrawal of draft guidance for industry on Electronic Records; Electronic Signatures, Electronic Copies of Electronic Records," *Fed Regr* 68 (23), 5645 (4 February 2003).
3. FDA. "Draft Guidance for Industry on 'Part 11, Electronic Records; Electronic Signatures—Scope and Application;' Availability of Draft Guidance and Withdrawal of Draft Part 11 Guidance Documents and a Compliance Policy Guide," *Fed Regr* 68 (37), 8775–6 (25 February 1997).
4. Snyder LR, Kirkland JJ. *Introduction to modern liquid chromatography*, 2nd ed., New York, Wiley-Interscience, 1979.
5. Ahuja S, Dong MW. *Handbook of pharmaceutical analysis by HPLC*, Amsterdam, Elsevier Academic, 2005.
6. Thurston CG. LIMS/instrument integration computing architecture for improved automation and flexibility. *Am Lab* 2004; Sep. 15–19.
7. Tejero J, Fish M. Internet delivery of LIMS via the application service provider model. *Am Lab* 2002; Sep. 32–8.
8. Avery G, McGee C, Falk S. Implementing LIMS: a how-to guide. *Anal Chem* 2000;72:57A–62A.

9. FDA. Guidance for Industry. PAT—A Framework for Innovative Pharmaceutical Development, Manufacturing, and Quality Assurance. http://www.fda.gov/cder/guidence/6419fnl.htm
10. Friedli D, Kappeler W, Zimmermann, S. Validation of computer system: practical testing of a standard LIMS. *Pharmaceut Acta Helv* 1998;72:343–8.

3

STATISTICAL MODELING IN PHARMACEUTICAL RESEARCH AND DEVELOPMENT

ANDREA DE GAETANO, SIMONA PANUNZI, BENOIT BECK, AND BRUNO BOULANGER

Contents

3.1 INTRODUCTION

The new major challenge that the pharmaceutical industry is facing in the discovery and development of new drugs is to reduce costs and time needed from discovery to market, while at the same time raising standards of quality. If the pharmaceutical industry cannot find a solution to reduce both costs and time, then its whole business model will be jeopardized: The market will hardly be able, even in the near future, to afford excessively expensive drugs, regardless of their quality.

Computer Applications in Pharmaceutical Research and Development, Edited by Sean Ekins.
ISBN 0-471-73779-8

In parallel to this growing challenge, technologies are also dramatically evolving, opening doors to opportunities never seen before. Some of the best examples of new technologies available in the life sciences are microarray technologies or high-throughput-screening. These new technologies are certainly routes that all pharmaceutical companies will follow. But these new technologies are themselves expensive, time is needed to master them, and success is in any case not guaranteed. So, by mere application of new technology costs have not been reduced, and global cycle time continues to extend while the probability of success remains unchanged.

One key consideration that should be kept in mind is that the whole paradigm for discovering and developing new drugs has not changed at all in the mind of the scientists in the field. The new technologies have been integrated to do the same things as before, but faster, deeper, smaller, with more automation, with more precision, and by collecting more data per experimental unit. However, the standard way to plan experiments, to handle new results, to make decisions has remained more or less unchanged, except that the volume of data, and the disk space required to store it, has exploded exponentially.

This standard way to discover new drugs is essentially by trial and error. The "new technologies" approach has given rise to new hope in that it has permitted many more attempts per unit time, increasing proportionally, however, also the number of errors. Indeed, no breakthrough strategy has been adopted to drastically increase the rate of successes per trial and to integrate the rich data into an evolving system of knowledge accumulation, which would allow companies to become smarter with time. For most new projects initiated, scientists start data production from scratch: The lessons they have learned, or they think they have learned, from previous projects are used only as a general cultural influence; they do not materially determine the continuing development of successive projects.

This possibly slightly pessimistic portrait of the current status of research in the life sciences contrasts sharply with the progression of technology and development changes achieved in other industrial areas. As an example, consider aeronautics. New airplanes today are completely conceived, designed, optimized, and built with computer models (in fact mathematical and statistical models), through intensive simulations. Once a new plane is constructed, it will almost surely fly on its first trial, even if fine-tuning may still be needed. In this industry, each attempt produces one success. If we were to translate the current paradigm of discovery and development of new drugs into aeronautics terms, we could think of many metallurgists with great personal expertise in metallurgy, who, using vague notions of aerodynamics and resistance of materials, assemble large numbers of "candidate planes," each a complex arrangement of metal pieces. Each "candidate plane" is then tested under real conditions, by attempting to fly it from a number of likely take-off surfaces and in different meteorological conditions: The very few that do not crash are finally called "planes." The configuration of the many candidate planes that crashed is examined, so as to avoid repeating the same kinds of error in the future, but each metallurgist has his or her own way to read the facts and draw conclusions for future assemblage instead of consulting or hiring a specialist in aerodynamics or materials. The theory here would be that a plane is, finally, a large collection of pieces of metal, all assembled together! So why would other kinds of expertise be needed, besides those closely linked to metallurgy? In this vision of the business, the more new planes one wants to launch, the more metallurgists one needs, and the process could even be accelerated if one could buy new-technology machines that automatically build and assemble large numbers of different pieces of metal.

In the aeronautics industry, when an experiment is envisaged, for example, testing the resistance of a particular piece, the goal of the experiment is first of all that of verifying and refining the computer model of that piece to answer a fundamental question: Does the model behave like the real piece, or what changes are needed to make the model behave like the piece? Once adequately tuned, the model forecasts will then be used to understand how to optimize the resistance of the piece itself, until the next comparison between model and reality is done. After a few such iterations, the final piece is fully checked for quality purposes and will almost surely be found to be the right one for the job at hand. Translating the pharmaceutical approach to an experiment into aeronautics terms produces a somewhat different picture: A piece is built, which should satisfy quality checks, and an experiment is done to evaluate the resistance of the piece. If the test fails, as it is very likely to do, the piece is thrown away and the metallurgist is asked to propose a new piece by next week.

This caricaturized image of the process of discovery and development of new drugs has been drawn to highlight the pivotal role that models (simplified mathematical descriptions of real-life mechanisms) play in many R&D activities. In the pharmaceutical industry, however, in-depth use of models for efficient optimization and continuous learning is not generally made. In some areas of pharmaceutical research, like pharmacokinetics/pharmacodynamics (PK/PD), models are built to characterize the kinetics and action of new compounds or platforms of compounds, knowledge crucial for designing new experiments and optimizing drug dosage. Models are also developed in other areas, as for example in medicinal chemistry with QSAR-related models. These can all be defined as mechanistic models, and they are useful. But in these models, the stochastic noise inherent in the data, the variability that makes biology so much more different from the physical sciences, is not as a general rule appropriately taken into account.

On the other side, many models of a different type are currently used in the biological sciences: These can be envisaged as complicated (mathematical) extensions of commonsense ways to analyze results when these results are partially hidden behind noise, noise being inescapable when dealing with biological matters. This is the area currently occupied by most statisticians: Using empirical models, universally applicable, whose basic purpose is to appropriately represent the noise, but not the biology or the chemistry, statisticians give whenever possible a denoised picture of the results, so that field scientists can gain better understanding and take more informed decisions. In the ideal case, as in regulated clinical trials, the statistician is consulted up front to help in designing the experiment, to ensure that the necessary denoising process will be effective enough to lead to a conclusion, positive or negative. This is the kingdom of empirical models.

The dividing line between empirical models and mechanistic models is not as clear and obvious as some would pretend. Mechanistic models are usually based on chemical or biological knowledge, or the understanding we have of chemistry or biology. These models are considered as interpretable or meaningful, but their inherent nature (nonlinearity, high number of parameters) poses other challenges, particularly once several sources of noise are also to be adequately modeled. For these reasons empirical approaches have been largely preferred in the past. Today, however, the combination of mathematics, statistics, and computing allows us to effectively use more and more complex mechanistic models directly incorporating our biological or chemical knowledge.

The development of models in the pharmaceutical industry is certainly one of the significant breakthroughs proposed to face the challenges of cost, speed, and quality, somewhat imitating what happens in the aeronautics industry. The concept, however, is not that of adopting just another new technology, "modeling." The use of models in the experimental cycle changes the cycle itself. Without models, the final purpose of an experiment was one single drug or its behavior; with the use of models, the objective of experiments will be the drug and the model at the same level. Improving the model will help understanding this and other drugs and the experiments on successive drugs will help improving the model's ability to represent reality. In addition, as well known in the theory of experimental design, the way to optimally conceive an experiment depends on the a-priori model you have. If you have very little a priori usable information (i.e., a poor model), then you will need many experiments and samples, making your practice not very cost effective. This is a bonus few realize from having models supporting the cycle: The cost, speed, and effectiveness of studies can be dramatically improved, while the information collected from those optimized experiments is itself used to update the model itself. Modeling is the keystone to installing a virtuous cycle in the pharmaceutical industry, in order to successfully overcome approaching hurdles. This, of course, requires us to network with or to bring on board modelers that are able to closely collaborate with confirmed drug hunters.

Using the mathematically simple example of Gompertz tumor growth, this chapter discusses the relationship between empirical and mechanistic models, the difficulties and advantages that theoretical or mechanistic models offer, and how they permit us to make safe decisions and also to optimize experiments. We believe there is an urgent need to promote biomathematics in drug discovery, as a tool for meaningfully combining the scientific expertise of the different participants in the discovery process and to secure results for continuing development. The key is to move, whenever meaningful, to mechanistic models with adequate treatment of noise.

3.2 DESCRIPTIVE VERSUS MECHANISTIC MODELING

According to Breiman [1], there are two cultures in the use of statistical modeling to reach conclusions from data. The first culture, namely, the data modeling culture, assumes that the data are generated by a given stochastic data model, whereas the other, the algorithmic modeling culture, uses algorithmic models and treats the data mechanism as unknown. Statistics thinks of the data as being generated by a black box into which a vector of input variables x (independent variable) enter and out of which a vector of response variables y (dependent variable) exits. Two of the main goals of performing statistical investigations are to be able to predict what the responses are going to be to future input variables and to extract some information about how nature is associating the response variables to the input variables.

We believe that a third possible goal for running statistical investigations might be to understand the foundations of the mechanisms from which the data are generated or going to be generated, and the present chapter is focused on this goal.

To understand the mechanism, the use of modeling concepts is essential. The purpose of the model is essentially that of translating the known properties about the black box as well as some new hypotheses into a mathematical representation. In this way, a model is a simplifying representation of the data-generating mechanism under investigation. The identification of an appropriate model is often not easy and may require thorough investigation. It is usual to restrict the investigation to a parametric family of models (i.e., to a set of models that differ from one another only in the value of some parameter) and then use standard statistical techniques either to select the most appropriate model within the family (i.e., the most appropriate parameter value) with respect to a given criterion or to identify the most likely subfamily of models (i.e., the most likely set of parameter values). In the former case the interest is in getting point estimates for the parameters, whereas in the latter case the interest is in getting confidence regions for them.

The way in which the family of models is selected depends on the main purpose of the exercise. If the purpose is just to provide a reasonable description of the data in some appropriate way without any attempt at understanding the underlying phenomenon, that is, the data-generating mechanism, then the family of models is selected based on its adequacy to represent the data structure. The net result in this case is only a descriptive model of the phenomenon. These models are very useful for discriminating between alternative hypotheses but are totally useless for capturing the fundamental characteristics of a mechanism. On the contrary, if the purpose of the modeling exercise is to get some insight on or to increase our understanding of the underlying mechanism, the family of models must be selected based on reasonable assumptions with respect to the nature of the mechanism. As the fundamental characteristics of the mechanism are often given in terms of rates of change, it is not unusual to link the definition of the family to a system of differential equations. As the mechanisms in biology and medicine are relatively complex, the systems of differential equations used to characterize some of the properties of their behavior often contain nonlinear or delay terms. It is then rarely possible to obtain analytical solutions, and thus numerical approximations are used.

Whenever the interest lies in the understanding of the mechanisms of action, it is critical to be able to count on a strong collaboration between scientists, specialists in the field, and statisticians or mathematicians. The former must provide updated, rich, and reliable information about the problem, whereas the latter are trained for translating scientific information in mathematical models and for appropriately describing probabilistic/stochastic components indispensable to handling the variability inherently contained in the data generation processes. In other words, when faced with a scientific problem, statisticians and biomathematicians cannot construct suitable models in isolation, without detailed interaction with the scientists. On the other hand, many scientists have insufficient mathematical background to translate their theories into equations susceptible to confrontation with empirical data. Thus the first element of any model selection process within science must be based on close cooperation and interaction among the cross-functional team involved.

When there is a relative consensus about the family of models to use, the data must be retrieved from available repositories or generated with a well-designed experiment. In this chapter, animal tumor growth data are used for the representation of the different concepts encountered during the development of a model and its after-identification use. The data represent the tumor growth in rats over a period of 80 days. We are interested in modeling the growth of experimental tumors subcutaneously implanted in rats to be able to differentiate between treatment regimens. Two groups of rats have received different treatments, placebo and a new drug at a fixed dose. So in addition to the construction of an appropriate model for representing the tumor growth, there is an interest in the statistical significance of the effect of treatment. The raw data for one subject who received placebo are represented as open circles in Figure 3.1. For the considered subject, the tumor volume grows from nearly 0 to about 3000 mm^3.

A first evaluation of the data can be done by running nonparametric statistical estimation techniques like, for example, the Nadaraya–Watson kernel regression estimate [2]. These techniques have the advantage of being relatively cost-free in terms of assumptions, but they do not provide any possibility of interpreting the outcome and are not at all reliable when extrapolating. The fact that these techniques do not require a lot of assumptions makes them

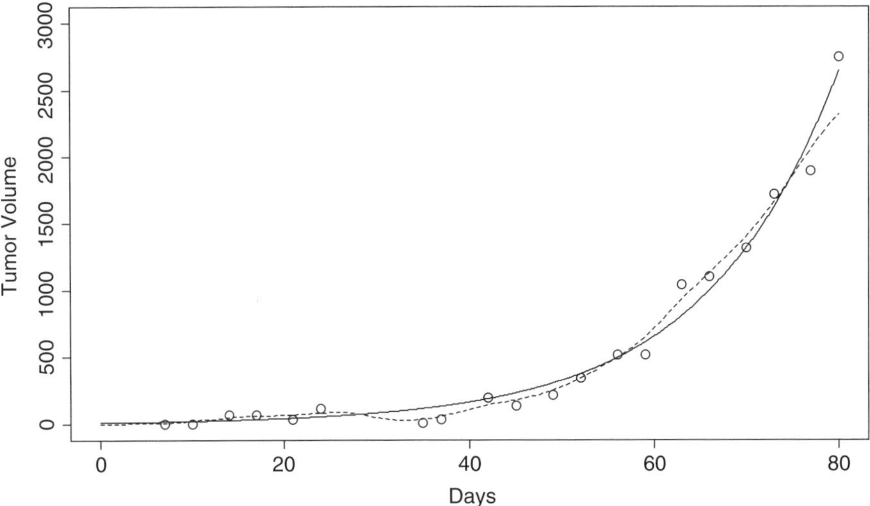

Figure 3.1 Time course of implanted tumor volume for one experimental subject (Control) and associated fitted model curves (solid line, exponential model; dashed line, nonparametric kernel estimate).

relatively close to what algorithm-oriented people try to do. These techniques are essentially descriptive by nature and are useful for summarizing the data by smoothing them and providing interpolated values. The fit obtained by using the Nadaraya–Watson estimate on the set of data previously introduced is represented by the dashed line in Figure 3.1. This approach, although often useful for practical applications, does not quite agree with the philosophical goal of science, which is to understand a phenomenon as completely and generally as possible. This is why a parametric mechanistic modeling approach to approximate the data-generating process must be used.

When looking at the presented data, it would be reasonable, as a first approximation, to imagine using a parametric family of models capturing the potential exponential growth of the tumor volumes. Although certainly reasonable from a physiological point of view, the selection of the exponential family is, at this stage, only based on the visual identification of a specific characteristic exhibited by the data, in this case, exponential growth. The exponential parametric family is mathematically fully characterized by the family of equations $V(t) = \alpha \exp(\lambda t)$. A particular model is fully specified by fixing the values for its two parameters α and λ. Note that it is particularly important to quantitatively study the change in behavior of the different models in terms of the parameters to have a good understanding of constraints existing on the parameters. In this case, for example, both parameters must be positive. To fit the model on the observed data, statistical techniques must be applied. These techniques attempt to optimize the selection of the parameter value with respect to a certain criterion. The ordinary least-squares optimization algorithm (see Section 3.3) has been used to get parameter estimates. Although this model has been selected essentially on the basis of the observed data structure, it is possible to try to give an interpretation of the model parameters. However, the interpretation of the parameters is only done after fitting the curve, possibly because of similar experiences with the same model used on other phenomena, which generate similar types of data. Up to this point, the interpretation is not at all based on known scientific properties of the data-producing mechanism built into the model. Note that again a similar a posteriori interpretability search is obviously not possible in the case of a nonparametric fit. For the exponential family of models, the first parameter might be interpreted as the tumor volume at time zero whereas the second might likely represent the tumor growth rate. The problem with the model identified from the exponential family is that mathematically the tumor growth will continue up to infinity, which from a physiological point of view is very difficult to accept and to justify. In other words, the very form of the mathematical model as such, independently of any recorded data, is incompatible with physiology as we know it. The mathematical analysis of the model behavior, abstracting from any recorded data, should be part of any serious modeling effort directed to the understanding of a physiological mechanism and should precede the numerical fitting of the model to the available data. This qualitative model analysis seeks to establish, first of all, that the model equations do admit a solution (even if we cannot explicitly derive one) and that this solution is unique. Secondly, the solution must have a set of desirable properties that are typical of the behavior of physiological systems, for example, they are bounded, positive, of bounded variation, stable with respect to the parameters and to the initial conditions. Finally, these solutions must exhibit or fail to exhibit some characteristic patterns, like oscillations whose period may depend on some parameter, or, more interestingly, may become established or change regime depending on some "bifurcation" parameter value. As noted before, in the absence of the possibility of actually deriving an explicit solution, given the complexity of the differential formulation, qualitative analysis seeks to characterize the unknown analytical solution, leaving to numerical techniques the actual computation of a close approximation to the unknown solution.

After having used a (simple) model formulation with some plausible meaning and a behavior matching the observed data structure, the next step in the quest for a good model is to go back to the selection of an appropriate family, this time operating a selection not only with reference to the apparent data structure but also incorporating some known or presumed quantitative properties of the mechanism under investigation. The investigation of tumor growth on which we concentrate in this chapter falls in fact into the broad topic of growth curve analysis, which is one of the most common types of studies in which nonlinear regression functions are employed. The special characteristics of the growth curves are that the exhibited growth profile generally is a nonlinear function of time with an asymptote; that random variability associated to the data is likely to increase with size, so that the dispersion is not constant; and finally, that successive responses are measured on the same subject so that they will generally not be independent [3]. Note that different individuals may have different tumor growth rates, either inherently or because of environmental effects or treatment. This will justify the population approach presented in Section 3.7.

The growth rate of a living organism or tissue can often be characterized by two competing processes. The net increase is then given by the difference between anabolism and catabolism, between the synthesis of new body matter and its loss. Catabolism is often assumed to be proportional to the quantity chosen to characterize the size of the living being, namely, weight or volume, whereas anabolism is assumed to have an allometric relationship to the same quantity. These assumptions on the competing processes are translated into mathematics by the following differential equation:

$$\frac{\mathrm{d}\mu}{\mathrm{d}t}(t) = \beta\mu(t)^{K+1} - \alpha\mu(t)$$

where $\mu(t)$ represents the size of the studied system in function of time. Note that this equation can be reformulated as follows:

$$\frac{\mathrm{d}\mu}{\mathrm{d}t}(t) = -\frac{\gamma}{K}\mu(t)\left(\left(\frac{\mu(t)}{\alpha}\right)^{K} - 1\right),$$

which has $\mu(t) = \alpha(1 + K\exp(-\gamma(t - \eta)))^{-1/K}$ as general solution. The curve represented by this last equation is commonly named the Richards curve. When K is equal to one, the Richards curve becomes the well-known logistic function. If the allometric factor in the relationship representing the catabolism mechanism is small, that is, K tends to 0, then the differential equation becomes

$$\frac{\mathrm{d}\mu}{\mathrm{d}t}(t) = -\gamma\mu(t)\log\left(\frac{\mu(t)}{\alpha}\right)$$

thanks to the relation $\exp(x) = \lim_{K\to 0}(1 + Kx)^{1/K}$. The general solution of this differential equation is now given by $\mu(t) = \alpha\exp(-\exp(-\gamma(t - \eta)))$, and is called the Gompertz curve. Note that, contrary to the logistic function, the Gompertz curve is not symmetric about its point of inflection. The Gompertz growth curve is certainly the principal model used in the analysis of the time courses of tumor volume growth. The model can be reparameterized as follows:

$$\frac{\mathrm{d}V}{\mathrm{d}t}(t) = aV(t) - bV(t)\log(V(t)), \quad V(0) = V_0$$

where V [mm^3] is the volume of the tumor, t [days] is time, a [days^{-1}] is the rate of growth, and b [days^{-1}] is the rate of degradation. The parameter vector $\theta = (a, b, V_0)^T$ will belong to some domain, $\theta \in \Theta \subset \mathrm{R}^3$, where the ^{T} indicates vector or matrix transposition, and ∇ is the real line. With the new notation, the solution of the differential equation is given by

$$V(t) = \exp\left(\frac{a}{b} - \left(\frac{a}{b} - \log V_0\right)\exp(-bt)\right).$$

The diagram in Figure 3.2 shows the model for the parameter value $\theta^* = (0.4, 0.04, 0.3)^{\mathrm{T}}$. From now on we will always indicate the parameter as $\theta = (a, b, V_0)^{\mathrm{T}}$. The sigmoidal behavior of the model is evident. The Gompertz curve has an asymptote given by $\exp(a/b)$. This curve can in fact be thought of as describing initial exponential growth that is increasingly damped as the size increases, until it eventually stops. Indeed, this can be easily deduced by using the Taylor expansion $\exp(-bt) \cong 1 - bt + \frac{b^2t^2}{2} - \frac{b^3t^3}{6} + \frac{b^4t^4}{24} \ldots$ for the internal exponential in the Gompertz solution:

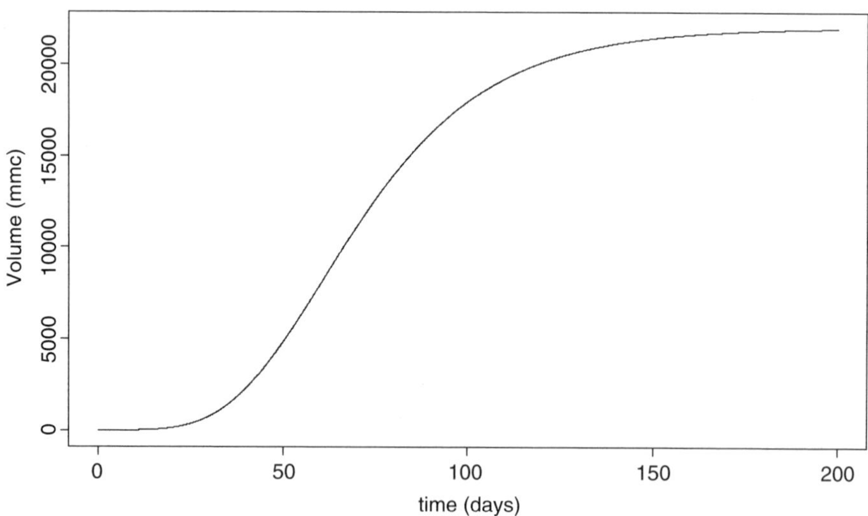

Figure 3.2 Example of Gompertz growth curve for parameter value $\theta^* = (0.4, 0.04, 0.3)^T$.

$$
\begin{aligned}
V(t) &= \exp\left(\frac{a}{b} - \left(\frac{a}{b} - \log V_0\right)\exp(-bt)\right) \\
&\cong \exp\left(\frac{a}{b} - \left(\frac{a}{b} - \log V_0\right)(1 - bt)\right) \\
&= V_0 \exp\left((a - b \log V_0)t\right) \\
&= \alpha \exp(\lambda t)
\end{aligned}
$$

The different curves obtained by increasing the number of terms in the Taylor expansion are represented in Figure 3.3 on top of the Gompertz curve itself. The exponential growth model can thus be now justified not only because it fits well the data but also because it can be seen as a first approximation to the Gompertz growth model, which is endowed with a mechanistic interpretation, namely, competition between the catabolic and anabolic processes.

3.3 STATISTICAL PARAMETER ESTIMATION

Once the model functional form has been decided upon and the experimental data have been collected, a value for the model parameters (point estimation) and a confidence region for this value (interval estimation) must be estimated

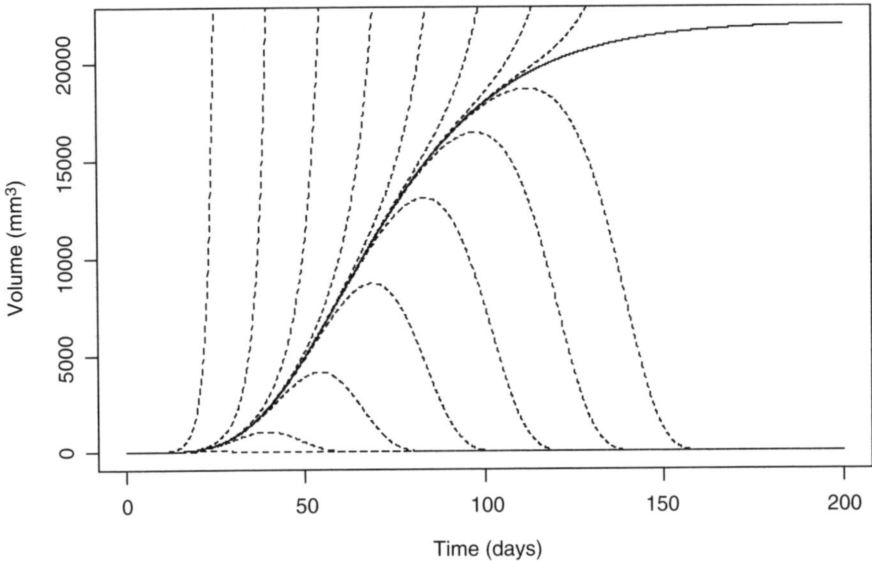

Figure 3.3 Approximations of the Gompertz growth curve based on Taylor expansion for the internal exponential term.

from the available data. We will follow as an example the application of the principle to a real-life situation in which nine experimental subjects (rats) have been inoculated in the ear with a small tumor. Five of the rats have not been treated with any drug, whereas four have received a novel antitumoral treatment. The goal of the experiment is, of course, that of verifying whether the treatment is effective in reducing tumor growth rate.

Our first goal is to retrieve a good approximation of the true value θ^* by means of some operation on the sample of observations, the *point estimate* of θ^*.

The heuristic reasoning is as follows. Suppose we were able to quantify how good a parameter is with respect to the available data, that is, suppose we were to obtain a value of merit as a function of data and parameters. The data are given and cannot be changed, but we can change the presumed parameter value so as to maximize the merit. Maximizing our merit function, we would find the best possible parameter value for the given data. Instead of a merit function it is usually more convenient to use a *loss function*, which is the opposite of a merit function in that it quantifies how badly a parameter value performs. We will then want to *minimize* our loss with respect to the parameter to find the best possible parameter value. As a loss function, Carl Friedrich Gauss between the late eighteenth and early nineteenth centuries formalized the use of the sum of squared residuals [4]. In its simplest form, the ordinary least squares criterion (OLS) prescribes as a loss function the sum of the squared "residuals" relative to all observed points, where the residual relative to each observed point is the difference between the observed and predicted value at that point. Clearly, if the model resulting from a certain parameter value tends to closely predict the actually observed values, then the residuals will be small and the sum of their squares will also be small, so the loss will be small. Conversely, a bad or unacceptable value of the parameter will determine a model that predicts values very far from those actually observed, the residuals will be large and the loss will be large [3, 5, 6]. We may suppose, in general, to have a nonlinear model with a known functional relationship

$$y_i = u(\mathbf{x}_i;\theta^*) + \varepsilon_i,\ E[\varepsilon_i] = 0,\ \theta^* \in \Theta, \tag{3.1}$$

where y_i is the ith observation, corresponding to a vector $\mathbf{x}_i$ of independent variables, where θ^* is the true but unknown parameter value belonging to some acceptable domain Θ, where u is the predicted value as a function of independent variables and parameter, and where ε_i are true errors (which we only suppose for the moment to have zero mean value) that randomly modify the theoretical value of the observation. We may rewrite the model in vector form as

$$\mathbf{y} = \mathbf{u}(\mathbf{X}, \theta^*) + \varepsilon,\ E[\varepsilon] = 0,\ \theta^* \in \Theta. \tag{3.1'}$$

Because the independent variable values are fixed for the problem, we may simplify notation by looking at $\mathbf{u}$ as a function of the variable $\boldsymbol{\theta}$: From now on we will therefore write $\mathbf{u}(\mathbf{X}, \boldsymbol{\theta})$ as $\mathbf{u}(\boldsymbol{\theta})$.

The ordinary least-squares estimate (OLSE) $\hat{\boldsymbol{\theta}}$ of $\boldsymbol{\theta}^*$ minimizes (globally over $\boldsymbol{\theta} \in \Theta$)

$$S(\theta) = [\mathbf{y} - \mathbf{u}(\theta)]^T [\mathbf{y} - \mathbf{u}(\theta)] = \mathbf{e}^T \mathbf{e} = \sum (y_i - u_i)^2. \tag{3.2}$$

Supposing $\mathbf{D} = \mathrm{Cov}(\boldsymbol{\varepsilon})$ to be known, we would possibly improve our estimation procedure by weighting more those points of which we are more certain, that is, those whose associated errors have the least variance, taking also into account the correlations among the errors. We may then indicate with $\hat{\boldsymbol{\theta}}$ the weighted least-squares estimator (WLSE), which is the value of $\boldsymbol{\theta}$ minimizing

$$S(\theta) = [\mathbf{y} - \mathbf{u}(\theta)]^T \mathbf{D}^{-1} [\mathbf{y} - \mathbf{u}(\boldsymbol{\theta})] = \mathbf{e}^T \mathbf{D}^{-1} \mathbf{e}, \tag{3.3}$$

where $\mathbf{e}$ is the vector of "residuals" $[\mathbf{y} - \mathbf{u}(\boldsymbol{\theta})]$.

In the case in which the errors are independent of each other their covariances will be zero, and if they also have the same variance, then $\mathbf{D} = \sigma^2 \mathbf{I}$, with the constant σ^2 being the common variance and $\mathbf{I}$ being the identity matrix. In this case, the same $\boldsymbol{\theta}$ minimizing (Eq. 3.3) would also minimize (Eq. 3.2) and the OLSE can therefore be seen as a particular case of the WLSE.

For our sample application we assume that the points are measured with independent errors and equal variance. We may thus fit the data points minimizing $\mathbf{e}^T \mathbf{e}$, after which we may estimate σ^2 as $s^2 = \mathbf{e}^T \mathbf{e}/(n-1)$.

To produce the needed model estimate $\mathbf{u}(t, \boldsymbol{\theta})$ at each time and for each tested value of the parameter $\boldsymbol{\theta}$ we may be lucky and have an explicitly solvable model, so that we directly compute $\mathbf{u}$, or less lucky, which is a more frequent occurrence. In fact, instead of an explicit formula for $\mathbf{u}$ we often have only a differential relation expressing the rate of change of $\mathbf{u}$ in time, given some initial value $\mathbf{u}(0)$. In this case we compute the approximate value of $\mathbf{u}(t, \boldsymbol{\theta})$ by numerical integration, with any one of a wide choice of algorithms, such as for example a fixed-step fourth-order Runge–Kutta procedure, or a more complicated variable-step, variable-order scheme [7, 8]. In our search for the optimum parameter value, minimizing the loss function, we again may use any one of a vast array of optimization schemes with varying requirements, convergence rates, and difficulty of implementation. Typically, either a simplex algorithm (which does not require or depend on the numerical computation of derivatives of the loss with respect to the parameters) or a more efficient, derivative-based nonlinear nonconstrained quasi-Newton variable metric optimization algorithm may be used [7], with a stopping criterion based on the convergence of either loss function or parameter value.

Sample fits of observed volumes at different times (open circles) and their OLS-predicted time course (solid line) can be seen for a few of the subjects in Figure 3.4, a–d; the OLS estimates of the parameter values for all subjects are reported in Table 3.1.

Once we have obtained our point estimate, we can ask ourselves what confidence we place in this estimate, how likely it would be, in real life, that actual parameter values differ from the values we have estimated.

3.4 CONFIDENCE REGIONS

The standard way to answer the above question would be to compute the probability distribution of the parameter and, from it, to compute, for example, the 95% confidence region on the parameter estimate obtained. We would, in other words, find a set of values I_θ such that the probability that we are correct in asserting that the true value $\boldsymbol{\theta}^*$ of the parameter lies in I_θ is 95%. If we assumed that the parameter estimates are at least approximately normally distributed around the true parameter value (which is asymptotically true in the case of least squares under some mild regularity assumptions), then it would be sufficient to know the parameter dispersion (variance-covariance matrix) in order to be able to compute approximate ellipsoidal confidence regions.

However, it is not generally possible to compute exactly the dispersion of the estimates in the case of nonlinear problems. What we can do is use approximate expressions whose validity is good in a small neighborhood of the true value of the parameter. In the present section we will assume that the model is not too far from linearity around the optimum found.

Suppose $\mathbf{D} = \mathrm{Cov}(\boldsymbol{\varepsilon})$, known. Indicate with $\hat{\boldsymbol{\theta}}$ the weighted least-squares estimator (WLSE), that is, let $\hat{\boldsymbol{\theta}}$ minimize $S(\boldsymbol{\theta}) = [\mathbf{y} - \mathbf{u}(\boldsymbol{\theta})]^T\mathbf{D}^{-1}[\mathbf{y} - \mathbf{u}(\boldsymbol{\theta})] = \mathbf{e}^T\mathbf{D}^{-1}\mathbf{e}$.

Expanding $\mathbf{u}$ in Taylor series around the true $\boldsymbol{\theta}^*$ and neglecting terms of second and higher order we may write $\left(\text{writing } \mathbf{U}. = \left.\frac{\partial \mathbf{u}}{\partial \boldsymbol{\theta}}\right|_{\theta=\theta^*}\right)$, we have $\hat{\theta} \cong [\mathrm{U}.^T\mathrm{D}^{-1}\mathrm{U}.]^{-1}\,\mathrm{U}.^T\,\mathrm{D}^{-1}\,\varepsilon + \theta^*$ We observe that the WLSE estimator $\hat{\theta}$ is approximately unbiased (in a small neighborhood of θ^*), and $Cov(\hat{\theta}) = E\left((\hat{\theta} - E(\hat{\theta}))(\hat{\theta} - E(\hat{\theta}))^T\right) \cong [\,\hat{\mathrm{U}}.^{\mathrm{T}}\mathrm{D}^{-1}\hat{\mathrm{U}}.]^{-1}$, where we have obviously denoted $\hat{\mathbf{U}}. = \left.\frac{\partial \mathbf{u}}{\partial \boldsymbol{\theta}}\right|_{\theta=\hat{\theta}}$.

If we believe that $\mathbf{D} = \sigma^2\,\mathrm{diag}(\mathbf{u})$, that is, that errors are independent and proportional to the square root of the predicted value, then $\mathbf{D}^{-1} = \mathrm{diag}(1/u_i)/\sigma^2$, where we may further approximate this result by estimating

$$\sigma^2 \cong s^2 = \frac{1}{(n-1)}\sum \frac{(y_i - u_i)^2}{u_i} \text{ at the optimum.}$$

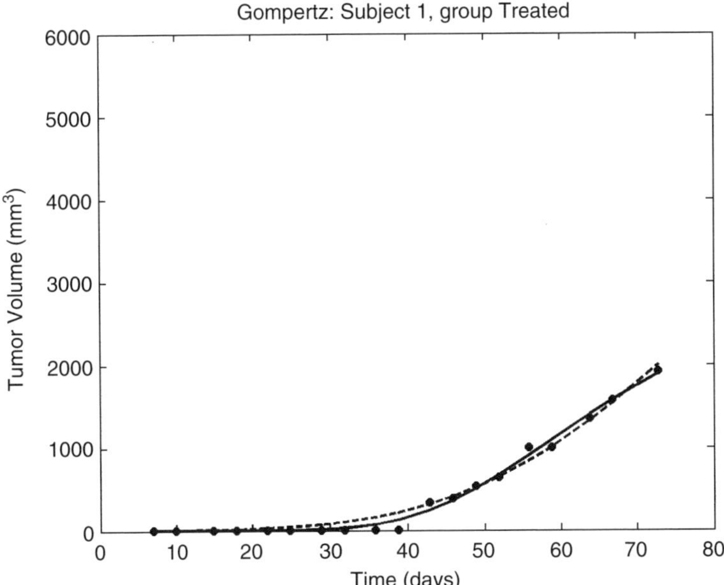

Figure 3.4a Observed (open circles), single-subject OLS-predicted (solid line), and population estimation (L&B90)-predicted (dashed line) time-volume points for *subject 1* (Treated).

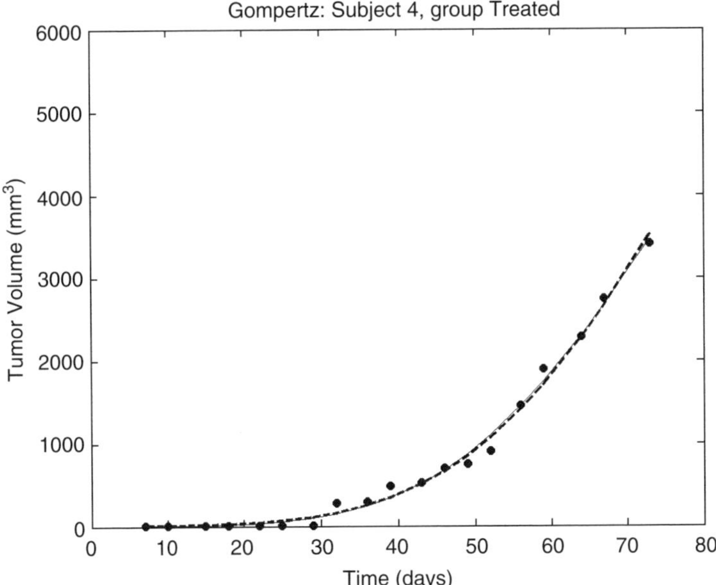

Figure 3.4b Observed (open circles), single-subject OLS-predicted (solid line), and population estimation (L&B90)-predicted (dashed line) time-volume points for *subject 4* (Treated).

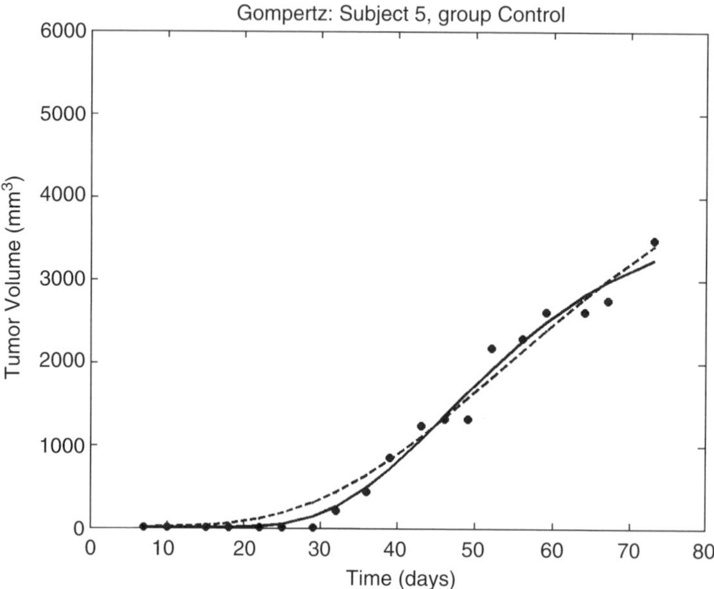

Figure 3.4c Observed (open circles), single-subject OLS-predicted (solid line), and population estimation (L&B90)-predicted (dashed line) time-volume points for *subject 5* (Control).

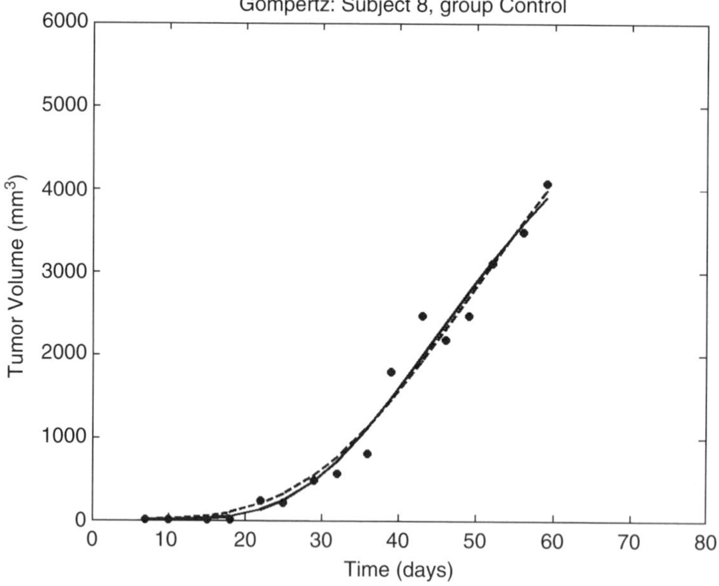

Figure 3.4d Observed (open circles), single-subject OLS-predicted (solid line), and population estimation (L&B90)-predicted (dashed line) time-volume points for *subject 8* (Control).

TABLE 3.1 Single-subject OLS Parameter Estimates

Subject	Treatment	A	b	V_0
1	1	0.050225	3.11E-12	51.13972
2	1	0.047986	8.8E-09	59.89137
3	1	0.048241	6.3E-11	51.20751
4	1	0.056145	5.18E-11	59.00714
5	0	0.330552	0.038063	1
6	0	0.384246	0.038479	1.000004
7	0	0.287166	0.036333	14.94381
8	0	0.377056	0.04155	1
9	0	0.184559	0.019011	24.10613

It is now immediate to compute approximate confidence intervals for any single parameter component from its estimated standard error. In Table 3.2, the individual OLS estimation results for *subject 9* are reported. Standard errors for all parameter components have been computed as the square roots of the diagonal elements of the parameter dispersion matrix. Parameter variability has also been expressed as coefficients of variation (percent size of standard error with respect to the estimated value). From the correlation matrix of parameter estimates it is evident how in our example the estimates of parameters a and b are very highly correlated: This means that, in order to explain the observed data set, if we entertain the hypothesis of a slightly higher growth rate we must simultaneously accept a slightly higher death rate; otherwise, the observations are no more compatible with the model.

It is interesting to see what shape the confidence regions take when we consider more than one parameter component at the same time. In fact, the high correlation between the estimates of a and b would indicate that we could change them together, in the same direction, without greatly changing the overall loss, but that altering their relative size would quickly cause major departures of the model from the observations.

A first approach to the definition of the confidence regions in parameter space follows the linear approximation to the parameter joint distribution that we have already used: If the estimates are approximately normally distributed around θ^* with dispersion $[\mathbf{U}.^T \mathbf{D}^{-1} \mathbf{U}.]^{-1}$, then an approximate $100(1-\alpha)\%$ confidence region for θ^* is

$$\left\{\boldsymbol{\theta} \middle| \left(1/ps^2\right)\left(\boldsymbol{\theta}-\hat{\boldsymbol{\theta}}\right)^T \left[\mathbf{U}.^T\mathbf{D}^{-1}\mathbf{U}.\right]\left(\boldsymbol{\theta}-\hat{\boldsymbol{\theta}}\right) \le F^{\alpha}_{p,n-p}\right\},$$

where p is the number of parameters, n the number of available independent observations, and $F^{\alpha}_{p,n-p}$ is the critical value of the Fisher's F-distribution at the α critical level with p and $(n-p)$ degrees of freedom. As this approximation is valid asymptotically, so the regions will cover the correct $(1-\alpha)$ confidence level asymptotically. For varying α, these confidence regions are

TABLE 3.2 Complete Fit Results for *Subject 9*

R^2	0.985944
Degrees of Freedom	16
Error Variance	15110.7
Error St.Dev.	122.926
Akaike Inform Crit	185.575
Schwartz B.I.C.	188.408

Hessian Matrix

	bi_a	bi_b	bi_V_0
bi_a	6.5029e+006	−4.1363e+007	2250.7
bi_b	−4.1363e+007	2.6391e+008	-14068
bi_V_0	2250.7	-14068	0.86104

Parameter Dispersion Matrix

	bi_a	bi_b	bi_V_0
bi_a	0.0016129	0.00021734	−0.66495
bi_b	0.00021734	2.9346e-005	−0.088646
bi_V_0	−0.66495	−0.088646	292.13

Parameter Correlation Matrix

	bi_a	bi_b	bi_V_0
bi_a	1	0.999	−0.96872
bi_b	0.999	1	−0.95739
bi_V_0	−0.96872	−0.95739	1

Parameter Point Estimates, Standard Errors, and Coefficients of Variation

$a = 0.18456 \pm 0.040161$ (21.76%)
$b = 0.019011 \pm 0.0054172$ (28.495%)
$V_0 = 24.106 \pm 17.092$ (70.903%)

shaped like multidimensional ellipsoids, which are the contours of the asymptotic multivariate normal density function of $\hat{\boldsymbol{\theta}}$. We may further approximate this distribution by taking $\hat{\mathbf{U}}$. in place of $\mathbf{U}$. (i.e., by computing the jacobian at $\hat{\boldsymbol{\theta}}$ instead of $\boldsymbol{\theta}^*$).

A second approach considers that the regions of equivalent parameter values must enclose parameters for which the loss function is nearly the same or at any rate less different than some threshold. In other words, the equivalence regions should take the form $\{\boldsymbol{\theta}|S(\boldsymbol{\theta}) \le c\ S(\hat{\boldsymbol{\theta}})\}$ for some appropriate constant $c > 1$. Note that in this case the shape of the regions would not necessarily be ellipsoidal, or even convex: In fact, we might postulate in general the existence of multiple minima surrounded by disjoint equivalence neighborhoods, the union of which would make up an equivalence region. More commonly, regions of this type (called "exact" confidence regions) may be distorted to a degree given by the nonlinearity of the model around the optimum. If we could compute the probability associated to one such region, then we could speak of a statistical confidence region. Again, we may resort to an approximation considering $\hat{\boldsymbol{\theta}}$ to be sufficiently near $\boldsymbol{\theta}^*$, so that we may use $\hat{\mathbf{U}}.$ in place of $\mathbf{U}.$: In this case the Taylor expansion of $S(\hat{\boldsymbol{\theta}})$ around $\boldsymbol{\theta}^*$ would allow us to write

$$S(\boldsymbol{\theta}^*) - S(\hat{\boldsymbol{\theta}}) \cong (\boldsymbol{\theta}^* - \hat{\boldsymbol{\theta}})^T \hat{\mathbf{U}}.^T \hat{\mathbf{U}}.(\boldsymbol{\theta}^* - \hat{\boldsymbol{\theta}})$$

so that an approximate $100(1 - \alpha)\%$ confidence region would be

$$\left\{ \boldsymbol{\theta} \middle| S(\boldsymbol{\theta}) \le S(\hat{\boldsymbol{\theta}}) \left(1 + \frac{p}{n-p} F^{\alpha}_{p,n-p} \right) \right\} \quad \text{or} \quad \left\{ \boldsymbol{\theta} \middle| \left(\frac{S(\boldsymbol{\theta})}{S(\hat{\boldsymbol{\theta}})} - 1 \right) \frac{n-p}{p} \le F^{\alpha}_{p,n-p} \right\}$$

Although asymptotically these regions are the same, for finite n there may be substantial differences: Figure 3.5 shows the confidence regions for the

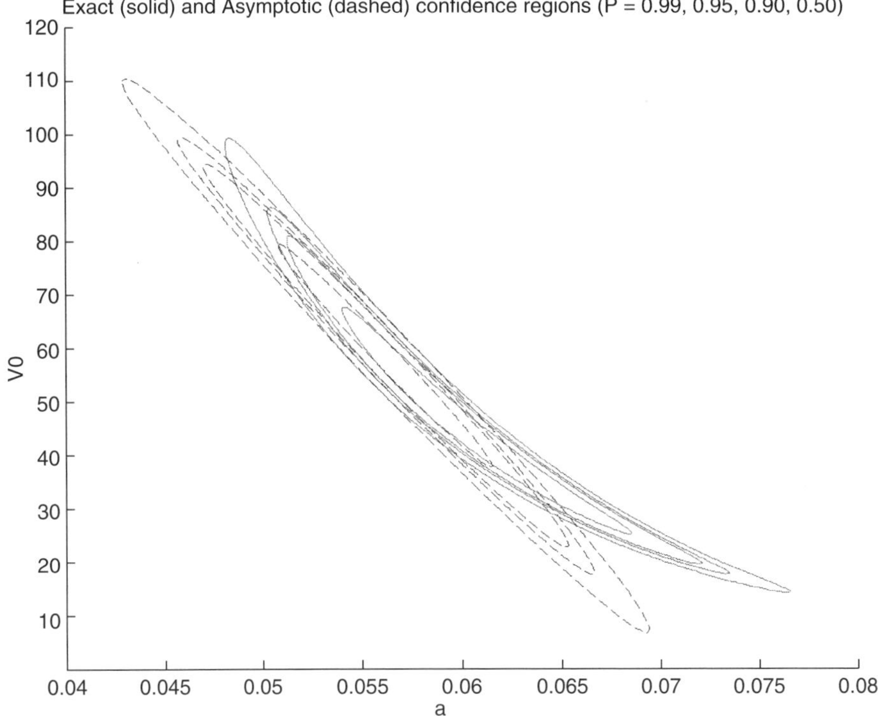

Figure 3.5 Confidence regions for the a and V_0 parameter estimates for *subject 4* (Treated).

estimates of parameters a and V_0 obtained for *subject 4*, conditional on the relative estimated value of b. It can be seen how the exact confidence regions (for 50%, 90%, 95%, and 99% probability) are distorted with respect to the corresponding asymptotic regions. The oblique elongation both in the asymptotic and in the exact regions depends on the strong correlation between parameter estimates for a and V_0.

3.4.1 Nonlinearity at the Optimum

We have seen how different approximate methods for constructing confidence regions for the parameters can be employed, once we believe that a linear approximation is warranted. The problem now is that of deciding that this is indeed the case. To this end, it is useful to study the degree of nonlinearity of our model in a neighborhood of the forecast. We refer the reader to the general treatment by Seber and Wild [9], relating essentially the work of Bates and Watts [5, 10, 11]. Briefly, there exist methods of assessing the maximum degree of intrinsic nonlinearity that the model exhibits around the optimum found. If maximum nonlinearity is excessive, for one or more parameters the confidence regions obtained applying the results of the classic theory are not to be trusted. In this case, alternative simulation procedures may be employed to provide empirical confidence regions.

3.5 SENSITIVITY ANALYSIS

Once a model has been fitted to the available data and parameter estimates have been obtained, two further possible questions that the experimenter may pose are How important is a single parameter in modifying the prediction of a model in a certain region of independent variable space, say at a certain point in time? and, moreover, How important is the numerical value of a specific observation in determining the estimated value of a particular parameter? Although both questions fall within the domain of sensitivity analysis, in the following we shall address the first. The second question is addressed in Section 3.6 on optimal design.

The goal here is to determine the (relative) effect of a variation in a given parameter value on the model prediction. Let $\mathbf{y} = \mathbf{u}(\mathbf{X}, \boldsymbol{\theta}) + \boldsymbol{\varepsilon}$ be the considered model, with $\mathbf{y} \in \nabla^m$ and $\boldsymbol{\theta} \in \Theta \subset \nabla^q$. We study the sensitivity of the modeling function $\mathbf{u}$ with respect to the parameter $\boldsymbol{\theta}$ by means of the (absolute) sensitivity coefficient, which is the partial derivative $\frac{\partial \mathbf{u}(\mathbf{X},\boldsymbol{\theta})}{\partial \boldsymbol{\theta}}$, or by means of the normalized sensitivity coefficient $\xi(\mathbf{X},\boldsymbol{\theta}) = \frac{\boldsymbol{\theta}}{\mathbf{u}(\mathbf{X},\boldsymbol{\theta})} \frac{\partial \mathbf{u}(\mathbf{X},\boldsymbol{\theta})}{\partial \boldsymbol{\theta}}$. The normalization serves to make sensitivities comparable across variables and parameters. In this context, by sensitivity we would mean the proportion of model value change due to a given proportion of parameter change. Absolute and normalized sensitivity coefficients can be computed analytically or approximated numerically. Figure 3.6a shows the time course of the absolute sensitivity coefficients of the Gompertz model with respect to the parameters, which can be computed analytically:

$$\frac{\partial V(t)}{\partial a} = \frac{\partial}{\partial a}\left(e^{\frac{a}{b}\left(\frac{a}{b} - \log V_0\right)e^{-bt}} \right) = \frac{V(t)}{b}\left(1 - e^{-bt}\right);$$

$$\frac{\partial V(t)}{\partial b} = \frac{\partial}{\partial b}\left(e^{\frac{a}{b}\left(\frac{a}{b} - \log V_0\right)e^{-bt}} \right) = V(t)\left[\left(\frac{a}{b} - \log V_0\right)te^{-bt} - \frac{a}{b^2}\left(1 - e^{-bt}\right)\right];$$

$$\frac{\partial V(t)}{\partial V_0} = \frac{\partial}{\partial V_0}\left(e^{\frac{a}{b}\left(\frac{a}{b} - \log V_0\right)e^{-bt}} \right) = \frac{V(t)}{V_0} e^{-bt}.$$

Figure 3.6b shows the same sensitivity coefficients expressed as a percentage of their maximum value. From these graphs it is apparent (without much

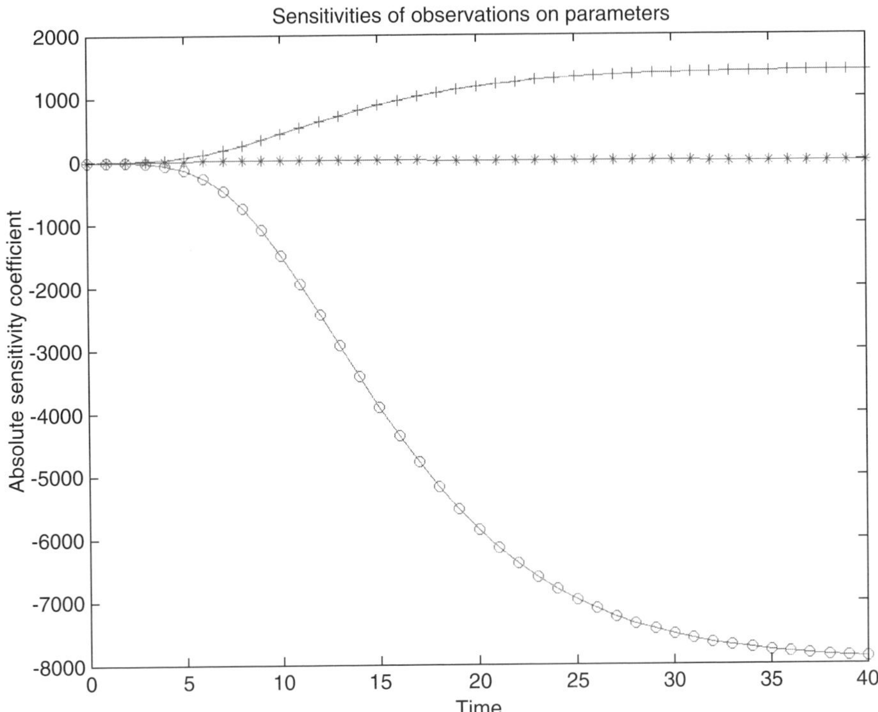

Figure 3.6a Absolute sensitivity coefficients of the Gompertz model. Each curve portrays the time course of the sensitivity of the model to a specific parameter: a (+), b (open circles), and V_0 (*).

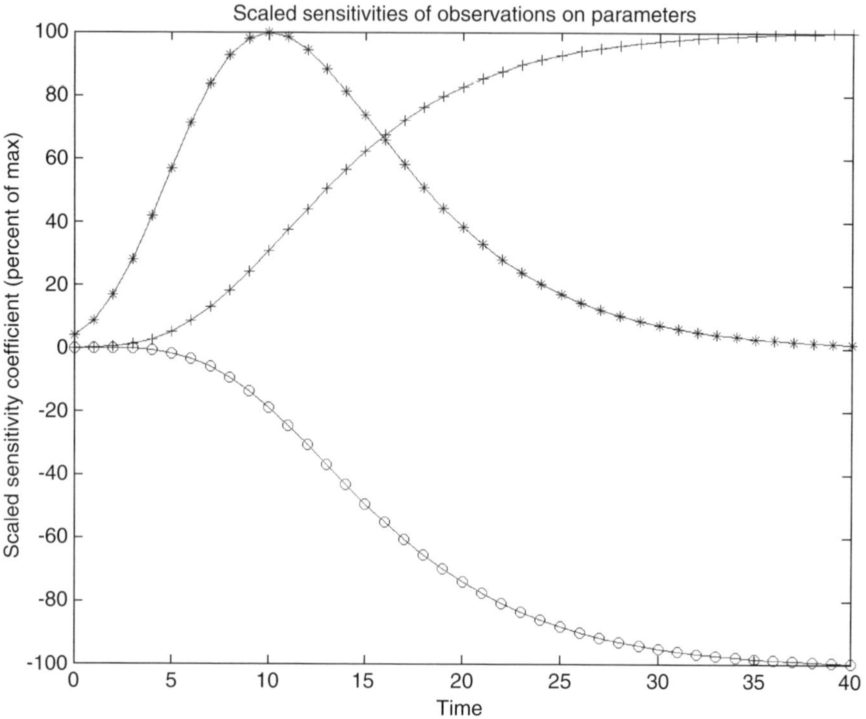

Figure 3.6b Rescaled sensitivity coefficients: a (+), b (open circles), and V_0 (*).

surprise, given the model formulation), that at time zero only the V_0 parameter influences model output. On the other hand, as time progresses, V_0 rapidly loses importance and growth and decay parameters a and b prevail in determining (much larger) variations in predicted volume, each in the expected direction (with a increasing and b decreasing expected volume). We note that model output derivatives with respect to the parameters may well be computed numerically, for example, when no closed form solution of the model itself is available.

An alternative approach [12, 13] is the following: n values for the parameter θ are generated randomly, according to some specified distribution over an acceptable domain Θ, giving rise to a parameter value matrix $\Theta_{n\times q}$ with columns $\Theta_{.j}$ corresponding to the randomly generated values for the parameter component θ_j. The model output is computed for some specified $\mathbf{X}$ of interest and for each generated value of $\theta=(\Theta_{i.})^T$, producing a model value matrix $\mathbf{U}_{n\times m}$, whose n rows $\mathbf{U}_{i.}$ are given by $(\mathbf{U}_{i.})^T = \mathrm{u}(\mathrm{X},(\boldsymbol{\Theta}_{i.})^T)$. The (Spearman nonparametric or Pearson parametric) Monte Carlo correlation coefficient (MCCC) matrix $\mathbf{R}_{m\times q}$ is then computed between the generated values of $\boldsymbol{\theta}$ and the obtained values of $\mathbf{u}$; in other words, $\mathbf{R} = (r_{kj})$ where r_{kj} is the

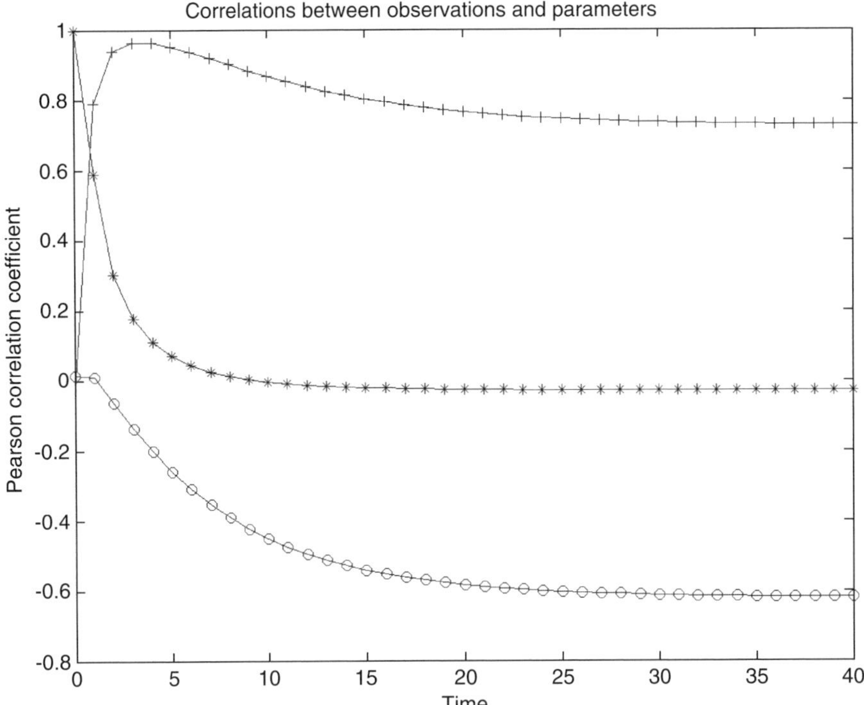

Figure 3.6c Sensitivity analysis: correlations of time points with parameter values. Each curve refers to one model structural parameter: a (+), b (open circles), and V_0 (*).

correlation coefficient between columns $\mathbf{U}_{.k}$ and $\mathbf{\Theta}_{.j}$. It is intuitive that the higher the correlation coefficient r_{kj}, the higher the importance of variations of θ_j in producing variations of u_k. Figure 3.6c shows the time course of the Pearson MCCC between V and the three model parameters for such a Monte Carlo simulation with $n = 10{,}000$, having generated values for the three parameters out of uniform distributions respectively on the intervals [0.9, 1.1], [0.165, 0.195], [0.55, 0.65].

We note in passing that there is a different (less expensive) way to generate simulated parameter values, the latin hypercube sampling scheme, in which a square grid over parameter space is constructed (from a set of small intervals for each parameter), and the cells of the p-dimensional grid are appropriately sampled so as to have exactly one sample in each possible combination of 1-dimensional parameter intervals. The main advantage of this scheme is that the required number of samples does not grow as fast as a regular Monte Carlo sampling from the joint distribution of the parameters as the number of parameters increases.

In our case, it is evident that, independently of the absolute values taken, even qualitatively the shapes of the time courses of the MCCC and of the classic sensitivity coefficients do not seem to agree.

The influence of parameter a on tumor size, as judged from classic sensitivity analysis, seems to increase monotonically to a plateau, reaching about 50% of its effect no sooner than *day 13*; conversely, MCCC indicates a fast increase of effect of parameter a up to a peak at about *day 3* or *4*, with a subsequent decrease and attainment of the plateau from above.

From the sensitivity diagrams it would appear that the influence of parameter V_0 is small at the beginning, peaks over the range approximately between 8 and 12 days, and slowly fades, being still evident at 20 days; conversely, the MCCC study would indicate its maximal effect at the very beginning of the experiment, with a subsequent fast monotonic decrease to essentially zero within 5 days.

The qualitative differences of the behavior of parameter b under sensitivity or MCCC analyses are less obvious, even if its (negative) influence on volume size seems to increase faster according to MCCC.

In the described MC simulation, the action of several simultaneous sources of variation is considered. The explanation of the different time courses of parameter influence on volume size between sensitivity and MCCC analyses lies in the fact that classic sensitivity analysis considers variations in model output due exclusively to the variation of one parameter component at a time, all else being equal. In these conditions, the regression coefficient between model output and parameter component value, in a small interval around the considered parameter, is approximately equal to the partial derivative of the model output with respect to the parameter component.

On the other hand, MCCC considers the influence of the variation of one parameter on model output in the context of simultaneous variations of all other parameters. In this situation, r_{jk} is smaller than 1 in absolute value and its size depends on the relative importance of the variation of model output due to the parameter of interest and the variation of model output given by the sum total of all sources (namely, the variability in all structural parameter values plus the error variance).

In our example, for very small times the theoretical influence of b (given by its sensitivity coefficient) grows more slowly than the theoretical influence of a, while the theoretical influence of V_0 (initially the only effective one) increases much more slowly than those of either a or b. Assembling these separate effects we have a combined situation in which the practical influence of a (measured by its MCCC) rises quickly while overcoming the influence of V_0, peaks when a is the only effective parameter, then decreases to reach a steady level as the action of b also asserts itself.

It would therefore seem that whereas standard sensitivity analysis only gives indications on theoretical single-parameter effects, MCCC would be able to quantify the effective impact that a parameter variation has in real life. However, it is crucial to correctly control the different amounts of variability (ranges for a uniform distribution, variances for a normal distribution) that we assign to the several parameters in computing MCCCs. If the arbitrarily chosen variability for parameter p_1 is small with respect to the variability chosen for parameter p_2, then the effect of p_2 will obviously overshadow the effect of p_1 in the MCCC computation. This will actually give rise to a different shape of their relative time courses. Furthermore, in the case of significant population correlation among parameter values, the MC simulation should make use of nonzero covariances in parameters when generating the parameter sample. Ideally, parameter variabilities should be assigned so as to reflect experimentally observed parameter dispersion.

Because this is often difficult, and indeed sometimes the whole point of the MCCC is to have an idea of what might be observed in hypothetical circumstances, extreme caution must be exercised in extrapolating the MCCC results.

These considerations lead us naturally to the question of how to estimate the population dispersion of the Gompertz parameters out of a given sample of growing tumors, in particular when data may not be as plentiful as we might desire.

3.6 OPTIMAL DESIGN

One further question that has a substantial impact on the application of modeling techniques to biomedical problems is the choice of the design. Suppose that in our Gompertz tumor growth example we wanted to decide, given the results of some pilot experiments, when it is most useful to observe the tumor volume. In other words, we wish to choose the time points at which we obtain tumor volume observations in order to maximize the precision of the resulting parameter estimates.

These considerations are important when, for example, a repetitive estimation process must be conducted (say, over several different inoculated tumors), and when each observation has a relevant cost, so that the goal is that of maximizing the information obtained from a (minimum) number of observations.

Although several design optimization criteria exist, the obvious approach is to choose the time points so as to minimize the parameter estimate dispersion (variance-covariance) matrix, which in our case, for ordinary least-squares estimation, is approximated by the inverse of the Fisher information matrix (FIM) at the optimum. Our criterion therefore becomes to "maximize" in some sense, the FIM. Depending on the specific objective we pose for ourselves, we might want to maximize one of the eigenvalues of the FIM, thus obtaining maximum precision on one parameter; maximize its trace (the sum of the eigenvalues); or maximize its determinant (the product of the eigenvalues). This last method, called D-optimal design (D as in determinant) is possibly the most widely utilized method of optimal design, and we provide here an example of its application.

Suppose we want to find optimal sampling times for either a three-sample, an eight-sample, or a twelve-sample experiment. The key idea is to obtain a large artificial sample of values of the parameter appropriately distributed and for each value of the parameter to maximize the determinant of the FIM with respect to the choice of times. To each such parameter value there will correspond therefore a choice of 3 (or 8 or 12) sampling times that will maximize the FIM under the hypothesis that the parameter value is actually equal to the one considered. We can then build a histogram showing the frequency with which sampling times have been chosen as optimal and use this empirical distribution of optimal sampling times to pick the times that we consider most appropriate for the next experiments.

To apply the above method, we must decide the distribution of parameter values to explore. One immediate answer would be to impose on the parameters an appropriate joint probability distribution, but this would require us to know it, or at least to have a reasonable idea of what it might be.

A different strategy is the following: Suppose that we have some preliminary observations. For instance, suppose that only *subject 4* has been observed. Given the observations for *subject 4*, we obtain an estimate $\boldsymbol{\theta}^\wedge$ of the parameters of the Gompertz model, as well as an estimate s^2 of the error variance σ^2. These estimates summarize all the information we can use. Now we can generate many artificial samples simply by adding to the theoretical predictions, computed from a Gompertz model with parameter $\boldsymbol{\theta}^\wedge$, random normal noise of variance s^2. If we then estimate a parameter value θ_r from each one of the r samples, we have an empirical distribution of θ that is, asymptotically, exactly the distribution of estimated values of θ , under the hypothesis that the true value is the generating value $\boldsymbol{\theta}^\wedge$ and that the observation error variance is s^2.

As an example, we have applied the above strategy using the observations from *subject 4* as our pilot sample. Figures 3.7, 3.8, and 3.9 report the obtained frequency distributions of sampling times for 3, 8, and 12 sampling times, respectively, as well as their cumulative distributions. A choice of optimal sampling times may be made by splitting into $(n + 1)$ equal parts the cumulative probability thus obtained and using the n critical time points defining the splits: These are indicated by the thin vertical lines in the cumulative distribution graphs.

In our case we note that the most important observations for parameter estimation are the initial one (determining, more than any of the others, the likely value of the parameter $V0$) and the last one, which is the most informative observation on the combination of values of parameters a and b.

3.7 POPULATION MODELING

Suppose we had established that the Gompertz model does reliably describe the growth of a particular tumor form and that we wish therefore to estimate

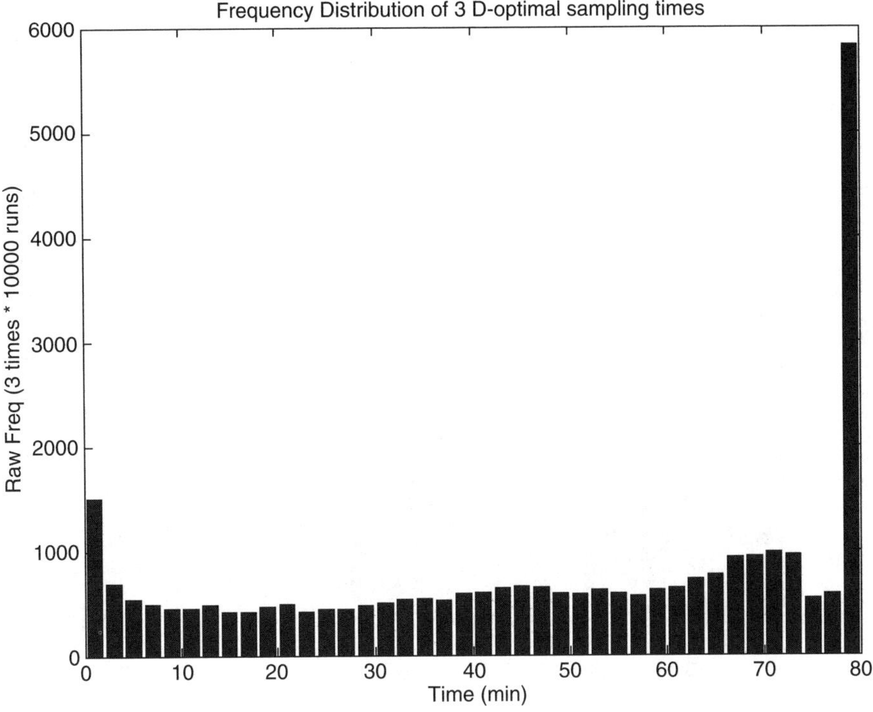

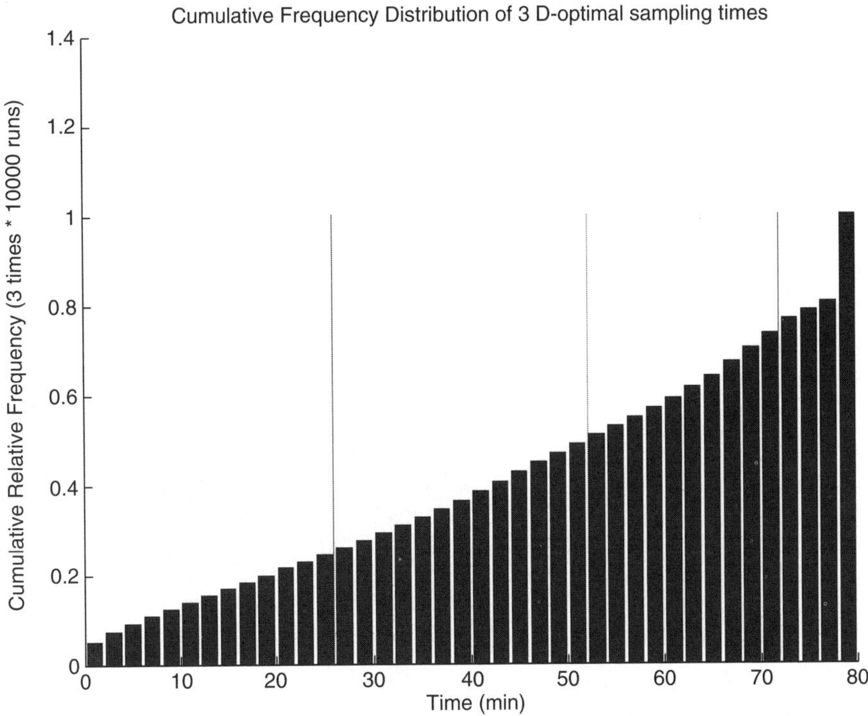

Figure 3.7 Frequency and cumulative frequency distributions of 3D-optimal sampling times for the Gompertz model, given the observations for *subject 4*. Vertical lines split the cumulative empirical distribution into equal probability regions.

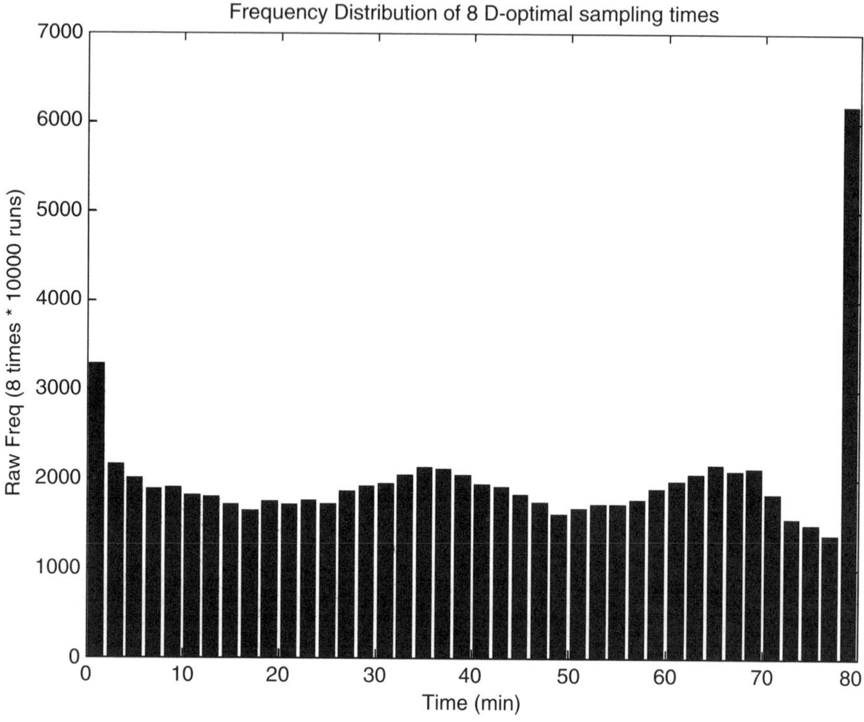

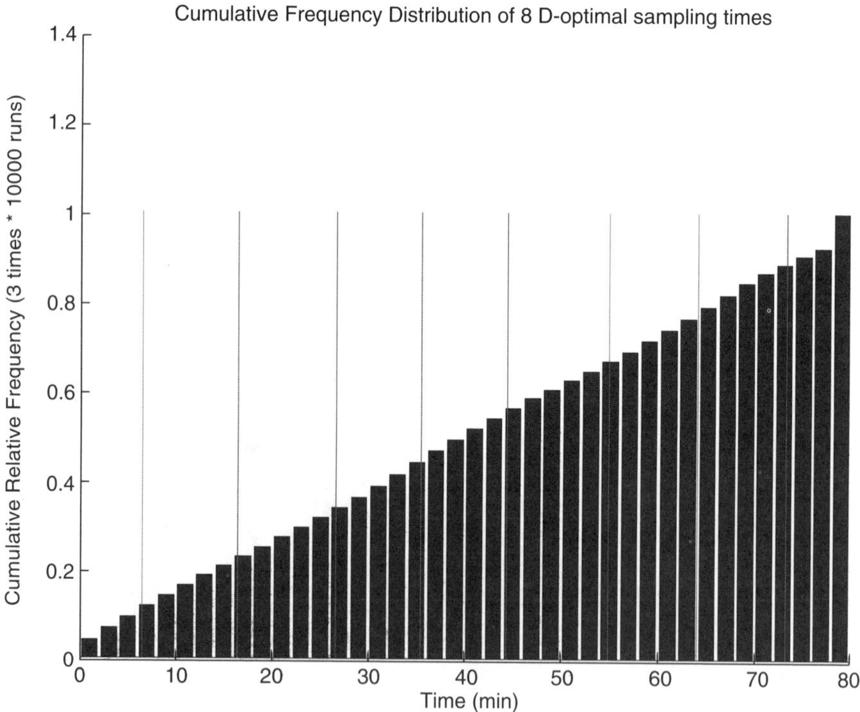

Figure 3.8 Frequency and cumulative frequency distributions of 8D-optimal sampling times for the Gompertz model, given the observations for *subject 4*. Vertical lines split the cumulative empirical distribution into equal probability regions.

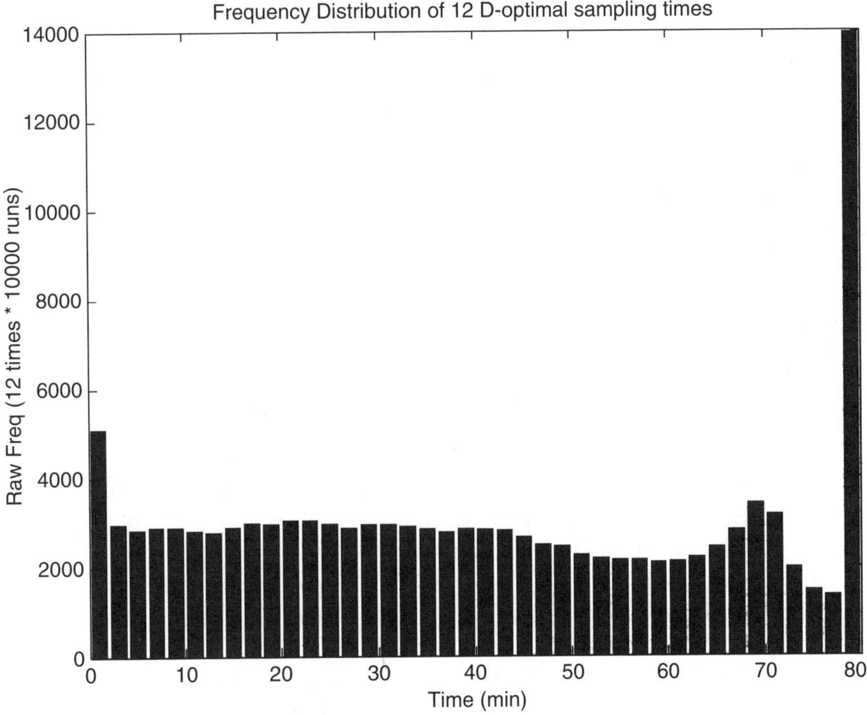

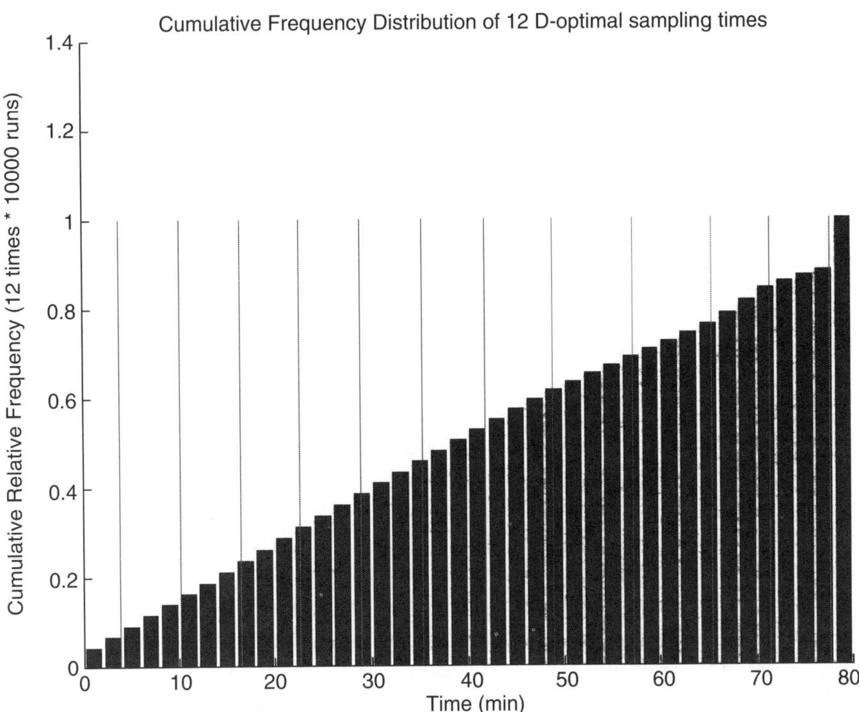

Figure 3.9 Frequency and cumulative frequency distributions of 12D-optimal sampling times for the Gompertz model, given the observations for *subject 4*. Vertical lines split the cumulative empirical distribution into equal probability regions.

the a, b, and V_0 parameters in a population of experimentally interesting tumors. More specifically, we are now interested in evaluating the effect of a specific drug on tumor growth in a population of rodents.

The standard way to proceed would be to fit the model to the data relative to each experimental unit, one at a time, thus obtaining a sample of parameter estimates, one for each experimental tumor observed. The sample mean and dispersion of these estimates would then constitute our estimate of the population mean and dispersion. By the same token, we could find the mean and dispersion in the "Control" and "Treated" subsamples.

There are two problems with the above procedure, however. The first is that it is not efficient, because the intersubject parameter variance it computes is actually the variance of the parameters between subjects plus the variance of the estimate of a single-subject parameter. The second drawback is that often, in real-life applications, a complete data set, with sufficiently many points to reliably estimate all model parameters, is not available for each experimental subject. A frequent situation is that observations are available in a haphazard, scattered fashion, are often expensive to gather, and for a number of reasons (availability of manpower, cost, environmental constraints, etc.) are usually much fewer than we would like.

It should be kept in mind that it would be a severe mistake to simply fit the model by least squares (ordinary or weighted) on the aggregated observations obtained from different experimental units. A simple linear regression example may explain why: Suppose that, in a hypothetical experiment designed to evaluate the correlation between a variable x and a variable y, the six experimental units depicted in Figure 3.10 all have a negative correlation between x and y, in other words, that $y = mx + q$, with m negative. Suppose further that the different experimental units all have high average y for high average x. If we were to fit all points from this experiment together we would estimate a very significantly positive linear coefficient m in our y versus x model, instead of the common negative m that all experimental units share.

What we need instead is a "population" method whereby we can estimate simultaneously, on the aggregated data, the model structural parameters, their population dispersion matrix, and the error variance. This method will then be able to incorporate information even from subjects for whom only relatively meager data sets are available. After the pioneering applications of a specific nonlinear mixed effects model (NONMEM) in pharmacokinetics by Sheiner et al. in the early 1980s [14], a well-developed literature on general nonlinear mixed effects (NLME) algorithms is now available [2, 15, 17]. We will now consider the following algorithm published by Lindstrom and Bates in 1990 (L&B90, reference 18).

Let y_{ij} denote the jth response, $j = 1, \ldots, n_i$, for the ith individual, $i = 1, \ldots, m$ taken at a set of conditions x_{ij} that in this case correspond to the set of temporal time. The function $f(\beta, x)$ represents the model relationship between y and x, where β is the vector of parameters of dimension $p \times 1$. Although the functional form f of the model is common to all individuals, the parameter β

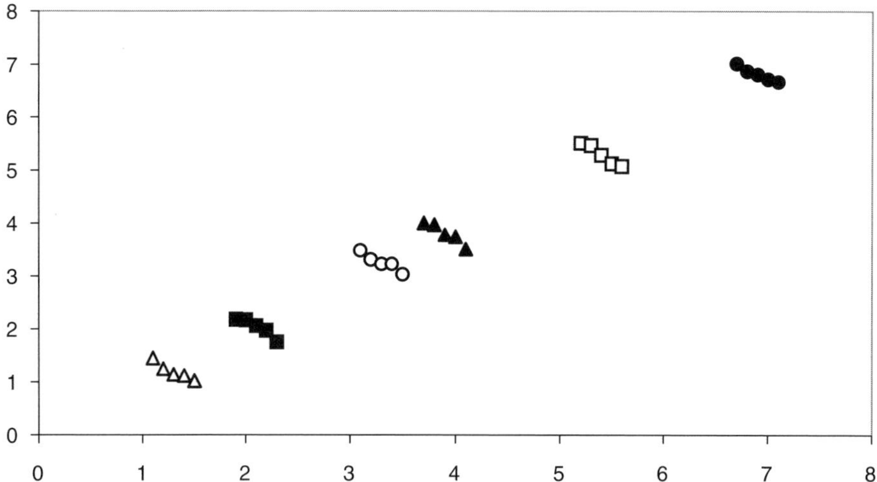

Figure 3.10 Illustrative example of linear regression between two artificial variables for six experimental units. For each unit, denoted by a different graphical symbol, a closely packed set of five observations with negative slope is measured. The whole data set, if fitted naively, would show a very significant positive slope.

may vary across the individuals. A vector $p \times 1$ of parameters β_i is therefore specified for each subject. The mean response for individual i depends on its regression parameters β_i so that $E(y_{ij}|\beta_i) = f_i(x_{ij}, \beta_i)$.

Let us define the following two-stage model:

Stage 1 (intraindividual variation)
In the first stage let the jth observation on the ith individual be modeled as follows:

$$y_{ij} = f_i(\beta_i, x_{ij}) + e_{ij}, i = 1, \ldots, m, j = 1, \ldots, n_i$$

where the function f is a nonlinear function of the subject-specific parameter vector β_i, x_{ij} is the observed variable, e_{ij} is the normally distributed noise term, m is the total number of subjects and n_i is the number of observations for the ith subject.

Stage 2 (interindividual variation)
In the second stage the subject-specific parameter vector is modeled as:

$$\beta_i = g(\beta, b_i) = \beta + b_i, b_i \sim N(0, \mathbf{D})$$

where β is a p-dimensional vector of fixed population parameter, b_i is a k-dimensional random effect vector associated with the ith subject (not varying with j), and D is its general variance-covariance matrix.

Let us suppose that the error vector is distributed as

$$e_i | b_i \sim N(0, R_i(\xi, \beta_i))$$

where the variance-covariance matrix may well depend on the specific individual parameters. This can be written as

$$e_i = R_i^{1/2}(\xi, \beta_i)\varepsilon_i,$$

where ε_i has mean zero, covariance matrix I_{ni}, and is independent of b_i, and $R_i^{1/2}(\xi, \beta_i)$ is the Cholesky decomposition of $R_i(\xi, \beta_i)$. The first stage of the model can be therefore written as:

$$y_i = f_i(\beta_i, x_i) + R_i^{1/2}(\beta_i, \xi)\varepsilon_i, \; i = 1, \ldots, m. \tag{3.4}$$

Lindstrom and Bates argue that a Taylor series expansion of (Eq. 3.4) around the expectation of the random effects $b_i = 0$ may be poor. Instead, they consider linearizing (Eq. 3.4) in the random effects about some value b_i^* closer to b_i than its expectation 0.

In particular, retaining the first two terms of the Taylor series expansion about $b_i = b_i^*$ of $f_i(\beta_i, x_i)$ and the leading term of $R_i^{1/2}(\beta_i, \xi)\varepsilon_i$, it follows that

$$\begin{aligned} y_i = f_i\{g(\beta, b_i^*), x_i\} + F_i(\beta, b_i^*)\Delta_{b_i}(\beta, b_i^*)(b_i - b_i^*) + \\ R_i^{1/2}(\beta, b_i^*, \xi)\varepsilon_i, i = 1, \ldots, m \end{aligned} \tag{3.5}$$

where $F_i(b, b_i^*)$ is the $(n_i \times p)$ matrix of derivatives of $f_i(\beta_i)$ with respect to β_i evaluated in $\beta_i = g(\beta, b_i^*)$, and $\Delta_{b_i}(\beta, b_i^*)$ is the $(p \times k)$ matrix of derivatives of $g(\beta, b_i)$with respect to b_i evaluated in $b_i = b_i^*$. Defining the $(n_i \times k)$ matrix $Z(\beta, b_i) = F_i(\beta, b_i)\Delta_{b_i}(\beta, b_i)$ and $e_i^* = R_i^{1/2}(g(\beta, b_i^*), \xi)\,\varepsilon_i$, $i = 1, \ldots, m$ (Eq. 3.5) can be written as

$$y_i = f_i\{g(\beta, b_i^*), x_i\} - Z_i(\beta, b_i^*)\; b_i^* + Z_i(\beta, e_i^*)b_i + b_i^*, \; i = 1, \ldots, m$$

It follows that for b_i close to b_i^* the approximate marginal mean and covariance of y_i is:

$$E(y_i) = f_i\{g(\beta, b_i^*), x_i\} - Z_i(\beta, b_i^*)b_i^*, \; i = 1, \ldots, m$$
$$Cov(y_i) = Z_i(\beta, b_i^*)DZ_i^T(\beta, b_i^*) + R_i(\beta, b_i^*, \xi) = V_i(\beta, b_i^*, \omega), i = 1, \ldots, m$$

where ω is the vector of parameters consisting of the intraindividual covariance parameter ξ and the distinct elements of D.

The following exposition of the L&B90 algorithm differs from the original in order to allow greater generality. In particular, Lindstrom and Bates describe their iterative algorithm under the following restrictive conditions: (i) that the interindividual regression function $g(\beta, b_i)$ is linear in β and in b_i and (ii) that the intraindividual covariance matrix $R_i(\beta_i, \xi)$ does not depend on β_i (and hence on b_i), but rather depends on the subject i only as far as its dimension. Our exposition offers a more general formalization of the problem, letting the functional form linking the fixed effects and the random effects be arbitrary and allowing a more general structure for the variance-covariance matrix of the error vector.

The L&B90 algorithm proceeds in two alternating steps, a penalized nonlinear least-squares (PNLS) step and a linear mixed effects (LME) step.

In the PNLS step the current estimates of D and ξ are fixed and the conditional modes of the random effects b and the conditional estimates of the fixed effects β are obtained minimizing the following objective function:

$$\sum_{i=1}^{m}\left(\begin{array}{l}\log\left|\hat{\mathbf{D}}\right| + b_i^T\hat{\mathbf{D}}^{-1}b_i + \log\left|R_i\left(\hat{\beta}_0,\hat{b}_{i,0},\hat{\xi}\right)\right| + \left[y_i - f_i\left\{g\left(\beta,b_i\right)\right\}\right]^T \\ R_i^{-1}\left(\hat{\beta}_0,\hat{b}_{i,0},\hat{\xi}\right)\left[y_i - f_i\left\{g\left(\beta,b_i\right)\right\}\right]\end{array}\right)$$

where $\hat{\beta}_0$ and $\hat{b}_{i,0}$ are some previous estimates of β and b_i.

Let $\hat{\beta}$ and $\hat{b}_i$ denote the resulting estimates.

The LME step updates the estimates of D, β and ξ minimizing:

$$\sum_{i=1}^{m}\left(\log\left|V_i\left(\hat{\beta},\hat{b}_i,\omega\right)\right| + r_i^{*T}\left(\beta,\hat{b}_i,\hat{\beta}\right)V_i^{-1}\left(\hat{\beta},\hat{b}_i,\omega\right)\ r_i^{*}\left(\beta,\hat{b}_i,\hat{\beta}\right)\right)$$

where

$$r_i^{*}\left(\beta,\hat{b}_i,\hat{\beta}\right) = \left[y_i - f_i\left\{g\left(\beta,\hat{b}_i\right)\right\}\right] + Z_i\left(\hat{\beta},\hat{b}_i\right)\hat{b}_i.$$

The process must be iterated until convergence and the final estimates are denoted with $\hat{\beta}_{LB}$, $\hat{b}_{i,LB}$, and $\hat{\omega}_{LB}$. The individual regression parameter can be therefore estimated by replacing the final fixed effects and random effects estimates in the function g so that:

$$\hat{\beta}_{i,LB} = g\left(\hat{\beta}_{LB},\hat{b}_{i,LB}\right) = \hat{\beta}_{LB} + \hat{b}_{i,LB}$$

Confidence intervals

If the approximation (Eq. 3.5) is assumed to hold exactly we can derive the usual asymptotic results. The $\hat{\beta}_{LB}$ estimator is asymptotically normal with mean β and covariance matrix

$$\Sigma_{LB} = \left(\sum_{i=1}^{m} X_i^T\left(\beta,\hat{b}_{i,LB}\right)V_i^{-1}\left(\beta,\hat{b}_{i,LB},\omega\right)X_i\left(\beta,\hat{b}_{i,LB}\right)\right)^{-1} \quad (3.6)$$

and an estimate $\hat{\Sigma}_{LB}$ may be obtained by evaluation of (Eq. 3.6) at the final estimates of β and ω with estimated standard errors calculated as the square roots of the diagonal elements.

We applied the algorithm to our sample of five Control and four Treated subjects, parameterizing the model so as to have general coefficients a, b, and V_0 (applicable to all subjects, whether treated or control), plus differential

TABLE 3.3 Population Parameter Estimates

$\hat{\sigma}^2 = 23214.1985$.

Fixed Effects

a	b	V_0	Delta_a	Delta_b
0.40517	0.042632	0.3055	−0.17573	−0.00576

Random Effects

Subject	Treatment	bi_a	bi_b	bi_V_0
1	1	0.00636	−0.01122	0.01222
2	1	0.01028	−0.01046	0.01484
3	1	0.00096	−0.01161	−0.01639
4	1	0.02586	−0.01083	0.00686
5	0	−0.03957	0.00005	−0.01211
6	0	−0.00421	−0.00311	0.00668
7	0	−0.02901	0.00532	−0.00047
8	0	0.00746	0.00344	0.00633
9	0	−0.01757	0.00440	−0.00999

Fixed Effect Covariance Matrix

	a	b	V_0	diff_a	diff_b
a	0.000974	0.000108	−0.00855	−0.00032	−1.69E-05
b	0.000108	2.87E-05	−0.00109	−2.42E-05	−1.71E-05
V_0	−0.00855	−0.00109	0.092512	0.001494	0.000113
diff_a	−0.00032	−2.42E-05	0.001494	0.000442	1.76E-05
diff_b	−1.69E-05	−1.71E-05	0.000113	1.76E-05	3.60E-05

Random Effect Variance-Covariance Matrix

	bi_a	bi_b	bi_V_0
bi_a	0.00079	−0.00001	−0.00043
bi_b	−0.00001	0.00007	0.00013
bi_V_0	−0.00043	0.00013	0.00023

effects Delta_a and Delta_b, applicable to the Treated subjects only. The parameter estimates are reported in Table 3.3. We note that treatment produces a large difference (−0.17 over 0.40, i.e., about minus 42%) in the coefficient a, describing the initial growth rate of the tumor, and a small difference (−0.006 over 0.043, i.e., about minus 14%) in the coefficient b, which is responsible for the saturation of tumor growth. The significance of these differences may be assessed by using the estimated standard errors for the difference parameters (0.021 and 0.006, respectively). Whereas the coefficient a is highly significantly different from zero (using either the t-distribution or the normal approximation to the appropriate t-test, given the large number of degrees of freedom), the coefficient b is not significantly different from zero. The conclusion is that, in our series, treatment appears to highly significantly affect growth rate of the tumor, slowing it down, whereas it does not appear to influence the saturation of growth as time progresses.

Sample graphs are reported in Figure 3.4, a–d, where some of the studied subject's observed volumes are reported together with single-subject OLS-predicted time courses (solid lines) and population-estimated time courses (using the subject's conditional modes). It can be seen how in some subjects (see for instance Fig.3.4, a and c) OLS would predict a faster-saturating time course than L&B, because the single-subject estimate is "stabilized," in the population approach, by the combined effect of all remaining subjects.

REFERENCES

1. Breiman L. Statistical Modeling: the two cultures. *Stat Sci* 2001;16:199–231.
2. Venables WN, Ripley BD. *Modern applied statistics with S-Plus, statistics and computing* Springer Verlag, 1996.
3. Lindsey JK. *Nonlinear models in medical statistics*, Oxford Statistical Science Series 24, 2001.
4. Gauss CF. Anzeige: Theoria Combinationis Observationum Erroribus Minimis Obnoxiae: Pars prior. *Goettingische gelehrte Anzeigen* 1821;32:313–18.
5. Bates DM, Watts DG. *Nonlinear regression analysis and applications*, New York, Wiley, 1988.
6. Draper RD, Smith D. *Applied regression analysis*, New York, Wiley, 1987.
7. Lambert JD. *Numerical methods for ordinary differential equations*, New York, John Wiley, 1993.
8. Press WH, Flannery BP, Teukolsky SA, Vetterling WT. *Numerical recipes in C. The art of scientific computing.* Cambridge, Cambridge University Press, 1994.
9. Seber GAF, Wild CJ, *Nonlinear regression.* New York, Wiley, 1989.
10. Bates DM, Hamilton DC, Watts DG. Calculation of intrinsic and parameter-effects curvatures for nonlinear regression models. *Commun Stat Simul Comput* 1983;12:469–77.
11. Bates DM, Watts DG. Relative curvature measures of nonlinearity. *J R Stat Soc B* 1980;42:1–25.
12. Blower SM, Dowlatabadi H. Sensitivity and uncertainty analysis of complex models of disease transmission: an HIV model, as an example. *Int Statistical Rev* 1994;62:229–43.
13. Iman RL, Helton JC, Campbell JE. An approach to sensitivity analysis of computer models: Part II—Ranking of input variables, response surface validation, distribution effect and technique synopsis. *J Quality Technol* 1981;13:232–40.
14. Sheiner LB, Beal SL. Evaluation of methods for estimating population pharmacokinetic parameters. II. Biexponential model and experimental pharmacokinetic data. *J Pharmacokinet Biopharm* 1981;9:635–51.

15. Davidian M, Giltinan DM. *Nonlinear models for repeated measurement data.* Chapman & Hall/CRC, 1995.
16. Pinheiro JC, Bates DM. Approximations to the loglikelihood function in the nonlinear mixed effects model. *J Comput Graphical Stat*, 1995;4:12–35.
17. De Gaetano A, Mingrone G, Castagneto M. NONMEM improves group parameter estimation for the minimal model of glucose kinetics. *Am J Physiol* 1996;271: E932–7.
18. Lindstrom MJ, Bates DM. Nonlinear mixed effects models for repeated measures data. *Biometrics*, 1990;46:673–87.

PART II

UNDERSTANDING DISEASES: MINING COMPLEX SYSTEMS FOR KNOWLEDGE

4

DRUG DISCOVERY FROM HISTORIC HERBAL TEXTS

Eric J. Buenz

Contents

4.1 INTRODUCTION

The ultimate goal of drug discovery is to identify novel compounds that have the potential to elicit biological effects. High-throughput screening allows an amazingly quick and relatively economic method to accomplish this goal [1]. The rate at which high-throughput systems are improving is remarkable, and it is likely that in the future the rate of these improvements will be even

Computer Applications in Pharmaceutical Research and Development, Edited by Sean Ekins.
ISBN 0-471-73779-8

greater [2]. Many of the chapters in this text describe clever ways to improve and develop compounds to examine in high-throughput screens.

Yet these high-throughput systems do lack certain abilities [3]. Fortunately, there are techniques to address these deficiencies. One of the most appealing approaches to managing the challenges of high-throughput screening is ethnobotany—the study of how people use plants [4]. However, ethnobotany is labor intense, and much of the knowledge regarding plant use is lost to modern-day healers [5]. Luckily, for thousands of years explorers and expatriates have documented the use of plants as medicines. Thus much of this lost knowledge remains in historic herbal texts [6]. Recent advancements in bioinformatics have made it possible to examine these texts in a high-throughput fashion, identifying plants, for a specific illness, that have yet to be examined in the current literature [7, 8]. Using this technique to augment classic high-throughput screening ultimately can result in a highly efficient drug discovery system in which plants to be screened are selected based on purported medicinal properties rather than random testing.

This chapter begins with a survey of the challenges of high-throughput screening, followed by a background in medicinal ethnobotany. The application of historic herbal texts as a resource is then addressed, and an outline of a bioinformatics system developed to facilitate high-throughput analysis of the historic texts is discussed. Finally, this chapter posits the future of mining historic herbal texts for novel drugs.

4.2 CHALLENGES OF HIGH-THROUGHPUT SCREENING

There are two principal challenges inherent to high-throughput screening. Although these two deficiencies are not fatal to high-throughput screens, mitigating these challenges results in a more efficient screening process.

Hits identified in high-throughput screening are not always effective in vivo. Many high-throughput screening approaches use cell-free systems. There are advantages to this simplified technique for drug discovery. For example, biological systems have compensatory mechanisms that can obscure readouts. Creating a specific biochemical pathway ex vivo to analyze in a high-throughput fashion allows for the examination of that pathway in isolation. However, directly relating identified drug leads in these artificial systems to a cell-based system is sometimes not possible. For example, using a nominal system to screen for novel HIV therapeutics has resulted in a number of identified hits of target compounds. However, when these target compounds were tested in a cell-based system they did not perform as in the cell-free system [9].

Selection of the compounds examined in high-throughput screening is not targeted. High-throughput screening excels at examining the efficacy of combinatorial derivatives. Yet, before the combinatorial derivatives are examined, lead compounds must be identified [10]. Although broad-based screens of natural products have resulted in successful chemotherapeutics such as taxol [11], these approaches are not targeted with previous knowledge. Applying known information regarding the use of a plant as medicine allows a more elegant and pointed approach.

4.3 MEDICINAL ETHNOBOTANY

Plants, as well as other organisms, have been developing defense mechanisms since the beginning of time [12]. These defense mechanisms are important for the existence of many organisms, yet these mechanisms are critical for plants because plants generally are not mobile, although the creatures dining on them are. Thus plants have developed secondary metabolites, agents that confer a selective advantage but are not essential for life processes. These secondary metabolites deter organisms from eating the plants, resulting in a selective advantage for the plant [13].

For thousands of years adept humans have been using these secondary metabolites as medicines [14]. Thus, although a plant may contain a compound that deters an animal from eating the plant, that same compound may selectively induce cell death in tumor cells at a lower dose. This situation is apparently the case with the chemotherapeutic taxol [11]. Through a presumed system of trial-and-error experimentation, knowledge regarding the medicinal uses of plants has been accumulated by several past populations [15]. This accumulated knowledge is traditional medicine knowledge, and medicinal ethnobotany is the study of how people, employing years of trial-and-error knowledge, use the plants as medicines.

The best example of using this knowledge in drug discovery is the identification of Prostratin. While working in Samoa to identify plants with potential chemotherapeutic properties, Dr. Paul Cox documented the use of *Homalanthus nutans* for the treatment of hepatitis [16]. Surprisingly, when extracts of this plant were incidentally examined for anti-HIV properties, the extract appeared effective for treatment of HIV [17]. Eventually, this compound was shown to be effective at activating the latently infected T-cell pool [18]. Importantly, this population of cells is a principal reason for HIV persistence [19].

Working with traditional healers is a thrilling experience. These individuals are frequently excited that someone is interested in their knowledge. Figure 4.1 shows the author working with a traditional healer in Samoa collecting the medicinal plant *Atuna racemosa*. This healer's excitement that someone was interested in her knowledge was so great that she was first in line to package samples for analysis.

Yet the reasons behind this healer's excitement are lamentable. There is a lack of interest in traditional medicine from the younger generation, and as a result there is a generational loss of traditional medicine knowledge [20]. For example, the two individuals that identified Prostratin as an antiviral have since passed away, and it is likely that an individual performing the

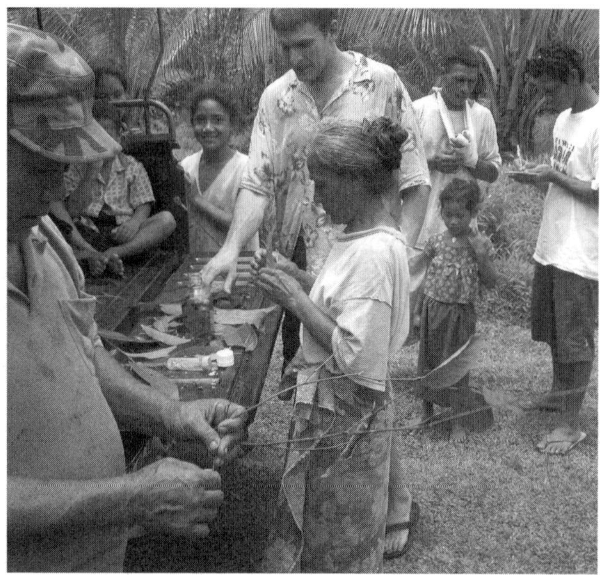

Figure 4.1 Collecting a medicine plant in Samoa. Ethnobotanical work involves working with healers to identify the medicinal uses of plants. Although this work is laborious, traditional medicine healers are frequently excited to share their knowledge.

same study today would not identify *H. nutans* as an antiviral candidate specimen.

Fortunately, for many years, expatriates, explorers, and missionaries have recorded this lost information in herbal texts [7]. Because of these individuals' diligence in recording the uses of certain plants, it is possible to identify novel agents by mining historic herbal texts. However, manual extraction of information from these texts can be laborious. Using a bioinformatics-based approach to mine these historic texts allows for a high-throughput system to identify new leads and resurrect lost traditional medicine knowledge [8].

4.4 HERBAL TEXTS

Historic herbal texts can be considered both works of art and troves of information. Many of the original copies of the texts still available were hand copied and corrected as deemed necessary by the transcriptionist [21]. Frequently, the images accompanying the text descriptions were ornately hand painted. Often, these images contain such intricate detail that it is possible to accurately identify the genus and species of the plant described. For example, Figure 4.2 shows the illustration of the common pineapple from the 400-year-old *Ambonese Herbal*.

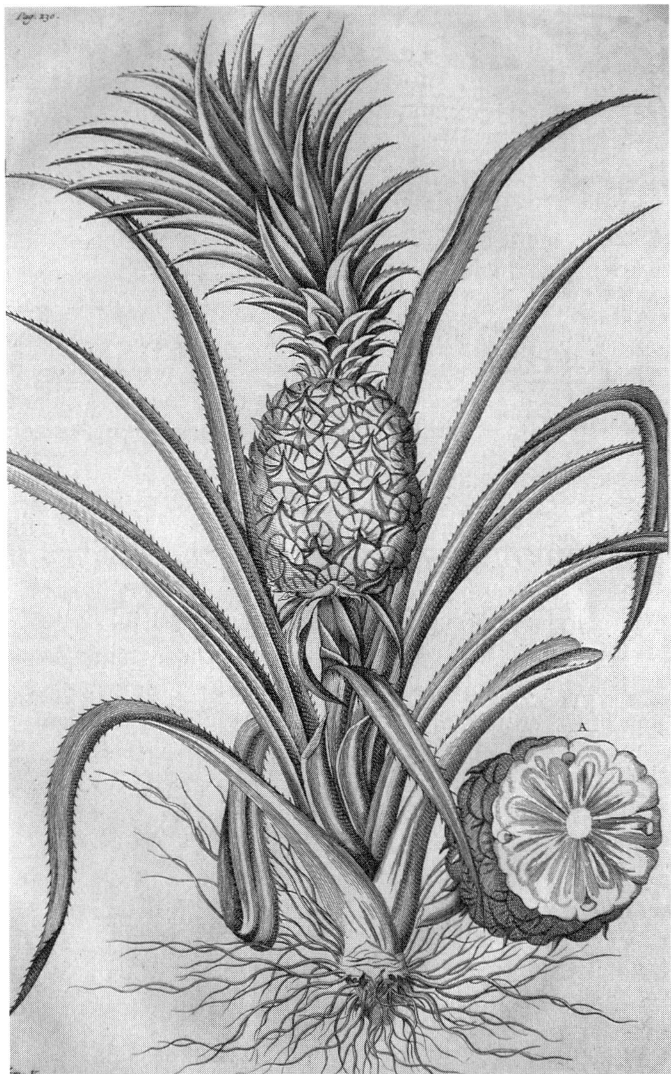

Figure 4.2 Nearly 400 years ago G. E. Rumphius was stationed on the island of Ambon in Indonesia. This figure shows his rendition of the common pineapple in the *Ambonese Herbal*. Frequently, the illustrations in historic herbal texts are detailed enough to accurately identify the plant described in the text.

There are many historic herbal texts throughout the world, some dating back as far as 3000 B.C. However, the ancient Greeks were the first to create herbal texts with enough detail to accurately identify the plant and ailment treated. Thus texts from around 500 B.C. and later are the only texts able to be examined for new drug leads [22]. The advent of mass printing systems (ca. 1500 A.D.) resulted in increased popularity and diversity of historic herbal texts [23]. The uniformity of the script in these works makes them particularly well suited for scanning into an electronic format. Many of these texts are held in national repositories in places ranging from the National Library of Medicine (Bethesda, MD, USA) to the Vatican Biblioteca (Rome, Italy).

Unfortunately, there is little doubt that some of the plants identified in these texts are extinct. The story of the silphium plant illustrates this loss of plant material (Appendix). Although the events driving the loss of plant resources are not exactly known, this loss is a concern for drug discovery [24]. Certain drugs, such as the phorbol ester Prostratin, would likely never have been included in a high-throughput screening assay today—generally phorbol esters are believed to be tumorigenic, yet interestingly, Prostratin is not [17].

4.5 HIGH THROUGHPUT WITH COMPUTER ASSISTANCE

Although manual extraction of information from herbal texts is straightforward (Fig. 4.3A), the work is labor intense and requires many areas of expertise (Fig. 4.3B). Historians must provide context for the language. Botanists are necessary to update the names and correctly identify the plants discussed. Physicians and biomedical scientists are required to extrapolate the potential pharmacological function of the plant compounds used to treat a certain disorder in the text. Luckily, the use of bioinformatics to extract this information can be more efficient than manual extraction [7].

Our group has worked to fashion a high-throughput system allowing for the rapid extraction of information from historic herbal texts. This system has only recently been made possible with the latest advancements in bioinformatics and technology [25]. Figure 4.3C outlines the application of these recent advancements and the role they play in extracting information from historic texts. Currently, it is not possible to streamline these functions seamlessly. Rather, data from each entity are collected, and then the next step in the sequence is initiated. Thus data collected from the SNOW-MED [26] analysis of the historic herbal must be queried in the NAPRALERT™ database [27]. Clearly, these resources are not the only available options. For example, W3 Tropicos (http://mobot.mobot.org/W3T/Search/vast.html) would likely assist in validating plant names, just as the International Plant Names Index (http://www.ipni.org/index.html) does for our system.

Developing a fully automated script will only be possible once all links of the process are available in the proper formats to receive these queries. The system we have developed is presented in Figure 4.4. Details of each component of the highlighted system are described below.

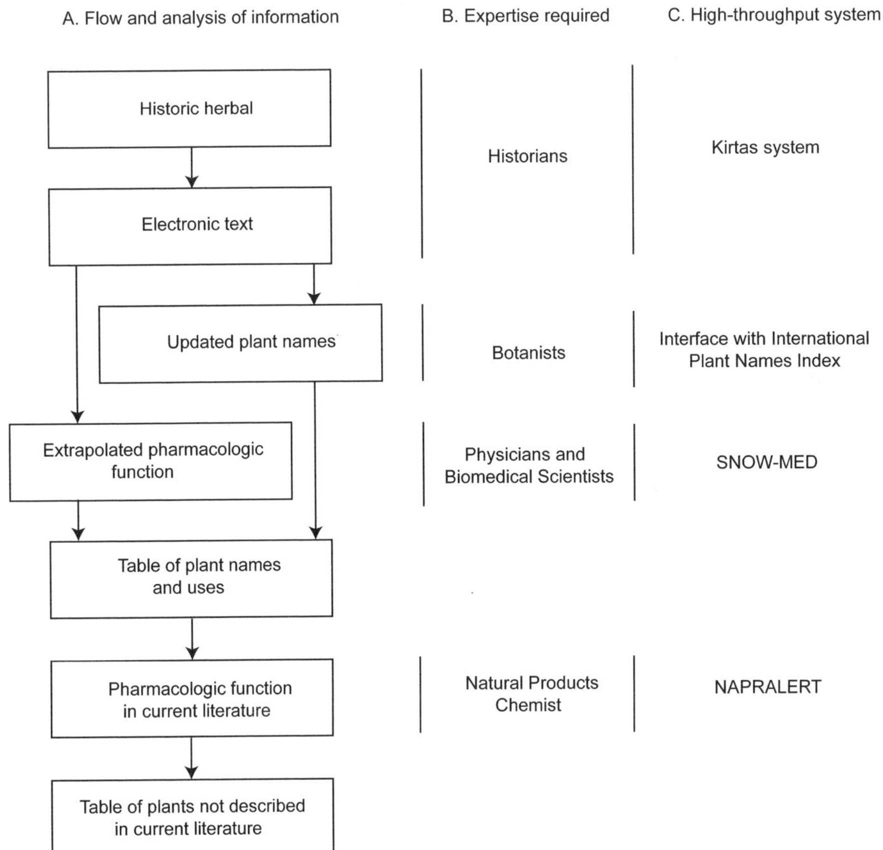

Figure 4.3 (A) The methods for choosing plants to examine from historic herbal texts are straightforward. (B) Yet a range of expertise is necessary to accurately identify plants and their purported uses. (C) A number of recent advancements in technology have allowed high-throughput examination of historic herbal texts.

4.5.1 Kirtas System

Foremost it is critical to move the historic herbal text into an electronic format. This process can be very time consuming [28]; however, it is essential for two reasons. First, these historic texts are rare and having them in an electronic format facilitates increased access for the collaborating groups. Second, the volume of information is difficult to handle when the data are not in an electronic format. We have recently employed the Kirtas system (Fig. 4.5) to move a number of texts into electronic format. We have yet to formally address the precision of the scanned-in documents; however,

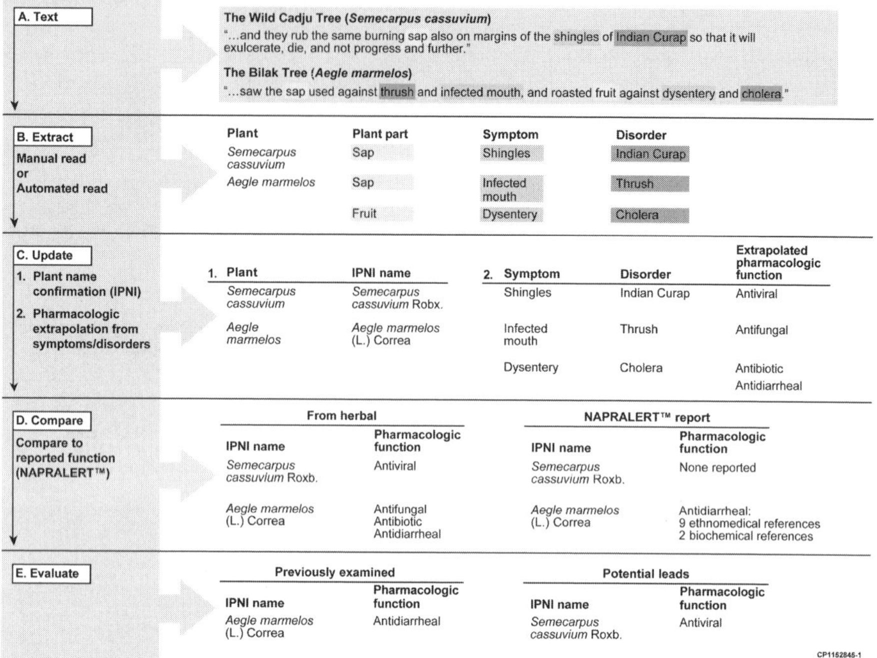

Figure 4.4 The general protocol for information extraction from an herbal text (A–E) is paired with case examples from our work with the *Ambonese Herbal* by Rumphius. (A) Text is digitized. (B) Through either manual reading or automated extraction the plant name(s), plant part(s), and symptoms or disorders are identified. (C) These extracted data are then updated (as necessary) to reflect current names of the plants, using the International Plant Names Index (IPNI), and the pharmacological function(s) of the described medicinal plants are extrapolated from the mentioned symptoms and disorders. (D) The current botanical names are queried against a natural products database such as the NAPRALERT™ database to determine whether the plant has been previously examined. (E) Differential tables are generated that separate the plants examined in the literature from plants that may warrant further examination for bioactivity. (Adapted from *Trends in Pharmacological Sciences*, with permission.) See color plate.

preliminary analysis suggests that this approach will provide a high-throughput system to move these texts into electronic format.

4.5.2 International Plant Names Index

As more is known regarding plant taxonomy, plant names change. Because the rules used to define how plants are named imply certain relationships [29]

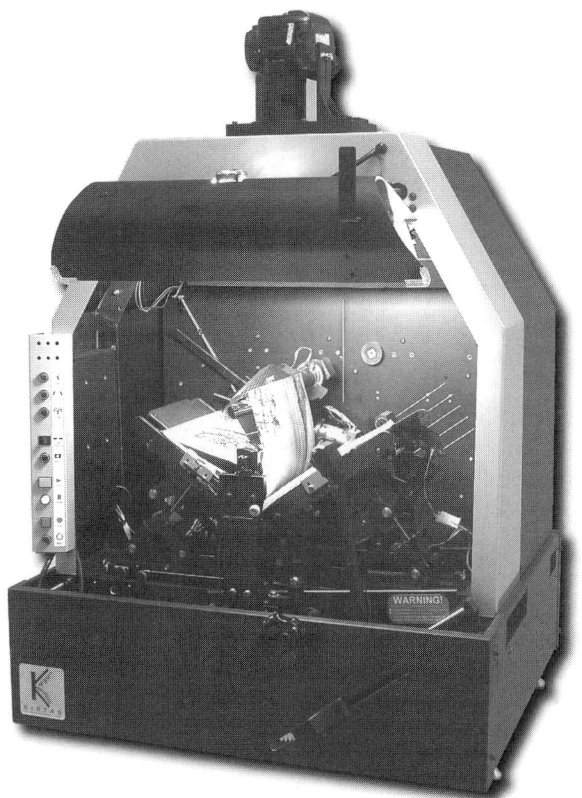

Figure 4.5 The Kirtas APT BookScan 1200 allows for the automated scanning of historic herbal texts into electronic format. (Image supplied by Lisa Stasevich, Kirtas Technologies.)

and allow interrelationships between different species to be determined [30], updating the plant names used in the analysis of herbal texts is important. As a result of this importance, the methods used to assign plant names are well defined [31] and there is an established protocol to change a plant name [32].

Nonetheless, these changes in plant names can be difficult to manage. Fortunately, there are a number of databases that provide correlations between historic names and the current names of these plants. We have chosen to use the International Plant Names Index for our analysis [33]. By querying this database we are able to either validate the name of the plant in the historic text or, more frequently, to update the plant name to the current name.

4.5.3 SNOW-MED

We have developed a system based on SNOW-MED to extract medical information from herbal texts. SNOW-MED is a semantic index that recognizes relationships between groups of words [26]. For example, the semantic map for *thrush* is related to *yeast*, *infection*, and *microbe*. Although this system may eventually allow a potential pharmacological function to be extrapolated, we are currently using the system to simply extract disorders from the text. We have used the Mayo Vocabulary Server to perform this data mining [34, 35].

4.5.4 NAPRALERT™

Incorporating the Kirtas system with the International Plant Names Index and SNOW-MED allows movement of the historic text into an electronic format, identification of current plant names, and identification of the symptoms treated with the plants. To complete the mining of historic herbal texts for novel drug leads we use the Natural Products Alert (NAPRALERT™) database to compare the information extracted from the historic herbal text to the reports of plant use in the current literature. The NAPRALERT™ database provides a summary of plants' ethnopharmacological use, biochemical activities, and isolated compounds [27]. By querying each plant (with the current plant name) it is possible to identify any reports in the current literature regarding the plant. As an example, Table 4.1 shows the NAPRALERT™ output for *Cycas rumphii*.

4.6 CURRENT CHALLENGES AND FUTURE DIRECTIONS

It is possible to extract novel drug leads from historic herbal texts. However, manual extraction techniques are laborious. The automated extraction system we have developed makes it possible to identify potential novel drug leads in a high-throughput fashion.

The prospect of using historic herbal texts as a tool to resurrect lost traditional medicine knowledge and to identify new drugs is exciting. However, there are six significant challenges that need to be addressed to increase the efficiency of this system:

1. Identification of historic herbal texts. There are thousands of herbal texts in the world. Many of them are rare and unknown to our modern repositories. Identifying the location of these texts and the language in which the texts are written would allow a clearer outlook for the future of this field.

2. Quantified evaluation of drugs that could have been identified in herbal texts. It would be a valuable assessment to quantify the number of pharmaceuticals that have been described with the correct purported uses in an herbal text. A project of this nature would incorporate selecting a historic

TABLE 4.1 Biological Activities for Compounds of *Cycas rumphii*

Activity	Plant Part	Assay	Concentration	Model	Result	Location	Reference
Antifungal	Dried leaf	Agar plate	Undiluted	*Aspergillus fumigatus*	Active	India	T11794
Antifungal	Dried leaf	Agar plate	Undiluted	*Aspergillus niger*	Active	India	T11794
Antiyeast	Dried leaf	Agar plate	Undiluted	*Candida vaginalis*	Active	India	T11794
Aromatase inhibition	Dried leaf	Tumor assay	75% Ethanol extraction 12.5 mg/ml	System to predict antitumor activity	Active	USA-FL	K21397

To generate this table NAPRALERT™ was queried for all biological activities of *Cycas rumphii*. The results of the Reference section correspond to the NAPRALERT™-coded references.

herbal text, or a group of texts, and identifying plants described in the texts that have ultimately resulted in a pharmaceutical.

3. *Effective movement of herbal texts into electronic format.* We have used a single system to move herbal texts into an electronic format. This system has worked well for texts printed after the era of mass printing. However, there are many texts that were written before 1600 A.D. It is likely that there are other mechanisms to complete the task of moving historic herbal texts into an electronic format. For example, the Missouri Botanical Gardens has manually scanned a number of historic herbal texts into electronic format [28].

4. *Proof-of-concept through new pharmaceuticals.* We have generated preliminary data suggesting that one of Rumphius's purported pharmaceuticals does have the medicinal properties described. However, it has not been shown that the active compound is novel. Examining other plants identified in historic herbal texts for their purported medicinal properties may ultimately show that novel pharmaceuticals can be developed by mining historic herbal texts.

5. *Translation into English.* Many of these herbal texts are in languages other than English. Regrettably, the semantic mapping systems are only appropriate for English texts. Certainly, as electronic translation programs improve, it will become possible to mine texts written in other languages.

6. *The loss of plants described in texts.* There is a loss of both traditional medicine knowledge and plant resources for traditional medicine use [24]. The loss of traditional medicine knowledge is regrettable; however, mining historic herbal texts provides a way to resurrect that information. In contrast to the loss of traditional medicine knowledge, the loss of biodiversity is permanent. For example, The Living Planet Index suggests a 37% loss of biodiversity between 1970 and 2000 [36], and pictures of ecological devastation are all too common (Fig. 4.6). It is usually assumed that this loss of biodiversity is inextricably tied to development; however, recent work has suggested this assumption to be false [24]. Thus, to prevent the loss of other species like silphium, ecologically sustainable development is critical.

4.7 CONCLUSION

The techniques for drug discovery are developing at an astonishing rate. However, there are certain challenges facing the current systems of drug development. The use of ethnobotanical information provides additional information regarding the potential pharmacological functions of plants. Yet there is a generational loss of traditional medicine knowledge, and ethnobotanical investigation is labor intensive. The use of bioinformatics to extract information from historic herbal texts provides an efficient method of identifying potential novel plant-based lead compounds.

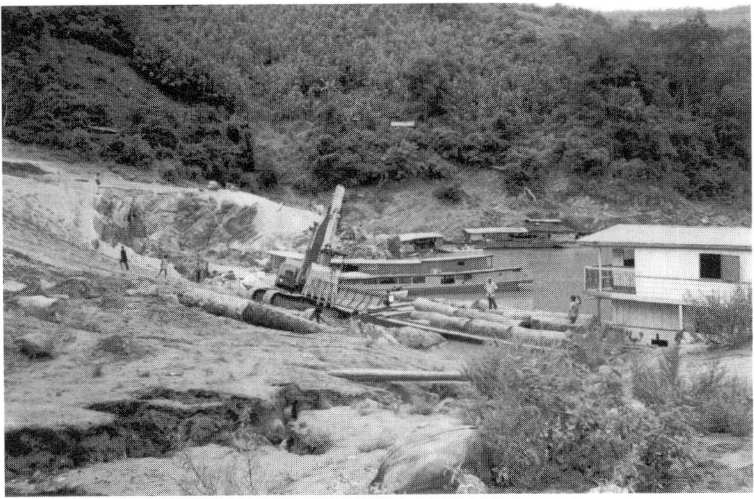

Figure 4.6 Nonsustainable logging in Laos is an example of the current loss of biodiversity.

Employing herbal texts as a resource for drug discovery holds significant promise. Yet this technology is in its infancy, and there are a number of challenges to overcome. Fortunately, many of these challenges are being addressed in different disciplines. In the future, incorporation of these multidisciplinary advancements will allow high-throughput mining of historic herbal texts to supplement high-throughput screening as a method for drug discovery.

4.8 APPENDIX. THE EXTINCTION OF SILPHIUM

Because not all of the species in the world are known, it is difficult to determine the exact rate of species extinction. Unfortunately, there are plants with medicinal properties that have gone extinct. The first case of a medicinal plant extinction documented in an herbal text is silphium [37].

Silphium was originally discovered in what is now Libya after a mysterious black rain fell around 600 B.C. This plant subsequently spread throughout the region [38] and became valuable because of the particular taste of meat from animals that fed on it. Silphium was also a highly effective medicine. The dried sap of the plant could be used on a variety of disorders from fevers and warts to hair loss. Because of the broad uses of the plant, and a reported inability to cultivate it [38], silphium became highly prized. Because the plant was difficult to find naturally, Julius Caesar held on to nearly a ton of the dried resin in the Roman treasury [39]. Eventually, the lack of supply drove the value of the plant resin so high that the Roman Empire declared a monopoly on silphium. Soon after, because of the scarcity of the plant and the Roman decree, silphium literally became worth its weight in gold. Ultimately, the combination of scarcity and high price led to the extinction of silphium.

ACKNOWLEDGMENTS

I am indebted to Moses Rodriguez, Charles Howe, and Brent Bauer, Mayo Clinic College of Medicine, Rochester, MN, for their support of this project. The help of Holly Johnson, Institute for Ethnomedicine, National Tropical Botanical Gardens, Kalaheo, HI, provided with the NAPRALERT™ database is appreciated. John Riddle, North Carolina State University, Raleigh, NC, has provided great insight into the history of herbal texts. Without the botanical expertise of Timothy Motley, The New York Botanical Gardens, Bronx, NY, this project would never have been possible. Finally, I would like to thank Peter Elkin, Mayo Clinic College of Medicine, Rochester, MN, for his assistance with the Mayo Vocabulary Server.

This work was supported by Mary Kathryn and Michael B. Panitch and the Mayo Clinic College of Medicine Department of Complementary and Integrative Medicine.

REFERENCES

1. Davis AM, Keeling DJ, Steele J, Tomkinson NP, Tinker AC. Components of successful lead generation. *Curr Top Med Chem* 2005;5:421–39.
2. Bodovitz S, Joos T, Bachmann J. Protein biochips: the calm before the storm. *Drug Discovery Today* 2005;10:283–7, 2005.
3. Rachakonda S, Cartee L. Challenges in antimicrobial drug discovery and the potential of nucleoside antibiotics. *Curr Med Chem* 2004;11:775–93, 2004.
4. Balick MJ. Ethnobotany and the identification of therapeutic agents from the rainforest. *Ciba Found Symp* 1990;154:22–31; discussion 32–9.
5. Cox PA. Will tribal knowledge survive the millennium? *Science* 2000;287:44–5.
6. Riddle JM. History as a tool in identifying "new" old drugs. *Adv Exp Med Biol* 2002;505:89–94.
7. Buenz EJ, Johnson HE, Beekman EM, Motley TJ, Bauer BA. Bioprospecting Rumphius's Ambonese Herbal: Volume I. *J Ethnopharmacol* 2005;96:57–70.
8. Buenz EJ, Schnepple DJ, Bauer BA, Elkin PL, Riddle JM, Motley TJ. Techniques: Bioprospecting historical herbal texts by hunting for new leads in old tomes. *Trends Pharmacol Sci* 2004;25:494–8.
9. Chapman RL, Stanley TB, Hazen R, Garvey EP. Small molecule modulators of HIV Rev/Rev response element interaction identified by random screening. *Antiviral Res* 2002;54:149–62.

10. Boldi AM. Libraries from natural product-like scaffolds. *Curr Opin Chem Biol* 2004;8:281–6.
11. Wani MC, Taylor HL, Wall ME, Coggon P, McPhail AT. Plant antitumor agents. VI. The isolation and structure of taxol, a novel antileukemic and antitumor agent from *Taxus brevifolia. J Am Chem Soc* 1971;93:2325–7.
12. Gunaydin K, Savci S. Phytochemical studies on *Ruta chalepensis* (Lam.) Lamarck. *Nat Prod Res* 2005;19:203–10.
13. Bruno M, Piozzi F, Rosselli S. Natural and hemisynthetic neoclerodane diterpenoids from scutellaria and their antifeedant activity. *Nat Prod Rep* 2002;19:357–78.
14. Van Gils C, Cox PA. Ethnobotany of nutmeg in the Spice Islands. J *Ethnopharmacol* 1994;42:117–24.
15. Pearn J. The world's longest surviving paediatric practices: Some themes of Aboriginal medical ethnobotany in Australia. *J Paediatr Child Health* 2005;41:284–90.
16. Cox PA. Saving the ethnopharmacological heritage of Samoa. *J Ethnopharmacol* 1993;38:181–8.
17. Gustafson KR, Cardellina JH 2nd, McMahon JB, Gulakowski RJ, Ishitoya J, Szallasi Z, Lewin NE, Blumberg PM, Weislow OS, Beutler JA et al. A nonpromoting phorbol from the samoan medicinal plant *Homalanthus nutans* inhibits cell killing by HIV-1. *J Med Chem* 1992;35:1978–86.
18. Williams SA, Chen LF, Kwon H, Fenard D, Bisgrove D, Verdin E, Greene WC. Prostratin antagonizes HIV latency by activating NF-κB. *J Biol Chem* 2004;279:42008–17.
19. Bailey J, Blankson JN, Wind-Rotolo M, Siliciano RF. Mechanisms of HIV-1 escape from immune responses and antiretroviral drugs. *Curr Opin Immunol* 2004;16:470–6.
20. Lee R, Balick M, Ling D, Brosi B, Raynor W. Special Report: cultural dynamism and change—an example from the Federated States of Micronesia. *Economic Botany* 2001;55:9–13.
21. Van Arsdall A. *Medieval herbal remedies. The old English Herbarium and Anglo-Saxon medicine*. Routledge, Boca Raton, 2002.
22. Opsomer C. *Index de la pharmacopee du ler au Xe siecle.* Olms-Weidmann, 1989.
23. Riddle JM. Theory and practice in medieval medicine. *Viator* 1974;5:157–184.
24. Buenz EJ. Country development does not presuppose the loss of forest resources for traditional medicine use. *J Ethnopharmacol* 2005;100(1–2):118–123.
25. Roberts PM, Hayes WS. Advances in text analytics for drug discovery. *Curr Opin Drug Discov Devel* 2005;8:323–8.
26. Wang AY, Sable JH, Spackman KA. The SNOMED clinical terms development process: refinement and analysis of content. *Proc AMIA Symp*: 2002;845–9.
27. Loub WD, Farnsworth NR, Soejarto DD, Quinn ML. NAPRALERT: computer handling of natural product research data. *J Chem Inf Comput Sci* 1985, 25:99–103.

28. Jackson S. Classic herbal texts brought into the digital age. *HerbalGram* 2003;60:30–7.
29. Stuessy TF. Taxon names are not defined. *Taxon* 2000;49:231–3.
30. Moore G. Should taxon names be explicitly defined? *Bot Rev* 2003;69:2–21.
31. Greuter W, McNeill J, Barrie FR, Burdet H-M, Demoulin V, Filgueiras TS, Nicolson DH, Silva PC, Skog JE, Trehane P, Turland NJ, Hawksworth DL. *International Code of Botanical Nomenclature (St. Louis Code),* Vol. 138. Konigstein, Koeltz Scientific Books, 2000.
32. Lawrence GHM. *Taxonomy of vascular plants.* Macmillan, 1951.
33. *The International Plant Names Index*, Published on the Internet http://www.ipni.org. 2004.
34. Elkin PL, Bailey KR, Ogren PV, Bauer BA, Chute CG. A randomized double-blind controlled trial of automated term dissection. *Proc AMIA Symp* 1999;62–6.
35. Elkin PL, Ruggieri AP, Brown SH, Buntrock J, Bauer BA, Wahner-Roedler D, Litin SC, Beinborn J, Bailey KR, Bergstrom L. A randomized controlled trial of the accuracy of clinical record retrieval using SNOMED-RT as compared with ICD9-CM. *Proc AMIA Symp* 2001;159–63.
36. WWF. *Living Planet Report 2004.* World Wildlife Fund for Nature, Gland, Switzerland, 2004.
37. Parejko K. Pliny the Elder's Silphium: First Recorded Species Extinction. *Conservation Biol* 2003;17:925–7.
38. Hort AT. *Theophrastus: enquiry into plants.* Cambridge, MA, Harvard University Press, 1968.
39. Rackham HT. *Pliny: natural history.* Cambridge, MA, Harvard University Press, 1950.

5

CONTEXTUALIZING THE IMPACT OF BIOINFORMATICS ON PRECLINICAL DRUG AND VACCINE DISCOVERY

DARREN R. FLOWER

Contents

5.1 INTRODUCTION

One should not lightly dismiss the importance of serendipity in the history of drug discovery. In this context, the tale of the antiallergy drug Intal is particularly interesting [1]. The toothpick plant (*Ammi visnaga*) originates in the

Computer Applications in Pharmaceutical Research and Development, Edited by Sean Ekins.
ISBN 0-471-73779-8

eastern Mediterranean and has, since antiquity, been used as a folk treatment for renal colic. First isolated from the fruit of the *Ammi visnaga* in 1879, khellin, which is still in use as a treatment for angina, was found to induce smooth muscle relaxation and have interesting bronchodilatory effects in asthma. In 1955, chemists at Benger Laboratories began studying khellin analogs as potential treatments for asthma, screening compounds against a guinea pig asthma model. At this point, asthmatic physician Roger Altounyan joined the research team. Altounyan (1922–1987) was born in Syria and subsequently received medical training in the UK. As children, he and his siblings acted as the inspiration for the Walker family, characters in Arthur Ransome's "Swallows and Amazon" novels. Working at Benger Laboratories, Altounyan tested hundreds of khellin analogs on himself, investigating their relative prevention of his allergic reaction to inhaled guinea pig dander. One analog, K84, significantly reduced his symptoms. In 1963, a contaminant—later identified as sodium cromoglycate—proved highly active. Early in 1965, Altounyan identified a compound—the 670th compound made over nine years—which worked for several hours; clinical trials began in 1967. The compound functions through mast cell stabilization, preventing the release of inflammatory mediators. Marketed as Intal, the drug, which has strong prophylactic properties, is used in numerous forms to treat asthma, rhinitis, eczema, and food allergy.

Charming, and, indeed, alarming, though this story seems, it happily undermines current notions of "proper" drug discovery. It gainsays the use of animal models, emphasizing, much to the delight of antivivisectionists, the necessity of direct human testing, and, as we began by saying, it highlights the importance of good fortune and serendipity in the process of discovering new medicines; as an old adage has it: An ounce of luck is worth a pound of cleverness. Today, of course, such practices are deemed utterly inconscionable: The modern pharmaceutical industry spends millions of person-hours and billions of dollars increasingly to systematize drug discovery. For example, the top 10 pharmaceutical companies spent nearly $36 billion on research and development (R&D) in 2003, though possibly rather more on the "D" than on the "R." This is all with the intention of finally eliminating the requirement for luck. Receptor-orientated, mechanism-driven research has replaced targetless pathologies as the primary focus of the discovery process. Sophisticated medium- and high-throughput synthesis and in vitro screening technologies have largely displaced individual "hand-crafted" assays. Increasingly also, sophisticated techniques of data management and prediction have begun to play their part. Of these, arguably, bioinformatics has been the most visibly successful. The discovery of marketable novel chemical entities (NCEs)—that is, new patentable drugs and medicines—is, for the pharmaceutical industry, the principal fountainhead of sustained and sustainable prosperity. Preclinical drug discovery typically starts by identifying initial lead compounds, which are then optimized into candidate drugs that then enter clinical trials. But before a new drug can be developed, one needs to find the targets of drug action, be that a cell surface receptor, enzyme, binding protein, or other kind of protein or nucleic acid. This is the domain of bioinformatics.

5.2 SO WHAT EXACTLY IS BIOINFORMATICS?

The word "bioinformatics" has been in common usage since the early 1990s, and it means, as words sometimes do, different things to different people. A simple, straightforward, yet comprehensive definition is not readily forthcoming. One of the better attempts summarizes the discipline as "the application of informatics methods to biological macromolecules." Forming a more inclusive description remains challenging. Why should this be? It is partly because the nature of bioinformatics is constantly changing or, at least, constantly growing: You cannot easily put a name to it because you cannot pin it down long enough. The scope and focus of bioinformatics is constantly developing and expanding to encompass more and more new areas of application. However, it is clear that bioinformatics concerns itself with medical, genomic, and biological information and supports both basic and clinical research. Bioinformatics develops computer databases and algorithms for accelerating, simplifying, and thus enhancing, research in bioscience. Within this, however, the nature and variety of different bioinformatics activities are hard to quantify. Bioinformatics is as much a melting pot of interdisciplinary techniques as it is a branch of information science: It operates at the level of protein and nucleic acid sequences, their structures, and their functions, using data from microarray experiments, traditional biochemistry, as well as theoretical biophysics.

The growth of bioinformatics is a clear success story of the incipient informatics revolution sweeping through bioscience. Although bioinformaticians may not find themselves quite as employable as they did five years ago, nonetheless computational biologists at all levels have reimagined themselves under this compelling brand; many computational biologists desire to shelter under the bioinformatics umbrella and thus access enhanced funding. The services of bioinformaticians are in demand by canny biologists of many flavors. As new genomes are sequenced we wish to know all manner of things: where sites of posttranslational modification are, the subcellular location of protein, whether a protein will be a substrate for certain enzymes, or what a particular pK_a is for an enzyme active site residue. The list is endless. Addressing all of this experimentally would be prohibitive in terms of time, labor, and resources. The only answer is recourse to a bioinformatics solution.

Bioinformatics focuses on analyzing molecular sequence and structure data, molecular phylogenies, and the analysis of postgenomic data, such as generated by genomics, transcriptomics, and proteomics. Bioinformatics seeks to solve two main challenges. First, the prediction of function from sequence, which can be performed with global homology searches, motif database searches, and the formation of multiple sequence alignments. Second, the prediction of structure from sequence, which may be attempted with secondary structure prediction, threading, and comparative, or so-called homology, modeling. It is also an implicit assumption that knowledge of a structure facilitates prediction of function. In reality, all predictions of function rely on identifying similarity between sequences or between structures. When this similarity is very high, and thus is intrinsically reliable, then useful inferences may be drawn, but as similarity falls away any conclusions that are inferred become increasingly uncertain and potentially misleading.

Within pharmaceutical research, bioinformatics typically equates to the discovery of novel drug targets from genomic and proteomic information. Bioinformatics can be subdivided into several complementary areas: gene informatics, protein informatics, and system informatics. Gene informatics, with links to genomics and microarray analysis, is concerned, inter alia, with managing information on genes and genomes and the *in silico* prediction of gene structure. A key component of gene informatics is gene finding: the relatively straightforward searching, at least conceptually if not always practically, of sequence databases for homologous sequences with, hopefully, similar functions and analogous roles in disease states. Protein informatics concerns itself with managing information on protein sequences and has obvious links with proteomics and structure-function relationships. Part of its remit includes the modeling of three-dimensional structure and the construction of multiple alignments. The third component concerns itself with the higher-order interactions rather than simple sequences and includes the elaboration of functional protein-protein interactions, metabolic pathways, and control theory. Thus another, and increasingly important, role of bioinformatics is managing the information generated by microarray experiments and proteomics and drawing from it data on the gene products implicated in disease states. The key role of bioinformatics is, then, to transform large, if not vast, reservoirs of information into useful, and useable, information.

Bioinformatics relies on many other disciplines, both as a source of data and as a source of novel techniques of proven provenance. It forms synergistic links with other parts of bioscience, such as genomics, as both consumer and vendor. In the era of high-throughput technologies, bioinformatics feeds upon many data-rich disciplines. Yet it also provides vital data interpretation and data management services, allowing biologists to come to terms with the postgenomic data deluge rather than being swept away by it. Bioinformatics is still largely concerned with data handling and analysis, be that through the annotation of macromolecular sequence and structure databases or through the classification of sequences or structures into coherent groups.

Prediction, as well as analysis, is also important. Conceptually, the difference is clear, but it is seldom properly appreciated. Risk is associated with predictions, but there should not be any significant risk associated with an analysis. To put it rather simply: Prediction is about making informed, educated guesses about uncertain, untested events, whereas analysis is about identifying relationships among known, certain data. However, despite the steady increase in studies reporting the real-world use of prediction algorithms, there is still an ongoing need for truly convincing validations of the underlying approach. Why should this be? Prediction, like all forms of forecasting, is prone to error and is seldom foolproof. The same, however, is also true of all human activities, experimental science included. Predictions made by informatics are seldom perfect, but neither are predictions about the weather or stock market forecasts. People live happily with inaccuracies in both, but many dog-in-a-manger scientists will have nothing to do with theoretical or informatics predictions. "It's not perfect. It's therefore trash! How can I trust it?" they say, yet trust implicitly their own inherently error-prone and discombobulating experiments, and expect others to trust them also. In physics, accurate and insightful prediction is the goal, and people are genuinely excited by the convergence of observation and theory. The use of prediction in biosciences should indeed be managed appropriately: Healthy skepticism is one thing, but mean-spirited polemics are quite another. There is no doubt that bioinformatics has delivered, perhaps not what its early proponents had promised or even what they privately envisaged, but delivered it certainly has. We shall see abundant evidence of its success here and elsewhere in this book. Yet, it is as well to remember that atavistic attitudes still persist and such assertions must continue to be contested. Although it is clear that more accurate prediction algorithms are still required, for such new techniques to be useful routinely they must be tested rigorously for a sufficiently large number of cases that their accuracy can be shown to work to statistical significance.

How then is this seeming dilemma to be addressed? What is required is more than just new algorithms and software; it requires the confidence of experimentalists to exploit the methodology and to commit laboratory experimentation. Despite the best efforts of programmers and software engineers, the use of many bioinformatics tools remains daunting for laboratory-based bioscientists. Use of these methods must become routine. It is not only a matter of training and education, however. These methods must be made accessible and robust. We have come to a turning point, where a number of technologies have obtained the necessary level of maturity: postgenomic strategies on the one hand and predictive computational methods on the other. Progress will occur in two ways. One will involve closer connections between bioinformaticians and experimentalists seeking to discover new drugs. In such a situation, work would progress through a cyclical process of using and refining models and experiments, at each stage moving closer toward a common goal of effective, cost-efficient drug and vaccine development. The other way is the devolved model, in which methods are made accessible and used remotely via web-based technology.

Moreover, there is a clear and obvious need for experimental work to be conducted in support of the development of accurate *in silico* methods. Bioinformaticians, like all other scientists physical or biological or social, need quality data to work with. Informaticians cannot exist merely on the detritus dropped from the experimentalists' table. Rather, experiments must be conducted that specifically address the kind of predictions that bioinformaticians need to make. The ability to combine in vitro and *in silico* analysis allows us to improve both the scope and the power of our predictions, in a way that would be impossible with literature data alone. If we wish to predict sites of posttranslational modification or accurate protein subcellular locations, we need to conduct properly designed, comprehensive initial experiments specifically for that purpose. To ensure that we produce useful, quality *in silico* models and methods, and not the opposite, we need to value the predictions generated by bioinformatics for themselves and conduct experiments appropriately. The potential benefits are obvious: Better data generate better predictive methods and thus routinely improved biologically important predictions. In this way predictions can become stable and reliable tools fully integrated into the process of drug discovery.

5.3 THE STUFF OF BIOINFORMATICS

Bioinformatics makes a series of synergistic interactions with both client disciplines (computer science, structural chemistry, etc) and with disciplines that act in the role of customer (genomics, molecular biology, and cell biology). Bioinformatics is concerned with activities such as the annotation of biological data (genome sequences, for example) and classification of sequences and structures into meaningful groups and seeks to solve two main challenges: the prediction of function from sequence and the prediction of structure from sequence. Put simply, bioinformatics deals with the similarity between macromolecular sequences, typically made manifest in global sequence searches using software such as FastA [2] or BLAST [3]. Bioinformatics seeks to identify genes descended from a common ancestor, which share a corresponding structural and functional propinquity. The assumption underlying is thus an evolutionary one: Functionally similar genes have diverged through a process of random mutation that results in evolutionarily more distant sequences being less and less similar to each another. The chain of inference that connects similarity to common function is complex. Thus successful functional assignment necessitates significant biological context. Such context is provided by databases: implicit context present as archived sequences and explicit context present as annotation.

5.3.1 Databases

Databases are the lingua franca—the common language—of bioinformatics. Although the kind of data archived may vary, nonetheless, the use, creation, and manipulation of databases remains the most critical feature of modern-day bioinformatics, both as a discipline in its own right and as a support for current biological science. Available biological data banks are currently proliferating; they now require their own database just to catalog them [4]. Databases began by simply storing the sequences and structures of genes and proteins. Soon, however, databases such as Swiss-Prot began to add biological context in the form of annotation, the fundamental character of which is well illustrated by the observation that currently only around 15% of the Swiss-Prot database is actually sequence. The remaining 85% is annotation: literature cross-references, descriptions of biological context, and illustrative notes. Rationalizing this mountain of biological data is now beyond the scope of individuals and requires both a global effort and an ever-increasing degree of automation. Automation, however, carries a heavy price. Functional annotation in protein sequence databases is often inferred from observed similarities to homologous, annotated proteins. This can lead to errors, particularly when sequence similarity is marginal. As a result, it is widely believed that there are now substantial numbers of incorrect annotations throughout commonly used databases [5]. Moreover, this problem can be compounded by the Markovian process of "error percolation" [6], whereby the functional annotations of similar proteins may themselves have been acquired through chains of similarity to sets of other proteins. Such chains of inference are seldom recorded, so it is generally impossible to determine how a particular database annotation has been acquired. Such a situation leads to an inevitable deterioration of quality and poses an ongoing threat to the reliability of data as a consequence of propagating errors in annotation. Although curators continually strive to address such errors, users must be constantly on their guard when inferring function from archived data.

However, bioinformatics is never still, and databases, like other aspects of the discipline, have moved on. Databases now encompass entities as diverse as whole genome sequences, transcriptomic and proteomic experiments, and a diversity of other kinds of experimental measurements and derived biological properties. From a pharmaceutical target-discovery perspective, arguably the most important type of derived data are discriminators of protein family membership. A variety of different analytical approaches have been used to create such discriminators, including regular expressions, aligned sequence blocks, fingerprints, profiles, and hidden Markov models (HMMs) [7]. Each such descriptor has different relative strengths and weaknesses, and thus produces databases with very different characters. Such discriminators are deposited in one of the many primary motif databases (i.e., PROSITE or PRINTS) or secondary motif databases such as SMART or INTERPRO. An underlying assumption of such databases is that a protein family can be identified by one or more characteristic sequence patterns. Such patterns are identified in three ways: first, by direct inspection of aligned protein sequences; second, by using unaligned sequences as input to programs such as MEME, which can perceive statistically significant patterns automatically; or third, from aligned sequence with a motif identification approach such as PRATT. Motif databases thus contain distilled descriptions of protein families that can be used to classify other sequences in an automated fashion.

5.3.2 Multiple Alignment

At the heart of bioinformatics is the multiple sequence alignment. Its uses are legion: prediction of three-dimensional structure, either through homology modeling or via de novo secondary structure prediction; identification of functionally important residues; undertaking phylogenetic analysis; and also identification of important motifs and thus the development of discriminators for protein family membership. The accuracy of many techniques, such as those just mentioned, is heavily dependent on the accuracy of multiple sequence alignments. The building of a multiple sequence alignment begins with the identification of a sequence/structure corpus. The definition of a protein family, the key step in annotating macromolecular sequences, proceeds through an iterative process of searching sequence, structure, and motif databases to generate a sequence corpus, which represents the whole set of sequences within the family. In an ideal case, this should contain all related sequences and structures related to the seed sequence of interest. The process is iterative and brings together the results of three types of searches: global sequence searches; such as BLAST, FastA, or a parallel version of Smith–Waterman; searches against motif databases such as InterPro or PRINTS; and searches for similar three-dimensional structures using full model searches, such as DALI, or topology searches, such as TOPS. Once a search has converged and no more reliable sequences can be added, then the final corpus has been found and a multiple alignment can be constructed.

5.3.3 Gene Finding

Much of the success of bioinformatics rests on its synergistic interactions with genomic and postgenomic science. The current, putative size of the human genome has been revised down from figures in excess of 100,000 to estimates closer to 40,000 genes. Most recently, a number closer to 20,000 has been suggested [8]. Clearly, the size of the human genome and the number of genes within it remain just estimates. Thus the ability to accurately identify genes remains an unsolved problem, despite rapid progress in recent years. When dealing with entire genome sequences, the need for software tools, able to automate the laborious process of scanning million upon million of base pairs, is essential. When we move from the genome to the proteome, gene finding becomes protein finding and an order of magnitude more difficult. The proteome is, however, much larger, principally through the existence of splice variants [9], but also because of the existence of protein-splicing elements (inteins) that catalyze their own excision from flanking amino acid sequences (exteins), thus creating new proteins in which the exteins are linked directly by a peptide bond [10]. Other mechanisms include posttranslational modifications, cleavage of precursors, and other types of proteolytic activation. The proteome varies according to the cell type and the functional state of the cell, and it shows characteristic perturbations in response to disease and external stimuli. Proteomics as a scientific discipline is relatively new but is based on rather older techniques, combining sophisticated analytical methods, such as 2D electrophoresis and mass spectrometry, with bioinformatics. Thus proteomics is the study of gene expression at a functional level. Genomic identification of genes is, however, the beginning rather than the end. Distinct proteins have different properties and thus different functions in different contexts. Identifying, cataloging, and characterizing the protein complement within the human proteome will thus prove significantly more challenging than annotation of the genome.

5.4 FINDING TARGETS FOR THERAPEUTIC INTERVENTION

An important recent trend has been the identification of "druggable" targets. Databases of nucleic acid and protein sequences and structures have now become available on an unparalleled, multigenomic scale. To capitalize on this, attention has focused on the ability of such databases accurately to compare active sites across a range of related proteins, and thus allow us to select and validate biological targets, to control drug selectivity, and verify biological hypotheses more precisely. What is a druggable receptor? This is dependent on the drug of interest: The properties required of a short-acting drug are very different from that of long-acting, orally bioavailable medicine. The G protein-coupled receptor (GPCR) is an archetypal "druggable" target, with its small, hydrophobic, internal binding site and crucial physiological roles. By "druggable" we mean proteins exhibiting a hydrophobic binding site of defined proportions, leading to the development of drugs of the right size and appropriate physicochemical properties. The term druggable relates both to the receptor structure and also to the provenance of a protein family as a source of successful drug targets. Estimates put the number of druggable receptors somewhere in the region of 2000 to 4000 [11]. Of these, about 10% have been extensively examined to date, leaving many, many receptors left to explore. Beyond the human genome, there are other "druggable" receptors now receiving the attention of pharmaceutical companies. Bacteria, fungi, viruses, and parasites are all viable targets for drug intervention. As the number of antibiotic-resistant pathogens increases, the hunt for new antimicrobial compounds, and thus the number of "druggable" microbial receptors, will also expand.

Set the task of discovering new, previously unknown "druggable" receptors, how would we go about it? In particular, how would we find a GPCR? The first step toward functional annotation of a new GPCR sequence usually involves searching a primary sequence database with pairwise similarity tools. Such searches can reveal clear similarities between the query sequence and a set of other sequences in the database. An ideal result will show unequivocal similarity to a well-characterized protein over its whole length. However, an output will regularly reveal no true hits. The usual scenario falls somewhere between these extremes, producing a list of partial matches that will either be to uncharacterized proteins or have dubious annotations. The difficulty lies in the reliable inference of descent from a shared ancestor and thus extrapolation to a common biological function. The increasing size of sequence databases increases the probability that relatively high-scoring, yet random, matches will be made. Even if a verifiable match is made, it is difficult for pairwise similarity methods to distinguish paralogs from orthologs. Moreover, low-complexity matches can dominate search outputs. The multidomain nature of proteins is also a problem: When matching to multidomain proteins, it is not always clear which domain corresponds to the search query. Thus achieving trustworthy functional assignments remains a daunting problem, and it has become common practice to extend search strategies to include motif- or domain-based searches of protein family databases, such as PRINTS or INTERPRO. Because family discriminators can detect weaker similarity, and can usefully exploit the differences between sequences as well as their similarities, searching family databases can be more sensitive and selective than global sequence searching. Bioinformatics can help in validation through the design and analysis of high-throughput testing, such as targeted transcriptomic experiments.

5.5 BIOINFORMATICS AND VACCINE DISCOVERY

Immunoinformatics is a newly emergent subdiscipline within the informatic sciences that deals specifically with the unique problems of the immune system. Like bioinformatics, immunoinformatics complements, but never replaces, laboratory experimentation. It allows researchers to address, in a systematic manner, the most important questions in the still highly empirical world of immunology and vaccine discovery.

The first vaccine was discovered by Edward Jenner in 1796, when he used cowpox, a related virus, to build protective immunity against viral smallpox in his gardener's son. Later, Pasteur adopted "vaccination"—the word coined by Jenner for his treatment (from the Latin *vacca*: cow)—for immunization against any disease. In 1980, the World Health Organisation declared that worldwide vaccination had freed the world of smallpox. A vaccine is a molecular or supramolecular agent that induces specific, protective immunity (an enhanced adaptive immune response to subsequent infection) against microbial pathogens, and the diseases they cause, by potentiating immune memory and thus mitigating the effects of reinfection. It is now widely accepted that mass vaccination, which takes into account herd immunity, is the most efficacious prophylactic treatment for contagious disease. Traditionally, vaccines have been attenuated or "weakened" whole pathogen vaccines such as BCG for TB or Sabin's polio vaccine. Issues of safety have encouraged other vaccine strategies to develop, focusing on antigen and epitope vaccines. Hepatitis B vaccine is an antigen—or subunit—vaccine, and many epitope-based vaccines have now entered clinical trials. A generally useful polyepitope vaccine might contain several T cell epitopes and several B cell epitopes, plus nonproteinaceous "danger signals," and may be a synthetic vaccine or a natural antigen, delivered as a protein, via live viral vectors, or as raw DNA, possibly accompanied by administration of an adjuvant, a molecule or preparation that exacerbates immune responses.

However, despite their practical and societal value, vaccines remain only a small component of the global pharmaceutical market ($5 billion out of $350 billion sales in 2000). The vaccine market is dominated by just four large manufacturers: GlaxoSmithKline, Aventis Pasteur, Wyeth, and Merck & Co. There is, however, a strong resurgence of interest in vaccines, with a growing cluster of small vaccine companies and biotech firms, led by Chiron.

Vaccinology and immunology are now at a turning point. After centuries of empirical research, they are on the brink of reinventing themselves as a genome-based, quantitative science. Immunological disciplines must capitalize on an overwhelming deluge of data delivered by high-throughput, postgenomic technologies, data that are mystifyingly complex and delivered on an inconceivable scale. High-throughput approaches are engineering a paradigm shift from hypothesis to data-driven research. Immunovaccinology is a rational form of vaccinology based on our growing understanding of the mechanisms that underpin immunology. It too must make full use of what postgenomic technologies can deliver.

Hitherto, bioinformatics support for preclinical drug discovery has focused on target discovery. Reflecting the economics, support for vaccines has not flourished. As interest in the vaccine sector grows, this situation is beginning to alter. There have been two main types of informatics support for vaccines. The first is standard bioinformatics support, technically indistinguishable from support for more general target discovery. This includes genomic annotation, not just of the human genome, but of pathogenic and opportunistic bacterial, viral, and parasite species. It also includes immunotranscriptomics, the application of microarray analysis to the immune system. The other type of support is focussed on immunoinformatics and addresses problems such as the accurate prediction of immunogenicity, manifest as the identification of epitopes or the prediction of whole protein antigenicity. The immune system is complex and hierarchical, exhibiting emergent behavior at all levels, yet at its heart are straightforward molecular recognition events that are indistinguishable from other types of biomacromolecular interaction. The T cell, a specialized type of immune cell mediating cellular immunity, constantly patrols the body seeking out foreign proteins originating from pathogens. T cells express a particular receptor: the T cell receptor (TCR), which exhibits a wide range of selectivities and affinities. TCRs bind to major histocompatibility complexes (MHCs) presented on the surfaces of other cells. These proteins bind small peptide fragments, or epitopes, derived from both host and pathogen proteins. It is recognition of such complexes that lies at the heart of both the adaptive, and memory, cellular immune response. The binding of an epitope to a MHC protein, or a TCR to a peptide-MHC complex, or an antigen to an antibody, is, at the level of underlying physicochemical phenomena, identical in nature to drug-receptor interactions. Thus we can use techniques of proven provenance developed in bioinformatics and computational chemistry to address these problems. Immunogenicity manifests itself through both humoral (mediated through the binding of whole protein antigens by antibodies) and cellular (mediated by the recognition of proteolytically cleaved peptides by T cells) immunology. Whereas the prediction of B cell epitopes remains primitive, or depends on an often-elusive knowledge of protein structure, many sophisticated methods for the prediction of T cell epitopes have been developed [12].

We have reached a turning point where several technologies have achieved maturity: predictive immunoinformatics methods on the one hand and post-genomic strategies on the other. Although more accurate prediction algorithms are needed, covering more MHC alleles in more species, the paucity of convincing evaluations of reported algorithms is a confounding factor in the take-up of this technology: For immunoinformatics approaches to be used routinely by experimental immunologists, methods must be tested rigorously for a large enough number of peptides that their accuracy can be seen to work to statistical significance. To enable this requires more than improved methods and software; it necessitates building immunoinformatics into the basic strategy of immunological investigation, and it needs the confidence of experimentalists to commit laboratory work on this basis.

The next stage will come with closer connections between immunoinformaticians and experimentalists searching for new vaccines, both academic and commercial, conducted under a collaborative or consultant regime. In such a situation, work progresses cyclically using and refining models and experiments, moving toward the goal of effective and efficient vaccine development. Methods that accurately predict individual epitopes or immunogenic proteins, or eliminate microbial virulence factors, will prove to be crucial tools for tomorrow's vaccinologist. Epitope prediction remains a grand scientific challenge, being both difficult, and therefore exciting, and of true utilitarian value. Moreover, it requires not only an understanding of immunology but also the integration of many disciplines, both experimental and theoretical. The synergy of these disciplines will greatly benefit immunology and vaccinology, leading to the enhanced discovery of improved laboratory reagents, diagnostics, and vaccine candidates.

5.6 CHALLENGES

Just as the pharmaceutical industry is faced with seemingly intractable problems of addressing rapidly diminishing time to market as well as ever-escalating regulatory constraints, so bioinformatics is seeking to answer equally difficult questions, albeit ones more technical in nature. How does bioinformatics integrate itself with the burgeoning world of systems biology, with immunology, with neuroscience? How will it cope with large amounts of data generated by an array of postgenomic high-throughput technologies: genomics, proteomics, microarray experiments, and high-throughput screening? How will it deal with SNPs and polymorphism and manipulate the even greater volume of data inherent within personalized medicine and pharmacogenomics? However, arguably the most pressing need is to effectively move beyond cataloging individual data items, be they sequences, structures, genomes, or microarray experiments, and to explore the inherent interrelationships between them. People have spoken for some time now about data mining genomes. Other "–omes" now abound: transcriptomes, proteomes, metabolomes, immunomes, even chemomes. We could add another, all-encompassing "–ome": the "infome," which goes beyond the narrow confines of sequence or structure data and is, in the widest sense, the sum of all biological and chemical knowledge. It is a goal that challenges the growth of knowledge management as it seeks to treat this huge, heterogeneous volume of data. There are currently two main practical thrusts to this endeavor: text mining and ontologies. The pharmaceutical company is one of the few organizations that can, within molecular science, hope, through its intrinsic scale and willingness to invest in the future, to pursue such an objective.

Text mining is, superficially at least, abstracting data from the literature in an automated manner. Much of the data that goes into sequence and structure databases, is, because of the requirements of journal editors and the largesse of publicly funded genome sequencers, deposited directly by their authors. However, much of interest—the results of tens of thousands of unique experiments stretching back over the decades—is still inaccessible and hidden away, locked into the hard copy text of innumerable papers. As the scientific literature has moved inexorably from paper to an electronic on-line status, the opportunity arises of interrogating automatically with software. Despite the effort expended, not to mention the establishment of text mining institutes, the results have not been that remarkable. The goal is doubtless a noble and enticing one, but so far little of true utility has been forthcoming. People—indeed people in some number—are still an absolute necessity to properly parse and filter the literature.

Research into so-called ontologies is also currently very active. Ontologies can be used to characterize the principal concepts in a particular discipline and how they relate one to another. Many people believe they are necessary if database annotation is to be made accessible to both people and software, but also in facilitating more effective and efficient data retrieval. The well-known "Gene Ontology" consortium, or GO, defines the term ontology as: ". . . 'specifications of a relational vocabulary'. In other words they are sets of defined terms like the sort that you would find in a dictionary, but the terms are networked. The terms in a given vocabulary are likely to be restricted to those used in a particular field, and in the case of GO, the terms are all biological." Should one wish to find all G protein-coupled receptors in a sequence set, be it a database or an annotated genome, then searching with software that can recognize that such proteins might be labeled as "GPCR" or "opsin" or "7TM protein" or even as "transmembrane protein" would be helpful in identifying all targets. This is a somewhat trivial example, but it illustrates both the potential utility of ontologies and also the potential pitfalls. For example, "transmembrane protein" would include all GPCRs, but many other proteins as well; after all, up to 30% of a genome will be membranous. This "toy" ontology uses a set of synonyms to identify the same core entity: "GPCR" = "G protein-coupled receptor", etc. Relationships exist that relate, hierarchically, concepts together: An "opsin" is a form of "GPCR." However, more serious ontologies require semantic relations with a network, graph, or hierarchy that specifies not just how terms are connected but also how they are related at the level of meaning. Unless this is undertaken properly, even the toy ontology outlined above would become both meaningless and without utility.

The GO definition is quite distinct from other meanings of the word. A dictionary defines an ontology as:

> 1. A science or study of being: specifically, a branch of metaphysics relating to the nature and relations of being; a particular system according to which problems of the nature of being are investigated; first philosophy. 2. A theory concerning the kinds of entities and specifically the kinds of abstract entities that are to be admitted to a language system.

In artificial intelligence (AI), an ontology is an explicit specification of a concept. In the context of AI, an ontology can be represented by defining a set of representational terms. In such an ontology, definitions associate named entities (e.g., classes, relations, or functions) with human-readable text that describes the associated meaning; the interpretation and use of terms are likewise constrained. Others dismiss ontologies as little more than restricted vocabularies. The point is that ontology should be either useful or interesting or both. How one distinguishes between a good ontology and a poor ontology is more difficult.

Arguably, the other great challenge for informatics is to integrate itself with science conducted on a global scale while at the same time addressing science conducted on the most local level. One global challenge is provided by peer-to-peer computing (the sharing of resources between computers, such as processing time or spare storage space), what is generally known as screen-saver technology. Internet-based peer-to-peer applications position the desktop at the center of computing, enabling all computer users to participate actively in the Internet rather than simply surfing it. Another global strand involves the emergent grid. Grid computing is a fundamental shift in the economic and collective nature of computing. It promises that the differing needs of high-performance computing can be integrated seamlessly. High performance—sometimes erroneously labeled supercomputing—delivers ultrafast teraflop processing power and terabyte storage. Many bioinformatics problems—mainly, but not exclusively, computer-intensive simulations—cry out for this previously unattainable performance: atomistic simulation of drug-receptor binding for virtual screening purposes; simulations of protein-protein interaction for genome annotation; dynamic simulation of protein folding; numerical simulation of primary and secondary metabolism, gene regulation, and signaling, to name but a few. This is, however, only skimming the surface: Only when these techniques become common will their full usefulness become apparent.

Grid computing is thus an ambitious worldwide effort to make this a reality. It visualizes an environment in which individual users can access computers and databases transparently, without needing to know where they are located. The grid seeks to make all computer power available at the point of need. Its name is an analogy to the power transmission grid: Should you wish to switch on a light or run a domestic refrigerator, it is not necessary to wait while current is downloaded first. Early steps have been faltering yet show promise. Thus far, some large-scale science has been conducted through distributed global collaborations enabled by the Internet. A feature of such collaborative enterprises is their need to access large data collections and large computing resources and to undertake high-performance visualization. Clearly, a much improved infrastructure is needed to grid computing. Scientists will need ready access to expensive and extensive remote facilities, including routine access to teraflop computers.

The local level is epitomized on the one hand by laboratory information management systems and local data architectures and on the other by electronic laboratory notebooks. Like all science, bioinformatics must make but also use data. Data sharing is a particular issue for biological science as it fully engages with high-throughput data generation. As transcriptomics, proteomics, and metabolomics generate data on an unprecedented scale, making such data fully transparent on the local level of e-notebooks is the essential first step in making it available to the wider world.

Although operating on vastly different scales, the challenges exhibited by both the local and the global level share an important degree of commonality: Both require transparent data sharing and anonymous advanced interoperability. As user requirements and underlying IT are constantly changing, true progress sometimes seems just as elusive as it ever was. Newly created data, produced on an industrial scale by factory biology, as well as historical data still locked away in the hard copy, or even soft copy, literature, must be made available corporation-wide or worldwide in an accessible, useable form for the benefit of all. We see in this the convergence of both global and local computing issues but also the potential utility of text mining and ontologies to build a degree of semantic understanding into the infrastructure itself. Consider this: A medical scientist records a single clinical observation on a palmtop device, which is copied to a central database via a wireless LAN and is integrated with like information from a hundred other observers, together with data extracted from a 40-year-old microbiology journal, thus allowing a bioinformatician to run a dynamic metabolomic simulation of host-pathogen interactions. This in turn informs critical decision making within an antibiotic discovery project. Such a reality, manifest as routine, is still someway off, but the concept is nonetheless compelling.

5.7 DISCUSSION AND CONCLUSION

Genomics has transformed the world. Or, rather, it has altered the intellectual landscape of the biosciences: Its implications suggest that we should be able to gain access to information about biological function at a rate and on a scale previously inconceivable. Of course, our hopes and expectations remain unfulfilled. Like Watson and Crick's 1953 structure of DNA, the complete sequencing of the human genome has simply suggested more questions than it answers: It is the beginning not the end. What we can conceive of still far exceeds what can actually be done. Experimental science is playing catch-up, developing postgenomic strategies that can exploit the information explosion implicit within genomics. Biology remains at risk of being overwhelmed by the deluge of new data on a hitherto unknown scale and complexity. The trick is to pull out the useful and discard the worthless, yielding first knowledge and then true understanding and the ability to efficiently manipulate biological systems.

One of the tasks of modern drug research is to evaluate this embarrassment of riches. Can we reduce incoherent data into usable and comprehensible information? Can we extract knowledge from this information? How much useful data is locked away in the literature? Can we ultimately draw out understanding from the accumulation of knowledge? One way that we can attack this problem is through computer-based informatics techniques, including bioinformatics. This is not meant, of course, to replace human involvement in the process. It is merely a powerful supplement compensating for an area where the human mind is relatively weak: the fast, accurate processing of huge data sets. Bioinformatics has already made significant contributions to drug discovery and has begun to do the same for vaccines.

Bioinformatics requires people. It always has, and probably always will. To expect informatics to behave differently from experimental science is, at best, hopeful and overly optimistic and, at worse, naive or disingenuous. Experimental science is becoming ever more reliant on instrumental analysis and robotics, yet people are still required to troubleshoot and to make sense of the results. Much the same holds for bioinformatics: We can devolve work that is routine to automation—scanning genomes, etc.—but people are still needed to ensure such automation works and to assess the results. New methods need to be developed and their results used and applied. There is only so much that putting tools on the desktops of experimentalists can achieve, useful though this is in both a tactical and a strategic sense. Annotation and reannotation is, and should be, a never-ending occupation. For that which we automate, sensible and useful ontologies still need to be built and verified. The dynamic interplay between people and algorithms remains at the heart of bioinformatics. Long may it be so: That's what makes it fun.

Academic bioinformaticians often forget their place as an intermediate taking, interpreting, and ultimately returning data from one experimental scientist to another. There is a need for bioinformatics to keep in close touch with wet laboratory biologists, servicing and supporting their needs, either directly or indirectly, rather than becoming obsessed with their own recondite or self-referential concerns. Moreover, it is important to realize, and reflect upon, our own shortcomings. Central to the quest to achieve automated gene elucidation and characterization are pivotal concepts regarding the manifestation of protein function and the nature of sequence-structure and sequence-function relations. The use of computers to model these concepts is limited by our currently limited understanding, in a physicochemical rather than phenomenological sense, of even simple biological processes. Understanding and accepting what cannot be done informs our appreciation of what can be done. In the absence of such an understanding, it is easy to be misled, as specious arguments are used to promulgate overenthusiastic notions of what particular methods can achieve. The road ahead must be paved with caution and pragmatism. The future belongs, or should belong, to those scientists who are able to master both computational and experimental disciplines.

ACKNOWLEDGMENTS

I should like to thank all my colleagues, past and present, whose attitudes and opinions have helped to shape my views of drug and vaccine discovery.

REFERENCES

1. Edwards AM, Howell JBL. The chromones: history, chemistry and clinical development. A tribute to the work of Dr R. E. C. Altounyan. *Clin Exp Allergy* 2000;30:756–74.
2. Lipman DJ, Pearson WR. Rapid and sensitive protein similarity searches. *Science* 1985;227:1435–41.
3. Altschul SF, Madden TL, Schaffer AA, Zhang J, Zhang Z, Miller W, Lipman DJ, Gapped BLAST and PSI-BLAST: a new generation of protein database search programs. *Nucleic Acids Res* 1997;25:3389–402.
4. Discala C, Benigni X, Barillot E, Vaysseix G. DBcat: a catalog of 500 biological databases. *Nucleic Acids Res* 2000;28:8–9.
5. Linial M. How incorrect annotations evolve—the case of short ORFs. *Trends Biotechnol* 2003;21:298–300.

6. Gilks WR, Audit B, De Angelis D, Tsoka S, Ouzounis CA. Modeling the percolation of annotation errors in a database of protein sequences. *Bioinformatics* 2000;18:1641–9.
7. Attwood TK. The role of pattern databases in sequence analysis. *Brief Bioinform* 2000;1:45–59.
8. International Human Genome Sequencing Consortium. Finishing the euchromatic sequence of the human genome. *Nature* 2004;431:931–45.
9. Ji H, Zhou Q, Wen F, Xia H, Lu X, Li Y. AsMamDB: an alternative splice database of mammals *Nucleic Acids Res* 2001;29:260–3.
10. Perler FB. InBase: the Intein Database. *Nucleic Acids Res* 2002;30:383–384.
11. Hopkins AL, Groom CR. The druggable genome. *Nat Rev Drug Discov* 2002;1:727–30.
12. Flower DR. Towards *in silico* prediction of immunogenic epitopes. *Trends Immunol* 2003;24:667–74.

6

SYSTEMS APPROACHES FOR PHARMACEUTICAL RESEARCH AND DEVELOPMENT

SEAN EKINS AND CRAIG N. GIROUX

Contents

6.1 INTRODUCING SYSTEMS BIOLOGY AND SYSTEMS PHARMACOLOGY

There is rarely one target for a disease, and drug design strategies are increasingly focused on multiple targets [1]. Developing effective treatments that do not interfere with other biological pathways is therefore difficult. However, there are ways to assess this impact beyond the target protein. One approach is to measure many parameters under well-defined conditions, analyze with computational biology methods, and produce a model that may also help to understand the likely side effects [2]. High-throughput screening data are routinely generated early in drug discovery for molecules of interest to determine biological activities toward both the desirable and undesirable targets

Computer Applications in Pharmaceutical Research and Development, Edited by Sean Ekins.
ISBN 0-471-73779-8

and to understand their physicochemical properties. Higher-content biological data are also generated after cells or animals are treated with a molecule and the levels of metabolites, genes, and proteins are determined. The combination of the reductionist approach for a molecule binding to one or more particular proteins with the global effect on metabolism, gene expression, and transcription as a whole system is therefore important for understanding efficacy and toxicity. Systems biology aims to quantify all of these molecular elements of a biological system and integrate them into graphical models [3]. Systems perspectives have been applied in most scientific fields such that "studying biology as an integrated system of genetic, protein, metabolite, cellular, and pathway events that are in flux and interdependent" has become a catch-all definition. Systems biology therefore requires the integration of many different scientific areas and complex data types to result in a complete picture and ultimately can be used to derive valuable knowledge. The evolution of systems biology approaches has been recently described to show the convergence of mainstream "data-rich" molecular biology and data-poor systems analysis [4]. The systems approach can be applied beyond pharmaceutical research to areas such as nutrigenomics, as the human diet consists of complex mixtures of molecules that are likely to impact gene responses. Such an approach is useful in understanding the risk-benefit analysis of bioactive foods. Biomarkers will also be required to determine effects that predict chronic effects of molecules we are exposed to [5]. Within systems biology there are simultaneously growing computational fields, such as computational molecular biology [6], the modeling of genetic and biochemical networks [7] that covers aspects from alignment of sequences, modeling activity of genes, gene expression, cell cycle regulation, proteomics, and others.

Systems biology can therefore be considered as the application of systems theory to genomics as well as the creation of an understanding of the relationships between biological objects. We are therefore seeing a shift in focus from molecular characterization to an understanding of functional activity in genomics. Systems biology provides methods for understanding the organization and dynamics of the genetic pathways [8]. The major focus of systems biology to date has been statistics and database generation [9]. Systems pharmacology describes the integrated responses resulting from complex interactions between molecules, cells, and tissues. Such studies are important because isolated molecules and cells in vitro do not display all of the properties possessed in vivo reflected by the function of intact tissues, organs, and organ systems.

A systems level approach can be used to address three questions: What are the parts? How do they work? How do they work together to perform their biological function? The application of systems approaches to physiology has not been widely accepted, however. Although within physiology departments physiology and integrative research were recognized as key components of the NIH road map, the importance of interdisciplinary research to generate systems models has also been stressed previously [10]. Systems approaches have been applied to make use of the vast amounts of qualitative and quantitative biological data collated in the various databases along with network-building algorithms. These can be used to build predictive signatures for diseases following treatment of cell or tissues with molecules. Similarly, microarray data from cells or animals treated with drugs can also be used to generate pathway maps or gene network signatures [11–14]. An early attempt to illustrate the many levels of relationships between genetics and physiology was made by Palsson [15], who captured and linked process databases from genes to proteins, to whole cells. Although biological systems contain many nonlinear processes that are continually interacting, a reductionist viewpoint is to treat parallel systems as an engineering process [16]. A systems-based approach has also been suggested for protein structural dynamics and signal transduction [17]. Simple protein networks can display complex behavior. For example, proteins in gene regulatory networks and signal transduction pathways show cooperative responses including allosteric protein conformational changes [17].

Numerous methods are used to connect information from functional genomic studies to biological function. Cluster analysis methods have traditionally been used for inferring the correlation between genes and have been integrated with existing information on biological pathways to reconstruct novel biological networks [18]. At least three theoretical methods for understanding all the genes and proteins exist: (1) kinetic models of small isolated circuits [19, 20], (2) gene expression arrays [21], and (3) a suggested ensemble approach using Boolean networks of genes that can be modeled as on-off alongside microarrays that enable the measurement of sophisticated dynamical features or real gene networks [22]. Systems biology approaches have been applied to understanding the network responses of DNA-damaging agents as well as other drugs. Most studies work with yeast, using large experiments with multiple treatments and hundreds of microarrays that can also use mutant strains. Using networks to describe cellular responses to damage helps account for different levels of influence in the cells. It is suggested that network responses may dictate the efficiency of DNA repair, genome stability and viability after damage. Small perturbations can therefore have more distant effects, and it is also likely because of redundancy that multiple proteins can have the same effect. A network approach may help researchers connect the many genes and proteins implicated in damage response [23]. The systems pharmacology approach includes *in silico* biology, biological pathways, disease modeling, and medical physiology incorporating cell and organ models.

6.2 SYSTEMS BIOLOGY: COMMERCIAL APPLICATIONS

A recent review has described the numerous commercial concerns that are involved in systems biology by providing either software or services [24]. Large, curated interaction databases combined with powerful analytical and network building tools are commercially available from companies like GeneGo Inc. (MetaCore™), Ariadne Genomics Inc. (Pathway Studio), Ingenuity Inc. (Pathways Analysis™), and Jubilant Biosys (PathArt™) that cover human metabolism, regulation, and signaling (Table 6.1). Currently there are hundreds of pathway databases, but they lack uniform data models and access, making pathway integration difficult (see the Pathway resource list, http://cbio.mskcc.org/prl). These tools can readily enable the visualization of global cellular mechanisms that drive the differences in gene expression by overlaying these data on the networks to discover relationships in such complexity. To date these approaches have been applied to modeling nuclear hormone receptor interactions [25], the generation of compound-related gene network signatures [26], and combining networks with metabolite prediction tools [27]. These systems pharmacology methods have a role in drug discovery when combined with the other computational and empirical approaches to identify biomarkers and understand interindividual variability in response to drugs [28, 29].

Several companies such as Gene Network Sciences [30], Entelos [31], and BioSeek [32] have emerged in recent years that focus on simulating cellular pathways, organs, whole cells, or whole diseases. Gene Network Sciences has developed an approach to predicting how external perturbations to the genetic and protein pathways of cells change cell and disease phenotypes, together with the molecular profiles underlying the altered phenotypes. They use a two-pronged approach of (1) inferring unknown pathway relationships from experimental data (inference modeling can both identify new and confirm existing biological relations with approaches based on reverse engineering, machine learning algorithms, and data-mining techniques) and (2) creating mechanistic dynamic simulations of known pathways. The mechanistic modeling approach implements known biology via dynamical simulations of pathways, cells, and organ- and tissue-level models. This approach determines the mechanism of action, biomarkers, and tissue specificity of new chemical entities, enhancing the accuracy of the predictive outputs. These mechanistic simulations are proposed to facilitate the rapid testing of "what if" hypotheses and become increasingly accurate through iteration with validation experiments. To date this company has described modeling the human cancer cell [30], using the Diagrammatic Cell Language to create a network model of interconnected signal transduction pathways and gene expression circuitry that control human cell proliferation and apoptosis. This model included receptor activation and mitogenic signaling, initiation of cell cycle, and passage of checkpoints and apoptosis. The efficacy of various drug targets was evaluated with this model, and experiments were performed to test the predictions.

A second company in this arena, Entelos, has over the past decade developed numerous disease PhysioLabs. These include comprehensive disease maps that are connected by validated mathematical equations, a knowledge management infrastructure with links to papers and documentation, and

TABLE 6.1 Network Building and High-Throughput Data Analysis Tools

Software	Website	Description of function and network algorithms used for gene network visualization	References
MetaDrug	http://www.genego.com	Prediction of metabolism and toxicology with rules and QSAR models. Analysis of high-throughput data on networks and static maps. Autoexpand, analyze network algorithms	27, 89–91
MetaCore	http://www.genego.com	Analysis of high-throughput data on networks and static maps Analyze network, shortest paths, direct interactions, autoexpand, analyze transcriptional regulation, self regulations, and expand by one interaction	11, 42–48, 89, 92
PathwayAnalysis	http://www.ingenuity.com/	Analysis of microarray data Direct interactions	12, 93–96
PathArt	http://www.jubilantbiosys.com/	Analysis of microarray data Shortest path and the alternative paths between any two components	97
PathwayStudio	http://www.ariadnegenomics.com/	Analysis of microarray data Direct interactions, shortest path, common targets or common regulators	98–101

TABLE 6.1 *Continued*

Software	Website	Description of function and network algorithms used for gene network visualization	References
Osprey	http://biodata.mshri.on.ca/osprey/servlet/Index	Network building software. One Circle, Concentric, Dual Ring, Spokes, Spoked Dual Ring	102
GeneWays	http://geneways.genomecenter.columbia.edu/	Network building software Direct interactions	68
CellDesigner	http://celldesigner.org/	A process diagram editor	103
GRAPHVIZ	http://www.graphviz.org/	Network building software. 2D-scaling	32, 66
Cytoscape	http://www.cytoscape.org/	Network building software Spring embedded layout, hierarchical layout, circular layout	104
BioTapestry	http://labs.systemsbiology.net/bolouri/soft ware/BioTapestry/	Interactive tool for building, visualizing, and simulating genetic regulatory networks	105
Pajek	http://vlado.fmf.uni-lj.si/pub/networks/pajek/	Network building software Random networks, shortest paths. Many options for network building	106
VisAnt	http://visant.bu.edu/	Network building software Relaxing layout	107, 108
GenMAPP	http://www.genmapp.org/	For viewing and analyzing gene expression data on MAPPS representing biological pathways and any other grouping of genes Tools for custom map drawing	109, 110

finally a complete virtual research workbench. This latter component allows the selection of virtual patients, targets, and the performance of simulations. To date they have produced an asthma model, a cardiac model, an obesity model, a rheumatoid arthritis model, and an adipocyte model that have been used with a number of pharmaceutical partners (Table 6.2).

BioSeek has analyzed a limited number of genes in cultured primary endothelial cells and used this model to assess different treatments. Seven proteins under four perturbing conditions could capture pathways for 25 different proteins. The networks were captured by multidimensional scaling using Graphiz. The overall approach is called BioMAP and represents a method to simplify systems biology [32, 33]. Other companies (such as Icoria and BG Medicine) have already generated or are generating large complex data sets and using network type visualization for analysis. These platforms are suggested to enable discovery scientists to analyze data streams from gene expression, biochemical profiles, and quantitative tissue analysis and to map them into biological pathways useful for biomarker identification for disease areas such as diabetes, obesity, and liver injury.

An alternative approach to the use of complex data sets for the evaluation of drug- and chemical-induced changes in cellular pathways has been taken by several companies, including Rosetta Inpharmatics [34], GeneLogic [35], and Iconix[36], which have established large chemogenomic databases comprised of a broad spectrum of perturbations to the genetic network that are obtained by chemical or mutational insult. In this approach, the gene expression profile of exposure to a test pharmaceutical compound is compared against the reference profiles in the compendium database. Pattern-matching algorithms are then applied to predict the expression signature and cellular pathways that are affected by the new drug [37, 38]. For new compounds that have been identified by target-based screening, this approach could identify secondary or "off-target" pathways and thus indicate potential adverse effects of the drug. In addition, this approach may be particularly useful for new compounds identified by phenotypic screening with high-throughput screening cell-based assays or for similar situations in which the drug target is not immediately evident [39].

6.3 APPLICATIONS OF GENE NETWORK AND PATHWAY TOOLS

Pathway and gene network tools have found numerous applications for understanding gene and protein expression in various circumstances, whether during disease or after treatment with a particular molecule. A recent review has described the tools for building biological networks that can be used for the analysis of experimental data in drug discovery [40]. The putative applications include target identification, validation, and prioritization. The methods available can be used to define toxicity biomarkers and for lead optimization

TABLE 6.2 Pharmaceutical Companies and Their Systems Biology Portfolios of Commercial Software and Collaborations Based on Press Releases, Posters at Scientific Meetings and Information on Vendor Websites

Company	Network Tools	Disease Models	Ontologies	Systems Biology Collaborations
Astra Zeneca		EOM	BW	BG, MIT
Bayer	JPA	EAM	EG	
Bristol-Myers Squibb	GGMC	EOM		
Eli Lilly				Lilly Systems Biology (Singapore)
Glaxo-Smith-Kline	IPA, GGMC, JPA		BW	BG
Johnson & Johnson	IPA, GGMC	ECM, EOM, GNS		
Merck	IPA			ISB
Novartis	JPA			BG
Organon	GGMC	ERAM		
Pfizer	IPA	EAM		
P&G	GGMC			
Roche	IPA, BSS	TBAG		
Sanofi-Aventis	IPA	EAM		
TNO	GGMC			GGMC
Wyeth	IPA			

Companies may have either accessed these technologies or continue to use them as standalone or integrated with proprietary technologies. These portfolios may be in addition to internal software efforts that are likely to be ongoing.

Abbreviations: BG, BG Medicine; EAM, Entelos Asthma Model; ECM, Entelos Cardiac model; EOM, Entelos Obesity Model; ERMA, Entelos Rheumatoid Arthritis Model; GGMC, GeneGo MetaCore; GNS, Gene Network Systems Oncology Model; IPA, Ingenuity Pathway Analysis; JPA, Jubilant PathArt, ISB, Institute for Systems Biology, Massachusetts Institute of Technology's Computational and Systems Biology Initiative. The Bio-Analytics Group ("TBAG") and BIOSoftware Systems ("BSS"); EG, Electric Genetics eVoke.

or candidate selection. Clinical data can also be analyzed and may be useful to provide new indications for marketed drugs or as a means to perform postmarketing studies.

One of the few instances where systems biology research from a major commercial concern (namely Proctor and Gamble) has been published concerns a study using gene expression data to identify stress response networks in *Mycobacterium tuberculosis* before and after treatment with different drugs [41]. The research combined the KEGG and BioCyc protein interaction databases with previously published expression data and a k-shortest path algorithm. It was found that networks for isoniazid and hydrogen peroxide indicated a generic stress response that highlighted unique features. The authors suggested that differential network expression can be used to assess drug mode of action with similar networks indicating similar mechanisms [41]. A second recently published study combined microarray expression data from HeLa cells with Ingenuity pathways software to understand the expression of DBC2. The authors were able to find two networks that had at least 50% of the genes that were affected by DBC2 expression. These corresponded to cell cycle control, apoptosis, and cytoskeleton and membrane trafficking [12]. Several other applications of this software have also been published (Table 6.1).

A growing number of studies to date presented as meeting abstracts have used MetaCore software for genomic and proteomic data analysis. Yang et al. used a proteomic analysis to examine the targets of oxidative stress in brain tissue from the PS1/APP mouse model for Alzheimer disease and visualized these targets as a network and highlighted the proteins that are oxidatively modified [42]. Waters et al. integrated microarray and proteomic data studies with pathway analysis and network modeling of epidermal growth factor signaling in human mammary epithelial cells and identified new cross talk mediators Src and matrix metalloproteinases as responsible for modification of the extracellular matrix [43]. Lantz et al. studied protein expression in rats exposed to arsenic in utero. Twelve proteins involved in signal transduction, cytoskeleton, nuclear organization, and DNA repair were differentially expressed and could be readily connected as a network to identify the potential involvement of RAC1, Pyk2, CDC42, JNK, and occludins as sites of action for arsenic [44]. Nie et al. produced a gene signature for nongenotoxic carcinogens after establishing a database of more than 100 hepatotoxicants and used a stepwise exhaustive search algorithm. Ultimately, six genes were selected to differentiate nongenotoxic carcinogens from noncarcinogens [45]. A mouse emphysema model treated with elastase was used to show 95 genes that were differentially expressed after 1 week [46]. These data were analyzed with pathway maps and gene networks to show that the principal nodes of gene regulation were around the vitamin D receptor, Ca^{2+}, MMP13, and the transcription factors c-myc and SP1. The myometrial events in guinea pigs during pregnancy were studied, using gene expression, signaling and metabolic maps, and gene networks to provide a global and comprehensive analysis for visualizing and understanding the dynamics of myometrial activation [47]. Further work from the same group has focused on G proteins, showing increased GTPase activity during pregnancy in guinea pigs, an effect also seen with estradiol [48]. The data in this study were visualized on metabolic maps and gene networks.

An algorithm for the reconstruction of accurate cellular networks (ARACNe) was recently described and used to reconstruct expression profiles of human B cells. ARACNe identifies statistically significant gene-gene coregulation and eliminates indirect interactions. Using 336 expression profiles after perturbing B cell phenotypes, a network was inferred. MYC appeared in the top 5% of cellular hubs, and the network consisted of 40% of previously identified target genes [49]. HCN-1A cells treated with different drugs were used to produce a compendium of gene signatures that was used to generate "sampling over gene space" models with random forests, linear discriminant analysis, and support vector machines. This approach was then used to classify drug classes, potentially representing a novel method for drug discovery as it discriminates physiologically active from inactive molecules and could identify drugs with off-target effects and assign confidence in their further assessment [38].

With a similar compendium-based comparative approach, the oxidative stress-inducing potential of over 50 new proprietary compounds under investigation at Johnson and Johnson was predicted from their matching gene expression signatures [50]. This study is particularly informative in that it was able to distinguish distinct mechanisms of action for diverse hepatotoxicants, all of which similarly resulted in oxidative stress, an adverse cellular condition. Initial successes such as this example suggest that gene expression signatures have potential utility in the detection of presymptomatic clinical conditions and in the molecular diagnosis of disease states. The ability to group patients who share a common disease phenotype or set of clinical symptoms by their gene expression signature is a critical milestone in achieving the goal of personalized and predictive medicine [51].

Numerous mechanisms have been proposed for hypertension, and subsequently there are many microarray studies with large amounts of data but little new information on mechanism to date. Therefore more complete sets of data and integration that may contribute to better therapeutic outcome and disease prevention are needed [52]. Ninety-two genes associated with atherosclerosis were used to generate a network with KEGG and Biocarta previously. Thirty-nine of these genes are in pathways containing at least three atherosclerosis genes, which represented 16 biological and signaling pathways with 353 unique genes. Numerous genes not previously associated with atherosclerosis were indicated on the network [53]. In contrast, the use of the commercially available tool MetaCore with this gene list enabled the mapping of 89 genes on networks, and 68 of these genes were on maps, with only three missing from this mapping. This set of genes was then used with the analyze networks algorithm to generate multiple networks. The network with the largest G-score (Fig. 6.1A, 35.72, $p = 6.1e^{-61}$) was different from that with the highest p-value (Fig. 6.1B, 13.44, $p = 2.7e^{-77}$). The former contained APOE and APOA1 as central hubs and also mapped onto the GO processes for cholesterol homeostasis ($p = 10e^{-14}$) and cholesterol metabolism ($p = 6.4e^{-13}$), whereas the latter had NF-κB as a hub gene and mapped to the inflammatory response ($p = 1.6e^{-16}$) and the immune response ($3.4e^{-10}$). There were several genes that were absent from the initial gene list identified in the original publication [53] but appear on either network including C/EBPα, EDNRβ, C/EBP, CRP, Brca1, CYP27B1, CYP2C8, PSAP, Calreticulin, Serglycin, MAPK7, MAPK1/3, α 2M, APP, Amyloid β, and Matrilysin. These may represent future genes to be assessed for their importance in hypertension.

Understanding the gene networks that can be generated in cells or whole organisms by single compounds enables the generation of signature networks [11]. Numerous recent studies have generated microarray data after treatment with xenobiotics (Table 6.3) that can be used with network and pathway database tools. Many other examples that have been recently summarized could also be used in this way [54]. For example, the anticancer activity of tanshinone IIA was evaluated against human breast cancer MCF-7 cells, and the changes in gene expression were evaluated over 72h with a microarray containing over 3000 genes [55]. The resultant data for 65 genes that were either significantly up- or downregulated were used as an input for MetaCore, and 48 of these genes were able to be used for network generation. The analyze networks algorithm was then used to generate multiple networks. The best G-score was 31.29 and $p = 6.24\ e^{-40}$ (Fig. 6.2A), whereas the best p-value network had a G-score of 13.17, $p = 3.41e^{-47}$ (Fig. 6.2B). The Gene ontology processes were mapped to these, and for the best G-score network cell adhesion $p = 6.29e^{-07}$ was the most significant, although the majority of genes were involved in the cell cycle $p = 1.32e^{-05}$ or apoptosis $p = 3.44e^{-05}$. The best p-score network indicated a role in the cell cycle $p = 1.33e^{-12}$, as over 30% of the genes were involved in this process. In both networks there were numerous genes that were not significantly up- or downregulated but nonetheless are present on these statistically significant networks. This type of approach has been taken for another anticancer drug, Tipifarnib, a non-peptidomimetic competitive farnesyltransferase inhibitor used for treatment in acute myeloid leukemia [56]. Gene expression analysis in three cell lines and blast cells from patients indicated a common set of 72 genes that were mapped onto cell signaling, cytoskeletal, immunity, and apoptosis pathways with Ingenuity Pathways Analysis [56]. Another published method has previously used GO annotations and correspondence analysis to generate a map of genes in human pancreatic cancer [57]. It is likely that an approach like this combining high-content data with curated databases and gene networks may be applicable to analysis of other diseases and available therapeutic treatments.

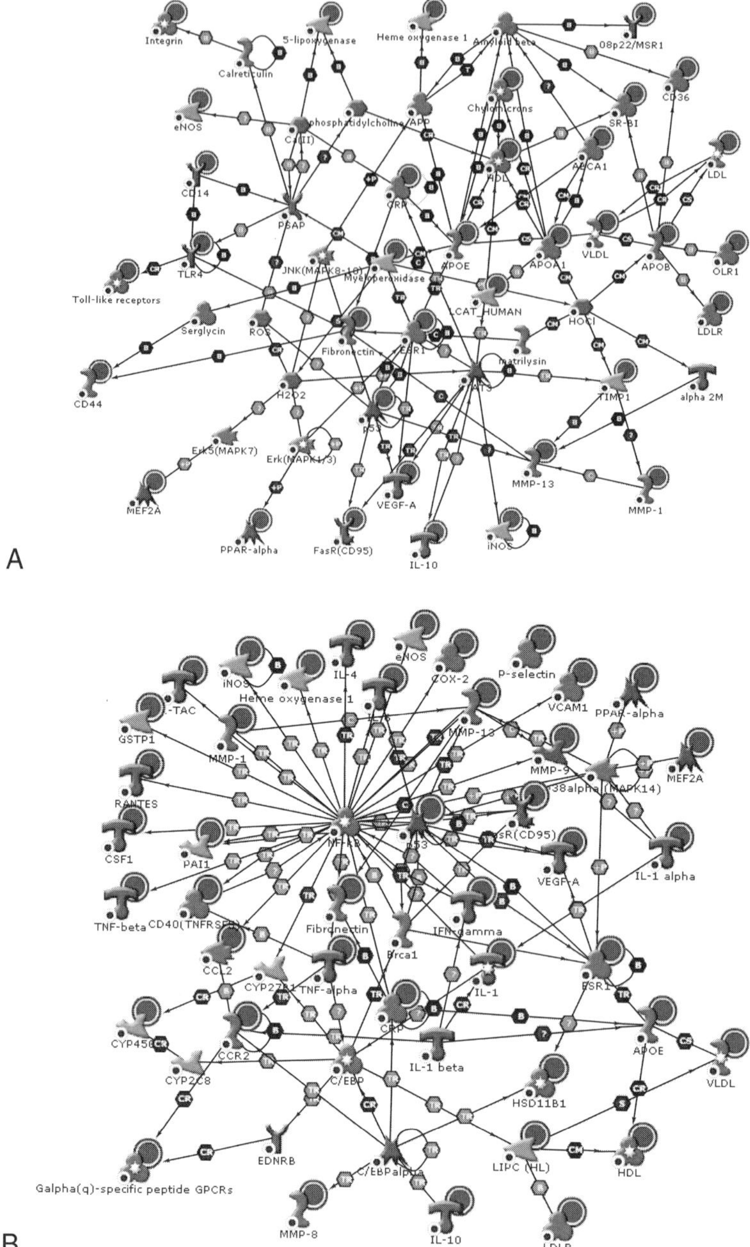

Figure 6.1 Gene interaction networks for atherosclerosis generated with the gene list from Ghazalpour et al. [53] with MetaCore™ (GeneGo, St. Joseph, MI). A. best G-score. B. best p value. The interaction types between nodes are shown as small colored hexagons, e.g., unspecified, allosteric regulation, binding, cleavage, competition, covalent modification, dephosphorylation, phosphorylation, transcription regulation, transformation. When applicable, interactions also have a positive or negative effect and direction. Ligands (purple) linked to other proteins (blue), transfactors (red), enzymes (orange). Genes with red dots represent the members of the original input gene list. See color plate.

TABLE 6.3 Literature Data That Could Be Used to Create Compound Signature Networks

Compounds	Tissue Source	Microarray type	Compounds	Data Availability	Reference
Docetaxel (Taxotere) Estramustine	Human prostate cancer cells PC3 and LNCaP	Affymetrix U133A	2 nmol/l Docetaxel 4 μmol/l Estramustine combination of 1 nmol/l Docetaxel and 2 μmol/l Estramustine for 6, 36 and 72 h	Gene name, accession number and fold change data in a manuscript table	111
Taxotere Capecitabine (Furtulon)	Human prostate cancer cells PC3 and LNCaP	Affymetrix U133A	2 nM Taxotere, 110 μM capecitabine combination of 1 nM taxotere and 50 μM capecitabine for 6, 36 and 72 h	Gene name, accession number and fold change data in a manuscript table	112
Nobiletin	Human HepG2 cells	Acegene human oligo chip subset A	10–3 M	Gene name	113
Allopregnanolone	Rat hippocampal neurons	Cell Cycle GEArray Q series, version 1	500 nM	Gene name and fold change on a bar chart	114
Palmitate	Human hepatic Huh-7	Custom	150 μM for 24 and 48 h	Gene name, fold change as accession number, tables	115
Letrozole Anastrozole Tamoxifen	MCF-7aro	Affymetrix U133A	200 nmol/l Letrozole 1 μmol/l Anastrozole 1 μmol/l Tamoxifen	Gene symbol, GenBank identifier, gene name, ratio as a table	13

TABLE 6.3 *Continued*

Compounds	Tissue Source	Microarray type	Compounds	Data Availability	Reference
Tanshinone IIA	MCF-7	HO4 ExpressChip	0.25 μg/ml Tanshinone IIA	Gene name, Unigene symbol and Unigene identifier, fold change	55
N-Hydroxy-4-acetylaminobiphenyl Benzo[*a*]pyrene diol epoxide	Human TK6 lymphoblastoid	Custom	*N*-Hydroxy-4-acetylaminobiphenyl 10 μM for 27 h Benzo[*a*]pyrene diol epoxide 10 μM for 1 h	Gene name, gene symbol, gene bank accession fold change in a table All data available online	116
Estradiol Medroxyprogesterone acetate	Human microvascular endometrial endothelial cells	Affymetrix U133A	E2 10^{-8} M, MDA 10^{-7} M for 48 h	Gene name, fold change	117
Genistein Daidzen Glycitein 17β-Estradiol	MCF-7	Custom	Genistein 10 μM Daidzen 10 μM Glycitein 10 μM 17β-Estradiol 10 nM	Gene name, Accession number, fold change in table	118
17β-Estradiol	Human endometrium	Affymetrix U133A	17β-Estradiol 1 nM	Gene name, Gene symbol, Accession number, fold change in table	119
Δ-9-tetrahydrocannabinol	4T1-stimulated lymph node cells from mice	GEArray Q series mouse TH1, Th2, Th3 array membranes	50 mg/kg Δ-9-tetrahydrocannabinol	Gene name, accession number and fold change in table	120

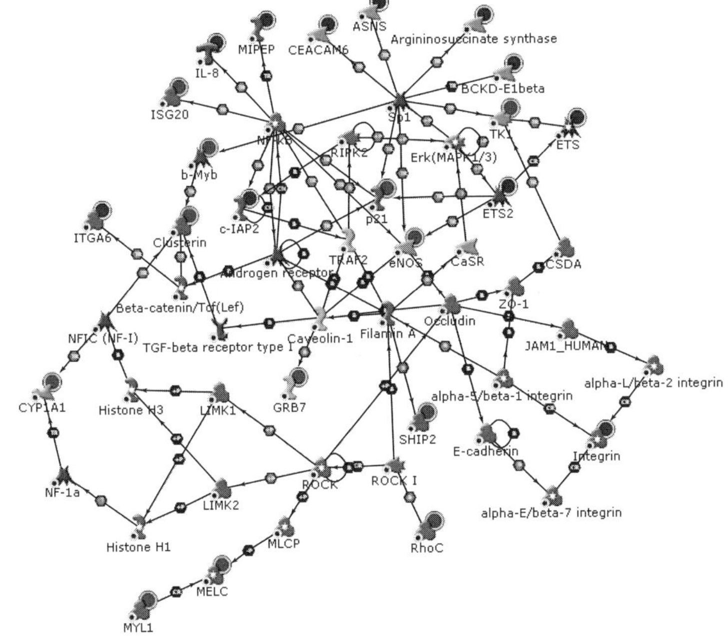

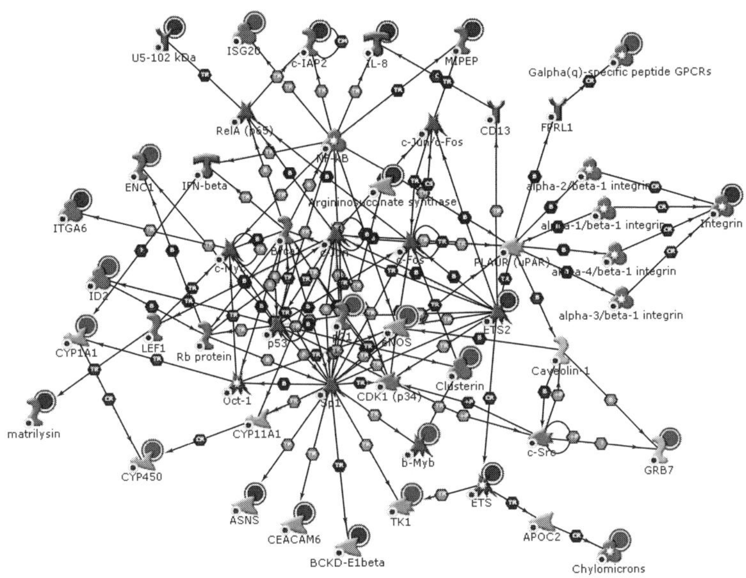

Figure 6.2 Gene interaction networks for tanshinone IIA-treated MCF-7 cells for 72h [55] were generated with MetaCore™ (GeneGo). A. best G-score. B. best p value. The interaction types between nodes are shown as small colored hexagons, e. g., unspecified, allosteric regulation, binding, cleavage, competition, covalent modification, dephosphorylation, phosphorylation, transcription regulation, transformation. When applicable, interactions also have a positive or negative effect and direction. Ligands (purple) linked to other proteins (blue), transfactors (red), enzymes (orange). Genes with red dots represent the members of the original input gene list that were upregulated, whereas blue dots represent downregulated genes. See color plate.

6.4 DATA UTILIZATION, EXTRACTION, AND STANDARDS

Currently the NIH road map is driving a systems biology agenda, with academia and government trying to facilitate this. Systems biology at the moment is significantly dominated by genomic experimental data and networks, and it is perhaps telling that the NIH and FDA have access to virtually all commercially available network-building software and databases. The FDA has released a guidance for industry on the use of pharmacogenomics data for drug safety evaluation and is actively working to establish reference data standards in this area [58]. The National Institute of General Medical Sciences supports systems biology research for the areas that are central to its mission of supporting basic biomedical research and focuses on developing new computational approaches to biomedical complexity. Besides the government, the biotechnology industry and pharmaceutical companies are major stakeholders in research progress and in utilizing the government investment in the most effective manner [24]. To date, however, the pharmaceutical industry in the majority of cases has concentrated on the acquisition of technologies and collaborative agreements with companies and academia, rather than expending significant resources in developing them internally. The pharmaceutical industry is thought likely to learn from engineering-based industries that have worked on open software standards and models to enable their integration and use by many groups. Consortia such as those facilitated by ESCHER (http://www.escherinstitute.org/) and funded by the US government have enabled an open source software repository. The Defense Advanced Research Projects Agency (DARPA) sponsored a workshop, Tool and Software Infrastructure in Systems Biology Workshop, (Arlington, VA, February 17–18, 2005) that suggested we will see the development of a similar independent organization for applying open standards for systems biology. The involvement of DARPA is hence indicative of the strategic importance of computational models and systems biology in general for the health sciences. An international consortium is developing a Systems Biology Markup Language (SBML) and a cross-platform Systems Biology Workbench (SBW) to facilitate integration of different data types and algorithms into a common computational environment for systems analysis [59, 60]. The SBW platform is integrated with the BioSPICE cellular modeling platform, a current DARPA initiative. A modular approach to model development would ensure that each drug company could advance those models that preceded it, and this would be a considerable advantage over each company developing proprietary tools.

With the considerable output of high-throughput screening one would expect this type of data to be combined with that from genomic and chemoinformatic studies. For example, large databases of high-throughput screening content are available either in companies internally or from vendors such as CEREP. These data can be used for QSAR modeling or for producing a spectrum or profile at a single concentration [61], representing a way to compare molecules and their biological profiles [54]. Ideally it would be useful to know the interactions of a molecule with all proteins, but this is only currently possible with microarray type approaches and is highly dependent on many other factors. Metabolomic data from metabolite profiling that measures many metabolites in parallel to provide information on the complex regulatory circuits must also be integrated with other data for systems biology. The metabolites can be plotted as networks with nodes connected by edges describing relationships [62]. Constructing networks from metabolomics data is difficult as the structural identification of many uncharacterized endogenous metabolites is still ongoing [63]; however, the scale-free nature of networks may suggest it is possible.

It is essential to have as much pathway information as possible to build reliable and meaningful networks, and several companies are likely to have already integrated commercial databases with their own proprietary databases, network, and analysis tools. There is also currently an urgent need for data standards to facilitate future integration efforts [64]. BioPAX is one such standardization approach from the biopathways community to facilitate easy information retrieval from different pathway resources such as signal transduction, gene regulation, and interaction databases [65]. The continual extraction of a huge amount of information arising from whole-genome analyses is a significant challenge and requires powerful computational methods. An early application of Natural Language Processing (NLP) extracted data from MEDLINE and GO and generated tools for gene expression analysis called PubGene. When compared with the manually curated databases DIP and OMIM, PubGene captured 51% and 45% of gene pairs, respectively [66]. A second NLP-type analysis has focused on Alzheimer disease and used molecular triangulation with many data types to generate networks and search for genes that are close to known genes important for the disease. Another tool called GeneWays has been used to extract literature data and, interestingly, was used to compute a topology-subtracted p-value that corrects for being close to a highly connected node, which would normally give a highly significant raw p-value [67]. This approach combined genetic and molecular pathway information to identify further possible disease-related genes. GeneWays is an integrated system that combines automated selection of articles, or automated extraction of information using natural language processing. It analyzes interactions between molecular substances, drawing on many sources of information and inferring a consensus view of molecular networks. GeneWays is designed as an open platform, analyzing interactions between molecular substances by using many sources of information [68]. A further program, CoPub Mapper, identifies and rates copublished genes and keywords. This can be used to group genes from microarray data [69]. New semantic technologies (semantics describes the meaning of words) based on ontologies can be used to integrate knowledge that can be reused by different applications using technologies such as the BioWisdom software [70]. This offers the advantage of tying together different data sources by providing a common vocabulary using names and synonyms with associated properties. These NLP and semantic efforts are important as the amount of information generated both in the public arena and inside companies is increasing at a rapid pace such that manually curated databases will not be economical in the future and it will be critical to integrate the different names into a controlled vocabulary of objects across databases.

NLP systems are being developed to address the increasingly challenging problem of data mining for systems level content from the published literature, that is, integrating across the global expert database of biomedical research [71]. One recent approach to this problem was to develop a web-based tool, PubNet, that is able to visualize concept and theme networks derived from the PubMed literature [72].

As biomedical data resources become increasingly shared and virtual, a common web-accessible infrastructure is required to ensure effective communication among data warehouses (resource providers) and data miners (resource end users). To this end, the National Cancer Institute is developing the caCORE initiative, which provides a common infrastructure for cancer informatics [73]. The integration of molecular "omics" data with clinical data, often categorical or descriptive, is particularly problematic. One solution to this problem for systems toxicology is being developed by the National Institute of Environmental Health Sciences as the Chemical Effects in Biological Systems (CEBS) knowledge base [74]. Much more than a relational database, this computational platform requires development of both an object model that can integrate disparate toxicological and molecular data types and a controlled vocabulary to capture the information content of phenotypic descriptions [75, 76]. In the future, subdiscipline-specific informatics platforms, such as those described here for cancer and toxicology, will themselves need to be combined to enable a fully integrated biomedical systems biology perspective.

6.5 SYSTEMS BIOLOGY AND FUTURE HEALTH CARE

The emerging field of systems biology provides a conceptual framework on which to build an integrated computational model of the complex genetic network that mediates an individual's state of health. The tools to construct such an integrated biomedical systems model are being provided by new high-throughput "omics"-based methods followed by application of computational algorithms for forward and reverse engineering to the systems parameters captured by these molecular profiling technologies. The goal of this biomedical systems modeling is to provide a practical guide for predictive, preventive, and personalized medicine. It has been suggested that this systems approach represents a paradigm shift and that it will take 10–20 years of development and transition to achieve the ultimate goal of personalized medicine [3]. At the heart of this conceptual change is the understanding of normal and pathological processes as distinct states of genetics-based hierarchical networks [77]. One important insight that has already been realized is that biological networks from different levels of organization (e.g., metabolic, protein interactions, regulatory, cell interactions, tissue and organ interactions, and even populations of individuals) share the same global architecture [78, 79]. The small-world property of biological networks, the high degree of connectivity between nodes, has profound consequences for our understanding of drug targets and of intervention strategies to correct disease states. From this systems perspective, combinatorial therapeutic strategies, designed to reprogram cellular responses by changing the local architecture of the genetic network, are likely to be more effective than traditional single target-based drug interventions. Conversely, the effects of a given drug will be dependent on its interactions with the specific genetic network state of a given individual, that is, pharmacogenetic interactions will mediate the efficacy of drug treatment in personalized medicine.

Genetic network states are dynamic, both in response to environmental stimuli and as a result of stochastic noise in the genetic circuitry [80, 81]. Thus comprehensive time course data on the changes in gene expression profiles for healthy versus disease states will need to be collected to support predictive, dynamic network models of disease progression and for prognosis for therapeutic interventions. For example, numerous attempts are ongoing to create such databases of gene, regulatory, and biochemical networks for cellular signaling processes, for example, the Alliance for Cellular Signaling [82] and the Signal Transduction Knowledge Environment (http://stke.sciencemag.org/index.dtl).

Integrative genomics therefore has the potential for ultimately mapping causal associations between gene expression profiles and disease states of the underlying cellular networks [51]. The etiologies of complex adult diseases, such as cancer, diabetes, asthma, and neurodegenerative conditions are determined by multiplex gene-environment interactions. Thus the promise of toxicogenomic modeling of risk factors for environmentally responsive disease is of particular importance and has resulted in the establishment of the Environmental Genome Project by the National Institute of Environmental Health Sciences, to provide a focus for development of a systems toxicology perspective for personalized medicine [83]. This paradigm shift for the field of drug safety evaluation and predictive risk assessment is reflected in the significant efforts to fund research that integrates toxicology, systems biology, and genomics, including initiatives that extend from the database level up to the exchange of information between different fields [84].

One could argue that the increase in publications on systems biology is a result of the increased funding and conceptual interest in this rather than the success of groundbreaking new discoveries [85]. However, initial studies in synthetic biology [86] and in pathway engineering of mammalian genetic networks [87], albeit only in the discovery stage of development at present, promise to provide practical tools for reprogramming of the cellular networks that underlie health and disease avoidance. If tailored to the specific pharmacogenetic state of an individual [88], such a set of network intervention tools would define a new class of therapeutic drug and would enable a practical implementation of personalized medicine.

Current progress in systems biology suggests that predictive, network-based analytical approaches will continue to be developed at the interface of chemoinformatics and bioinformatics, generating a broad spectrum of applications ranging from drug target selection through clinical data analysis. Given the emphasis that we are currently seeing on systems approaches within academia and the pharmaceutical industry, systems-based technologies are likely to have an increasingly important role in enabling future advances in drug discovery and development.

ACKNOWLEDGMENTS

SE gratefully acknowledges the contributions of his colleagues at GeneGo Inc. in the development of the software described. CNG acknowledges research support from EHS Center Grant P30-ES-06639 from the National Institute of Environmental Health Sciences.

REFERENCES

1. Csermely P, Agoston V, Pongor S. The efficiency of multi-target drugs: the network approach might help drug design. *Trends Pharmacol Sci* 2005;26: 178–82.
2. Walgren JL, Thompson DC. Application of proteomic technologies in the drug development process. *Toxicol Lett* 2004;149:377–85.
3. Hood L, Heath JR, Phelps ME, Lin B. Systems biology and new technologies enable predictive and preventative medicine. *Science* 2004;306:640–3.
4. Westerhoff HV, Palsson BO. The evolution of molecular biology into systems biology. *Nat Biotechnol* 2004;22:1249–52.
5. van Ommen B. Nutrigenomics: exploiting systems biology in the nutrition and health arenas. *Nutrition* 2004;20:4–8.
6. Pevzner PA. *Computational molecular biology.* Cambridge: MIT Press, 2000.
7. Bower JM, Bolouri H, editors. *Computational modeling of genetic and biochemical networks.* Cambridge: MIT Press, 2001.
8. Wolkenhauer O. Systems biology: the reincarnation of systems theory applied in biology? *Brief Bioinform* 2001;2:258–70.
9. van der Greef J, Stroobant P, van der Heijden R. The role of analytical sciences in medical systems biology. *Curr Opin Chem Biol* 2004;8:559–65.
10. Strange K. The end of "naive reductionism": rise of systems biology or renaissance of physiology? *Am J Physiol Cell Physiol* 2005;288:C968–74.

11. Nikolsky Y, Ekins S, Nikolskaya T, Bugrim A. A novel method for generation of signature networks as biomarkers from complex high throughput data. *Toxicol Lett* 2005;158:20–9.
12. Siripurapu V, Meth J, Kobayashi N, Hamaguchi M. DBC2 significantly influences cell-cycle, apoptosis, cytoskeleton and membrane-trafficking pathways. *J Mol Biol* 2005;346:83–9.
13. Itoh T, Karlsberg K, Kijima I, Yuan YC, Smith D, Ye J, et al. Letrozole-, anastrozole-, and tamoxifen-responsive genes in MCF-7aro cells: a microarray approach. *Mol Cancer Res* 2005;3:203–18.
14. Nambiar S, Mirmohammadsadegh A, Doroudi R, Gustrau A, Marini A, Roeder G, et al. Signaling networks in cutaneous melanoma metastasis identified by complementary DNA microarrays. *Arch Dermatol* 2005;141:165–73.
15. Palsson BO. What lies beyond bioinformatics? *Nat Biotechnol* 1997;15:3–4.
16. Kitano H. Computational systems biology. *Nature* 2002;420:206–10.
17. Rousseau F, Schymkowitz J. A systems biology perspective on protein structural dynamics and signal transduction. *Curr Opin Struct Biol* 2005;15:23–30.
18. Cavalieri D, De Filippo C. Bioinformatic methods for integrating whole-genome expression results into cellular networks. *Drug Discov Today* 2005;10:727–34.
19. Wolf DM, Arkin AP. Motifs, modules and games in bacteria. *Curr Opin Microbiol* 2003;6:125–34.
20. McAdams HH, Arkin AP. Gene regulation: towards a circuit engineering discipline. *Curr Biol* 2000;10:R318–R20.
21. Butte A. The use and analysis of microarray data. *Nat Rev Drug Discov* 2002;1:951–60.
22. Kauffman S. A proposal for using the ensemble approach to understand genetic regulatory networks. *J Theor Biol* 2004;230:581–90.
23. Begley TJ, Samson LD. Network responses to DNA damaging agents. *DNA Repair (Amst)* 2004;3:1123–32.
24. Mack GS. Can complexity be commercialized? *Nat Biotechnol* 2004;22:1223–9.
25. Ekins S, Kirillov E, Rakhmatulin EA, Nikolskaya T. A novel method for visualizing nuclear hormone receptor networks relevant to drug metabolism. *Drug Metab Dispos* 2005;33:474–81.
26. Nikolsky Y, Ekins S, Nikolskaya T, Bugrim A. A novel method for generation of signature networks as biomarkers from complex high throughput data. *Toxicol Lett* 2005;158:20–9.
27. Ekins S, Nikolsky Y, Nikolskaya T. Techniques: Application of systems biology to absorption, distribution, metabolism, excretion, and toxicity. *Trends Pharmacol Sci* 2005;26:202–9.
28. Ekins S, Boulanger B, Swaan PW, Hupcey MAZ. Towards a new age of virtual ADME/TOX and multidimensional drug discovery. *J Comput Aided Mol Des* 2002;16:381–401.
29. Ekins S, Bugrim A, Nikolsky Y, Nikolskaya T. Systems biology: applications in drug discovery. In: Gad S, editor, *Drug discovery handbook*. New York: Wiley, 2005. p. 123–183.

30. Christopher R, Dhiman A, Fox J, Gendelman R, Haberitcher T, Kagle D, et al. Data-driven computer simulation of human cancer cell. *Ann NY Acad Sci* 2004;1020:132–53.
31. Defranoux NA, Stokes CL, Young DL, Kahn AJ. In silico modeling and simulation of bone biology: a proposal. *J Bone Miner Res* 2005;20:1079–84.
32. Plavec I, Sirenko O, Privat S, Wang Y, Dajee M, Melrose J, et al. Method for analyzing signaling networks in complex cellular systems. *Proc Natl Acad Sci USA* 2004;101:1223–8.
33. Butcher EC, Berg EL, Kunkel EJ. Systems biology in drug discovery. *Nat Biotechnol* 2004;22:1253–9.
34. Hughes TR, Marton MJ, Jones AR, Roberts CJ, Stoughton R, Armour CD, et al. Functional discovery via a compendium of expression profiles. *Cell* 2000;102:109–26.
35. Castle AL, Carver MP, Mendrick DL. Toxicogenomics: a new revolution in drug safety. *Drug Discov Today* 2002;7:728–36.
36. Ganter B, Tugendreich S, Pearson CI, Ayanoglu E, Baumhueter S, Bostian KA, et al. Development of a large-scale chemogenomics database to improve drug candidate selection and to understand mechanisms of chemical toxicity and action. *J Biotechnol* 2005;119:219–44.
37. Natsoulis G, El Ghaoui L, Lanckriet GR, Tolley AM, Leroy F, Dunlea S, et al. Classification of a large microarray data set: algorithm comparison and analysis of drug signatures. *Genome Res* 2005;15:724–36.
38. Gunther EC, Stone DJ, Rothberg JM, Gerwien RW. A quantitative genomic expression analysis platform for multiplexed in vitro prediction of drug action. *Pharmacogenomics J* 2005;5:126–34.
39. Hart CP. Finding the target after screening the phenotype. *Drug Discov Today* 2005;10:513–9.
40. Nikolsky Y, Nikolskaya T, Bugrim A. Biological networks and analysis of experimental data in drug discovery. *Drug Discov Today* 2005;10:653–62.
41. Cabusora L, Sutton E, Fulmer A, Forst CV. Differential network expression during drug and stress response. *Bioinformatics* 2005;21:2898–905.
42. Lu B, Soreghan BA, Thomas SN, Chen T, Yang AJ. *Towards global proteomic analysis in a PS1/APP mouse of Alzheimer's disease.* ACS. San Diego, 2005.
43. Waters KM, Shankaran H, Wiley HS, Resat H, Thrall BD. Integration of microarray and proteomics data for biological pathway analysis and network modeling of epidermal growth factor signaling in human mammary epithelial cells. *Keystone Symposia, 2005.*
44. Lantz RC, Petrick JS, Hays AM. Altered protein expression following in utero exposure to arsenic. Society of Toxicology, 2005.
45. Nie AY, McMillian MK, Leone AM, Parker JB, Piechta L-A, Bryant S, et al. A gene signature for non-genotoxic carcinogens. Society of Toxicology, 2005.
46. Meng Q, Waters KM, Malard JM, Lee KM, Pounds JG. Gene expression modifications in a mouse emphysema model induced by elastase. Society of Toxicology, 2005.
47. Mason CW, Swaan PW, Weiner CP. Gene Array Profiling of myometrial events during pregnancy: unlocking the universe of gene interactions using gene maps

and interactive networks. Society of Gynecological Investigation. Los Angeles, CA, 2005.

48. Weiner CP, Mason CW, Buhimschi C, Hall G, Swaan PW, Buhimschi I. Changes in uterine GTPase activity are not consistent with changes in expression of Gα subunits of heterotrimeric G-proteins: A potential mechanism for myometrial quiescence. Society of Gynecological Investigation. Los Angeles, CA, 2005.
49. Basso K, Margolin AA, Stolovitzky G, Klein U, Dalla-Favera R, Califano A. Reverse engineering of regulatory networks in human B cells. *Nat Genet* 2005;37:382–90.
50. McMillian M, Nie A, Parker JB, Leone A, Kemmerer M, Bryant S, et al. Drug-induced oxidative stress in rat liver from a toxicogenomics perspective. *Toxicol Appl Pharmacol* 2005;207:171–8.
51. Schadt EE, Lamb J, Yang X, Zhu J, Edwards S, Guhathakurta D, et al. An integrative genomics approach to infer causal associations between gene expression and disease. *Nat Genet* 2005;37:710–7.
52. Thongboonkerd V. Genomics, proteomics and integrative "omics" in hypertension research. *Curr Opin Nephrol Hypertens* 2005;14:133–9.
53. Ghazalpour A, Doss S, Yang X, Aten J, Toomey EM, Van Nas A, et al. Thematic review series: The pathogenesis of atherosclerosis. Toward a biological network for atherosclerosis. *J Lipid Res* 2004;45:1793–805.
54. Ekins S. Systems-ADME/Tox: Resources and network approaches. *J Pharmacol Toxicol Methods* 2006;53:38–66.
55. Wang X, Wei Y, Yuan S, Liu G, Lu Y, Zhang J, et al. Potential anticancer activity of tanshinone IIA against human breast cancer. *Int J Cancer* 2005.
56. Raponi M, Belly RT, Karp JE, Lancet JE, Atkins D, Wang Y. Microarray analysis reveals genetic pathways modulated by tipifarnib in acute myeloid leukemia. *BMC Cancer* 2004;4:56.
57. Busold CH, Winter S, Hauser N, Bauer A, Dippon J, Hoheisel JD, et al. Integration of GO annotations in Correspondence Analysis: facilitating the interpretation of microarray data. *Bioinformatics* 2005;21:2424–9.
58. FDA. Food and Drug Administration. Guidance for Industry, Pharmacogenomic Data Submissions. March 2005.
59. Hucka M, Finney A, Sauro HM, Bolouri H, Doyle JC, Kitano H, et al. The systems biology markup language (SBML): a medium for representation and exchange of biochemical network models. *Bioinformatics* 2003;19:524–31.
60. Sauro HM, Hucka M, Finney A, Wellock C, Bolouri H, Doyle J, et al. Next generation simulation tools: the Systems Biology Workbench and BioSPICE integration. *Omics* 2003;7:355–72.
61. Fliri AF, Loging WT, Thadeio PF, Volkmann RA. Biological spectra analysis: Linking biological activity profiles to molecular structure. *Proc Natl Acad Sci USA* 2005;102:261–6.
62. Fernie AR, Trethewey RN, Krotzky AJ, Willmitzer L. Metabolite profiling: from diagnostics to systems biology. *Nat Rev Mol Cell Biol* 2004;5:763–9.
63. Kell DB. Metabolomics and systems biology: making sense of the soup. *Curr Opin Microbiol* 2004;7:296–307.

64. Cary MP, Bader GD, Sander C. Pathway information for systems biology. *FEBS Lett* 2005;579:1815–20.

65. Luciano JS. PAX of mind for pathway researchers. *Drug Discov Today* 2005;10:937–42.

66. Jenssen TK, Laegreid A, Komorowski J, Hovog E. A literature network of human genes for high-throughput analysis of gene expression. *Nat Genet* 2001;28:21–8.

67. Krauthammer M, Kaufmann CA, Gilliam TC, Rzhetsky A. Molecular triangulation: bridging linkage and molecular-network information for identifying candidate genes in Alzheimer's disease. *Proc Natl Acad Sci USA* 2004;101: 15148–53.

68. Rzhetsky A, Iossifov I, Koike T, Krauthammer M, Kra P, Morris M, et al. GeneWays: a system for extracting, analyzing, visualizing, and integrating molecular pathway data. *J Biomed Inform* 2004;37:43–53.

69. Alako BT, Veldhoven A, van Baal S, Jelier R, Verhoeven S, Rullmann T, et al. CoPub Mapper: mining MEDLINE based on search term co-publication. *BMC Bioinformatics* 2005;6:51.

70. Gardner SP. Ontologies and semantic data integration. *Drug Discov Today* 2005;10:1001–7.

71. Krallinger M, Valencia A. Text-mining and information-retrieval services for molecular biology. *Genome Biol* 2005;6:224.

72. Douglas SM, Montelione GT, Gerstein M. PubNet: a flexible system for visualizing literature derived networks. *Genome Biol* 2005;6:R80.

73. Covitz PA, Hartel F, Schaefer C, De Coronado S, Fragoso G, Sahni H, et al. caCORE: a common infrastructure for cancer informatics. *Bioinformatics* 2003;19:2404–12.

74. Waters M, Boorman G, Bushel P, Cunningham M, Irwin R, Merrick A, et al. Systems toxicology and the Chemical Effects in Biological Systems (CEBS) knowledge base. *EHP Toxicogenomics* 2003;111:15–28.

75. Xirasagar S, Gustafson S, Merrick BA, Tomer KB, Stasiewicz S, Chan DD, et al. CEBS object model for systems biology data, SysBio-OM. *Bioinformatics* 2004;20:2004–15.

76. Fostel J, Choi D, Zwickl C, Morrison N, Rashid A, Hasan A, et al. Chemical Effects in Biological Systems—Data Dictionary (CEBS-DD): a compendium of terms for the capture and integration of biological study design description, conventional phenotypes and 'omics data. *Toxicol Sci* 2005;88:585–601.

77. Heath JR, Phelps ME, Hood L. NanoSystems biology. *Mol Imaging Biol* 2003;5:312–25.

78. Barabasi A-L, Oltvai ZN. Network biology: understanding the cell's functional organization. *Nat Rev Genet* 2004;5:101–13.

79. Giot L, Bader JS, Brouwer C, Chaudhuri A, Kuang B, Li Y, et al. A protein interaction map of *Drosophila melanogaster*. *Science* 2003;302:1727–36.

80. de Menezes MA, Barabasi AL. Fluctuations in network dynamics. *Phys Rev Lett* 2004;92:028701.

81. Raser JM, O'Shea EK. Noise in gene expression: origins, consequences, and control. *Science* 2005;309:2010–3.

82. Gilman AG, Simon MI, Bourne HR, Harris BA, Long R, Ross EM, et al. Overview of the Alliance for Cellular Signaling. *Nature* 2002;420:703–6.
83. Wilson SH, Olden K. The environmental genome project: phase I and beyond. *Mol Interv* 2004;4:147–56.
84. Henry CJ. Evolution of toxicology for risk assessment. *Int J Toxicol* 2003;22: 3–7.
85. Werner E. Meeting report: the future and limits of systems biology. *Sci STKE* 2005; 2005:pe16.
86. McDaniel R, Weiss R. Advances in synthetic biology: on the path from prototypes to applications. *Curr Opin Biotechnol* 2005;16:476–83.
87. Kramer BP, Fischer C, Fussenegger M. BioLogic gates enable logical transcription control in mammalian cells. *Biotechnol Bioeng* 2004;87:478–84.
88. Lash LH, Hines RN, Gonzalez FJ, Zacharewski TR, Rothstein MA. Genetics and susceptibility to toxic chemicals: do you (or should you) know your genetic profile? *J Pharmacol Exp Ther* 2003;305:403–9.
89. Ekins S, Bugrim A, Nikolsky Y, Nikolskaya T. Systems biology: applications in drug discovery. In: Gad SC, editor, *Drug discovery handbook*. New York: Wiley, 2005. p. 123–83.
90. Ekins S, Kirillov E, Rakhmatulin E, Nikolskaya T. A novel method for visualizing nuclear hormone receptor networks relevant to drug metabolism. *Drug Metab Dispos* 2005;33:474–81.
91. Ekins S, Andreyev S, Ryabov A, Kirilov E, Rakhmatulin EA, Bugrim A, et al. Computational prediction of human drug metabolism. *Exp Opin Drug Metab Toxicol* 2005;1:303–24.
92. Ekins S, Giroux CN, Nikolsky Y, Bugrim A, Nikolskaya T. A signature gene network approach to toxicity. *Toxicologist* 2005;84.
93. Kasamatsu A, Endo Y, Uzawa K, Nakashima D, Koike H, Hashitani S, et al. Identification of candidate genes associated with salivary adenoid cystic carcinomas using combined comparative genomic hybridization and oligonucleotide microarray analyses. *Int J Biochem Cell Biol* 2005;37:1869–80.
94. Zeng F, Schultz RM. RNA transcript profiling during zygotic gene activation in the preimplantation mouse embryo. *Dev Biol* 2005;283:40–57.
95. Paris D, Ait-Ghezala G, Mathura VS, Patel N, Quadros A, Laporte V, et al. Anti-angiogenic activity of the mutant Dutch A(beta) peptide on human brain microvascular endothelial cells. *Brain Res Mol Brain Res* 2005;136:212–30.
96. Lee TS, Eid T, Mane S, Kim JH, Spencer DD, Ottersen OP, et al. Aquaporin-4 is increased in the sclerotic hippocampus in human temporal lobe epilepsy. *Acta Neuropathol (Berl)* 2004;108:493–502.
97. Chen YF, Shin SJ, Lin SR. Ets1 was significantly activated by ERK1/2 in mutant K-ras stably transfected human adrenocortical cells. *DNA Cell Biol* 2005;24: 126–32.
98. Daraselia N, Yuryev A, Egorov S, Novihkova S, Nikitin A, Mazo I. Extracting human protein interactions from Medline using a full-sentence parser. *Bioinformatics* 2003;19.
99. Nikitin A, Egorov S, Daraselia N, Mazo I. Pathway studio—the analysis and navigation of molecular networks. *Bioinformatics* 2003;19:2155–7.

100. Donninger H, Bonome T, Radonovich M, Pise-Masison CA, Brady J, Shih JH, et al. Whole genome expression profiling of advance stage papillary serous ovarian cancer reveals activated pathways. *Oncogene* 2004;23:8065–77.

101. Yonan AL, Palmer AA, Smith KC, Feldman I, Lee HK, Yonan JM, et al. Bioinformatic analysis of autism positional candidate genes using biological databases and computational gene network prediction. *Genes Brain Behav* 2003;2:303–20.

102. Breitkreutz BJ, Stark C, Tyers M. Osprey: a network visualization system. *Genome Biol* 2003;4:R22.

103. Funahashi A, Morohashi M, Kitano H, Tanimura N. CellDesigner: a process diagram editor for gene-regulatory and biochemical networks. *BioSilico* 2003;1:159–62.

104. Shannon P, Markiel A, Ozier O, Baliga NS, Wang JT, Ramage D, et al. Cytoscape: a software environment for integrated models of biomolecular interaction networks. *Genome Res* 2003;13:2498–504.

105. Longabaugh WJ, Davidson EH, Bolouri H. Computational representation of developmental genetic regulatory networks. *Dev Biol* 2005;283:1–16.

106. Peri S, Navarro JD, Amanchy R, Kristiansen TZ, Jonnalagadda CK, Surendranath V, et al. Development of human protein reference database as an initial platform for approaching systems biology in humans. *Genome Res* 2003;13:2363–71.

107. Hu Z, Mellor J, Wu J, Yamada T, Holloway D, Delisi C. VisANT: data-integrating visual framework for biological networks and modules. *Nucleic Acids Res* 2005;33:W352–7.

108. Hu Z, Mellor J, Wu J, DeLisi C. VisANT: an online visualization and analysis tool for biological interaction data. BMC *Bioinformatics* 2004;5:17.

109. Dahlquist KD, Salomonis N, Vranizan K, Lawlor SC, Conklin BR. GenMAPP, a new tool for viewing and analyzing microarray data on biological pathways. *Nat Genet* 2002;31:19–20.

110. Doniger SW, Salomonis N, Dahlquist KD, Vranizan K, Lawlor SC, Conklin BR. MAPPFinder: using Gene Ontology and GenMAPP to create a global gene-expression profile from microarray data. *Genome Biol* 2003;4:R7.

111. Li Y, Hong X, Hussain M, Sarkar SH, Li R, Sarkar FH. Gene expression profiling revealed novel molecular targets of docetaxel and estramustine combination treatment in prostate cancer cells. *Mol Cancer Ther* 2005;4:389–98.

112. Li Y, Hussain M, Sarkar SH, Eliason J, Li R, Sarkar FH. Gene expression profiling revealed novel mechanism of action of Taxotere and Furtulon in prostate cancer cells. *BMC Cancer* 2005;5:7.

113. Ohnishi H, Asamoto M, Tujimura K, Hokaiwado N, Takahashi S, Ogawa K, et al. Inhibition of cell proliferation by nobiletin, a dietary phytochemical, associated with apoptosis and characteristic gene expression, but lack of effect on early rat hepatocarcinogenesis in vivo. *Cancer Sci* 2004;95:936–42.

114. Wang JM, Johnston PB, Ball BG, Brinton RD. The neurosteroid allopregnanolone promotes proliferation of rodent and human neural progenitor cells and regulates cell-cycle gene and protein expression. *J Neurosci* 2005;25:4706–18.

115. Swagell CD, Henly DC, Morris CP. Expression analysis of a human hepatic cell line in response to palmitate. *Biochem Biophys Res Commun* 2005;328:432–41.

116. Luo W, Fan W, Xie H, Jing L, Ricicki E, Vouros P, et al. Phenotypic anchoring of global gene expression profiles induced by *N*-hydroxy-4-acetylaminobiphenyl and benzo[*a*]pyrene diol epoxide reveals correlations between expression profiles and mechanism of toxicity. *Chem Res Toxicol* 2005;18:619–29.

117. Krikun G, Schatz F, Taylor R, Critchley HO, Rogers PA, Huang J, et al. Endometrial endothelial cell steroid receptor expression and steroid effects on gene expression. *J Clin Endocrinol Metab* 2005;90:1812–8.

118. Ise R, Han D, Takahashi Y, Terasaka S, Inoue A, Tanji M, et al. Expression profiling of the estrogen responsive genes in response to phytoestrogens using a customized DNA microarray. *FEBS Lett* 2005;579:1732–40.

119. Punyadeera C, Dassen H, Klomp J, Dunselman G, Kamps R, Dijcks F, et al. Oestrogen-modulated gene expression in the human endometrium. *Cell Mol Life Sci* 2005;62:239–50.

120. McKallip RJ, Nagarkatti M, Nagarkatti PS. Delta-9-tetrahydrocannabinol enhances breast cancer growth and metastasis by suppression of the antitumor immune response. *J Immunol* 2005;174:3281–9.

PART III

SCIENTIFIC INFORMATION HANDLING AND ENHANCING PRODUCTIVITY

7

INFORMATION MANAGEMENT—BIODATA IN LIFE SCIENCES

RICHARD K. SCOTT AND ANTHONY PARSONS

Contents

Computer Applications in Pharmaceutical Research and Development, Edited by Sean Ekins.
ISBN 0-471-73779-8

7.1 INTRODUCTION

It is the contention of the authors of this chapter that information management, data standards, and knowledge management form the three cornerstones of improving scientific productivity. Taking one of these away or choosing to ignore it will cause the overall strategy to fall down. Each discipline regularly receives substantial review, but historically there is no significant crossover. The latest "innovation" of systems biology attempts to provide a holistic approach to scientific research and development (R&D) [4], but it is often too challenging a task for large life sciences organizations to meld a multitude of niche disciplines together (e.g., chemistry, biology, genomics, physics, information management, performance computing, physiology, clinical data). Similarly, smaller organizations have neither the manpower nor the financial muscle to invest in fully integrated approaches to R&D [5].

7.2 INFORMATION MANAGEMENT—THE MISUNDERSTOOD COUSIN OF KNOWLEDGE MANAGEMENT

Information management and knowledge management (KM) are actually closely related [6, 7]. Information management acts as "glue," keeping data joined to people and processes. According to the pyramid model, data is too far down the tree as a raw material for information management (Fig. 7.1). Data itself is far more pervasive within an organization, spread between people (Fig. 7.2) according to the jigsaw model. Information management is actually all about connecting people to information (Fig. 7.3), people to technology (Fig. 7.4), and ultimately people to people (Fig. 7.5). Here is where KM is useful in helping to establish communities of best practice (CoPs), which are of extreme value. The organization of CoPs is a real challenge, as the "what's in it for me" factor comes into play. Some people like to keep their cards close to the chest, but what they don't realize is knowledge is not power but the aggregation of knowledge through networks of sharing is.

A well-developed knowledge and information management strategy ultimately helps facilitate decision making [8]. Information models also help to visualize and interpret patterns in complex data. A well-implemented information management strategy allows us to ask questions of data—Can we do it? Why did we succeed? Why did we fail? [7]. Professor Needham, sadly no longer with us, once asked of computers and technology when it would be that we could ask questions like "Show me the film of the girl who rides off into the sunset on the back of a horse with her lover" (http://www.admin.cam.ac.uk/news/dp/2003030401). Likewise, collaborators should be able to share results, ask questions, generate information, and make decisions based on analysis of relevant information. If only people would. The truth is that we are still very bad at this because of the "three big reasons," namely, resistance to change, internal politics, and bureaucracy [9].

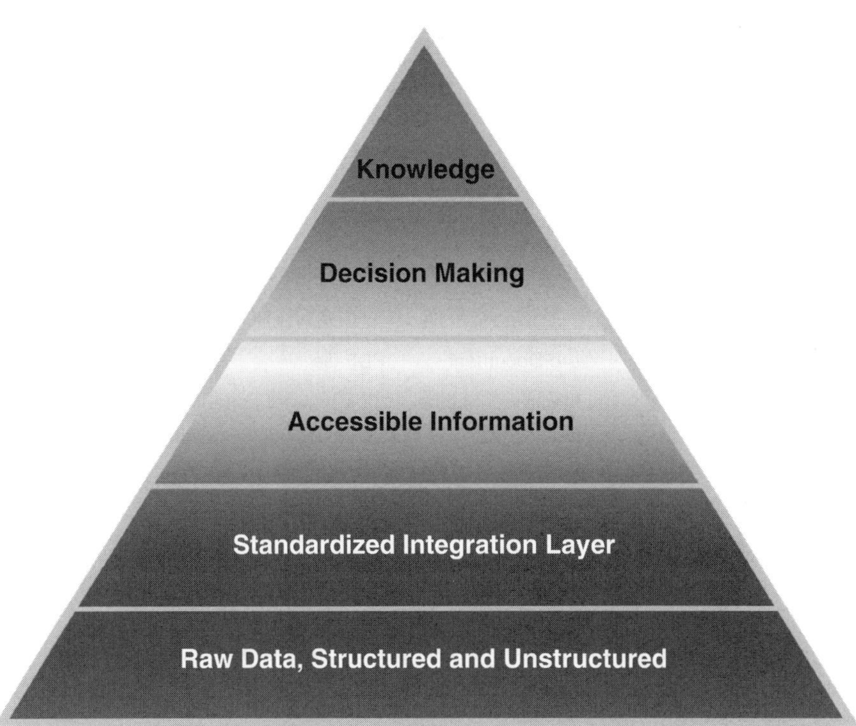

Figure 7.1 The pyramid model.

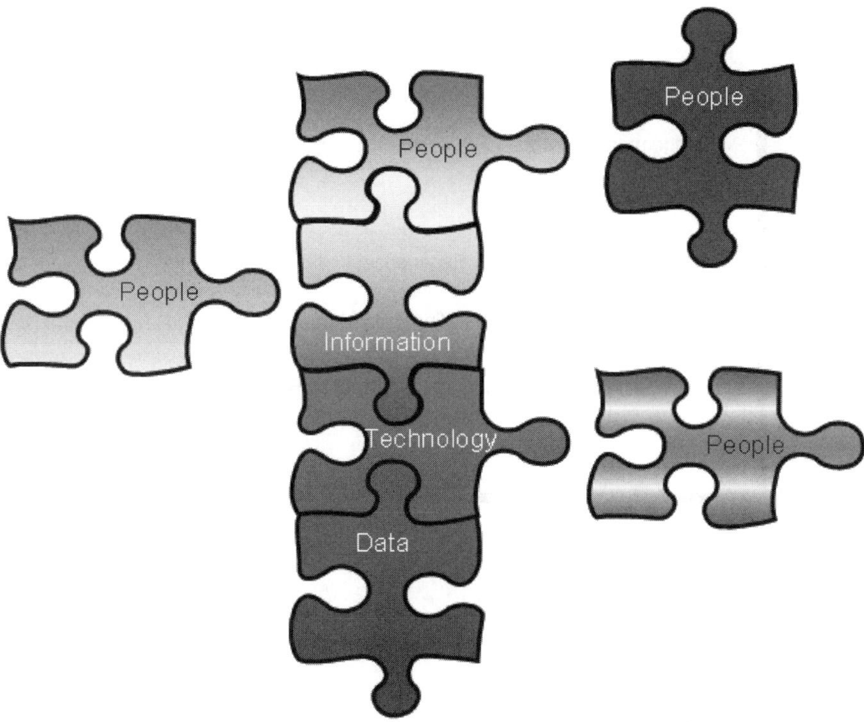

Figure 7.2 The jigsaw model.

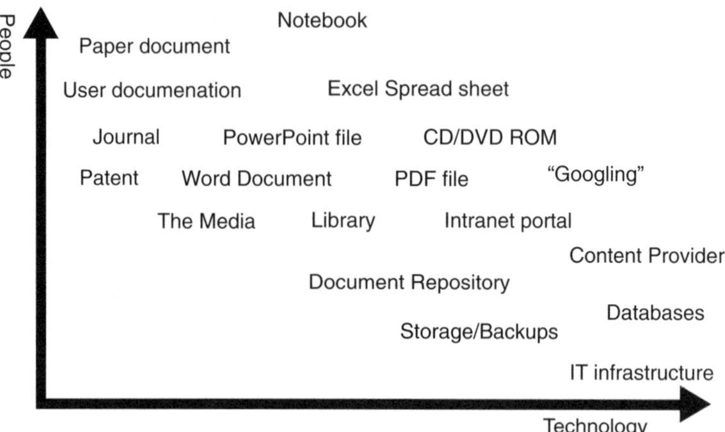

Figure 7.3 Connecting people to information.

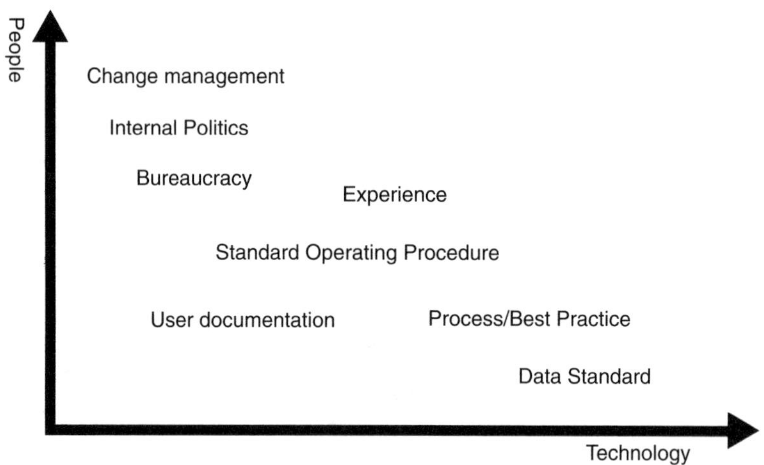

Figure 7.4 Connecting people to technology.

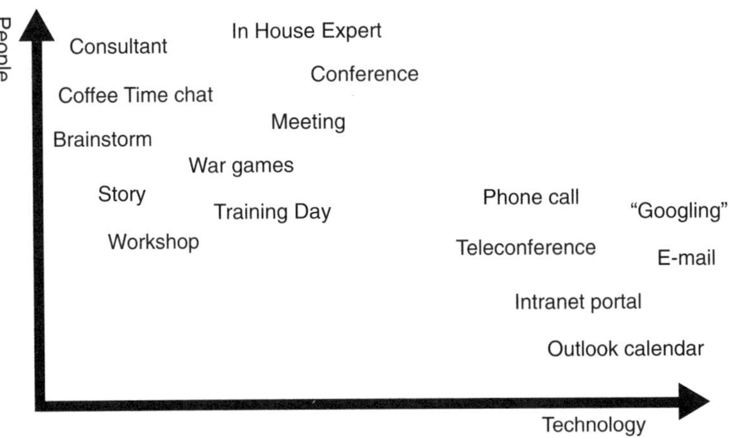

Figure 7.5 Connecting people to people.

Typically, funding to embark on information and/or knowledge management initiatives within the life sciences only occurs after a serious failure within the business, such as a project failure or a withdrawal of a medicine from the market. Recently, COX-2 programs across the industry are under close scrutiny since the highly publicized withdrawal of Vioxx [10]. Of course, there has been no withdrawal of aspirin, paracetamol, alcohol, or tobacco products, which are well known as toxic.

The marriage of information and KM should ideally allow us to change the outcome and learn. Successful outcomes are repeated, become part of best practice, and are further refined. Mistakes and failures are understood, reduced, and form part of a diagnostic early warning system to help reduce costs and improve success [11]. An example here is Pharmamatrix, which has been so successful for Pfizer; it does a billion intersections between diseases, targets, and therapeutic agents. Some organizations are now grasping this concept and attempting to dig down into the various information silos and come up with new medicines [12]. Once you begin to share data and knowledge, you must also begin to enumerate or evaluate the impact of this "new" seam of information [13, 14].

7.3 DATA INTEGRATION STANDARDS

Data in raw form is simply noise. The pyramid in Figure 7.1 has a hidden foundation—this is the data noise of an organization! Normalized data is in graveyards—accessibility is key, as is being able to infer relationships between data types. Transference of bones from one graveyard to another generally results in loss of value or addition of soil (so yet more noise). Data is generally badly managed, a mess that requires standards. There is a tacit desire for data standards from the community, but these efforts are, sadly, poorly supported by vendors and customers. There is still a cottage industry mentality to building software tools and components [15] despite the positive impact of Open-Source initiatives [16]

Raw data is almost always incomplete, being highly dependent on the data production platform and often localized to a platform or regional database. Applications (and processes) generate data. However, applications often use proprietary data types and cannot parse data types from other third-party applications. It is important to consider that there are translation issues plus the host of reasons stated below in the requirements for data standards.

The life science community wants tools and toolkits, but no major software vendor is prepared to make the investment for fear of short-term loss of market share. Many companies disappeared in merger and acquisitions who embraced the vision of integrated and interoperable components such as Synomics, Cherwell, Netgenics, Synopsis, etc. These companies were too early to market when the community was still content to use legacy vertical applications. To bypass the problems associated with a lack of data standards, some new companies wrap legacy applications with "sticky" interfaces, such as SciTegic and Inforsense. This allows the chaining together of discrete processes to form often complex workflows, usually bringing together a range of vendor applications to manipulate the data.

As stated on the OMG (Object Management) website (http://www.omg.org/), a lack of data standards results in data conversions, loss of information, lack of interoperability, etc. Current standards du jour are XML (Extensible Markup Language) [17], LSID (Life Sciences Identifiers), and now the RDF (Resource Description Framework) from the W3C (World Wide Web Consortium), which is extensible though hard to implement. Substantial work on OO (Object Oriented) modeling of life science data types takes place at the OMG's LSR (Life Sciences Research) group—this is discussed below.

7.4 WHAT STATE IS THE INFORMATION COMMUNITY IN?

The state of health of the biology informatics sectors (bioinformatics, proteomics, metabolomics, etc.) is perhaps better than cheminformatics; this is due primarily to a history of legacy technology in cheminformatics versus homegrown tools in the virgin territory in bioinformatics [15, 16]. Open source is still not mature enough yet for people to move to the new "application killers." Vertical lock-in is still present in the life sciences market, although as stated above new companies are emerging that try to connect data and applications horizontally.

7.5 APPROACHES TO INFORMATION MANAGEMENT

7.5.1 Brute Force

Buy a really big digger and lots of dynamite and mine everything. This systematic approach is taken by organizations that have to resources to build the plant, buy the equipment, staff the building, and pay for all the infrastructure, hardware, and software licenses. It is the Big Pharma equivalent of opencast mining. Vast amounts of genes are screened for upregulation, thousands of proteins isolated, hundreds of pathways elucidated, dozens of targets selected, millions of compounds screened, tens of millions of data points and activity determinations taken. Compound inventory and registration is tightly controlled. All data is deposited in either a single data warehouse or is federated across each data silo. Entire departments are responsible for the collection, storage, backup, and retrieval of data. More and more data is deposited—legacy documents are scanned and captured. Everything is audited and date stamped. Compliance and good governance are the watchwords of the business. Data security and integrity is paramount. Nothing is left to chance, and the machinery itself becomes part of the massive process of R&D. This approach is highly efficient with massive throughput but is very slow to dismantle and reinvent itself. The costs of failure in late-stage development can be very high but are offset by current product revenues.

7.5.2 Small Scale

Do geophysics analysis, take samples, predict where to dig, mine on a smaller scale. This is the approach taken by prospectors who may have stumbled upon something that looks like gold and have only a small amount of resources to extract the value. This is the biotechnology equivalent of the Welsh gold mines—small scale, very high value if successful but more likely to go broke first. A single target or single lead compound may be present, small highly targeted libraries are screened, a few hundred compounds that are similar to the lead compound are made by hand (or purchased) for testing. Any activity is then pursued, but when selectivity is not found, the compound (and often target) is dropped and the prospector moves on. Data storage is in local drives, paper documents, and folders. Most legacy information is simply lost or archived. Most of the business-critical information resides in the heads of employees. Transfer of data and information to prospective bigger partners is done on an ad hoc basis. Some important data sets are generated by skunkworks and never see the light of day.

Chance (or serendipity as embittered biotech CEOs like to call it) plays a major factor in the successful outcome of an R&D program. External forces in the marketplace can make or break small companies; hence the environment is highly volatile and subject to change rapidly.

These two information management approaches are at the extreme ends of the scale. In reality, most organizations have strengths in certain areas (such as barcoding and full sample life cycle) but are still dealing with the issues of data extraction from the collated information. Information management is rarely seen as a strategic investment, and local communities (or individuals) build their own collection of solutions to store and extract value from the data they generate.

The skill in information management is to develop communities of best practice using technologies that are accessible by both data producers and consumers.

This is why data standards and knowledge management are so important to information management.

7.6 APPROACHES TO KNOWLEDGE MANAGEMENT

7.6.1 Stamp Collecting

Measuring, scorecards, metrics, portal hit counters, and e-mail traffic are all good statistics to justify the position of a KM practitioner, but how do you measure the way a business changes its approach to R&D? The only metric that stockbrokers are interested in are revenue generated by products on the market, the pipeline of products in the clinic (and estimated future revenues), and remaining time on patents (prediction of drop in revenue). It can be difficult to find secondary markers for innovative success (such as publications and patents) in an industry known for its secrecy [18]. A KM practitioner will look for value creation in "hard" and "soft" benefits to the business. Hard benefits are more easily recognized by most companies. These are benefits such as improved revenue stream, shorter time to market, better efficiency in process, and protection of intellectual property. Soft benefits are less obvious in their impact to the business. These are benefits such as better communication, idea generation, and innovation, improved response time to market conditions, and improved access to information. Recognizing the value of soft benefits is equally as important as hard value, as these keep the business competitive in the marketplace [13, 14]. True knowledge management should therefore empower innovation and creativity.

7.6.2 Reality Shift

Good knowledge management practice is like an innovative technology—It is disruptive in the sense that it should challenge the status quo and change the way we go about our work. The strategic goal (gold?) of the business should be clearly understood—*We are here to bring new highly profitable medicines to market for areas of high unmet medical need.* Keeping a close eye not only on your competitors but also on your collaborators and complementors provides a valuable source of information—No organization can assimilate all information and data alone, despite the not-invented-here mentality [19]! Positive feedback is the most important force in the network economy to change culture. Information and data are far more accessible in a positive environment, so knowledge management must provide a mechanism for reward as well as a framework for building teams (or communities of best practice) [20]. Knowledge management sees people as sources of information intellectual capital, an important difference in comparison with information management, where most information is *inhuman* (electronic, paper, data media, etc). Connecting the human to the inhuman information mines has two simple requirements—keep it real, and keep it simple. Users of information/knowledge management systems will accept nothing else (unless you threaten them!) [21].

If you embrace standards, it will avoid technology lock-in and make migration and change easier to deal with. This is why information management and data standards are so important to knowledge management

7.7 APPROACHES TO DATA INTEGRATION STANDARDS

7.7.1 OMG, I3C (RIP) LSIT, and W3C

In the approaches to data standards, the authors make no apology for using the OMG's life science research group as a structured approach to building new data standards (as both authors have a wealth of experience in bringing standards to the market via this organization [22, 23]). As only a handful of readers will be conversant with the OMG, here is a brief overview on how the OMG works to deliver standards to the life science community.

The OMG adopts and publishes "Interface" specifications. Specifications may also be chosen from existing products in competitive selection process. Any interface specifications are freely available to both members and nonmembers. Implementations must be available from an OMG member (either commercially or open source). The OMG is not a common object request broker architecture (CORBA)-only shop but uses many approaches to object-oriented modeling of complex data types. As data types are often industry specific, the OMG has specific domain task force (DTF) groups that deal with these specific types. Working groups are formed to address specific areas of interest within the task force. Of course, whenever there is potential for reuse of existing standards, it is positively encouraged!

The life sciences domain task force (LSR DTF) has several working groups: architecture and road map, biochemical pathways, cheminformatics, gene expression, sequence analysis, and single nucleotide polymorphisms.

Each working group has a corresponding chairperson who champions requests for proposals (RFPs) from any interested parties. The working group members identify key needs and help with the building of RFPs from a "boilerplate" standard document issued by the OMG. Anyone can submit a letter of intent (LOI) to respond to a RFP; however, to become a submitter, the organization must become an OMG member. A typical OMG standards adoption process is 20 months (Fig. 7.6). The gene expression RFP issued on March 10th 2000 and was an available specification on 16th Nov 2001 [24]

There are many products based on these life sciences standards, such as the aforementioned gene expression standard that is used in Rosetta Merck's Resolver product and the European Bioinformatics Institute's (EBI) Array-Express database. The LECIS (Laboratory Equipment Control Interface Specification) standard is used by Creon as part of their Q-DIS data standard support (note that one of the authors was the finalization task force chairperson for this standard).

There are many "open" tools out there, too—biomolecular sequence analysis standard (BSA) [25] is at the EBI in the form of Open BSA. The bibliographic query service standard (BQS) is also at the EBI as OpenBQS [26]. The macromolecular structure standard [27] is supported by the Protein Data Bank as the Open MM toolkit. You can implement (i.e., start writing code) as early as the first submission, without waiting for the final specification to be approved. It does help if you keep things modular, of course! The reason that LSR works is not technology but people—participation is essential for organizations, individuals, and evangelists. OMG's constitution is both fair and equitable—Having a well-defined process that is transparent in operation to allow open sharing of information is the key to its success. The reader is referred to references 28–30 for further information.

Of course, there are many other groups out there, all doing their own thing and occasionally interacting with other like-minded groups, such as the world

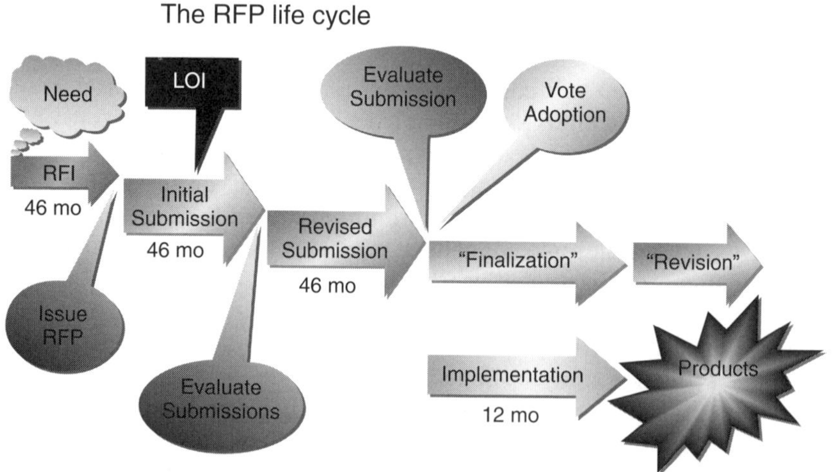

Figure 7.6 The request for proposals life cycle. Used with kind permission from David Benton, GSK. See color plate.

wide web consortium (W3C) that is encouraging the "semantic web" and LSIT (Life Sciences Information Technology Global Institute) trying to build "Good informatics practices." These groups come and go, for example, the I3C (Interoperable Informatics Infrastructure Consortium) that, like its website, no longer functions, but in the main, standards emerge with the backing of one or two major vendors and the consumers follow. Very rarely, the consumers rally together and force change upon the vendors. Finally, government bodies enforce mandatory changes that we struggle to comply with (just ask any CEO about Sarbanes–Oxley). The authors speculate what would happen if the FDA (Food and Drug Administration) stated that all electronic submissions had to be in XML for CFR 21 part 11 compliance (Title 21 Code of Federal Regulations, part 11)! This is why information management and knowledge management are so important to data standards.

7.8 BRINGING TOGETHER ALL THREE DISCIPLINES

Overcoming the "three big reasons" is the first milestone in bringing together information and knowledge management with data standards. This achievement should not be underestimated in importance. Many personal empires may fall as a consequence of this new way of mining the information landscape. Domain-specific knowledge is also critical and cross-domain knowledge even better. Finding the data architect who understands the process and workflow of a chemist is like mining for a rare gem among the seams of coal. These people are hard to find and harder to retain. As expert disciplines mature and become more accessible to younger scientists, then multiskilled employees will gradually filter upward. However, as this will take several years, the most widely used approach is to lure staff from a parallel organization into the business. The only downside is that new ways of thinking and innovation are now at a premium.

As with all successful projects, a small "proof-of-concept" pilot that addresses key stakeholder needs is the best way of gathering momentum to achieve lasting change and progress. [8] Fixing the time delay between compound submission and biology IC_{50} (inhibitory concentration at which 50% of the enzyme is inhibited) results has a better defined scope than building a "science Google" for all users.

7.9 ADVANCED MINING

Text mining is the bread-and-butter method used by researchers on a daily basis [31, 32]. If you ask researchers what they really want from information management, you might be surprised how often they wish for a "science Google" to mine for data. As beautiful and simple as this paradigm sounds, what lurks beneath the search page are all types of data, structured and unstructured—doing the science Google with knobs on requires measurement of relevancy, ontology, and taxonomies [33]. We are a long way off from this, despite the promise of RDF from the W3C. After all, can you really be sure that everything out there is uniquely defined?

There are several companies that are building ontology subsets of R&D information such as Biowisdom [34] and Cycorp on behalf of Big Pharma clients. Yet more companies provide the architecture and toolsets for companies to "build their own" ontologies such as Verity, APRSmartlogik, and Autonomy. The hope of these ontologies is that relevant (and related) information can be extracted from document repositories by using a range of user keyword or natural language queries. Image mining is also possible [35]. Companies such as Bioimagine and North Plains Systems provide technology to store, search, and retrieve image files. This can speed up the analysis of gels, tissues, and cells [36]. Finding undiscovered relationships between diverse data types such as text and images offers new potential in the mining for new medicines [37].

7.10 WHERE ARE THE REAL GOLD SEAMS OF DATA TO MINE?

There are really only three rules to information management and intelligence rules in organizations and academia.

1. CRIB—Card records in box
2. OGFAM—Optically guided finger access mechanism
3. EIFOB—Eyes in front of brains—the most important, of course

There are hidden gold mines under our noses—in house data becomes the "new lamps for old" on the tons of old clinical data from 50 years of R&D—but of course, none of it is electronically accessible. It is called a library! Many organizations have undertaken huge OCR (optical character recognition) projects to scan laboratory notebooks—some data even exists on microfilm and microfiche. As it is a legal requirement for a drug submission to provide provenance of scanned notebooks [38], paper, and microfilm, many businesses concentrate solely on the capture and verification of this data, rather than considering it a valuable resource to be remined.

Even on a relatively small subset of reused data, it is possible to license old medicines for new therapeutic applications and greatly reduce the costs of clinical development—many of these "reused" medicines have already passed muster for pharmacokinetic safety, so smaller-scale clinical trials are possible, saving considerable money (e.g., Arakis—soon to become Sosei). Even Sildenafil may have new indications [39]. There are huge potential reserves of information to mine in each and every large pharmaceutical company!

There are new seams to be mined, too—with changes in data access for clinical data, a voluntary clinical data disclosure scheme to publish the clinical data on websites may provide savvy information managers with valuable therapeutic insights [40, 41].This scheme is so far voluntary, but one day could this become compulsory? This would provide a whole new "gold rush" that was last seen after the publication of the human genome [42–44]. In the early years there were thought to be about a 100,000 active genes, but now this number is down to 25,000 active genes in a human, of which a small number are druggable (http://www.esi-topics.com/nhp/2004/march-04-AndrewHopkins.html).

7.11 TECHNOLOGY AS FACILITATOR

Using hardware tends to speed things up and produces more data, and grid computing is a good example of this [45]. This sort of hardware is no good for legacy data (e.g., 50 years of physical data storage, notebooks, and Microfilm). Using the experience of other domains outside life sciences is a worthwhile exercise. Banking, for example, is 10 years ahead (or pharma is 10 years behind) in adopting new technology to improve efficiency and foster innovation [46, 47]. The life sciences sector is cautious in adopting technology because of the intellectual value of the data it produces. Security is still a major issue for decision makers, despite the technology itself being possibly safer than online banking.

7.12 PRACTICALITIES

Assuming you have data under control (the description and format), how do you store it? Data is increasing at a rate greater than Moore's law. In 1965, Gordon Moore of Intel predicted that the density of transistors in integrated circuits would double every two years. The press called it Moore's law, and it has continued to be the case for nearly four decades. Freely available public data competes with curated "top-up charges" data, plus the in-house-generated data (which is never shared). There are at least three ways of providing storage solutions—SAN (storage area network), DAS (direct attached storage), and NAS (network attached storage)—with costs closely related to storage volume. Another issue is that data volumes are so huge now that they can no longer be indexed overnight. In a globally connected 24×7 network this equates to 12 hours.

Storage is one of the biggest challenges of biodata. If you wish to keep all raw data, ensure that your infrastructure and support and grow in pace with the raw data. If you only want to keep the relevant data, ensure your that business rules are able to filter the raw data properly—that is, do not lose anything vital. Banks spend far greater proportions of their profits on servers and data storage than large pharmaceutical companies. On such a large scale, even floor space and cooling can become major issues for data centers.

As well as hardware architecture for storage, software also plays a significant role. Data can be stored as flat files, indexed files, relational files, binary files, or any other electronic format, structured or unstructured. The life sciences industry has in the main chosen relational database management systems (RDBMS) using software such as ORACLE or (to a lesser extent) DB2. There are, of course, certain types of data that do not lend themselves well to storage in an RDBMS. For these cases, specialist software exists—such as Lion Biosciences' SRS (Sequence Retrieval Service) for biological sequence information. Even the KM industry uses a range of software for storage of data (see Table 7.1). Whereas other industries have precompetitive sharing of computer resources [40] (often where the data itself is non-IP sensitive), Big Pharma and biotech do not want large amounts of data being distributed on networks outside of their firewall. The issues of "IP on the Internet" [41] are still poorly understood by many budget holders who fund the acquisition of high-performance computing technology.

7.13 SUMMARY

Data production will continue to increase year on year as the life sciences continue to industrialize and scale up R&D process. Spending on data storage and data centers will increase in parallel with data production, putting pressure on the development of new approaches to data mining, sharing, and analysis. Much of the strain will be taken up by distributed performance computing and services within each organization, rather than across multiple organizations. Many companies will still choose to bring expertise in house rather than license in platforms for intelligent data mining, for fear of loss of IP. As long as a religious fear of data security and integrity persists, there is limited scope for precompetitive collaboration between the major pharmaceutical companies or between biotech small- to medium-sized enterprises. Perhaps the greatest untapped public available resource will be the clinical data published on corporate websites. This could pave the way for old drugs to be used in new indications, saving time and money for everyone involved.

7.14 CONCLUSION

Improving scientific productivity is not simply down to information management alone. Nor is knowledge management alone going to increase the number of new medicines reaching the marketplace. Standards initiatives are only driven by the need to avoid chaos and reduce data loss, not by compliance or

TABLE 7.1 A Selected List of Some KM Platforms

Group	Website	KM Platform	Explicit XML Support	Open Source
TheBrain	http://www.thebrain.com/	BrainEKP	No	No
Ipdeo	http://www.ipedo.com/	XML Intelligence Platform	Yes	No
Agilience	http://www.agilience.net/	Agilience EPS	Yes	No
J.B. Dietrich	http://www.jbdietrich.com	Mandarax and Oryx	Yes	Yes
Spotfire	http://www.sptofire.com	DecisionSite	Yes	No
Verity	http://www.verity.com	K2 Enterprise	Yes	No
Convera	http://www.convera.com	RetrievalWare	Yes	No
Autonomy	http://www.autonomy.com	IDOL server (plus interfaces)	Yes	No
Entopia	http://www.entopia.com	Quantum	No	No
KnowledgeBase	http://www.knowledgeBase.net	KnowledgeBase	No	No

governance. Combining all three disciplines provides a basic framework for success, upon which the vision of systems biology can be built. The business model of buying bigger diggers to mine for the increasingly more difficult to find gold nuggets is not sustainable. Similarly, the model of small-time prospectors panning the streams relies too much on luck rather than judgment. In the life sciences information landscape, mining must respond far more rapidly to new advances in both technology and working practice, or we will be swamped in the mountains of data waste. In an industry that is slow to adopt change, the courage to apply a new way of thinking is needed if we are indeed to improve our productivity in turning data ore into precious medicines.

ACKNOWLEDGMENTS

The authors would like to thank Dr. David Benton of GSK for his kind permission for reuse of the RFP image.

REFERENCES

1. Donnelly B. Data integration technologies: an unfulfilled revolution in the drug discovery process? *Biosilico* 2003;1:59–63.
2. Blumberg R, Atre S. The problem with unstructured data. *DM Rev* 2003.
3. Helfrich JP. Knowledge management systems: coping with the data explosion. *Biosilico* 2004;2:8–11.
4. Henry CM. Systems Biology. *Chemical & Engineering News* 2003;81:45–55.
5. Aderem A. Systems biology: its practice and challenges. *Cell* 2005;121: 511–13.
6. Peitsch M. Knowledge management and informatics in drug discovery, *Biosilico* 2004;2:394–6.
7. Newman V. *The Knowledge Activist's Handbook.* Oxford, Capstone Publishing Ltd.
8. Scott RK. Exploiting Knowledge Management in Drug Discovery R&D: Extracting value from Information. *Current Opinion in Drug Discovery* 2004;7:314–17.
9. Conference Meeting: Boosting R&D Productivity. The *Smart Pharma Forum* 8th October 2002.
10. Horton R. Vioxx, the implosion of Merck, and aftershocks at the FDA , *The Lancet* 2004;364:1995–6.
11. Zimmerman KA. Learning from success . . . and failure: Pharmaceuticals make the most of knowledge management. *KMWorld* 2003;12.
12. Lipinski C, Hopkins A. Navigating chemical space for biology and medicine, *Nature* 2004;432:855–61.
13. Koch C. Why doesn't your ROI add up? You do the math. Technology payback review http://www.darwinmag.com/read/030102/roi.html

14. Daum JH. *Intangible Assets and value creation.* John Wiley & Sons 2002.
15. Stahl MT. Open-source software: not quite endsville, *Drug Discovery Today* 2005;10:219–22.
16. DeLano WL. The case for open-source software in drug discovery. *Drug Discovery Today* 2005;10;211–13.
17. Blumberg R, Atre S. Digging into the Web: XML, Meta Data and Other Paths to Unstructured Data. *DM Review Magazine* May 2003.
18. Helvey T, Mack R, Avula S, Flook P. Data security in Life Sciences research. *Biosilico* 2004;2:97–103.
19. Gershell LJ, Miller TA. Emerging unscathed? *Nature Reviews Drug Discovery* 2002;1:739.
20. Skyrme D. *Knowledge Networking: Creating the Collaborative Company.* Butterworth-Heinemann, 1999.
21. Krue S. Don't Make Me Think!: A Common Sense Approach to Web Usability. *Que*, 2001.
22. http://www.omg.org/cgi-bin/doc?dtc/01-12-07
23. http://www.omg.org/cgi-bin/doc?lifesci/2003-01-08
24. http://www.omg.org/cgi-bin/doc?dtc/02-02-05
25. http://www.omg.org/cgi-bin/doc?dtc/00-11-01
26. http://www.omg.org/cgi-bin/doc?dtc/01-04-05
27. http://www.omg.org/cgi-bin/doc?lifesci/00-11-01
28. http://www.omg.org/cgi-bin/doc?lifesci/00-12-18
29. http://www.omg.org/cgi-bin/doc?lifesci/00-12-17
30. http://www.omg.org/gettingstarted/payoff.htm
31. Krallinger M, Erhardt RA, Valencia A. Text-mining approaches in molecular biology and biomedicine. Drug Disc Today 2005;10:439–45.
32. Gieger C, Deneke H, Fluck J. The future of text mining in genome-based clinical research. *Biosilico* 2003;1:97–102.
33. Feldman R, Regev Y, Hurvitz E, Finkelstein-Landau M. Mining the biomedical literature using semantic analysis and natural language processing techniques *Biosilico* 2003;1:69–80.
34. Gardner SP. Ontologies and semantic data integration *Drug Discovery Today* 2005;10:1001–7.
35. Berlage, T. Analyzing and mining image databases *Drug Discovery Today* 2005; 10:795–802.
36. Müller H, Michoux N, Bandon D, Geissbuhler A. A review of content-based image retrieval systems in medical applications—clinical benefits and future directions. *International Journal of Medical Informatics* 2004;73:1–23.
37. Berger CR. Predictive Analysis Is Data Mining's Future BioIT world 2005, June 20, 2005 http://www.bio-itworld.com/newsitems/2005/06-05/06-23-05-news-oracle.
38. CFR 21 part 11 http://www.fda.gov/cder/guidance/5667fnl.htm
39. Dear M. Sildenafil for hypertension: Old drug, new use. *Drug Topics* 2005; Jul 11, http://www.drugtopics.com/drugtopics/article/articleDetail.jsp?id=169471

40. Carrol J. Trials on Trial. The Push for Clinical Data Disclosure, *Biotechnology Healthcare* 2004; Oct: 51–5.
41. Mullin R. Lilly to post clinical data. *Chem and Eng News* 2004;82:7.
42. Initial sequencing and analysis of the human genome. International Human Genome Sequencing Consortium. *Nature* 2001;409:860–921.
43. Venter JC, Adams MD, Myers EW, Li PW, Mural RJ, Sutton GG, Smith HO, Yandell M, Evans CA, Holt RA et al. The sequence of the Human Genome. *Science* 2001;291:1304–51.
44. Istrail S, Sutton GG, Florea L, Halpern AL, Mobarry CM, Lippert R, Walenz B, Shatkay H, Dew I, Miller JR, Flanigan MJ, Edwards NJ, Bolanos R, Fasulo D, Halldorsson BV, Hannenhalli S, Turner R, Yooseph S, Lu F, Nusskern DR, Shue BC, Zheng XH, Zhong F, Delcher AL, Huson DH, Kravitz SA, Mouchard L, Reinert K, Remington KA, Clark AG, Waterman MS, Eichler EE, Adams MD, Hunkapiller MW, Myers EW, Venter JC. Whole-genome shotgun assembly and comparison of human genome assemblies *Proc Natl Acad Sci U S A*. 2004;101:1916–21. Feb 9th 2004.
45. Scott RK. Assessing the impact of high-performance computing on the drug discovery and development process. *Drug Discovery Today* 2004;2:175–9.
46. Chang YT. Dynamics of Banking Technology Adoption: An Application to Internet Banking. CCP, University of East Anglia, September 2004. http://www.uea.ac.uk/~j106/IB.pdf
47. Rees P. A lively future for IT. Life Science IT, 2004; Spring: http://www.lifescienceit.com/lsitspr04rees.html.
48. CERN's Large Hadron Collider (LHC) project at http://lcg.web.cern.ch/LCG/
49. A survey of issues by World Intellectual Property Organisation (WIPO) at http://ecommerce.wipo.int/survey/index.html

8

CHEMOINFORMATICS TECHNIQUES FOR PROCESSING CHEMICAL STRUCTURE DATABASES

VALERIE J. GILLET AND PETER WILLETT

Contents

Computer Applications in Pharmaceutical Research and Development, Edited by Sean Ekins.
ISBN 0-471-73779-8

8.1 INTRODUCTION

The corporate database of a large pharmaceutical research and development organization represents a significant part of the company's intellectual property, containing the structures of very large numbers of molecules that the company has synthesized and tested. It is thus hardly surprising that much effort has gone into developing techniques to maximize the value of such an intellectual asset. *Chemoinformatics* is the name of the new discipline that has emerged to provide tools for the storage, retrieval, and processing of databases of chemical structures [1, 2]. Corporate chemical databases have traditionally stored machine-readable representations of two-dimensional (2D) chemical structure diagrams, but these are increasingly being augmented by the inclusion of atomic coordinate data that permit the description of molecules in three dimensions (3D). This chapter describes some of the computational tools that are available for the processing of database information, focusing on the representation and searching of 2D and 3D molecules and on selecting compounds for biological testing.

8.2 REPRESENTATION OF CHEMICAL STRUCTURES

Four main approaches have been suggested for the representation of chemical structures in machine-readable form: *fragment codes, systematic nomenclature, linear notations,* and *connection tables.*

A fragment code describes a molecule by its constituent fragment substructures, namely, the rings, functional groups, and linking carbon chains that are present. Such a description is ambiguous in that no information is provided as to the way that the individual fragments are interconnected, so that a given set of fragment substructures characterizes a class of molecules rather than an individual substance. This characteristic is, however, of use for the representation and searching of the generic chemical substances that occur in chemical patents [3, 4] and also for increasing the efficiency of substructure searching, as described in detail below. Systematic nomenclature has for a long time provided the basis for printed indexes to the chemical literature, such as those produced by Chemical Abstracts Service (CAS) [5, 6]. A systematic chemical name provides a unique and compact characterization of a single molecule; however, the lack of any explicit information as to the way in which the individual atoms are linked together means that names may require very substantial processing if they are to be of general use in chemical information systems. Similar comments apply to linear notations. A linear notation consists of a string of alphanumeric characters that provides a complete, albeit in some cases implicit, description of the molecule's topology. Notations, in particular the Wiswesser Line Notation, formed the basis for most chemical information systems in the 1960s and 1970s [7]; their role today is less important, but they are still frequently used, normally in the form of

SMILES (for Simplified Molecular Input Line Entry Specification) notations, as a compact molecular representation [8].

Present-day chemoinformatics systems are mostly based on connection table representations of molecular structure. A connection table contains a list of all of the atoms within a structure, together with bond information that describes the exact manner in which the individual atoms are linked together. Thus a complete and explicit description of the molecular topology is available for searching purposes, and connection tables now form the basis for most public and in-house chemical information systems. There are many ways in which a connection table can be represented in machine-readable form, but it is generally very easy to convert from one form of connection table to another. An example of a structure diagram and the corresponding chemical name, connection table, and SMILES is shown in Figure 8.1.

An important characteristic of a connection table is that it can be regarded as a *graph*, a mathematical construct that describes a set of objects, called *nodes* or *vertices*, and the relationships, called *edges* or *arcs*, that exist between pairs of the objects [9, 10]. The equivalence between a labeled graph and a connection table means that connection tables may be processed by using algorithms derived from graph theory, in particular the isomorphism algorithms that are used to identify structural relationships between pairs of graphs [11, 12].

8.3 SEARCHING 2D CHEMICAL STRUCTURES

Current chemical information systems offer three principal types of search facility. *Structure search* involves the search of a file of compounds for the presence or absence of a specified query compound, for example, to retrieve physicochemical data associated with a particular substance. *Substructure search* involves the search of a file of compounds for all molecules containing some specified query substructure of interest. Finally, *similarity search* involves the search of a file of compounds for those molecules that are most similar to an input query molecule, using some quantitative definition of structural similarity.

8.3.1 Structure Searching

Structure searching is the chemical equivalent of graph isomorphism, that is, the matching of one graph against another to determine whether they are identical. This can be carried out very rapidly if a unique structure representation is available, because a character-by-character match will then suffice to compare two structures for identity. However, connection tables are not necessarily unique, because very many different tables can be created for the same molecule depending upon the way in which the atoms in the molecule are numbered. Specifically, for a molecule containing N atoms, there are $N!$

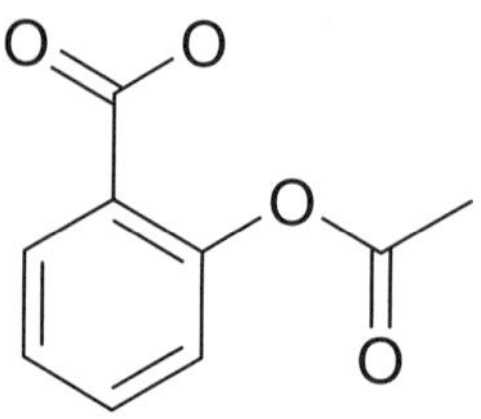

(a)

acetyl salicylic acid

(b)

```
-ISIS -   09270222202D

 13  13  0  0  0  0  0  0  0  0999  V2000
   -3.4639   -1.5375   0.0000 C   0  0  0  0  0  0  0  0  0  0  0  0
   -3.4651   -2.3648   0.0000 C   0  0  0  0  0  0  0  0  0  0  0  0
   -2.7503   -2.7777   0.0000 C   0  0  0  0  0  0  0  0  0  0  0  0
   -2.0338   -2.3644   0.0000 C   0  0  0  0  0  0  0  0  0  0  0  0
   -2.0367   -1.5338   0.0000 C   0  0  0  0  0  0  0  0  0  0  0  0
   -2.7521   -1.1247   0.0000 C   0  0  0  0  0  0  0  0  0  0  0  0
   -2.7545   -0.2997   0.0000 C   0  0  0  0  0  0  0  0  0  0  0  0
   -2.0413    0.1149   0.0000 C   0  0  0  0  0  0  0  0  0  0  0  0
   -3.4702    0.1107   0.0000 C   0  0  0  0  0  0  0  0  0  0  0  0
   -1.3238   -1.1186   0.0000 C   0  0  0  0  0  0  0  0  0  0  0  0
   -0.6125   -1.5292   0.0000 C   0  0  0  0  0  0  0  0  0  0  0  0
   -0.6167   -2.3542   0.0000 C   0  0  0  0  0  0  0  0  0  0  0  0
    0.1000   -1.1125   0.0000 C   0  0  0  0  0  0  0  0  0  0  0  0
  1  2  2  0  0  0  0
  6  7  1  0  0  0  0
  3  4  2  0  0  0  0
  7  8  1  0  0  0  0
  7  9  2  0  0  0  0
  4  5  1  0  0  0  0
  5 10  1  0  0  0  0
  2  3  1  0  0  0  0
 10 11  1  0  0  0  0
  5  6  2  0  0  0  0
 11 12  2  0  0  0  0
  6  1  1  0  0  0  0
 11 13  1  0  0  0  0
M END
```

the first atom is carbon

the bond between atoms 1 and 2 has order 2

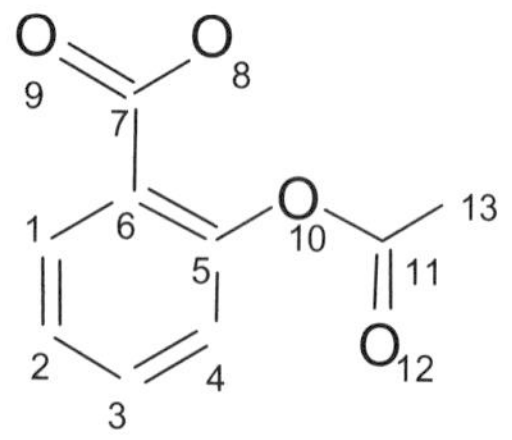

(c)

OC(=O)c1ccccc1OC(=O)C

(d)

Figure 8.1 Example of (a) a structure diagram, (b) systematic nomenclature, (c) connection table in MDL format (see URL http://www.mdli.com), and (d) SMILES for a molecule.

different ways of enumerating the atoms. The obvious algorithm for detecting the equivalence of two such variant representations hence involves the generation of all possible numberings of one molecule for comparison with the other; however, the factorial enumeration procedure is computationally infeasible for all but the smallest structures, unless some sort of heuristic can be invoked to reduce the number of possible atom-to-atom equivalences that must be considered [11, 12]. Two main approaches have been devised to overcome this problem in the chemical context.

The first of these involves the use of an algorithmic technique that can transform a connection table into a *canonical* form for the purposes of storage and retrieval. The best-known canonicalization scheme is that due to Morgan [13]: This algorithm defines a simple and elegant method for producing a unique numbering of the set of atoms in a connection table and forms the basis of the CAS Chemical Registry System, which has now been in operation for some four decades and which contains connection tables for some thirty million distinct chemical substances [5, 6]. The unique numbering is based on the concept of *extended connectivity*, an iterative procedure in which atom codes are derived that represent the numbers of atoms one, two, three, etc., bonds away from a given atom. The second, highly efficient, means of implementing structure search is to use a technique called *hashing*: A hashing function is a computational procedure that takes some data record and converts it to an address at which that record is stored. In the chemical structure context, the hash code is calculated from the atom and bond information in a connection table; the query structure then must undergo the detailed isomorphism search for an exact match for only those (hopefully) few molecules that have a hash code that is identical to its code [14].

8.3.2 Substructure Searching

Substructure searching is the chemical equivalent of the graph-theoretic problem of subgraph isomorphism, which involves determining whether a query graph is contained within another, larger graph [15] (Fig. 8.2). Subgraph isomorphism is known to be very demanding of computational resources, again involving factorial numbers of node-to-node comparisons, and substructure searching is hence normally effected by a two-level search procedure. In the first stage, a *screen search* is carried out to identify those few molecules in the database that match the query at the screen level, where a screen is a substructural fragment the presence of which is necessary but not sufficient for a molecule to contain the query substructure. These fragments are typically small, atom-, bond- or ring-centered substructures that are algorithmically generated from a connection table. The screen search involves checking each of the database structures for the presence of those screens that are present in the query substructure. In the second stage, each of the molecules that match the query in the screen search then undergoes a detailed *atom-by-atom* comparison with the query to determine whether the

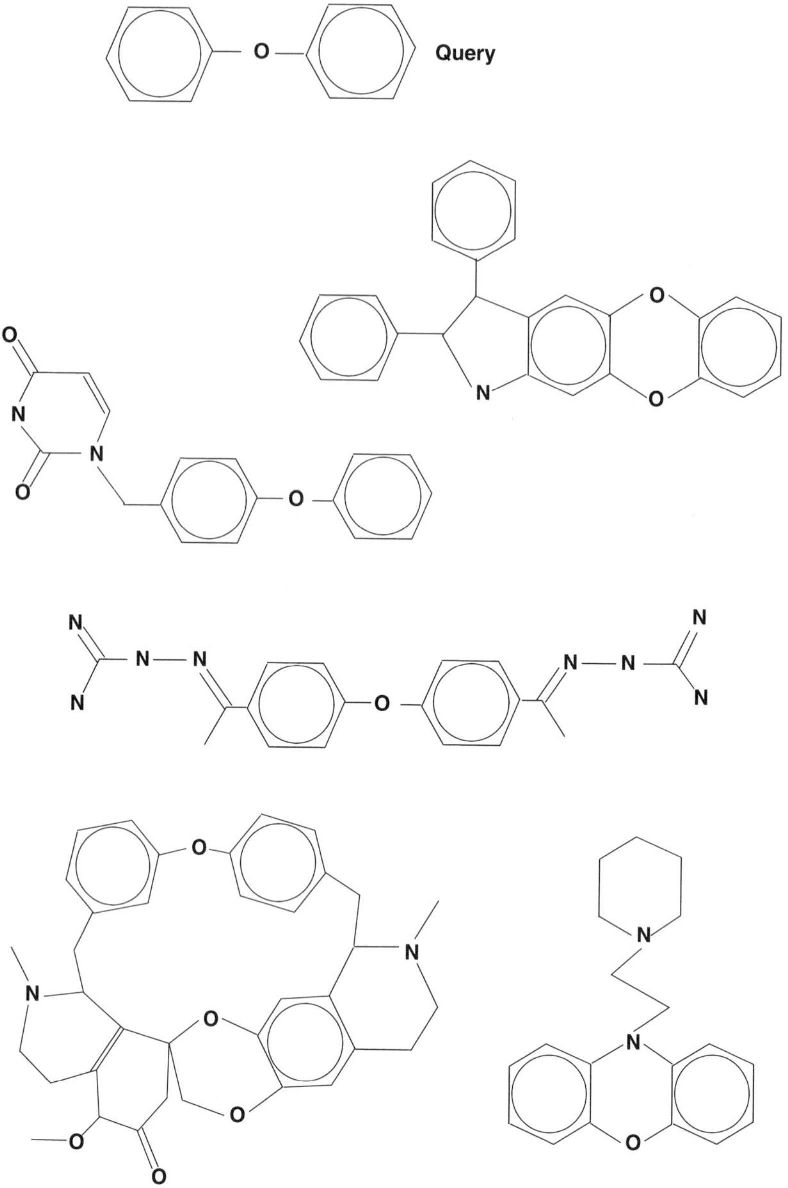

Figure 8.2 Example of a 2D substructure search. The search is for the diphenyl ether query substructure at the top of the figure, below which are shown five of the hits resulting from a search of the National Cancer Institute database of molecules that have been tested in the US government anticancer program (see URL http://dtp.nci.nih.gov/). This database is also used for the search outputs shown in Figures 8.3 and 8.4.

required substructure is present, this stage involving a subgraph isomorphism algorithm. The overall efficiency of the search will depend on the *screenout*, that is, the fraction of the database that is eliminated by the screening search, and there has accordingly been considerable interest in the development of algorithmic techniques for the selection of discriminating fragments that will give high screenout (see, e.g., Refs. 16, 17).

The fragments that have been chosen to act as screens are listed in a fragment coding dictionary. When a query or a new molecule is to be processed, the corresponding connection table is analyzed to identify those screens from the coding dictionary that are present in the structure. A database structure or query substructure is then represented by a fixed-length bit string, or *fingerprint*, in which the nonzero bits correspond to the screens that are present. An alternative approach involves the use of *superimposed coding* techniques in which each fragment is hashed to several bit locations; here, rather than having a predefined list of acceptable fragments, an algorithmic fragment definition (such as all chains containing 4 nonhydrogen atoms) is used to generate all fragments of that type in a molecule. Each of the resulting fragments is then input to the hashing procedure that switches on the set of bits associated with that hashcode.

Once the screen search has been completed, the second stage, atom-by-atom search, is carried out for just those few molecules matching at the screen level, that is, having a fingerprint in which bits are set at all the positions that have been set in the fingerprint describing the query substructure. This atom-by-atom search is normally applied to only a very small fraction of the connection tables in a database. The factorial nature of subgraph isomorphism means that there has been much interest in sophisticated heuristics that can minimize the computational requirements [15]. Of these, the most common is the subgraph isomorphism algorithm of Ullmann [18], which now provides the central component of many operational chemoinformatics systems.

8.3.3 Similarity Searching

Structure and substructure searching are very powerful ways of accessing a database, but they do assume that the searcher knows precisely the information that is needed, that is, a specific molecule or a specific class of molecules, respectively. The third approach to database searching, similarity searching, is less precise in nature because it searches the database for molecules that are similar to the user's query, without formally defining exactly how the molecules should be related (Fig. 8.3).

Similarity searching requires the specification of an entire molecule, called the *target structure* or *reference structure*, rather than the partial structure that is required for substructure searching. The target molecule is characterized by a set of structural features, and this set is compared with the corresponding sets of features for each of the database structures. Each such comparison enables the calculation of a measure of similarity between the

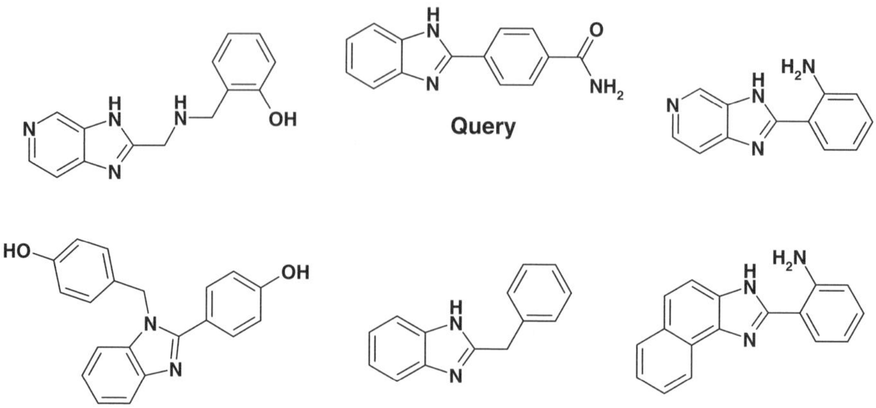

Query

Figure 8.3 Example of a 2D similarity search, showing a query molecule and five of its nearest neighbors. The similarity measure for the search is based on 2D fragment bit-strings and the Tanimoto coefficient.

target structure and a database structure, and the database molecules are then sorted into order of decreasing similarity with the target. The most similar molecules to the target structure, the *nearest neighbors*, are then displayed first to the user; accordingly, if an appropriate measure of similarity has been used, these nearest neighbors will be those that have the greatest probability of being of interest to the user. Since its introduction in the mid-1980s [19, 20], similarity searching has proved extremely popular with users, who have found that it provides a means of accessing chemical databases that is complementary to the existing structure and substructure searching facilities.

At the heart of any similarity searching system is the measure that is used to quantify the degree of structural resemblance between the target structure and each of the structures in the database that is to be searched. Willett et al. [21] provide an extended review of intermolecular structural similarity measures for database searching. The most common measures of this type are based on comparing the fragment bit-strings that are normally used for 2D substructure searching, so that two molecules are judged as being similar if they have a large number of bits in common. A normalized association coefficient, typically the Tanimoto coefficient, is used to give similarity values in the range of zero (no bits in common) to unity (all bits the same). Specifically, if two molecules have A and B bits set in their fragment bit-strings, with C of these in common, then the Tanimoto coefficient is defined to be

$$\frac{C}{A + B - C}.$$

Although such a fragment-based measure clearly provides a very simple picture of the similarity relationships between pairs of structures, it is both efficient (because it involves just the application of logical operations to pairs of bit-strings) and effective (in that it is able to bring together molecules that are judged by chemists to be structurally similar to each other) in operation.

Many other types of similarity measure have been described in the literature [22, 23]. One type of measure that is gaining increasing interest is the use of the maximum common substructure, or MCS, where the MCS between a pair of molecules is the chemical equivalent of a maximum common subgraph, that is, the largest subgraph common to a pair of graphs. The MCS for a pair of molecules thus represents the optimal superimposition of one molecule upon the other: This provides a very precise measure of the degree of similarity between them, but a measure that is far slower to compute than the simple fragment-based measures described above [24].

8.4 SEARCHING 3D CHEMICAL STRUCTURES

Thus far, we have considered the representation and searching of 2D structures, but the last few years have seen the development of comparable systems for the processing of 3D structures, for which atomic coordinate data are available. The traditional source of such data was the Cambridge Structural Database, which contains coordinate data for the approximately 330K molecules for which an X-ray crystal structure has been determined [25]. However, an X-ray structure is not available for many, perhaps most, of the molecules that are of interest in drug discovery, and this fact spurred the development of *structure-generation* programs that can convert a 2D connection table to a reasonably accurate 3D structure without the extensive computation required by approaches such as quantum mechanics, molecular dynamics, and molecular modeling [26]. The availability of such programs enables a pharmaceutical company to create an in-house database of 3D structures, and there is then a need for tools to search the resulting database. In particular, there is a need to identify those molecules that contain a user-defined *pharmacophore*, or *pharmacophoric pattern*, that is, the arrangement of structural features in 3D space necessary for a molecule to bind at an active site. An example of a pharmacophore, specifically an antileukemic pattern suggested by Zee-Cheng and Cheng [27], is shown in Figure 8.4.

Gund was the first person to recognize that pharmacophore searches could be effected by graph-based approaches [28]. In a 2D chemical graph, the nodes and edges of a graph are used to represent the atoms and bonds, respectively, of a molecule; in a 3D chemical graph, the nodes and edges are used to represent the atoms and interatomic distances, respectively. The presence or absence of a pharmacophoric pattern can then be confirmed by means of a subgraph isomorphism procedure in which the edges in a database structure

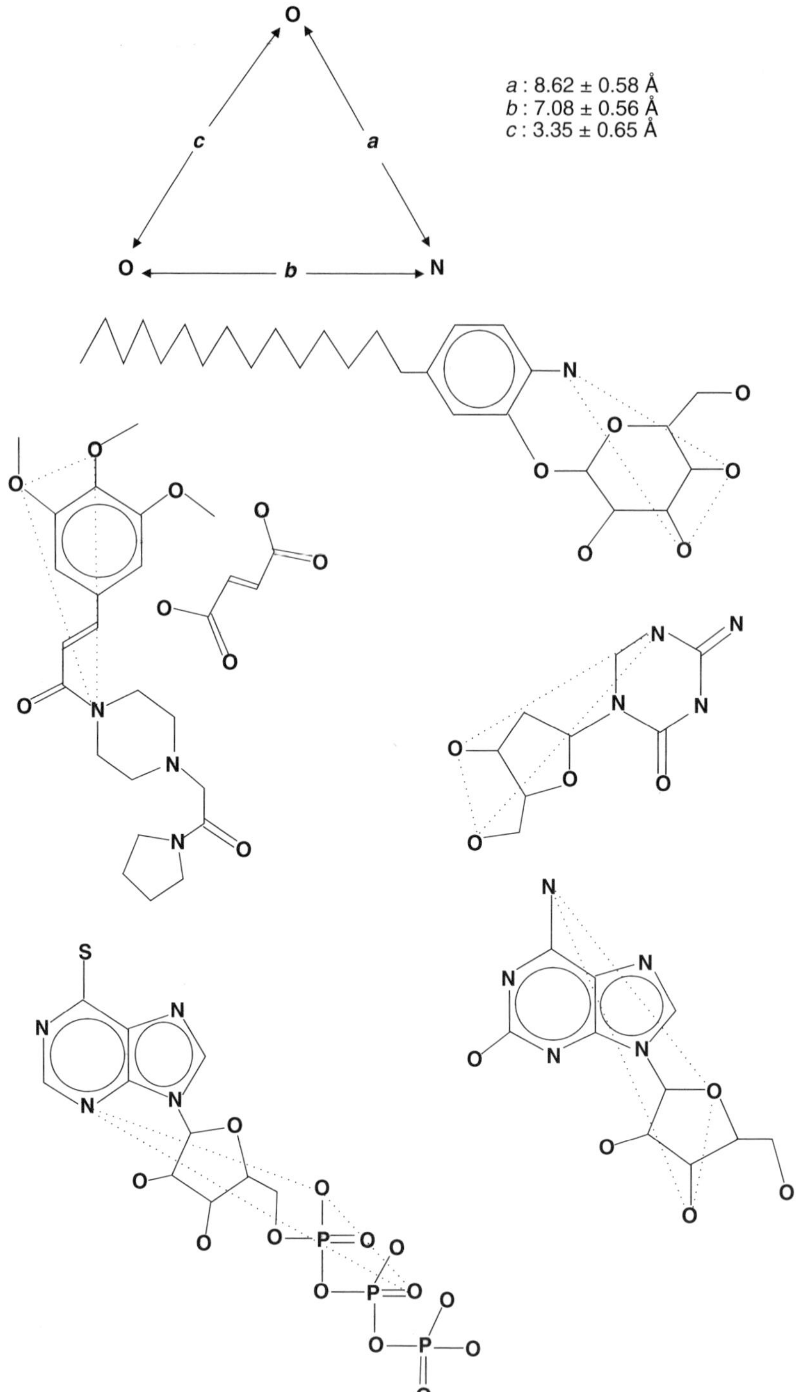

Figure 8.4 Typical hit structures for the antileukemic pharmacophore shown at the top of the page, with the presence of the pharmacophore in the retrieved molecules shown by dotted lines.

and a query substructure are matched if they denote the same interatomic distance (to within any user-specified tolerance such as ±0.5Å). As with 2D substructure searching, an effective screening mechanism is required if there is to be an acceptable response time for a search. The screens that are used for 3D substructure searching normally specify the presence within a molecule of two specific atoms separated by a distance that lies within an associated interatomic distance range. Analysis of the interatomic distances within a molecule is used to set the appropriate bits in a fingerprint, and then the time-consuming subgraph isomorphism search is applied to those molecules that match the query pharmacophore at the screen level [29, 30]. As an example, Figure 8.4 shows some of the hits from a 3D search for the antileukemic pharmacophore shown at the top of the figure: It will be seen that the hits encompass a wide range of structural types, while all containing the specified three atoms at distances within the allowed tolerances (as marked by the dotted lines).

Thus far, we have considered only rigid molecules, that is, structure representations that take no account of the flexibility that characterizes many molecules. A pharmacophore search is hence likely to miss large numbers of matching molecules that can adopt a conformation containing the pharmacophore but that are represented in the database by a low-energy conformation that does not contain this pattern. Two main approaches to flexible 3D searching have been described in the literature to overcome this problem and hence to increase the recall of pharmacophore searches. In the first, a flexible molecule is represented by some small number of carefully selected low-energy conformations, with these being generated either when the database is being built or at search time. The screening and subgraph isomorphism searches are then applied repeatedly to each of the conformations describing a molecule to determine whether any matches are present. The second approach involves a more extensive exploration of conformational space that is carried out at search time. The distance between a pair of atoms in a flexible molecule depends on the conformation that is adopted. The separation of a pair of atoms is hence conveniently described by a distance range, the lower bounds and upper bounds of which correspond to the minimum and maximum possible distances. The searching algorithms that are used for rigid 3D searching operate on graphs in which each edge denotes a single interatomic distance; these procedures require only minor modifications to enable them to process graphs in which each edge contains a distance range, thus allowing the retrieval of all molecules that could possibly adopt a conformation that contains a query pharmacophoric pattern [31]. However, a final search is required, after the subgraph matching, to ensure that the conformations retrieved are geometrically and energetically feasible. This means that the second approach is more time-consuming than the use of multiple conformations, but can result in still higher recall.

8.5 COMPOUND SELECTION

The previous sections have summarized the basic techniques available for searching chemical databases for specific types of query. Another important database application is *compound selection*, the ability to select a subset of a database for submission to a biological testing program. The selection procedure can be applied to in-house databases, to externally available compound collections, or to *virtual libraries*, that is, sets of compounds that could potentially be synthesized.

The development of automation techniques for compound synthesis and biological screening has resulted in a great increase in the rate at which compounds can be tested for activity. Thus high-throughput screening allows hundreds of thousands of compounds to be tested in a bioassay and combinatorial chemistry allows many hundreds of compounds to be synthesized in parallel. However, the vast size of chemistry space (it has been estimated that more than 10^{60} druglike compounds could potentially exist [32,33]) and the real costs associated with testing large numbers of samples mean that it is essential that screening sets are carefully designed. The design criterion that is applied depends on the intended use of the screening set and the information that is available concerning the biological end point.

Diverse compound sets are required for screening against a range of biological targets and for screening against a single target when little is known about the target. The rationale for diversity stems from the similar property principle [34, 35], which states that structurally similar compounds are likely to share the same activity. If this is so, then it should be possible to design a diverse subset of compounds that covers the same biological space as the larger set from which it is derived. Biased compounds sets are appropriate when the compounds are to be screened against a family of targets with related properties, for example, kinases or GPCRs. Such compound sets can be designed by placing restrictions on the chemistry space that compounds should occupy; however, it is still important to select a diverse subset of compounds from within the allowed space.

Diversity is also a key criterion in compound acquisition programs. In-house databases are typically biased collections with the coverage of chemistry space reflecting the therapeutic areas that a company has worked on during its lifetime. There are many companies that supply compounds for purchase, with the source of the compounds including both traditional and combinatorial synthesis, and pharmaceutical companies are now actively engaged in compound acquisition programs with the aim of filling the gaps in chemistry space that exist in their own collections. Such programs require methods for comparing datasets to enable the purchasing of compounds that are diverse with respect to the compounds that are already available internally.

When active compounds have already been found or when the 3D structure of the biological target is known, then focused or targeted sets are required.

The use of computational methods to select focused compound sets is often referred to as *virtual screening* [36]. Virtual screening techniques also include similarity searching and pharmacophore searching as already discussed in this chapter, machine-learning methods based on training sets of known active and inactive molecules, and protein-ligand docking methods. The rest of this chapter describes compound selection methods with particular emphasis on diversity and on methods for comparing compound sets.

Compound selection methods usually involve selecting a relatively small set of a few tens or hundreds of compounds from a large database that could consist of hundreds of thousands or even millions of compounds. Identifying the n most dissimilar compounds in a database containing N compounds, when typically $n << N$, is computationally infeasible because it requires consideration of all possible n-member subsets of the database, and therefore approximate methods have been developed as described below.

Several compound selection methods are based on calculating the pairwise similarities or dissimilarities of the compounds in the database. Methods for calculating the similarity between a pair of molecules were described above, and are typically based on the Tanimoto coefficient. When using a similarity coefficient such as the Tanimoto coefficient that returns values in the range zero to unity, dissimilarity is the complement of similarity ($1 - S_{TAN}$). When molecules are represented by their physicochemical properties, such as molecular weight, logP, molar refractivity, etc., then dissimilarity is often measured with Euclidean distance (following standardization of the properties). Whereas similarity and dissimilarity are properties of a pair of molecules, diversity is the property of a collection of molecules. A variety of different ways have been developed to assess the diversity of a set of molecules [34, 35]. Some are based on combining pairwise (dis)similarities, whereas other measures involve quantifying the amount of chemistry space that is covered by the compounds.

8.5.1 Dissimilarity-Based Compound Selection

Dissimilarity-based compound selection (DBCS) methods involve selecting a subset of compounds directly based on pairwise dissimilarities [37]. The first compound is selected, either at random or as the one that is most dissimilar to all others in the database, and is placed in the subset. The subset is then built up stepwise by selecting one compound at a time until it is of the required size. In each iteration, the next compound to be selected is the one that is most dissimilar to those already in the subset, with the dissimilarity normally being computed by the MaxMin approach [38]. Here, each database compound is compared with each compound in the subset and its nearest neighbor is identified; the database compound that is selected is the one that has the maximum dissimilarity to its nearest neighbor in the subset.

Sphere exclusion algorithms are closely related to DBCS methods. The basic algorithm operates by selecting a compound and then excluding from consideration all the compounds within an exclusion sphere centered on that compound [39, 40]. In one implementation of this basic idea (others are possible), the first compound is the one that is most dissimilar to all others in the database. In subsequent iterations, the next compound chosen is that remaining in the data set which is least dissimilar to the compounds already chosen. The algorithm continues until all compounds are either selected or excluded, and hence, in contrast to DBCS, it is not possible to specify the final size of the subset.

8.5.2 Cluster-Based Compound Selection

Clustering is the process of dividing a collection of objects into groups (or clusters) so that the objects within a cluster are highly similar whereas objects in different clusters are dissimilar [41]. When applied to databases of compounds, clustering methods require the calculation of all the pairwise similarities of the compounds with similarity measures such as those described previously, for example, 2D fingerprints and the Tanimoto coefficient.

Many different clustering algorithms have been developed. The techniques that are most commonly applied to compound selection include the Jarvis–Patrick method, and Ward's clustering. Jarvis–Patrick clustering [42] involves first generating a nearest neighbor list for each compound in the database. Compounds are then placed into the same cluster if they share some number of near neighbors, for example, two compounds may be placed in the same cluster if eight of their 14 nearest neighbors are in common. Jarvis–Patrick is a relatively fast clustering method; however, the basic algorithm can result in rather skewed clusters with a small number of very large clusters and a large number of singletons.

Ward's clustering is an agglomerative hierarchical clustering method in which smaller clusters of very similar molecules are embedded within larger clusters [43]. The method begins by placing each compound in its own cluster and then proceeds by merging the most similar clusters together in an iterative manner. Thus, in the first step the closest two compounds are merged into a single cluster; in the next step, the closest two clusters are merged; and so on. The process continues until all compounds are in a single cluster. At this point the clustering can be represented as a dendrogram as illustrated in Figure 8.5.

The next step is to choose a clustering level, which is equivalent to moving the dashed line up and down the dendrogram; in Figure 8.5, the dashed line represents a level in the hierarchy that consists of four clusters. Various methods are available for automatically determining an appropriate clustering level [44]. Once a database has been clustered, a diverse subset can be selected by choosing one or more compounds from each cluster. For a focused screening set, the compounds could be selected from clusters containing known actives.

Clustering methods are based solely on intermolecular similarities, and they hence provide a relative measure of the space covered by a data set rather

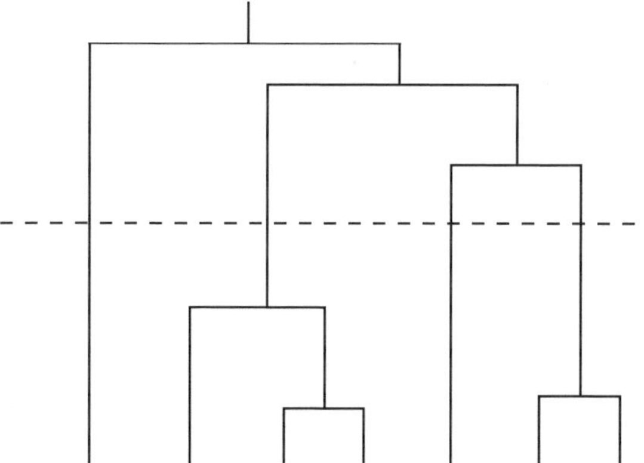

Figure 8.5 Example dendrogram representing an hierarchical clustering of a set of seven compounds.

than an absolute measure. This makes it difficult to compare data sets such as an in-house database and a database offered by a commercial vendor. The comparison would require that the databases are combined and then clustered as a combined unit. The degree of overlap in the two databases could then be assessed by examining the contents of each cluster. If a cluster is mainly occupied by compounds from one of the databases, this indicates a region of space where the databases differ. Thus a company may decide to augment its internal database by purchasing vendor compounds from clusters that are sparsely occupied by its own in-house compounds.

8.5.3 Partitioning Methods

Partitioning or *cell-based* methods provide an absolute measure of the chemical space covered by a collection of compounds. They are based on the definition of a low-dimensional chemistry space, for example, one based on a small number of physicochemical properties such as molecular weight, calculated logP, and number of hydrogen bond donors [45]. Each property defines an axis of the chemistry-space. The range of values for each property is divided into a set of bins, and the combinatorial product of all bins then defines the set of cells or partitions that make up the space.

When a chemistry space has been defined, a database can be mapped onto the space by assigning each molecule to a cell according to its properties and a diverse subset selected by taking one or more molecules from each cell; alternatively, a focused subset can be selected by choosing compounds from a limited number of cells, for example, from the cells adjacent to a cell occupied by a known active. The partitioning scheme is defined independently of the compounds that are mapped onto it, and so the space occupied by different data sets can be compared easily. Partitioning methods also allow voids or underrepresented regions of the space to be identified and can therefore be used for compound acquisition from external vendors.

Rather than using whole-molecule physicochemical properties, partitioning can also be based on sets of descriptors known as BCUTS that are calculated from matrix representations of a connection table [46, 47]. The diagonals of a matrix represent a property of each of the atoms such as atomic charge, atomic polarizability, and atomic hydrogen bonding ability. The off-diagonals are assigned the value 0.1 times the bond type if the atoms are bonded and 0.001 if the atoms are not bonded. The highest and lowest eigenvalues of each matrix are then extracted for use as descriptors.

8.5.4 Pharmacophore Fingerprints

Pharmacophoric fingerprints have also been widely used for compound selection [48]. They record the spatial arrangement of pharmacophoric features such as hydrogen bond donors, hydrogen bond acceptors, cations, anions, and aromatic and hydrophobic centers. Each bit in a three-point pharmacophoric fingerprint represents a particular triplet of features at specified distance ranges or bins. The pharmacophoric fingerprint for a 3D conformation of a molecule is constructed by identifying all the triplets of features and distances that exist in the conformer and setting the appropriate bits to "on" in the fingerprint. Flexibility is usually handled by generating an ensemble of conformers for a structure and taking the logical union (i.e., the Boolean "OR") of the fingerprints generated for each conformer to obtain a final ensemble fingerprint that represents the conformational space available to the molecule.

The pharmacophore fingerprints for a set of molecules can be combined into an ensemble pharmacophore that is the union of the individual fingerprints. The resulting fingerprint can then be used to measure total pharmacophore coverage; to identify pharmacophores that are not represented in the set of molecules; and to compare different sets of molecules. Thus, if the aim is to select a diverse set of compounds this would correspond to maximizing the coverage of pharmacophore triplets over all compounds in the subset. Pharmacophore fingerprints are also widely used in the design of focused screening sets, for example, the analysis of known active compounds can lead to the identification of *privileged substructures*, features that occur frequently within the known actives [49, 50]. In such cases, the criterion for selecting compounds would be to enrich the subset in compounds that contain the privileged features.

8.5.5 Optimization Methods

Optimization techniques can provide effective ways of sampling large search spaces, and hence several such methods have been applied to compound selection, for example, the use of Monte Carlo methods combined with simulated annealing [51, 52]. In the Monte Carlo method, the selection of a diverse subset proceeds as follows. An initial subset is chosen at random, and its diversity is calculated. A new subset is then generated from the first by replacing some of the compounds with others chosen at random. The diversity of the new subset is measured: If it is more diverse than the previous subset it is accepted for use in the next iteration; if it is less diverse, then the probability that it is accepted depends on the Boltzmann factor. The process continues for a fixed number of iterations or until no further improvement is observed in the diversity function.

An interesting diversity function that has been used for compound selection is based on computing the minimum spanning tree for the set of molecules [53]. A spanning tree is a set of edges that connect a set of nodes without forming any cycles. The nodes are the molecules in the subset, and each edge is labeled by the dissimilarity between the two molecules it connects. The minimum spanning tree is the spanning tree that connects all molecules in the subset with the minimum sum of pairwise dissimilarities. The diversity of the subset then equals the sum of the intermolecular similarities along the edges in the minimum spanning tree.

8.5.6 Computational Filters

Despite the initial enthusiasm for high-throughput screening, results from early runs were disappointing, with lower hit rates than expected, and the hits that were found often had properties that made them unsuitable as drugs (e.g., they were too large or too insoluble or they contained inappropriate functional groups). Thus it is now common to apply computational filters to eliminate undesirable compounds before performing compound selection.

To this end, medicinal chemists have compiled "bad lists" of substructures that can be used in substructure searches to identify and remove compounds that contain undesirable functional groups [54, 55]. Other commonly used filters are based on counts of structural features such as numbers of rotatable bonds and on physicochemical properties such as molecular weight and logP. These criteria have been in widespread use since the publication of the "rule of five" [56, 57]. The preferred route of administration of a drug is oral, and the rule of five suggests that oral absorption is unlikely for a molecule that violates two of the following criteria: molecular weight >500; number of hydrogen bond donors >5; number of hydrogen bond acceptors >10; calculated logP >5.0. These criteria provide powerful filters, but it is important to realize that there are always exceptional compounds that violate the rules but are still bioactive.

More sophisticated approaches have also been developed that aim to classify compounds as druglike or nondruglike [54, 58]. These methods generally involve the use of a training set of known drugs and nondrugs, with the classification methods including genetic algorithms, neural networks, and decision trees, inter alia. The algorithms "learn" classification rules from the data in the training set, with the rules being based on the molecular descriptors used to represent the compounds. Once the algorithms have been trained, the rules can be used to classify or score previously unseen compounds according to their likelihood of exhibiting druglike properties.

High-throughput screening is normally used to identify lead compounds rather than drug candidates. Lead compounds are typically weakly active and are subsequently optimized to improved their potency, selectivity, and physicochemical properties. The lead optimization process generally involves adding functionality to the compounds, which consequently results in an increase in the values of properties such as molecular weight and number of hydrogen bonding groups. Hence a recent focus has been on the prediction of lead-likeness rather than drug-likeness, especially when selecting screening sets [59, 60].

8.6 CONCLUSIONS

Chemoinformatics techniques are widely used to increase the cost-effectiveness of drug discovery programs, and in this chapter we have described some of the chemoinformatics approaches that have been developed for processing databases of 2D and 3D chemical structures. Many other chemoinformatics techniques are available, for example, for accessing databases of chemical reactions [61, 62], for correlating structure and activity with methods based on machine learning [63, 64], for docking ligands into the active sites of proteins for which a 3D X-ray crystal structure is available [65, 66], and for extending the 2D similarity searching methods described previously to the searching of 3D databases [50, 67]. Overviews of these, and other, approaches are provided by Leach and Gillet [1] and by Gasteiger and Engel [2]; however, it is hoped that the brief description that has been presented here will suffice to highlight the contributions that chemoinformatics can make to pharmaceutical research.

REFERENCES

1. Leach AR, Gillet VJ. *An introduction to chemoinformatics.* Dordrecht, Kluwer, 2003.
2. Gasteiger J, Engel T. *Chemoinformatics.* Weinheim, Wiley-VCH, 2003.
3. Barnard JM. *Computer handling of generic chemical structures.* Aldershot, Gower, 1984.
4. Berks AH. Current state of the art of Markush topological search systems. *World Patent Inf* 2001;23:5–13.
5. Weisgerber DW. Chemical Abstracts Service Chemical Registry System: history, scope, and impacts. *J Am Soc Inf Sci* 1997;48:349–60.

6. Fisanick W, Amaral NJ, Metanomski WV, Shively ER, Soukop KM, Stobaugh RE. Chemical Abstracts Service Information System. In: Schleyer P von R, Allinger NL, Clark T, Gasteiger J, Kollman PA, Schaefer HF and Schriener PR, editors, *Encyclopedia of computational chemistry*. Vol. 1. New York: John Wiley & Sons, 1998. p. 277–315.
7. Ash JE, Hyde E, *Chemical information systems*. Chichester, Ellis Horwood, 1975.
8. Weiniger D. SMILES, a chemical language and information system. 1. Introduction to methodology and encoding rules. *J Chem Inf Comput Sci* 1988;28:31–6.
9. Wilson R. *Introduction to graph theory*, 4th edition. Harlow, Longman, 1996.
10. Diestel R. *Graph theory*. New York, Springer-Verlag, 2000.
11. Read RC, Corneil DG. The graph isomorphism disease. *J Graph Theory* 1977;1:339–63.
12. Gati G. Further annotated bibliography on the isomorphism disease. *J Graph Theory* 1979;3:95–109.
13. Morgan HL. The generation of a unique machine description for chemical structures: a technique developed at Chemical Abstracts Service. *J Chem Docum* 1965;5:107–13.
14. Freeland RG, Funk SA, O'Korn LJ, Wilson GA. The CAS Chemical Registry System. II. Augmented connectivity molecular formula. *J Chem Inf Comput Sci* 1979;19:94–8.
15. Barnard JM. Substructure searching methods: old and new. *J Chem Inf Comput Sci* 1993;33:532–8.
16. Adamson GW, Cowell J, Lynch MF, McLure AHW, Town WG, Yapp AM. Strategic considerations in the design of screening systems for substructure searches of chemical structure files. *J Chem Docum* 1973;13:153–7.
17. Feldman A, Hodes, L. An efficient design for chemical structure searching. I. The screens. *J Chem Inf Comput Sci* 1975;15:147–52.
18. Ullmann, JR. An algorithm for subgraph isomorphism. *J ACM* 1976;16:31–42.
19. Carhart RE, Smith DH, Venkataraghavan R. Atom pairs as molecular features in structure-activity studies: definition and applications. *J Chem Inf Comput Sci* 1985;25:64–73.
20. Willett P, Winterman V, Bawden, D. Implementation of nearest neighbour searching in an online chemical structure search system. *J Chem Inf Comput Sci* 1986;26:36–41.
21. Willett P, Barnard JM, Downs, GM Chemical similarity searching. *J Chem Inf Comput Sci* 1998;38:983–96.
22. Sheridan RP, Kearsley SK. Why do we need so many chemical similarity search methods? *Drug Discov Today* 2002;7:903–11.
23. Bender A, Glen RC. Molecular similarity: a key technique in molecular informatics. *Org Biomol Chem* 2004;2:3204–18.
24. Raymond JW, Willett P. Maximum common subgraph isomorphism algorithms for the matching of chemical structures. *J Comput-Aided Mol Des* 2002;16:521–33.
25. Allen FH. The Cambridge Structural Database: a quarter of a million crystal structures and rising. *Acta Cryst B* 2002; B58:380–8.

26. Green DVS. Automated three-dimensional structure generation. In: Martin YC and Willett P, editors, *Designing bioactive molecules. Three-dimensional techniques and applications.* Washington DC, American Chemical Society, 1998;47–71.
27. Zee-Cheng KY, Cheng CC. Common receptor-complement feature among some anti-leukemic compounds. *J Pharm Sci* 1970;59:1630–4.
28. Gund P. Three-dimensional pharmacophoric pattern searching. *Prog Mol Subcell Biol* 1977;5:117–43.
29. Jakes SE, Willett P. Pharmacophoric pattern matching in files of 3-D chemical structures: selection of inter-atomic distance screens. *J Mol Graph* 1986;4:12–20.
30. Sheridan RP, Nilakantan R, Rusinko A, Bauman N, Haraki KS, Venkataraghavan R. 3DSEARCH: a system for three-dimensional substructure searching. *J Chem Inf Comput Sci* 1989;29:255–60.
31. Clark DE, Willett P, Kenny PW. Pharmacophoric pattern matching in files of three-dimensional chemical structures: use of smoothed bounded-distance matrices for the representation and searching of conformationally-flexible molecules. *J Mol Graph* 1992;10:194–204.
32. Valler MJ, Green DVS. Diversity screening versus focussed screening in drug discovery. *Drug Discov Today* 2000;5:286–93.
33. Hann MM, Leach AR, Green DVS. Computational chemistry, molecular complexity and screening set design. In: Oprea TI, editor, *Chemoinformatics in drug discovery*, Weinheim, Wiley-VCH, 2004;43–57.
34. Willett P. Computational methods for the analysis of molecular diversity. *Perspectives in Drug Discovery and Design* Vols 7/8. Dordrecht; Kluwer, 1997.
35. Lewis RA, Pickett SD, Clark, DE. Computer-aided molecular diversity analysis and combinatorial library design. In: Lipkowitz KB and Boyd DB, editors, *Reviews in Computational Chemistry. Vol. 16.* 2000;1–51.
36. Bohm H-J, Schneider G. *Virtual screening for bioactive molecules.* Weinheim: Wiley-VCH, 2000.
37. Lajiness MS. Molecular similarity-based methods for selecting compounds for screening. In: Rouvray DH, editor, *Computational chemical graph theory.* New York: Nova Science Publishers, 1990;299–316.
38. Snarey M, Terrett NK, Willett P, Wilton DJ. Comparison of algorithms for dissimilarity-based compound selection. *J Mol Graph Model* 1997;15:372–85.
39. Hudson BD, Hyde RM, Rahr E, Wood J, Osman J. Parameter based methods for compound selection from chemical databases. *Quant Struct-Act Relat* 1996;15:285–9.
40. Pearlman RS, Smith KM. Novel software tools for chemical diversity. *Perspect Drug Discov Des* 1998;9/10/11:339–53.
41. Downs GM, Barnard JM. Clustering methods and their uses in computational chemistry. In: Lipkowitz KB and Boyd DB, editors, *Reviews in Computational Chemistry,* Vol. 18. New York, VCH Publishers, 2002;1–40.
42. Jarvis RA, Patrick EA. Clustering using a similarity measure based on shared near neighbours. *IEEE Trans Comput* 1973; C-22:1025–34.

43. Ward JH. Hierarchical grouping to optimise an objective function. *J Am Stat Assoc* 1963;58:236–44.
44. Wild DJ, Blankley J. Comparison of 2D fingerprint types and hierarchy level selection methods for structural grouping using Ward's clustering. *J Chem Inf Comput Sci* 2000;40:155–62.
45. Lewis RA, Mason JS, McLay, IM. Similarity measures for rational set selection and analysis of combinatorial libraries: The diverse property-derived (DPD) approach. *J Chem Inf Comput Sci* 1997;37:599–614.
46. Pearlman RS, Smith KM. Metric validation and the receptor-relevant subspace concept. *J Chem Inf Comput Sci* 1999;39:28–35.
47. Cavallaro CL, Schnur DM, Tebben AJ. Molecular diversity in lead discovery: From quantity to quality. In: Oprea TI, editor, *Chemoinformatics in drug discovery*, Weinheim, Wiley-VCH, 2004;175–98.
48. Davies K. Using pharmacophore diversity to select molecules to test from commercial catalogues. In: Chaiken IM and Janda KD, editors, *Molecular diversity and combinatorial chemistry. Libraries and drug discovery.* Washington DC: American Chemical Society, 1996;309–16.
49. Mason JS, Pickett, SD. Partition-based selection. *Perspect Drug Discov Des*, 1997;7/8:85–114.
50. Mason JS, Morize I, Menard PR, Cheney DL, Hulme C, Labaudiniere RF. New 4-point pharmacophore method for molecular similarity and diversity applications: Overview of the method and applications, including a novel approach to the design of combinatorial libraries containing privileged substructures. *J Med Chem* 1999;42:3251–64.
51. Waldman M, Li H, Hassan M. Novel algorithms for the optimization of molecular diversity of combinatorial libraries. *J Mol Graph Model* 2000;18:412–26.
52. Agrafiotis DK. Stochastic algorithms for maximising molecular diversity. *J Chem Inf Comput Sci* 1997;37:841–51.
53. Hassan M, Bielawski JP, Hempel JC, Waldman M. Optimisation and visualisation of molecular diversity of combinatorial libraries. *Mol Diversity* 1996;2:64–74.
54. Walters WP, Murcko MA. Prediction of 'drug-likeness'. *Adv Drug Deliv Rev* 2002;54:255–71.
55. Leach AR, Bradshaw J, Green DVS, Hann MM, Delany JJ III. Implementation of a system for reagent selection and library enumeration, profiling and design. *J Chem Inf Comput Sci* 1999;39:1161–72.
56. Lipinski CA. Drug-like properties and the causes of poor solubility and poor permeability. *J Pharm Toxicol Methods* 2000;44:235–49.
57. Oprea TI. Property distributions of drug-related chemical databases. *J Comput-Aided Mol Des* 2000;14:251–264.55.
58. Clark DE, Pickett SD. Computational methods for the prediction of "drug-likeness". *Drug Discov Today* 2000;5:49–58.
59. Oprea TI, Davis AM, Teague SJ, Leeson PD. Is there a difference between leads and drugs? A historical perspective. *J Chem Inf Comput Sci* 2001;41:1308–15.
60. Hann MM, Leach AR, Harper G. Molecular complexity and its impact on the probability of finding leads for drug discovery. *J Chem Inf Comput Sci* 2001;41:856–64.

61. Ridley DD. Strategies for chemical reaction searching in SciFinder. *J Chem Inf Comput Sci* 2000;40:1077–84.
62. Chen L. Reaction classification and knowledge acquisition. In: Gasteiger J, editor, *Handbook of chemoinformatics*. Weinheim: Wiley-VCH, 2003;348–88.
63. Wilton DJ, Willett P, Mullier G, Lawson K. Comparison of ranking methods for virtual screening in lead-discovery programmes. *J Chem Inf Comput Sci* 2003;43:469–74.
64. Jorissen RN, Gilson MK. Virtual screening of molecular databases using a Support Vector Machine. *J Chem Inf Model* 2005;45:549–61.
65. Halperin I, Ma B, Wolfson H, Nussinov R. Principles of docking: an overview of search algorithms and a guide to scoring functions. *Proteins* 2002;47:409–43.
66. Taylor RD, Jewsbury PJ, Essex JW. A review of protein-small molecule docking methods. *J Comput-Aided Mol Des* 2002;16:151–66.
67. Schuffenhauer A, Gillet VJ, Willett P. Similarity searching in files of 3D chemical structures: analysis of the BIOSTER database using 2D fingerprints and molecular field descriptors. *J Chem Inf Comput Sci* 2000;40:295–307.

9

ELECTRONIC LABORATORY NOTEBOOKS

ALFRED NEHME AND ROBERT A. SCOFFIN

Contents

9.1 INTRODUCTION

Within a very short space of time—perhaps only the last 5 years, there has been an explosion of interest in electronic laboratory notebook systems in general, and particularly within the drug discovery community. In large part

Computer Applications in Pharmaceutical Research and Development, Edited by Sean Ekins.
ISBN 0-471-73779-8

it seems that this particular level of interest derives from the importance attached to both legal and regulatory issues within the pharmaceutical industry.

An electronic laboratory notebook system ("e-notebook" or "ELN") addresses several different areas that impact upon scientific productivity, including time efficiencies and communication of information.

Time spent in complying with regulatory and legal issues, for instance, completing the paper notebook write-up of an experiment, is time taken out of the lab and is therefore time not spent making new discoveries. Shortening the time taken to both set up new experiments and document experimental outcomes will therefore have a direct and positive impact on scientific productivity.

Communication between co-workers on a project tends to be good within the modern research organization—the use of electronic communications technologies such as instant messaging, voice over IP ("VoIP"), and video conferencing have even made this true at a global level. However, communications between different research groups, and between current and past colleagues (particularly where the colleagues have retired or moved to a different company) are not so clearly helped by these technologies. ELNs do address communications issues within project teams, research groups, and global research and development (R&D) organizations; ELN systems allow for passive and active communications, that is, users can search within the archive of past experiments to determine whether a particular experiment, or something similar, has been carried out before or information can be actively shared between research colleagues—using project folders as an example.

An additional aspect of the communication of information is the desire to increase the efficiency with which a researcher can work with the various service organizations that are typically found within a large Pharma organization. A good example of this is the use of centralized analytical chemistry facilities for purification and identification of synthesized product molecules. In this case, the typical workflow involves a medicinal chemist running a synthesis experiment, which results in a crude reaction product. The crude reaction product may be sent out to an analytical service for purification and identification of products. In the old paradigm, this would involve one or more paper forms being filled out in a multistep process. Each step involves the copying of the reaction drawing or an anticipated product molecule structure. The requests are then delivered, along with the physical sample, to the analytical group, who work up the materials, purify and identify the products, and generate an analytical report. This is then returned, usually in paper form, to the chemist, who has to cut out the relevant spectra, for example, and paste them into the paper notebook.

In the new paradigm involving the use of an ELN, the workflow is much simplified. The analytical requests are generated directly from the experimental write-up within the medicinal chemists' notebook. No copying or manual duplication is required. The request is then routed electronically to the analytical group; unfortunately, it is still necessary to physically transfer the samples also! After the analysis and identification of the products, a report is generated, again directly within the ELN, and this is routed back to the chemist to be directly incorporated into the experimental record.

Within this chapter we provide an assessment of the rationale behind the adoption of an ELN system, an overview of the current market for such systems, and the typical uses and key benefits for drug discovery to be derived from a successful implementation.

9.2 E-NOTEBOOK BACKGROUND AND HISTORY

Record keeping is a fundamental requirement for any serious research activity, and of course drug discovery and development is no different. In the case of drug discovery, there are a number of convergent requirements for keeping good scientific records:

- Intellectual property capture
  - Patenting
- Regulatory
- Knowledge management
  - Know-how and other intellectual capital

The requirements for regulatory approval and intellectual property management, and in particular the ability to file USPTO patent submissions, do place constraints on what systems can be applied for record keeping, but the good news is that there are no insurmountable barriers to these records being captured and managed electronically.

The history of the ELN within pharmaceutical research goes back to the 1980s and the growing role of both personal computers and centralized informatics systems. Since around 1978 when MDL (Molecular Design Limited) was founded, tools and applications have existed that could be used to capture experimental information more conveniently than the traditional paper notebook. These chemical information systems provided advantages in terms of task automation (e.g., stoichiometry calculations), legibility, portability (sharing of information across networks), and the ability to search research documents by text and/or chemical structure. In some sense these early systems were ELN systems, but there were some key shortcomings that needed to be addressed before they could be true replacements for a paper notebook records management system.

However, adoption of ELNs as a standard tool within corporate research was hampered by both the legal and regulatory requirements of the time. The FDA, the federal courts, and the USPTO were not really aligned to adoption of electronic records for NDA submission or for patent purposes. This was to start changing in the mid-1990s. In 1994 the FDA issued a draft set of rules for the acceptance of electronic records as part of NDA and other regulatory submissions. These rules became codified as law in 1995 and were issued as Code of Federal Regulations number 21 part 11 ("21CFR Part 11"; see also Chapter 26). Later the rules surrounding the use of electronic records for submission to the USPTO for patents, interferences, and other types of litigation were also codified, becoming 37CFR.

In 2000 the US government and other worldwide governments and authorities (e.g., UK government, European Central Court) issued new laws stating that all electronic records have the same validity and are subject to the same rules of evidence as paper records. This meant that electronic documents could be signed with digital signatures and would be treated exactly as a paper document with a "wet" signature.

9.2.1 Electronic Signatures

Key to the acceptance of electronic notebooks for intellectual property ("IP") and regulatory purposes is the implementation of a set of compliance rules and a related document management system. In the traditional paper notebook world, this consisted of a set of standard operating procedures ("SOPs") and a paper/microfiche archiving system. In the new electronic paradigm, this can also revolve around a paper-based records management system (so called "hybrid" systems) or may involve the use of e-signatures to validate the author and contents of an electronic record. e-signatures make use of advanced cryptography methods to create a unique digital "fingerprint" of a document and to capture information regarding the author of the document, the contents of the document, and optionally the date and time of signing of the document.

The process of creating an e-signature can be described graphically (Fig. 9.1a). The "E-Signature Applied" and "Witness Reviews and Signs" process steps can be further broken down (Fig. 9.1b). The finally stored record within the e-signature repository may be compared to an onion, it is a hash (or unique fingerprint), wrapped in an encrypted layer that identifies the author (and optionally the witness), which itself may be wrapped in a further encrypted layer that provides a digital timestamp (Fig. 9.1c).

To validate the record one proceeds as follows:

1. Decrypt the outer layer with the public key provided by the appropriate digital timestamp authority [1], validate the timestamp contents, and read the date/time information.
2. Extract the next layer, decrypt the contents with the public key provided by the witness, and check the contents.
3. Extract the next layer, decrypt the contents with the public key provided by the author, and check the contents. This is the hash code for the document generated when it was originally signed.

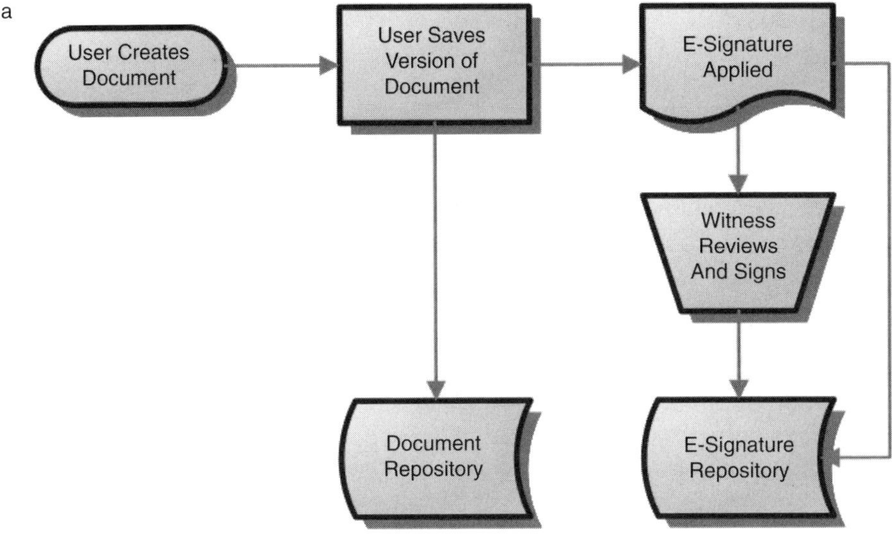

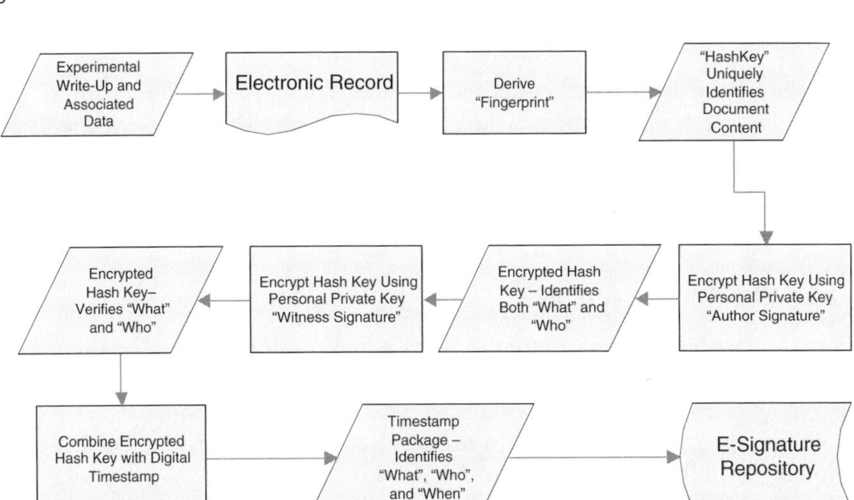

Figure 9.1 a. The process of creating an e-signature. b. The "E-Signature Applied" and "Witness Reviews and Signs" steps expanded. c. The stored record within the e-signature repository.

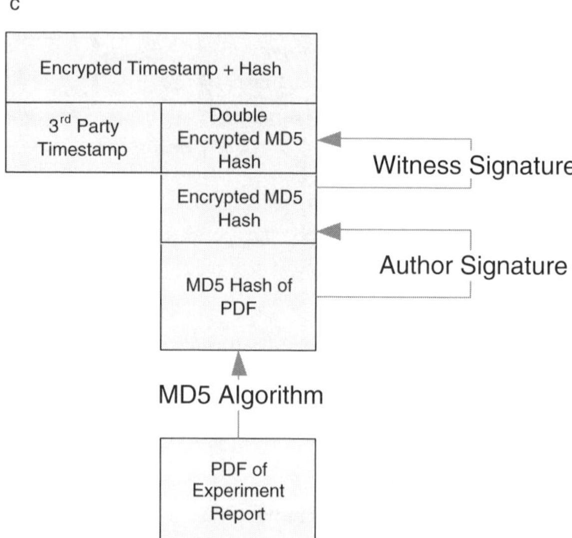

Figure 9.1 *Continued*

4. Derive a new hash code for the electronic record being validated, compare the two fingerprints, and if they are different, then the document contents have changed since the record was originally signed: The e-record is not valid. If the fingerprints match, then the content has not been changed: The e-record is valid.

9.2.2 ELN Implementations

Over the last 5 or 6 years there has been a marked increase in the number of companies implementing an ELN system within drug discovery. There has also been a corresponding increase in the number of companies providing commercial applications in this market sector (see Section 9.6 for more details). Initially this adoption of ELNs was done despite the "problem" of e-signatures, but lately more companies are moving to a fully electronic process, with the associated benefits that this proffers.

The first implementations of an ELN tended to be in-house developed applications, using standard and familiar components such as Microsoft Word, with chemical intelligence provided in the background by for example, ISIS from Elsevier MDL (http://www.mdli,com) or ChemDraw/ChemOffice from CambridgeSoft (http://www.cambridgesoft.com). An example of such a system, which is still in use today, is the TAN ("Template-Assisted Notebook") of Novartis. This is an example of a hybrid electronic notebook where the record management function is still handled through traditional paper and archiving methodologies. However, the benefits of increased legibility and enhanced searching are still present; the time savings and enhanced compliance associated with a fully electronic system typically will not be realized.

In 1999 CambridgeSoft released a desktop/personal version of an e-notebook, specifically targeted at medicinal chemistry; this incorporated reaction drawing and searching, automatic stoichiometry calculations, and simple procedure write-up using plain text. This system was adopted both by individuals, particularly in the academic community, and by small and medium-sized companies as an alternative to building an in-house hybrid system (Fig. 9.2).

This initial medicinal chemistry ELN was followed into the market by products such as the Arthur™ suite from Synthematix and the iELN system from Intellichem (both since acquired by Symyx), which were more oriented at reaction planning and process chemistry. The heavyweight of the traditional cheminformatics companies, Elsevier MDL, also released a system, called Élan, which combined a Word-based front end with their well-known ISIS chemical technology on the back end (Fig. 9.3).

All four of the companies mentioned above have continued to develop their presence in the ELN market, and, along with Creon/Waters, they

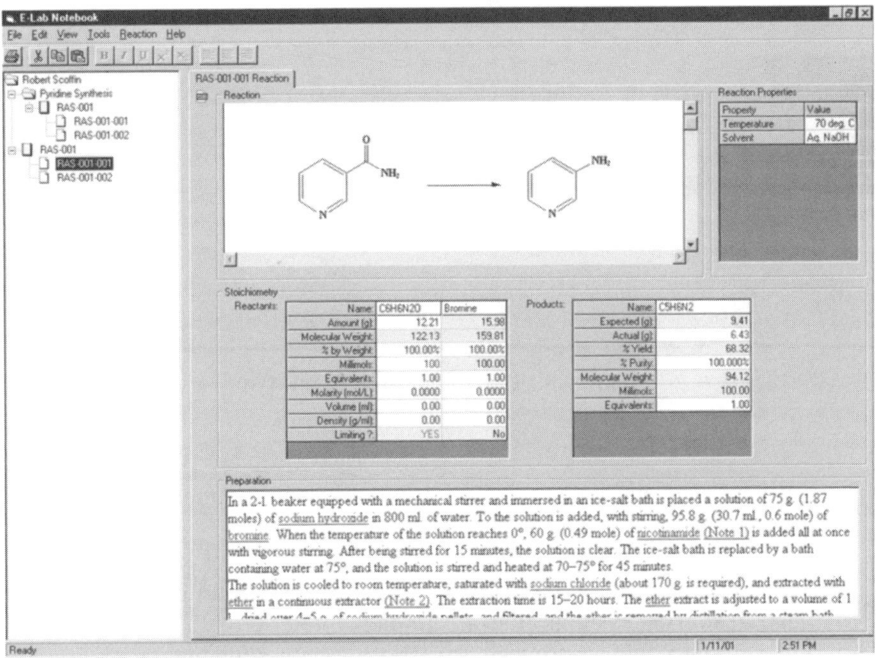

Figure 9.2 First release of e-notebook by CambridgeSoft.

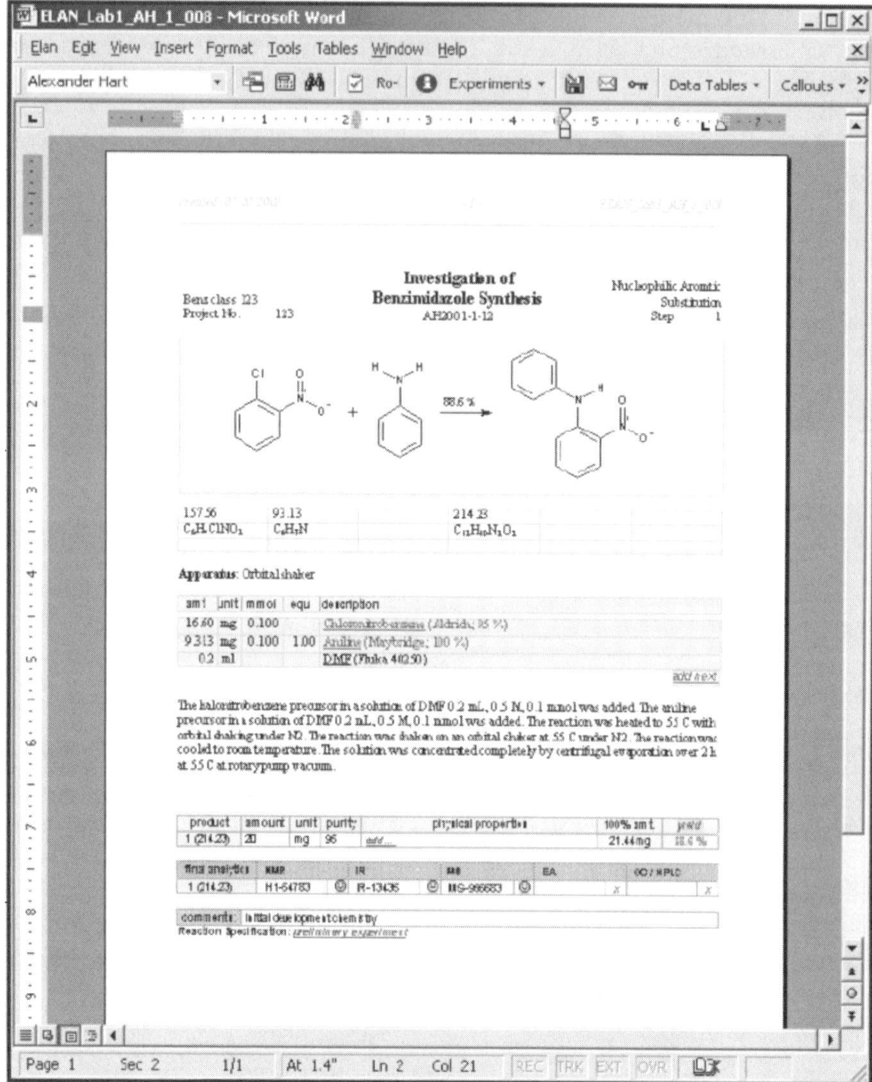

Figure 9.3 Élan screenshot from MDL.

probably represent more than 75% market share of commercially installed systems within drug discovery.

Today's ELN market is characterized by a number of niche providers, focusing their solutions on particular vertical markets, and general solution providers, delivering systems that are implemented across a broad range of disciplines. These two approaches are both very valid, having their own strengths and weaknesses. One trend that does seem to be emerging is a recognition by larger global pharmaceutical companies that a "one size fits all" policy does not always work for implementing an ELN system. There are a number of examples now of companies deploying ELN solutions from two, three, or more vendors. For example, the analytical group, process chemistry group, and discovery chemistry group may all decide to go with a more vertically oriented application in each of their business spaces. The key to making this approach successful is, then, strong systems integration capabilities from each of the individual solutions and a strong IP records management system on the back end.

9.3 WHAT EXACTLY IS AN E-NOTEBOOK?

One of the problems associated with reviewing the impact of ELNs within drug discovery is the issue of defining exactly what we mean when we talk about such systems. There are many possible definition frameworks that allow for conceptual or functional descriptions of typical systems, and we explore some of these in more detail below.

An ELN may be viewed as an enterprise software application that enables scientists to record chemical and biological data and to search and share their work with their colleagues, who can be on the other side of the globe. This simplistic definition is not sufficient to portray what real-world ELN applications do and how they have improved the productivity of scientists, engineers, and innovators. Therefore, a historical overview is useful to help understand the broader usefulness of ELN applications.

From the earliest days of recorded scientific research, scientists and engineers have used paper notebooks to record their experimental work. The paper notebook is a convenient medium for this purpose: It is widely available, was and still is ingrained in the educational culture of every country, and has proven acceptable and sufficient evidence for the protection of IP. Although paper notebooks serve the need of recording data, they fail to provide an efficient mechanism for sharing these data. At best, the content of a paper notebook is available to a small group of scientists working together in close proximity in a single geographical location. Another important drawback is that searching the contents of paper notebooks is impossible or at least a very tedious task.

The digital revolution of the past 20 years, coupled with the decrease in the price of communications technologies, brought about collaboration possibilities that revolutionized all industries. Most leading organizations, chemical and pharmaceutical companies being no exception, are now globally distributed. This can be seen by looking at organizations such as Pfizer, Merck and Co., or GlaxoSmithKline, all of whom have R&D sites in the US, Europe, and Asia-Pacific. This may also be seen the strong trend toward outsourcing of functions to, for example, India and China. Engineers, research scientists, manufacturing plant managers, and business decision makers often need to communicate on a daily or hourly basis. It is often said that "need is the mother of invention": The need for global collaboration and sharing of chemical data among chemical and pharmaceutical companies was the precursor to the birth of the idea of ELNs. In addition to global sharing of data and collaboration, and like many other transformations that moved to a digital medium, this metamorphosis brought about an array of additional functionalities that not only improved productivity but also could not exist in a paper notebook. For instance, a chemical name can be deduced from a chemical structure and vice versa, thanks to smart computer algorithms. In the paper notebook world, scientists had to rely on their memory and IUPAC nomenclature skills. To say that ELNs are simply electronic replacements of paper notebooks is therefore an understatement; ELNs add significant functional capabilities that are not possible in paper format.

So what is an ELN system? It depends who you ask, because what an ELN system can do very much depends on the medium and environment in which it is being used. Just as CRM (customer relationship management) applications are loosely defined, because they can be adapted to manage the workflow of hundreds of different business models, so well-designed ELN systems are similarly diffuse. In the case of ELNs the translation of "hundreds of different business models" is the broad spectrum of data types generated in laboratories and the unlimited ways in which scientists capture and organize scientific data, innovative ideas, and discoveries. A well-designed ELN system will be flexible and versatile enough to allow scientists to design their own data recording forms and extend the ELN application with software controls capable of capturing diverse laboratory data.

Now that we are close to appreciating what constitutes an ELN system, the natural questions that a scientist might ask are: What can an ELN system do for me? How does it improve my work? Can it be modified to accommodate my style and needs in recording data? Can it record any and all data that I have? And, importantly, can it protect my intellectual property?

The answers to these questions and others are now addressed in further depth.

9.3.1 Productivity and Return on Investment

A number of approaches have been made to justifying the implementation of IT systems within drug discovery, and ELN is no exception, although these systems do seem to have generated something of their own mythology in terms of return-on-investment ("ROI") and other justification methods. What is clear from our work with major pharmaceutical customers is that there is broad acceptance of the benefits to be accrued from implementation of an ELN. The areas of benefit at which the majority of customers have looked are:

- Time reduction and increased efficiencies
- Direct cost savings
- Enhanced communications
- Improved future discovery through knowledge-driven research
- Compliance

Time Reduction and Increased Efficiencies. Time reduction and the corollary of increased efficiencies appear to be the main factors driving the short-term benefits deriving from implementation of an electronic notebook system. The argument is fairly simple, and there are good data [1] to show that the benefits are real and realistic. Most studies and projects associated with implementation of ELN within a research discipline focus on the reduction in time taken to set up a typical experiment and to document the experiment once completed. Further time savings are evident when examining workflows such as report or patent preparation, or when thinking about time taken to needlessly repeat previously executed experiments.

A key factor in determining an ROI on the basis of increased efficiencies is to be able to apply metrics to the existing processes; commonly this requires measurement of the process before the implementation of a new system and then a corresponding measurement of the process after implementation. In the case of ELN systems, this information can also be supplemented through the use of the ELN database itself, for example, by looking at the number of completed experiments created per scientist per week. These data can then be compared with an historical analysis of data from paper notebook archives on scientific productivity by similar groups.

Typical data gathered within a drug discovery environment shows a measured time saving of approximately 1 hour per week per scientist when comparing the use of electronic and paper notebooks. This was translated to a financial payback of around 2 years, with a long-term ROI showing significant cost savings. One thing, though, that must be borne in mind when assessing figures like this is the different approaches that companies take to realizing the benefits: One approach is to use the efficiencies to reduce head count, that is, do the same amount of science with fewer people at lower cost. The second approach, which seems to be more common, is to carry out more research with the same number of people and therefore at the same cost. Thus in the latter case, the ROI that is calculated is of conceptual value but is not reflected in decreased costs.

Direct Cost Savings. One medium-sized biotech company in the US reported that almost 10% of the synthetic chemistry experiments being carried out within their discovery team were pure duplicates or were partial duplicates that could have benefited from knowledge and understanding of the prior experiments carried out within the company. By implementing an ELN system, this pure duplication of experiments can rapidly be brought to almost zero and the number of ill-informed experiments reduced. This has a clear direct cost saving in terms of chemicals and consumables, as well as a time saving and research efficiency gain, based on having scientists carry out potentially more productive experiments instead.

Enhanced Communications. In addition to the direct cost savings mentioned above, which derive from one aspect of enhanced scientific communication brought about through the use of an ELN system, there are other benefits falling into the area of enhanced communications. In one US West Coast major biotech company, we have observed scientists moving from creating PowerPoint slides and acetates into group meetings to working directly within the ELN environment, running through completed experiments, as well as proposing new directions to be taken, while directly capturing the information from the discussion in the electronic records management system. Not only does this provide efficiencies, it is also a key part of the creation of an electronic experimental record for IP purposes, showing the proposal of an initial idea, which is then reduced to practice, and hopefully in a "diligent" manner as prescribed by the USPTO regulations! As we will see in the section below on compliance, this provides an earlier "first-to-invent" date, which in the ultracompetitive environment of modern drug discovery could be a vital factor in determining which company gets to exploit a blockbuster.

Improved Future Discovery. One of the most talked-about benefits of an electronic notebook system, but one of the hardest to measure in any meaningful way, is the long-term aspect of applying past knowledge to future drug discovery programs, a so-called "knowledge-driven discovery" paradigm. Although the benefits of applying past knowledge to future activities is undoubted (this is after all what a lot of scientific research activity is founded upon), there are questions that are typically raised as to how much of this type of activity will realistically occur, and exactly what the difference between a world with an extensive knowledge base and one without would be. What seems to have the greatest influence on thinking here though is the FUD factor (fear, uncertainty, and doubt). The fear exists that those companies who invest in a high-quality knowledge-driven research strategy will be at a significant advantage over those who do not. This in itself may be enough to tip larger companies into some level of ELN implementation.

Compliance. There is a common approach, taken by companies looking at ELN systems, to view them as "risky"; this is mostly in comparison to what is seen as the gold standard of reliability and low risk, the paper notebook. In fact, there is an alternative approach to thinking about the implementation of an IP and regulatory records management system (which is just what a paper or electronic notebook is) that does take into consideration the risks associated with paper notebooks.

A key area in which this assessment of risk actually comes down in favor of the electronic notebook versus the paper notebook is in ensuring compliance with the standard operating procedure ("SOP") for signing and witnessing of experimental records. This SOP will typically dictate a maximum period between the completion of an experiment and the completion of the experimental write-up. The SOP may also dictate a maximum period between the author signing an experimental record to denote completion of the write-up and the application of a witness signature to provide third-party verification of the work having been carried out as specified.

It is in the last-mentioned step that a key weakness of a paper notebook system is found: having to take the physical notebook to a witness, or having to have a witness come to the author's office to witness experiments. This is a time-consuming process, and one result is that compliance with the SOP can be weak. At least one major pharmaceutical company has discovered potential projects in which noncompliance with the signing and witnessing SOP could have caused the loss of a major drug to a competitor through the loss of first-to-invent status, which is the key date used in granting of a US patent.

One way of addressing this specific weakness is to implement an electronic notebook system, deployed with e-signature capabilities. Typical e-signature modules provide the ability to derive an e-record from the experimental write-up (currently this is most often a derived PDF document) and then to collect author and witness e-signatures. Controls can be implemented such that witnesses are sent reminders of completed experiments requiring review and witnessing, or, in the most draconian examples, authors whose experiments are far from compliance with the appropriate SOP may be prevented from starting any new experiments until they are back in compliance. See the discussion above for more information on the use of e-signatures and the legal aspects and impacts of this technology.

9.4 ELN REQUIREMENTS AND CRITERIA

What do customers look for before they decide to adopt an ELN system? The companies that are implementing ELN systems can be reasonably divided at this point into large enterprises and small companies. Large enterprises, by the nature of the complexity of their operations, are the major driving force behind many of the software architectural decisions behind well-designed ELN systems.

Smaller companies tend to have fewer concerns around, for example, system scalability, global WAN performance, and complex systems integration. They are rather more driven by the "pure" functionality of the ELN that is addressing the specific scientific disciplines of interest. Key drivers in this sector of the market have been medicinal chemistry departments, where the obvious benefits of searching existing reactions by substructure and reaction transformations, the ability to automate stoichiometry calculations, the ability to load spectral information, etc. have made for easy adoption and clear and realizable benefits.

Customers who have used paper notebooks for as long as they can remember are at first uneasy about moving to an electronic format. Resistance to adoption almost always exists within an enterprise for several reasons that can be of a technical, political, or psychological nature. Therefore, customers have many requirements for an ELN system. Of paramount importance are the following issues.

9.4.1 Software Extensibility

One feature that almost all customers require is extensibility of the software for greater integration with legacy systems and other applications. Enterprises with large IT infrastructures do not change their legacy systems overnight. Corporate success relies on uninterrupted continuity and availability of information from many disparate sources and applications. It is essential that an ELN system seamlessly mesh with this sea of information coming from and flowing into different applications.

Software systems in general bring about extensibility through the use of interfaces. A software interface, usually published by the host application, can be thought of as a "contract" guaranteeing a particular behavior from the called system as long as the calling system agrees to pass appropriate information. This makes the communication between the host application (e.g., the ELN system) and the external software module (e.g., an add-in to the ELN system) possible. We will not delve deeper into how interfaces can be used to bring about extensibility. This is a large topic in itself that can be researched in advanced software engineering architecture books.

There are hundreds of different ways of integration scenarios between an ELN and another application. Described below are four recurring scenarios employed by many companies that describe how the extensibility of an ELN system makes it adapt to the business rules and workflow of a given company.

Compound Registration. A common step in a chemical synthesis experiment is the reaction of one or more existing molecules to form a desired product. This necessitates "selecting" molecules from a chemical database or repository and "registering" the target molecule into that same chemical database or repository.

Obviously a compound registration system is already a fundamental part of the informatics infrastructure for any pharmaceutical company. However, there is a powerful efficiency gain in not having scientists input information twice into different systems: the reaction information into the ELN and then the product molecules into the registration system. One would rather have a mechanism of pushing the product molecule information from the ELN to the registration system. The obvious corollary to this is to have the ability to retrieve compound information from the registration system and have it automatically entered into the ELN—an example would be for the scientist to enter a corporate ID ("XX-109567-A") and have the molecule structure appear within the reaction drawing in his/her notebook page.

User Authentication. User authentication is a vital required function, particularly for fully electronic systems, but one whose implementation varies widely from one company to another. Different companies may use different authentication mechanisms and technologies to validate their users, for example, Windows username, Oracle usernames, smartcards (such as SAFE-compliant cards provided by a trust authority), and biometrics. Typical enterprise ELN systems will delegate this authentication process to an external module that is customized to match the corporate IT infrastructure.

Experiment Naming and Numbering Systems. Different companies or different subgroups within a company may have an existing methodology for naming and numbering notebooks and experiments. Here, too, through the use of interfaces, the ELN system will often delegate the naming and/or numbering operations to an external module. This allows for easier transitions from legacy systems to an ELN, as well as ensuring compliance with business rules employed across the company. This is particularly important in situations where there are multiple ELN systems from different vendors, when having a central and independent "Experiment ID" service is crucial for ensuring consistent and nonduplicate experimental record identifiers.

Closing and Reopening of Experiments. Software interfaces can also be used to detect when an experiment is about to close and, before closing it, consult an external module that scans the experiment and other related information to make a decision on whether to accept and resume the closing operation or cancel out the closure.

In summary, the need to provide software hooks at different parts and process points of an ELN system is of paramount importance to allow optimal integration with other systems. Companies are unlikely to adopt an ELN system designed as a monolithic application; most certainly this is true for the larger pharmaceutical organizations. There is a still a place in the market for this kind of monolithic or vertically oriented application, but there is a consequent reduction in the broad applicability of the system, and the depth of benefits to be derived from its use.

9.4.2 Long-Term Document Preservation

Experiments may need to be viewed or presented 30 or 40 years after they are saved in a database. For instance, a lawyer may ask for experimental documents to defend a company in a product liability lawsuit. An important requirement here is that the document format should be independent of the application used to create the information, and that ideally the long-term archive format should not be based on a proprietary technology. This is a legitimate requirement for two simple reasons: (1) The proprietary application and technology might not support a document generated 30 or 40 years ago. (2) The company that owns this proprietary technology may not exist 30 or 40 years from now. This has driven the adoption of open and pseudo-open document formats for long-term archival purposes. The commonest format in use today is the Portable Document Format ("PDF"); this is only a pseudo-open format, as it is owned and defined by Adobe. However, there has recently been a move to create a more standard archival version of PDF—this is now ratified as ISO 19005-1 [2] or PDF/A. Further out in the future, there are moves to create an XML-based standard for archival records, a candidate for which might be a development of the Structured Vector Graphics (SVG) document format.

9.4.3 Software Vendor Reputation and Financial Health

Customers are right to carefully consider the financial stability of the software vendor offering the ELN system. Besides technical soundness, it is important to consider whether the software vendor will be in business in 10 years' time to support and enhance the ELN system. Is the vendor financially stable and likely to survive cyclical economic downturns and recessions?

9.4.4 Supported Data Formats

The ability to handle and view different data types is of paramount importance. For instance, a customer might want to extract a graph or a drawing from a laboratory instrument and save it in an experiment. Does the system allow the creation of a new user interface (UI) control that can be embedded in the ELN system to view that specific graph or drawing? Here software interfaces can help, and some existing ELN systems allow the embedding of new controls that can handle new data that are added into the ELN system. The new UI controls integrate seamlessly with the ELN and they look and feel to the user as though they are native to the application.

9.5 CASE STUDY

Unfortunately, because of legal considerations, it is not possible to fully describe an implemented system within a specifically named company. However, in this section we address some key issues that have arisen within one of our recent projects with a major Pharma company, some of the lessons from which are, we feel, broadly applicable to future projects.

9.5.1 Major Pharma—Broad R&D Rollout

Company X set out an initial project that addressed the ROI and benefits analysis of ELNs. This study was used to build several critical components for a successful project, including:

- Use-case scenarios
- Process change requirements
- Key ROI factors
- Go/no-go decision criteria

This project was slightly unusual, in that the success and ROI criteria were investigated and developed ahead of the rest of the project. This led to a project that had clear goals and milestones in terms of usability and performance, set out ahead of any review of available solutions. In addition, the project had measurable criteria for the impact that the system was having on the efficiency of the drug discovery process. These criteria were then also used to establish go/no-go criteria for the implementation project.

Once the criteria were clearly established, the project team reviewed available commercial solutions and started out on a serious of presentations from vendors. From the list of possible vendors, a short list was drawn up, in rank order, and pilot evaluations were carried out. In the pilot program the systems were deployed in a real-world environment to approximately 100 scientists worldwide.

Data gathered during the pilot evaluations was used for several purposes:

- To assess the performance and suitability of the systems
- To gather and refine user requirements for an eventual production deployment
- To further assess likely business impacts, process changes, training requirements, etc.
- To decide whether to go ahead with an ELN at all, and if so . . .
- . . . Whether to buy or build

Following on from successful completion of the evaluation phase, a commercial solution from one vendor was selected to be rolled out to the whole of R&D, one of the consequences of this decision being that complex requirements gathering needed to be done to assess the degree of customization required in biology, chemistry, analytical services, etc. This process was carried out through user surveys, driven by the core team (which was actually a slightly expanded version of the pilot evaluation team) and taking input from all functions and all global sites.

Project implementation, which is a collaborative effort between the corporate IT group and the selected vendor, is initially scheduled as a three-phase effort, phase one of which is nearing completion as we write this chapter.

Key lessons learned so far in the process, other than the amount of time and work required to develop an ELN system for 2500 scientists at 10 sites in 5 countries across 3 continents, are that setting out the success criteria up front allowed for a very focused selection process. Also, engaging a broad user community in all stages of the vendor selection, and using this engagement to build user requirements at an early stage, meant that there is a real sense of project ownership among users from the business as well as the IT department.

9.6 COMMERCIAL SOLUTIONS

There are an increasing number of solution providers who supply or claim to supply ELN systems. The products themselves can be categorized in a number of different ways, looking at, for example, packaged solutions versus bespoke systems, single-purpose systems versus flexible, open-architecture versus proprietary technology.

Within the drug discovery market, there are some clear market leaders; the companies involved, in one way or another and in strictly alphabetical order, are:

- Amphora Research Systems
- CambridgeSoft
- Contur
- Elsevier MDL
- IDBS
- Klee
- Rescentris
- Symyx
- Tripos
- Velquest
- Waters

As the ELN software market continues to develop and mature, there will undoubtedly be new entrants in the field, mergers, and acquisitions (such as IDBS's recent acquisition of their E-Workbook system from Deffinity and Symyx acquiring and merging Synthematics and Intellichem products). It also seems clear that some of the existing products and companies will not survive as we move from the initial phase of market development into a more mature and therefore commoditized situation. Currently systems are being developed and deployed at several thousand dollars "per seat," while it is clear that these applications, unlike the majority of other scientific applications, are day-to-day applications, similar to Microsoft Outlook. It is reasonable to speculate that the intense competition and drive to commoditization of the market will inevitably lead to a lowering of the per-seat cost of systems. We would therefore expect cost figures to come down closer to standard office software prices of a few hundred dollars per seat for a pervasive system across the whole of an R&D organization.

What has become clear is that adoption of ELN systems within drug discovery is an important and ongoing process. A number of market reports have been published predicting a "hockey stick" or explosive growth model for the market sector. We feel that this is a little unrealistic, as our experience shows that the ELN project cycle, particularly for larger pharmaceutical companies, can be very long. Among the top 10 pharmaceutical companies, it would not be unusual to see an initial 6- to 12-month project to assess the impacts for the company of adopting an ELN. This would typically be followed by a 6- to 12-month project to assess in-house development versus commercial acquisition, and in the latter case to review the available solutions and draw up a short list. This might then be followed by a 6- to 18-month initial development project, building customizations and systems integrations, ahead of a production deployment. Thus a best-case scenario might see an ELN project taking 18 months from inception to first production deployment. In the worst case this could be 3 years.

A consequence of this long project cycle is that the number of major customers deploying systems at any one time is relatively small.

REFERENCES

1. See, for example, Surety Inc. http://www.surety.com/
2. http://www.aiim.org/documents/standards/ISO_19005-1_(E).doc

10

STRATEGIES FOR USING INFORMATION EFFECTIVELY IN EARLY-STAGE DRUG DISCOVERY

David J. Wild

Contents

Computer Applications in Pharmaceutical Research and Development, Edited by Sean Ekins.
ISBN 0-471-73779-8

10.1 INTRODUCTION

Anyone who has worked for some time in the pharmaceutical industry has a story of how a successful drug was developed after a fortuitous coffee machine encounter between two or more scientists, or how a problem was not discovered until late-stage development because an important piece of information was missed.

A tragic example described in the literature tells of a 24-year-old woman who died in 2001 after participating in a research study involving administration of hexamethonium bromide by inhalation [1]. Despite the fact that there were concerns about the safety of the study, it went ahead because the literature found by the researchers demonstrated four reports involving 20 patients who appeared to show no adverse effects. However, the researchers failed to find several earlier publications indicating potential pulmonary complications. Further, a 1978 study on hexamethonium bromide failed to report adverse reactions that occurred during the study—a classic case of publication bias, the failure to report failures or unattractive results [2]. This story bears many similarities to the Challenger space shuttle tragedy forensically analyzed by Edward Tufte [3].

A more encouraging story is that of Exenatide, a type II diabetes drug marketed as Byetta by Eli Lilly, the product of a formal partnership between Eli Lilly and Amylin that reportedly resulted from a chance meeting at a conference between Amylin's founder and a scientist from Eli Lilly. Other well-known positive stories include the discovery of the antiviral properties of acyclovir as it was being developed as an anticancer drug and, of course, the discovery of a secondary effect of the unpromising angina drug Sildenafil citrate leading to the successful erectile dysfunction drug Viagra [4].

These stories are extreme cases of a pervasive issue in the life sciences: They tell of the benefit of a pertinent piece of information getting to the right person at the right time, or of the consequences of the failure to do so. Unpredictable and fortuitous events will always play their part in drug discovery, but those of us who design and build software tools and informatics frameworks for use in drug discovery have a great opportunity to maximize the use of information. To do so, however, many hurdles must be overcome: Drug discovery requires scientists to find ways of contextualizing and communicating information between distinct disciplines and widely dispersed geographic locations and cultures; recent technological developments such as high-throughput screening, microarray assays, and combinatorial chemistry have vastly increased the amount of information available without necessarily providing a clear way of using it effectively (something which has been dubbed *data overload* [5]); frequent mergers and acquisitions in the pharmaceutical industry create havoc for stable, coherent companywide information systems, and even in best-case situations information must be gleaned from a mixed set of sources.

We are thus dealing generally with large volumes of many kinds of information coming from diverse sources, with limited experience of how this information can most effectively be interpreted and applied. An example of the kinds of information that are required for a scientist to make a good decision at the chemistry follow-up stage in a modern drug discovery environment is illustrated in Figure 10.1. Currently, assembling the pieces of information necessary can resemble a game of Clue (Cluedo in Europe), with the amount of pertinent information being received being dependent on the scientist asking just the right questions of the right people and systems, the effectiveness of those people and systems in delivering it, and the scientist in turn linking the pieces of information correctly.

As a further issue, information technology efforts at pharmaceutical and large life science companies historically have not focused on research, and thus software solutions to research problems have been created on an ad hoc basis by individual groups within a company, resulting in research computing being very fragmented and heterogeneous [6]. With the exception of rudimentary biological data point and 2D chemical structure storage and retrieval,

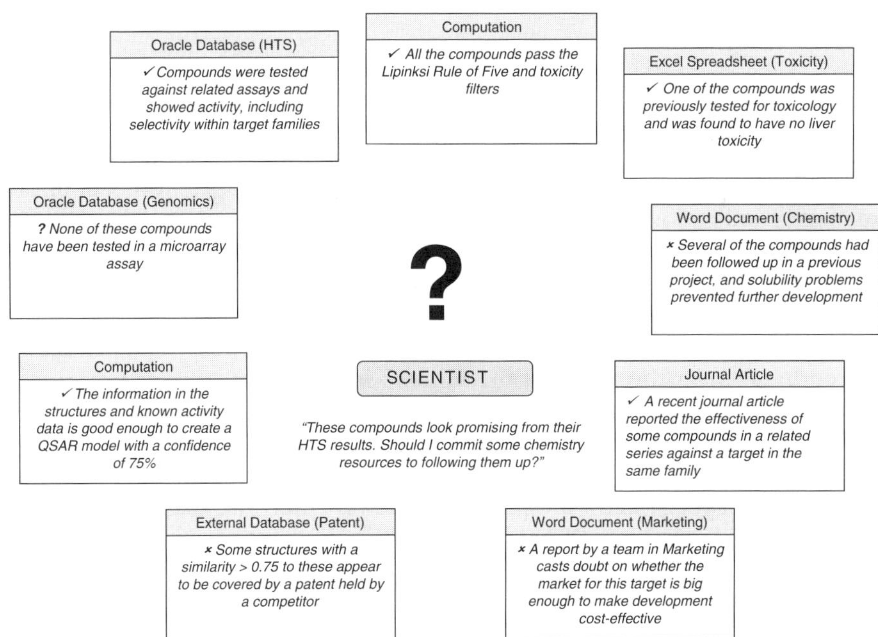

Figure 10.1 An example of the kinds of information needed by a scientist to make an effective decision about chemical follow-up. Note the variety of data sources, some of which might be unavailable to the scientist or which he or she may not be aware exists.

information systems are typically local to a laboratory or site and are domain bound (i.e., they are unavailable or not contextualized for others outside the immediate environment in which the information is generated). Although this situation has proved somewhat adequate, the previously mentioned explosion in the amount of data produced in early-stage drug discovery has made information aggregation (the collection of pertinent information into useful formats and delivery mechanisms) and data mining (tools and techniques for discovering knowledge from information) very high priorities in the life science industries.

10.2 KINDS OF INFORMATION BREAKDOWN

Before looking at some techniques for improving information use in this kind of environment and some encouraging technology trends that show promise for the future, it is pertinent to consider the kinds of information problems that frequently occur in early-stage drug discovery. They can be classified in various ways, but the one we shall use here delimits four groups: breakdowns in information *storage*, breakdowns in information *access*, breakdowns in information *use*, and *missed opportunities*.

10.2.1 Information Storage Breakdowns

Breakdowns in information storage occur when pertinent information is either not stored at all or is kept but without related information that is required to interpret it. For example, a column of assay results may be stored in an Oracle table, but without any cross-referencing to assay protocol information or indication of which values should be considered "active." The data are therefore rendered useless except to the person who stored the results.

A major area in which information storage breakdowns occur is with derived or metainformation. For example, decisions about whether to follow up compounds, observations about them, and so on are rarely systematically stored in electronic form. Most often, this kind of information is preserved, if at all, in reports and other higher-level documents usually circulated via e-mail and not permanently archived. Some companies are implementing "document searching" systems that allow reports to be searched, etc., but these have not yet gained widespread use. Newer enterprise searching systems such as *Google Desktop Search for Enterprise* (see http://www.google.com/enterprise/) may change this.

A very human kind of information storage breakdown referred to in the earlier anecdote is *publication bias*. This refers to the tendency of researchers to publish or otherwise make visible experimental results or conclusions that are considered a "success" or otherwise further the designs of the researcher but to discard results that are considered a failure (or at least to downplay them). Because of this, there is a tendency to preserve *positive information* (for example, compounds that show some activity against a target) and to discard *negative information* (for example, compounds that show no activity or that are excluded for chemical or pharmacological reasons). Furthermore, there is often an assumption that negative results do not provide useful information.

10.2.2 Information Access Breakdowns

Information access breakdowns occur when pertinent information has been stored but it either cannot be accessed for technical reasons or for some reason cannot be found in a meaningful or expedient manner for a particular application. Technical reasons can include legacy databases that are not connected with current systems, incompatibility issues between systems, problems of localized access (information can only be accessed within a site, a group or domain area, or even a personal computer), and authentication (people do not have the required authority to access information they need or cannot remember usernames and passwords).

Often overlooked but of no less importance, information access breakdowns often occur even when there is no underlying technical reason. Common causes are that it is not clear what system should be used to find a particular piece of information or that its absence on one system incorrectly implies that it is not available elsewhere. Even if a scientist knows which system to use to look for a piece of information, if the interface is not contextualized for her particular domain or project the information may be missed because it is presented in a fashion that is not familiar to the user. A problem that is harder to correct occurs when a person requires a piece of information but is unsure whether that information even exists at all.

10.2.3 Information Use Breakdowns

An information use breakdown occurs when a piece of information is successfully accessed but is not interpreted correctly. There can be a number of reasons for this: The meaning of data is incorrectly interpreted, a single piece of information is used when using a wider range of information would lead to different conclusions, lessons learned from one project are incorrectly applied to another, biases and preconceptions cloud the interpretation of the information, or "fuzzy" information is taken as concrete information. Examples include contrasting two molecules classified as "active" and "inactive" when their activities differ by only a statistically insignificant margin, mistaking a calculated logP value for an experimental one, or giving more weight to a single data point that indicates a desired conclusion than other data points that do not.

10.2.4 Missed Opportunities

Missed opportunities occur when it becomes clear that had a piece of information been available or used correctly at a particular point in time, a better decision could have been made than the one that was actually made at that time. Examples of missed opportunities are:

- A group of compounds is being followed up as potential drugs, but a rival company just applied for a patent on the compounds.
- A large amount of money is being spent developing a high-throughput screening assay for a target, but marketing research shows any drug is unlikely to be a commercial success.
- A compound tested in one therapeutic area shows some promise in another, but that information is never communicated to the right project team or group.

By definition they only become apparent with hindsight, so tackling missed opportunities involves historical analysis of information generation and use, and decisions made.

10.3 TECHNIQUES FOR QUICKLY IMPROVING INFORMATION USE

We shall shortly discuss long-term strategies for making better use of information and avoiding information breakdowns, but there are also some short-term "quick wins" that can be easily implemented and have been shown to yield a fast improvement in information use.

10.3.1 Understanding Current Information Flow and Use and Designing Software Accordingly

Techniques are available that enable software development teams to better understand the workflows and environments of users, and can be more generally applied to gain understanding of the current processes and functions (and thus the information needs) of different kinds of scientists working in a corporate or academic environment.

Contextual design is a flexible software design approach that collects multiple customer-centered techniques into an integrated design process [7]. The approach is centered around *contextual inquiry* sessions in which detailed information is gathered about the way individual people work and use systems and the associated information flow. The data from each contextual inquiry session are used to create *sequence models* that map the exact workflow in a session along with any information breakdowns, *flow models* that detail the flow of information between parties and systems (much akin to but less formal than a standard data flow diagram), *cultural models* that highlight cultural influences and pressures (such as management goals or personal preferences), *physical models* that map the physical layout of the environment in which the people are working, and *artifact models* that describe secondary items employed in the workflow. These models are then consolidated for multiple contextual inquiry sessions into one or several overall workflow models.

Interaction design [8] is based on the profiling of actual users into *personas*, which are stereotypes of individual users that are described as if they were real people. Primary personas are then formed that represent the distinct kinds of users of a system. Software is designed specifically for these personas, rather than anonymous "users," which tend to be much more influenced by the minds of programmers than real people. Interaction design can be used to understand much better the kinds of people that are involved in information flow within an organization, and what their goals and workflow scenarios are. Interaction design can be used in a complementary fashion with contextual design, particularly in the consolidation of models.

Usability testing [9] is a method of directly testing the effectiveness of software in interacting with real users. Volunteers are assigned domain-related tasks to accomplish using the software, and their efforts are recorded by an observer (and also possibly a video or audio tape). Breakdowns in the use of software (including information breakdowns) are assigned severity ratings, from critical to cosmetic, which can then be used to prioritize adjustments in the software. A small study with 5–10 participants is usually sufficient to highlight the most pressing issues.

Contextual design, interaction design, and usability testing have been applied to the effective deployment of web-based information tools at Pfizer [10]. The Pfizer study showed that contextual inquiry and usability testing sessions in particular were able to very quickly highlight breakdowns in the current systems and that when new versions of the software were released that included modifications based on the study, both the quantity of use and the satisfaction of the users increased significantly. The techniques can also be used to determine where the current gaps in information provision are, and to match these gaps with the capabilities of commercial software products.

10.3.2 Agile Software Development Methodologies

Despite its weaknesses (such as described in the 1975 collection of essays *The Mythical Man Month* [11]), the traditional software development life cycle (collect requirements, design, implement, test, deploy, maintain) has remained the standard framework for software development. However, in recent years it has become clear that the life cycle is not well suited to applications that are experimental in nature (i.e., where there is no precedent for the particular kind of application) or that exist in rapidly changing environments. This has led to the development of *agile methodologies* (also known as *lightweight methodologies* or *adaptive software development*), which are crafted to incorporate change and experimentation.

The most famous agile methodology is *extreme programming (XP)* [12], which introduces techniques such as *pair programming* (having programmers work in pairs for on-the-fly debugging and shared ownership of code), *unit testing* (writing tests before you write code, so developers get immediate feedback on whether code works), and *radical colocation* (encouraging developers to work together instead of individually). The XP approach emphasizes:

- Short development and release cycles (days or weeks instead of months) allowing fast response to changing business requirements, feedback from users and bugs, and continuous integration and testing of software revisions
- Simple design, with an emphasis on solving the problems at hand instead of attempting to forecast future needs, and constant refactoring to avoid software becoming cumbersome. Central to this is the idea that "code is cheap"—in fact, it is often cheaper to write code and throw it away if necessary than it is to engage in an extensive analysis process.
- Collective ownership—no programmer "owns" code, but a team will collaborate, possibly using pair programming, vetting each others' work.
- Onsite customers—a real user must sit with the team during the development process.

The great advantage of using agile methodologies is that software tools can be changed rapidly to meet new (or newly discovered) requirements and that if a "quick win" opportunity is located (for example, by contextual inquiry or usability testing), it can be implemented quickly with a high chance of success.

XP in particular has come in for valid criticism, particularly in that it makes budgeting for projects difficult and that it tends toward short-term solutions to problems. What appears to be happening is that XP and other agile techniques are influencing pharmaceutical software development without being adopted wholesale. For example, programming teams may be encouraged to take a "code is cheap" and code-sharing approach, but they are not necessarily taking the full steps to radical colocation or pair programming. In many ways, one of the biggest influences has been lending "permission" to programmers to develop code and build software to meet immediate scientific needs even if the software quickly becomes redundant or is replaced. The philosophy that software should be continually developed in response to changing scientific needs is generally a helpful one, at least for enabling informatics "quick wins."

10.3.3 Use of Commercial, Shareware, and Public Domain Searching and Data Mining Tools

A number of commercial vendors are producing programs that allow the exploration and organization of information from current heterogeneous sources, without the need to alter the underlying information frameworks.

One of the most prevalent data mining products in pharmaceutical research and development is Spotfire's *DecisionSite*. DecisionSite permits large multidimensional data sets to be visualized and explored through a variety of techniques such as the use of color, shape, and size of plotted points, filters, and interconnected plots. In recent years its life science-related functionality has expanded greatly, including integration with Oracle/SQL databases, prepackaged and customizable interfaces for life science applications (such as lead discovery and functional genomics), and statistical methods such as hierarchical clustering. DecisionSite's ability to draw data from a diverse set of sources and to work with other applications means that it can be used effectively in a wide variety of environments.

Several packages use a *workflow* or *pipelining* paradigm, in which existing applications and data sources are "tied" together so that, for example, the output of one application can be fed in as input to another. Notable examples of this approach are Scitegic's *Pipeline Pilot* (www.scitegic.com), Inforsense *Knowledge Discovery Environment* (www.inforsense.com), and Accusoft's *Visiquest* (www.accusoft.com). These products provide a graphical environment for the creation of workflows, which can then be encapsulated and included in other workflows (or in some instances published as web services). Once an application is "wrapped" for use in the package, then creation of workflows involving the application does not require programming skills.

A different approach is taken by IO-Informatics (www.io-informatics.com), whose *Sentient* product allows users to manage, analyze, compare, link, and associate data from heterogeneous sources. Instead of creating workflows, data sources and applications are aggregated "upfront" in a graphical user interface that allows many kinds of information to be viewed at once, and customized links and queries between them can also be created easily.

A more general tool is Google's *Desktop Search*, a version of Google's popular search engine that can be applied to the local search of files on a user's machine. The personal version of Desktop Search is available for free (desktop.google.com), but greatly enhanced functionality is given by *Google Mini* and the *Google Search Appliance* (www.google.com/enterprise), both of which allow intranet-accessible documents and files across an organization to be searched.

10.4 LONG-TERM APPROACHES TO INTEGRATED LIFE SCIENCE INFORMATICS

10.4.1 Integration of Tools and Data

Chemoinformatics and bioinformatics software companies are well aware of the demand for integrated informatics frameworks in life sciences industries and are producing a new wave of software in response, as well as overhauling their software philosophies and architectures [13]. Tripos (www.tripos.com) emphasizes what it calls "knowledge-driven chemistry," in which computational tools are woven into drug discovery scientific processes. It is collaborating with companies like Pfizer and Schering to develop systems such as ECIMS (Enhanced Chemistry Information Management System), which provides integrated registration, electronic notebook, and compound handling functions [14]. MDL (www.mdl.com) has launched a "Discovery Framework" called *Isentris* with the aim of providing an open and integrated set of applications and technologies that work cleanly with other technologies. Accelrys (www.accelrys.com) has assembled a similar framework called "Discovery Studio."

Electronic laboratory notebooks (ELNs), despite their slow uptake particularly in larger companies, are likely to be one of the main points of interaction between scientists and informatics systems, and there is thus much interest in how broad their functionality should be. ELN products are broadly split into two camps—discipline specific, which are highly tailored to a domain, often around vendors' other tools, and universal, which are designed to meet the basic notebooking needs of almost any laboratory work [15]. Other applications that require integration include Scientific Data Management Systems (SDMS), Laboratory Information Management Systems (LIMS), 2D and 3D chemical structure searching tools, biological, bioinformatics, genomic and proteomic database and analysis systems, data mining tools, and computational chemistry and biology applications.

Within a pharmaceutical company, whether or not an internal or commercial software solution is used, one can consider four layers of an effective information system, illustrated in Table 10.1. At the bottom, most fundamental level is the storage layer, which is concerned simply with the storage of all of the information that could potentially be of use in a manner that can be retrieved and searched reliably and efficiently. This does not necessarily mean that all information has to be stored in traditional databases—even publishing of a document on a corporate intranet site can be sufficient, so long as it is reliably accessible. It is also important to store as much metadata and related semantic information as possible—for example, a document containing data should contain enough information to explain its purpose, or one containing a chemical structure should ideally include tags to allow it to be substructure searched. The second layer is concerned with common interfaces to the data sources below it. For example, if one is searching for a protein sequence, there

TABLE 10.1 Four Layers of a Comprehensive Information Storage and Access System

Interaction	Software for information access and storage by humans, including e-mail, browsing tools, and "push" tools
Aggregation	Software, intelligent agents, and data schemas customized for particular domains, applications, and users
Interface	Common interfaces to stored information—there may be several for different kinds of information
Storage	Comprehensive information storage including semantics and metadata. May be in a single system or multiple systems

The layers should generally be implemented from the bottom to the top, including provision for change at each level.

should be a single way of specifying the query even if the data sources below require different mechanisms (SQL, Google search, proprietary format, and so on). The third layer involves aggregation, that is, the merging of sources and selection of information that is pertinent and contextualized for a particular domain, application, or user, including the use of "push" as well as browsing or "pull" models as discussed below. Finally, the interaction layer is the software that permits human interaction with the information, particularly access and storage of information. Software in this layer can include e-mail clients, web-based browsing tools, web servers, and customized applications.

With this four-layer model, it is important to establish a comprehensive framework at one level before investing too many resources in developing the next. Many information breakdowns occur because this is not done—a piece of software for retrieving information relevant to a particular project might be developed, but could be ineffective because not all relevant data sources can be searched and the ones that are available have many different access mechanisms. As each layer is developed, provision should also be made for change at that level, commensurate with the amount of technological change anticipated. For example, interfaces should be designed to allow expansion of the quantity and types of data sources in the storage layer without requiring change in the aggregation layer.

Three interrelated web technologies are likely to be important in the implementation of storage, interface, and aggregation layers: semantic and ontologic languages (XML, OWL, RSS), web services, and intelligent agents. These technologies are considered part of the next wave of Internet usage known as the *semantic web* [16, 17], which is concerned with the association of meaning with data on the Internet. The use of these three technologies will likely have a significant effect on the design of information systems and the way in which people interact with software over the next few years. The pervasiveness of the Internet browsing model means that most current life science software is typically passive, in that it waits for a user to initiate a search, computation, or other action through "browsing" to a particular database, web page, or system. However, as the amount of information available grows beyond human capacity to effectively organize, filter, and employ it, there will be a growing demand for "smart" software. In particular, software that attempts to intelligently discern relevant information for particular people and to *push* it to them (as opposed to waiting for them to *pull* information in the browsing model) could be of key importance.

XML (eXtensible Markup Language, see http://www.w3.org/XML/) is a markup language similar to HTML, but which conveys metadata (i.e., information about the data). XML tags can be included in HTML documents, wrapping around different kinds of data and describing its meaning: For example, a person's name might be represented in XML as <NAME> Fred Bloggs </NAME>, the NAME tags encapsulating the data and describing its type. In this way, information relevant to a particular application or web service (see below) can be automatically extracted from an HTML or pure XML document. XML can also be used as a standard file format. XML is designed to allow domain-specific subsets, and several subsets have been developed for life sciences, including *Chemical Markup Language* (CML) [18], and *Biomolecular Sequence Markup Language* (BSML, see http://www.bsml.org/) inter alia [19]. Further very recent developments of XML include languages for describing rules and ontologies on the web, thus enabling complex forms of knowledge representation. These languages, such as RDF and OWL, will greatly facilitate integration and processing of pharmaceutical information [20].

A by-product of XML is *RSS* [21], which popularly stands for *Really Simple Syndication*, although the origin of the acronym is disputed. RSS is a simple system for information aggregation, which involves websites creating a simple HTTP-accessible XML file that describes the articles available on the site. *RSS aggregators* can then run on users' machines and scour these XML files for the addition of new articles or pages that may be of interest to the user (e.g., by looking for keywords). RSS is interesting in that it gives the appearance of a push model (i.e., proactively finding and presenting information to a user) but it operates using a browsing model by repeatedly pulling the XML files from sites of interest. The potential use of RSS with CML for chemical structure searching has recently been considered [22].

Web services are an emerging way of aggregating and integrating data sources and software, and their use in the life sciences is described by Curcin et al. [23]. Web services allow software applications and data sources to be published on the Internet (or on intranets), thus making tools and data widely available with a standardized interface and facilitating the construction of applications that employ distributed resources and data to solve complex tasks. Three standards have emerged for creating web services: Web Services Description Language (WSDL) is an XML-based standard for describing web services and their parameters; Simple Object Access Protocol (SOAP) "wraps around" existing applications to map abstract interfaces in WSDL to their actual implementations; Universal Discovery, Description, and Integration (UDDI) effects the publishing and browsing of web services by user communities. Web services are gaining popularity in life sciences computing. Several bioinformatics service providers such as the European Bioinformatics Institute (EBI, http://www.ebi.ac.uk) have already made their tools available as web services. A number of life science software products are available that build on the web services model to enable the visual aggregation of data and applications, thus enabling nonprogrammers to work with the model, including the previously mentioned visual workflow products.

Intelligent agents [24, 25] are programs that exhibit a degree of autonomy in acting on behalf of another agent or a human being. Intelligent agents typically exhibit four properties: *autonomy* (they can act without direct external instruction), *social ability* (they can communicate with other agents or humans by an *agent communication language*), *reactivity* (they perceive their environment and react in a timely manner to changes in it), and *proactiveness* (they can take the initiative in acting, not necessarily just as a response to external stimulus). Intelligent agents are becoming quite widely used on the Internet, where they are more familiarly known as "bots" (short for knowledge robots), and are used for applications such as automated searching and news gathering. For example, bots are available that will continually scour auction websites such as eBay for items on a bidding wish list, phone you with reminders and notifications of events you request, or create your own "personal newspaper" from a variety of online sources [26]. To date, the application of intelligent agents in the life sciences has been limited, the most notable being sequence alerting systems such as *Swiss-shop* (see http://www.expasy.org/swiss-shop/) that provide personalized alerts when new protein sequences that match a user's specified interests are added to a database.

Once web service, XML, and agent frameworks are in place, it is not difficult to think up many intriguing applications. For example, a drug discovery scientist might set up an intelligent agent to automatically look for new compounds added to the corporate database by other scientists in a company. Once new compounds are found, the agent will request a virtual screening tool (made available as a web service) to computationally evaluate the docking of the new structures (represented in XML) against a selection of protein targets relevant to the scientist's project and to alert him or her by e-mail of any potential hits. A second agent might scour project reports generated by other project teams for results that might indicate some activity in his or her project. A third agent might automatically search conference proceedings and publications for key words related to the project. In this way, the chances of avoiding missed opportunities are reduced and fertile ground is laid for "serendipitous" discoveries, without overburdening scientists with information.

10.4.2 Issues for Software Developers

The ability of IT groups in the pharmaceutical industry to build effective information infrastructures in the medium- to long term is going to be dependent on a number of factors yet to be resolved. Particularly:

- If software solutions tend toward vendor-tied products (i.e., a high level of integration within tools offered by a particular vendor only) or toward cooperative integration in which software is developed around common standards. If the former is the case, companies are likely to be forced to opt for a particular vendor for life science software, and it will be difficult to integrate new algorithms and software into the framework. The movement toward web services and XML is strong in the software development industry in general, so the latter scenario is arguably more likely at this stage. However, this will require software companies to work together on standards and interfaces.
- The extent to which the current trend toward mergers and acquisitions continues in life sciences, and also the extent to which larger pharmaceutical companies outsource research and development to smaller companies. It may become necessary for rapid integration of systems between companies that had previously had no relationship at all, and for the secure integration of particular systems between collaborating companies.
- Whether life sciences informatics software ultimately becomes a commodity, with the commercial rewards for software companies being in packaging, integration, support, and deployment (in a similar way to the Linux community), and what impact the open source movement will have. In bioinformatics and chemoinformatics, open source, free software, and shareware are increasing in quantity, and it is becoming common for smaller software companies at least to release reduced-functionality versions of their software into the public domain at no cost.
- Whether the rate of introduction of disruptive new technologies (both scientific and computational) increases, decreases, or stays the same. Historically, this has tended to be phasic, with periods of rapid technological change and subsequent periods of absorption of the change. A continuing high rate of technological change will emphasize the need for rapid software development and continuous integration of new software and algorithms.
- Whether life sciences IT departments emphasize internal development or external licensing of software, and whether internal development is centralized or delocalized. This is clearly related to the level of homogeneity across an organization and is an issue generally held in tension between extremes. Centralized development and external licensing is attractive in that it allows for efficiency of scale and helps maintain

a homogeneous software environment, but it increases risk (in that a failure of a companywide project has a greater and costlier impact than a local one) and can make it difficult to respond quickly to changes in technology. Delocalized and internal software development can have lower development overheads and rapidly respond to changing environments but require higher level orchestration between groups and systems.

The current trend toward public domain and open source software is of particular interest, because, as noted above, it could lead to the partial commoditization of life science software. *Open source* refers to software where the source code is made freely available, with the intention that a large number of people will participate in the development of the software. The wider term *FOSS* (Free and Open Source Software) is also used to include software that is freely distributed but not in source code format. Advantages of the use of FOSS software in drug discovery include immediate product availability (usually a web download), independence from vendors, open standards, increase in competition, collaboration, and avoidance of reinvention by different vendors [27]. However, the FOSS software movement is still young, and care does need to be taken that companies abide by licensing (for example, the requirement that software produced that includes open source software should itself be open source) and understand the inherent risks and complexities [28]. Bioinformatics is the life science domain with the broadest range of FOSS software available, although other fields such as chemoinformatics are beginning to catch up. Some examples of such software are given in Table 10.2.

10.5 SUMMARY

In his book *Information Anxiety* [29], Richard Wurman calculates that a single issue of the *New York Times* contains more information than a seventeenth century Englishman would likely be exposed to in his entire lifetime. The reason the *New York Times* doesn't overwhelm us is that its information is expertly processed, edited, organized, prioritized, and presented in a consistent, easily digestible manner, so we can quickly select the information that is of most import to us. The vast increase in the volume of information generated and the number of information sources in early-stage drug discovery has not yet been balanced by processes that allow scientists to exploit the information in a similar fashion, with the result that information storage, access, and use breakdowns, as well as "missed opportunities," frequently hamper drug discovery and development efforts. There is therefore an urgent need to rethink strategies for storage, access, and use of information. Several "quick win" techniques have been presented in this chapter that can help improve the situation in the short term without altering underlying information frame-

TABLE 10.2 Examples of Some Popular Open-Source, Free and Shareware Life Science Products

Software	Function	Webpage
ArgusLab	Molecular modeling	http://www.planaria-software.com/
BioPerl	Perl tools for bioinformatics, genomics and life sciences; part of a wider bioinformatics open source initiative at http://www.open-bio.org	http://bio.perl.org/
Chime	Molecule viewer	http://www.mdl.com/products/framework/chime/
Chimera	Molecular modeling	http://www.cgl.ucsf.edu/chimera/
Chemistry Development Kit (CDK)	Java library for chemoinformatics and bioinformatics	http://almost.cubic.uni-koeln.de/cdk/
Ensembl	Automatic annotation and genome browser	http://www.ensembl.org
JMol	Molecule viewer	http://jmol.sourceforge.net/
Molecular Workbench	Molecular modeling education	http://workbench.concord.org/modeler/index.html
OpenBabel	Conversion of molecular file formats	http://openbabel.sourceforge.net/
Taverna	Workflow system for bioinformatics web services	http://taverna.sourceforge.net

More can be found at http://www.bioinformatics.org, http://www.open-bio.org, http://www.cheminformatics.org, and http://www.chemoinf.com.

works. For the medium- to long term, new strategies currently in their infancy will assist in the integration of information sources and for organizing, contextualizing, and "pushing" the most relevant information to scientists. The extent to which these strategies can be applied effectively will depend on the direction that life science software development takes, in particular the interoperability of software and the development of open standards.

REFERENCES

1. Ogilvie RI. The death of a volunteer research subject: lessons to be learned. *Can Med Assoc J* 2001;165:1335–7.
2. Savulescu J. Two deaths and two lessons: Is it time to review the structure and function of research ethics committees? *J Med Ethics* 2002;28:1–2.
3. Tufte ER. *Visual explanations*. 1997, Cheshire, CT: Graphics Press.
4. See http://en.wikipedia.org/wiki/Viagra
5. Mullin R. Dealing with data overload. *Chem Eng News* 2004;82:19–24.
6. Gardner SP, Flores TP. Integrating information technology with pharmaceutical discovery and development. *Trends Biotechnol* 1999;18:2–5.
7. Beyer H, Holtzblatt K. *Contextual design*. 1998, San Francisco: Morgan Kauffman.
8. Cooper A. *The Inmates Are Running the Asylum: Why High Tech Products Drive Us Crazy and How to Restore the Sanity*. 2nd ed. 2004,:, Indianapolis, IN: Sams.
9. Nielsen J. *Usability engineering*. 1993, San Diego: Academic Press.
10. Wild DJ. et al., Making Web Tools Work for Chemists, in 6th International Conference on Chemical Structures. 2002: Noordwijkerhout, NL.
11. Brooks FP. *The mythical man month*. 1975, Boston: Addison Wesley.
12. Beck K. *Extreme programming explained*. 2000, Boston: Addison Wesley.
13. Salamone S. Riding the New Wave. *Bio-IT World*, 2004(October): 42.
14. Green Pastures for Discovery Informatics. *Bio-IT World*, 2005(May): 38–44.
15. Rees P. In the lab: how to capture data to share. *Sci Comput World* 2004 (November/December): 10–14.
16. Berners-Lee T, Hendler J, Lassila O. The semantic web. *Sci Am* 2001;284:34–43.
17. Hendler J, Berners-Lee T, Miller E. Integrating applications on the semantic web. *J Inst Elect Eng Japan* 2002;122:676–80.
18. Murray-Rust P, Rzepa HS. Chemical Markup Language and XML Part I. Basic Principles. *J Chem Inform Comput Sci* 1999;39:928–42.
19. For a comprehensive list of XML subsets for the life sciences, see http://www.visualgenomics.ca/gordonp/xml/
20. Gardner SP. Ontologies and semantic data integration. *Drug Discov Today* 2005;10:1001–7.
21. A good introduction to RSS can be found at http://www.xml.com/pub/a/2002/12/18/dive-into-xml.html.

22. Murray-Rust P, Rzepa HS. Towards the chemical semantic web. An introduction to RSS. *Internet J Chem* 2003;6: Article 4.
23. Curcin V, Ghanem M, Guo Y. Web services in the life sciences. *Drug Discov Today* 2005;10:865–71.
24. Hendler J. Is there an Intelligent Agent in your future? Nature Web Matters, www.nature.com/nature/webmatters, 1999; (March 11).
25. Wooldridge M, Jennings N. Intelligent agents: theory and practice. *Knowledge Eng Rev* 1995;10.
26. For more information on these bots, see http://www.botknowledge.com/
27. DeLano W. The case for open-source software in drug discovery. *Drug Discov Today* 2005;10:213–17.
28. Stahl MT, Open source software: not quite endsville. *Drug Discov Today* 2005;10:219–22.
29. Wurman RS. *Information anxiety*. 1989; New York: Doubleday.

11

IMPROVING THE PHARMACEUTICAL R&D PROCESS: HOW SIMULATION CAN SUPPORT MANAGEMENT DECISION MAKING

ANDREW CHADWICK, JONATHAN MOORE,
MAGGIE A. Z. HUPCEY, AND ROBIN PURSHOUSE

Contents

Computer Applications in Pharmaceutical Research and Development, Edited by Sean Ekins.
ISBN 0-471-73779-8

The most exciting phrase to hear in science, the one that heralds new discoveries, is not "Eureka!" ("I found it!") but "That's funny. . . . "

—Isaac Asimov

11.1 INTRODUCTION

Much has been published about simulations of research and development (R&D), but in the area of research process improvement there are still many challenges. This chapter consists of two main parts, covering current approaches, which have met limited acceptance, and newer approaches aimed more directly at overcoming the most likely areas of cognitive difficulty that research managers face when making decisions on performance improvement.

11.2 THE BUSINESS PROBLEM, CURRENT APPROACHES, AND RESEARCH MANAGEMENT VIEWS

Setting the scene for original material, we:

1. Describe the pressures on the pharmaceutical industry to improve R&D performance, with emphasis on the earlier stages of R&D where irreversible choices are made
2. Cite highlights from previous literature on use of quantitative methods already widely used by R&D management
3. Explain the basis of decision analysis in R&D management applications, including the use of multiple criteria
4. Present verbatim comments from recent interviews with research managers on needs for organizational learning about processes and performance, which also reveal some common attitudes toward the use of IT support and simulation tools.

11.3 THE PERFORMANCE IMPROVEMENT CHALLENGE

The environment for pharmaceutical R&D is changing, with the main challenge stemming from decreasing R&D productivity. "R&D costs are increasing to a point that is just not sustainable and we need to ask ourselves just how long we can keep going like this" [1].

The number of new product approvals has fluctuated around 40 per year since about 1950, but the costs have grown exponentially above inflation, so that "the real issues lie in the cost base of the industry . . . therein lies the problem for which solutions should be sought by pharmaceutical companies and regulators" [2]. The costs of development are now so high—in the order of $1 billion per successful launch—that, according to ongoing surveys by Tufts University [3, 4], only around 30% of products repay their R&D costs, adjusted for inflation. The use of unprecedented targets increases project risk, yet, under increasing competition from generics and facing the market power of managed healthcare, drugs that are "me-too" cannot be sure of commanding a high price. Discovery groups, despite failing in at least four in five of their projects, are issuing increased numbers of drug candidates into development, but the success rates in drug development have not increased above at best one in ten [4]. On any recent analysis, there is a recognized problem with R&D productivity.

We know, from consulting to a wide range of pharmaceutical and biotech R&D groups, that managements are under strong pressure to achieve a breakthrough in their own company performance and, collectively, in industry performance. Ultimately this must be quantified as the long-run ratio between the value created by new products and the costs of R&D.

As R&D spending increases to a record share of revenue, many R&D management teams have started to appraise their own performance in decision making. None of the following simple recipes seems like the easy answers that they appeared to be to many companies (and consultancies) over the past 15 years:

- *Doing it faster* (at some point, the risks of hasty decisions may overwhelm the time saving)
- *Doing it more cheaply* (outsourcing contracts can face cost escalation, or painful and expensive break clauses when the real scope of work is discovered)
- *Doing it on a larger scale* (extending screening libraries, for example through combinatorial chemistry, without ensuring the purity or even correct identification of compounds may initially give the illusion of increased productivity but eventually just reduces the useful yield of leads from hits)

We have seen many recent attempts to improve the quality of compound collections so as to increase the signal-to-noise ratio in high-throughput screening. As automation increases the number of hits, research groups are attempting a right-first-time approach to lead optimization by eliminating unpromising series before new examples have to be synthesized. Making better predictions is now seen as a major challenge: from predictions that targets will be "druggable," through computational preselection of screening sets, to evaluation of high-throughput ADME or toxicology assays, animal models, biomarkers, and beyond.

In summary, the current emphasis in R&D management circles seems to be upon reducing risk, improving pipeline quality, and improving team accountability and communications between functional specialties and units.

The measures of success in this kind of improvement initiative are quite intangible. Scientists are used to working with numbers, but numbers that describe the overall team business performance are much harder to agree on than specific results from experiments: "The absence of formal valuation procedures often gives rise to informal procedures that can become highly politicized" [5]. The emphasis given to cycle time, attrition rates, screening volumes, unit cost saving, or other short- to medium-term metrics, can depend on who is in charge and on the prevailing fashion in R&D management circles. Relevant quantitative performance measures that are clearly linked to long-term value creation might perhaps remove some of the "office politics."

There is therefore a need to consider how to link scientific and business performance numbers in a way that is both transparent and soundly based. There has been much written but little agreed on about this important point.

11.4 QUANTITATIVE METHODS ALREADY APPLIED TO R&D PLANNING

Figure 11.1 shows different kinds of decisions important to preclinical research. Clearly, IT and simulation support are completely accepted at the lowest level of this diagram as ways of predicting molecular, cellular, organ, animal, or human properties, interactions, and responses (covered elsewhere in this volume). Therefore, scientists moving into leadership roles will very often be familiar with the strengths and weaknesses of such methods.

At a much higher strategic level of decision making, therapy area strategy, the choice of project and valuation within a portfolio has been addressed quantitatively for many years with the help of spreadsheets and more sophisticated decision support systems. These discount future costs and earnings back to present values and factor in risks, so that comparisons use "expected net present value," or eNPV. All pharmaceutical companies now have sophisticated portfolio management groups advising which projects to take into development, in-license and out-license. Specialized software products are available to help them assess and provide for aggregate resource demands over a range of disciplines, allowing for different probabilities of failure in different projects and at different stages of R&D, for example, Planisware as recently implemented at Genentech [6].

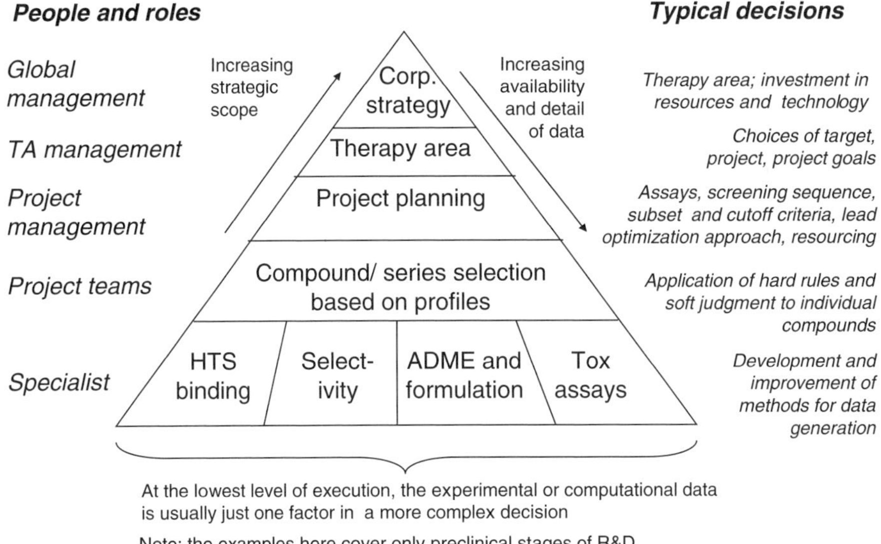

Figure 11.1 The hierarchy of strategic and operational decisions in preclinical research.

In interviews of R&D management during 2004, comments by research managers on portfolio management included:

> In the past, we were seduced by portfolio management tools.
>
> Algorithms placing value on commercial outcomes can be dangerous due to the enormous uncertainties. Past evaluations based on this method are necessarily incorrect. Now the approach is that if we benefit patients, money will follow.

Nevertheless, many companies have been using project valuation methods even from the early stages of drug discovery. Merck's CFO [7] has described application of financial theory in a Research Planning Model initiated in 1983. This was based on Monte Carlo analysis to assess R&D project risk and on financial option theory for assessment of collaboration investments. Her view even in 1993 was "Everywhere I look in the pharmaceutical industry today, I see increasing complexity and uncertainty. . . . [W]e make huge investments now and may not see a profit for 10 to 15 years. . . . [I]f I use option theory to analyze that investment, I have a tool to examine uncertainty and to value it." There is widespread recognition of this view of R&D as *creating options*. The product of research is "enabling information" that might be valuable if used for development of a product but carries no obligation to be used in that way, if research results disappoint. Projects deemed unpromising after such research can be terminated early to stop loss.

The best modeling framework for R&D options is, however, more contentious. The famous, or infamous, "Black–Scholes" formula [8], based on valuation of traded financial options, has in our view impeded the practical use of decision analysis methods by scientific managers:

> Much of the apparent complexity of current approaches to "real-options analysis" arises from the attempt to fit financial-option formulae to real-world problems. Usually this does not work since real-world options are often quite different from financial options. Option-pricing formulae are treated as a procrustean bed by academics: Either the real world is simplified beyond recognition or unwarranted assumptions are added to make the facts fit the theory. Neither approach satisfies managers.
>
> There is an alternative. Simple financial models can capture the essence of option value by directly incorporating managers' existing knowledge of uncertainty and their possible decisions in the future. This approach avoids the dangers of complex formulae and unwarranted assumptions, and gives a lot more management insight than black-box formulae while creating less opportunity for academic publications [9].

It is in the intermediate areas of Figure 11.1 that R&D managements most lack effective tools and support for decision making:

- Resourcing decisions on people and technology
- Formulation of specific R&D project plans, including choice of screening sequence

Below, we focus on aids to R&D project planning and process improvement, exploring the extent to which IT really can help managers to be more effective in decision making through simulation that fosters the ability to "look before you leap."

11.5 DECISION ANALYSIS APPROACHES RELEVANT TO R&D PLANNING AND IMPROVEMENT

R&D management tends to be dominated by a "project management" paradigm, and most organizations develop systems based upon standard project management software, for example, Microsoft Project®. This is very useful for project control, but of much less help in decision support. John Gittins claimed in 1997 [10] that very few pharmaceutical companies practice use of decision analysis in *planning* their work. Decisions tend to be made only for a baseline plan, and typically . . .

- *There is little or no capability to evaluate risk.* The robustness of the plan to key uncertainties is rarely assessed. Important risks in R&D development include unexpected trial results, delays, requirements to do unforeseen work, and changes in the market potential of products.

- There is no systematic approach to exploiting flexibility. Upper management tends to make decisions that are too fixed and does not communicate well the trade-offs that should be applied when the future is different from its central assumption. For example, those implementing decisions may receive a deadline for completion of a trial, rather than a target completion date with guidelines on the value of different completion dates to the business and how to respond accordingly.

We therefore consider how organizations address, or could better address:

1. Risk management
2. Flexibility achieved through maintaining options
3. Choices involving multiple criteria
4. Performance across multiple parallel projects, which amounts to *improving the R&D process*

11.5.1 Common First Steps to Risk Management

Organizations tend to focus on two risk management approaches:

- *Assessing risks under fixed policies.* Most project management packages allow for testing the effect on project outcomes of random variations in a range of basic properties of tasks. The simulation approaches discussed in Section 11.7 can extend this approach.
- *Optimizing while ignoring risks.* One may, for example, run a calculation to work out the resource allocations that will help a project to finish as soon as possible.

These two are normally carried out separately, although some organizations are now adopting a combined approach. There is a third and more effective approach: *optimization of outcome distributions.* Rather than optimizing merely the results in a base case, one can optimize according to a realistic distribution of outcomes. Parallel to optimizing a baseline project end date, one might optimize an *expected* project end date, or the date by which there is a 90% chance of the project ending. This capability is increasingly common in commercially available software; for example, OptTek System's OptQuest products provide such capabilities and are available in several well-known simulation packages, including AnyLogic, Arena, Crystal Ball, Promodel, and Simul8.

11.5.2 Valuing Flexibility Through Options Analysis

Even the optimization of outcome distributions does not normally take account of the value of flexibility (i.e., by reacting to project events and findings as they emerge, one can make better decisions for the future than could be made in advance of the project, "planning blind").

Options analysis is a technique that can deal with such contingencies. It is a form of decision analysis that includes chance variables, initially hidden, representing "states of nature" that can be uncovered, in whole or in part, through a decision to carry out research. Such research creates *options*—the ability to progress, or abandon, one of several courses of action. This research might be technical or market research, in applications of option analysis to R&D planning.

Options analysis reveals the value of making decisions about *investments in information* that can guide future judgment by revealing the true states of nature in time for the project team to react to them, exploiting them through further decisions. Such states of nature include manageable risks, for example, a competitor operating R&D in the same space. They also include unexpected favorable events, for example, an observation of a side-effect that turns out to be a whole new indication for treatment (cf. impotence or hair loss treatments).

In classic options analysis, one first creates an approximate version of the decisions and risks to be considered and then tries to *exactly* optimize the decision policies.

In a tiny fraction of cases, a quick formula can be used. For most cases, the analysis uses an "options tree," with one "leaf" per possible outcome. However, this falls prey to the "curse of dimensionality"—the number of leaves on the tree grows exponentially in the number of risk and decision dimensions considered. Thus only a limited, simple set of situations can be optimized in this way because one has to severely limit the decisions and risks that are considered. Tools available to help automate and simplify options analysis, widely used in pharmaceutical project evaluation, include Excel add-ons such as @RISK [11] and more graphically based solutions such as DPL [12]. Both of these support the creation and evaluation of decision trees and of influence diagrams; Figure 11.2 shows a simple example of each of these. A primer in applied decision theory is Clemen's book *Making Hard Decisions*; other sources may be found in the website of James Vornov, Director of Clinical Research at Guildford Pharmaceuticals, a recent convert to decision theory for options analysis [13].

A recent review of option models in drug development, co-authored by a biostatistician from AstraZeneca in Mölndal, Sweden [14], suggests that there has up to now been a lack of appreciation among pharmaceutical executives of the value that statistics could bring to the decision making process. This review quantifies the value of information that could terminate unsuccessful projects early and assesses the time-risk trade-off. It proves that projects split

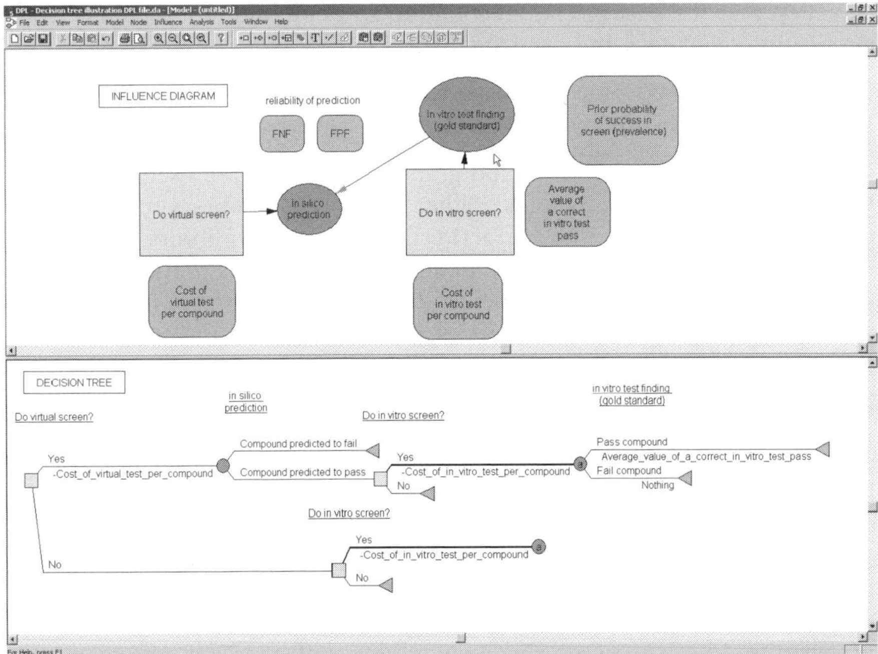

Figure 11.2 A decision tree, based on an associated influence diagram, can help organize and integrate information about risks and the way in which research work buys better information that allows choice of the options most likely to succeed. This example describes the relationship between *in silico* predictions and in vitro assay results for the same compound structures.

into many successive decision points run the least risk; running tasks in parallel, to save time elapsed, tends to increase work performed at risk. "The general rule is to terminate inferior projects as early as possible. The ideal is to find inexpensive tests of the weakest links."

A review of simulations in pharmaceutical R&D, focusing on the drug development process [15], commented that "the traditional approach to drug discovery and development is sequential, non-iterative and is carried out according to a plan-execute-evaluate principle. The approach of the future, however, is iterative, adaptive and is carried out according to a plan-execute-evaluate-replan-execute principle." Clinical trial simulation based on prior information on pharmacokinetics and pharmacodynamics can help managers to value alternative clinical trial designs based on assumptions about the trial population, the trial execution, and the effect of the drug in question.

Simulations may also be used to inform understanding of market dynamics and life cycle management and to aid in understanding the ways in which reference pricing and parallel trading may influence the best sequence of drug launches, and the best pricing negotiation strategy, within a region of communicating regulators and connected trade channels.

11.5.3 Choices Involving Multiple Criteria

In research, many quantitative and graphical methods are used in selecting between individual compounds, either as potential library of collection members or in filtering hits. Multicriteria approaches to library design typically seek to balance diversity and likelihood of favorable properties [16]. In early screening, the rules for choices between hits are part of a research process typically applied to diverse projects, whereas at the end of the discovery process compound choice commits to starting a single development project.

Development candidates must be measured against multiple performance criteria, including such aspects as potency, safety, and novelty. Conflict may be experienced between the criteria, in which improved performance in one criterion can only be achieved at the expense of detriment to another. In this situation—as is often the case for activity against bioavailability—a *trade-off* is said to exist between the objectives. A trade-off between potency and safety may also be present.

When trade-offs exist, no single compound will stand out uniquely as the optimum drug for the market, ranked first on all measures of performance. Rather, a *set* of compounds will be considered that, on current knowledge, span the optimal solution to the problem. These compounds are those for which there is no other compound that offers equivalent performance across all criteria and superior performance in at least one. In multicriteria decision analysis (MCDA) terminology, they are known as *Pareto-optimal* solutions. This concept is illustrated by the two-criteria schematic in Figure 11.3.

Elicitation of decision maker preferences may needed to reduce the set of Pareto-optimal compounds to a single candidate to be progressed.

Capture and use of decision maker preferences can be performed in advance of the search for compounds, during the search itself, or after the search has returned a Pareto-optimal set of compounds. In the past, it has been common for the relative importance of different criteria to be decided in advance, with these being expressed as a set of weightings. The performance of a candidate compound is then established as the weighted sum of performance across all individual criteria. The subsequent search—using this aggregated performance indicator as a guide—will return a single compound from the set of Pareto-optimal compounds that is optimal over the weighted combination of selection criteria.

This weighted-sum approach is conceptually simple but has a number of disadvantages:

- Decision makers may not be able to decide on an appropriate set of weights in advance.

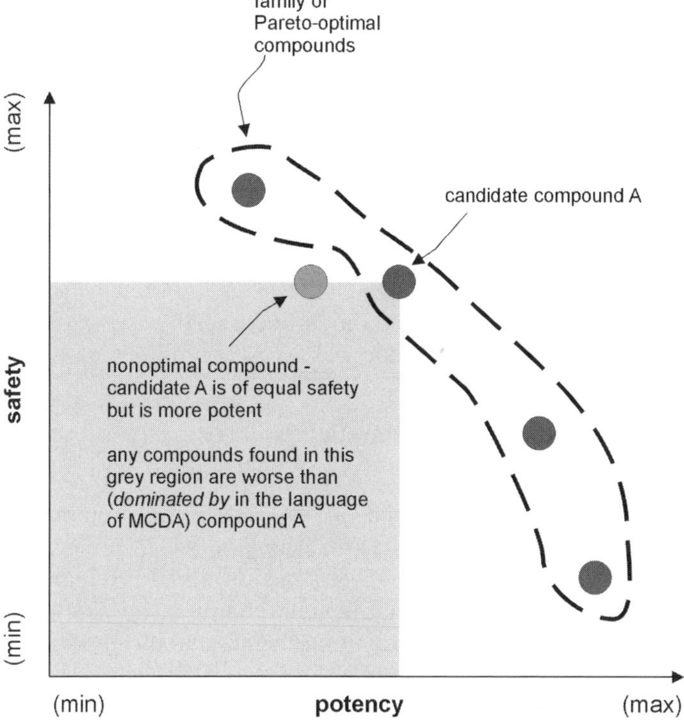

Figure 11.3 The relative values of multiple criteria can be assessed by establishing preference between pairs of examples; some examples will "dominate" others on two or more dimensions of choice.

- There is no consideration of project-specific trade-offs.
- The technique is sensitive to the precise choice of weights.
- The forced aggregation of criteria of different types and of different scales is nonintuitive and potentially misleading.
- The direct search for a global optimum may not uncover some of the Pareto-optimal solutions close to the overall optimum, which might be good trade-off solutions of interest to the decision maker.

It may be more appropriate for the decision-making team to express preferences after the need for trade-off between the different compounds found has become apparent via the search results. Visualization and quantitative analysis techniques can then be used to reveal the trade-offs in the problem, facilitating the choice of a single compound, or a candidate and one or more backups that have different risk profiles.

These so-called *Pareto-based* techniques do not force consolidation over multiple criteria in advance and aim to return a representation of the set of optimal compounds. They support discussion between team members who may have different views on the downstream impacts of different risk factors; perhaps, for example, one team member may know that there is a reliable biomarker for one potential side-effect. This would then mean that assessing this risk need not consume much development time and cost, and the risk factor can have a reduced weighting within the target product profile being evolved by the team.

Population-based search techniques, such as *evolutionary algorithms*, are natural choices for Pareto-based methods because they work with a set of interim, approximate solutions on the way to an overall optimum.

11.5.4 Choices Across Multiple Parallel Projects: "Process Improvement"

So far, we have been addressing decisions on projects and compounds of the type shown in Figure 11.1. As well as decisions on which project to do, and which specific targets and compounds to work on, there are important decisions on how to run the R&D projects in general; how to *operate and improve the R&D process*. This means "doing things right" as well as "doing the right things." Investments in research facilities and resources such as skilled people are made on a timescale even longer than the typical research project, and so there is a need to look ahead at the potential needs of multiple projects in at least one therapeutic area. Many companies also combine early discovery activities across multiple therapy areas because of the very capital-intensive nature of high-throughput screening, materials characterization, and high-end computational chemistry or biology. Such organizations then must decide not only on the capacity to be provided but also on the rules for allocating or prioritizing its use between different projects or project stages. For example, should all compounds screened have NMR spectra taken to confirm structure, or just those compounds that show initial signs of activity?

Relevant organizational research by Argyris [17] and others can be summarized through the concept of "double loop learning." This presents the need to step outside the routine process of how work is done and to start to change the goals and governing variables through which work is regulated. This might include such challenges as "Is increased volume better?" or "Are faster research time cycles consistent with high-quality decisions?"

Any formal models of the conduct of research work and success are often "soft" or "fuzzy" in nature, and so may be distrusted by those used to "hard" evidence. There is a particular distrust of opaque, "black box" solutions, and numerate managers rightly demand to see the detailed assumptions made in any decision analysis. The most controversial assumptions tend to be those about project future costs, chance of success, and potential value within drug discovery, and some senior managers still refuse to countenance this kind of quantification of performance or performance targets.

A decision analysis method, taking expectations over possible futures, gives a theoretically optimal recommendation; nevertheless, many managers will prefer to see a stochastic simulation because that gives them more confidence that they have a "feel" for the problem, based on examples of possible futures, rather than some kind of average view. However powerful in principle a decision support method might be, it will not help performance improvement unless the intended users—research teams and managers—see the point and trust the system to help their judgments.

11.6 RESEARCH MANAGEMENT VIEWS ON IMPROVEMENT, ORGANIZATIONAL LEARNING, AND THE POTENTIAL CONTRIBUTION OF IT SUPPORT

A recent survey of pharmaceutical research management attitudes toward learning and systematic improvement by Michael Aitkenhead at the Judge Institute, University of Cambridge (MBA dissertation, "Performance Management and Measurement in Drug Discovery Projects"), revealed how they see the real challenges of improving drug discovery performance. It also uncovered very mixed views on the usefulness of quantitative methods and decision support tools, as seen by practicing research managers. However, seven senior R&D leaders, in research, early development, and planning functions across three large pharmaceutical companies, all shared the same opinion that something is needed to achieve a more systematic approach to performance improvement:

> Industry has been looking for quick fix solutions for the last 10–15 years. Learning is not embedded in the culture—this is a business based on scientific endeavor with a core culture of individualism and "heroic individuals."
>
> The structure of the organization is not optimal to allow feedback. It can sometimes be very difficult to obtain an overview of the reasons for failure.
>
> Currently, no one (individual) knows what it is like to develop a drug (in its entirety).

These comments seem to argue for increased use of quantified decisions based on the accumulated evidence of the past, with support from IT and knowledge management; however, the same survey revealed views that:

> Scientists believe they are data driven—not true! They use data to confirm decisions they wish to take. Data is used selectively in support.
>
> Knowledge Management IT systems are not as pivotal as thought. Expertise arises from a network of people, and difficult problems are not solved by IT.

> Computers are no better than human judgments in early discovery; they don't possess creativity and innovative capacity.

It is clear that quantitative predictions of research performance, and models of possible improvements, are not well accepted by research managers. Two major barriers are the uncertainty that exists at early stages of R&D and the mix of repetition and variation between different projects.

These are essentially cognitive challenges, and therefore we need to understand where managers are most likely to need help in forming better judgments based on a mix of visual presentations that aid perception, support to quantitative reasoning, and simulations that avoid the danger of "black box" answers but instead permit risk-free experimentation with possible ways of working.

11.7 ADVANCES IN RESEARCH SIMULATIONS INTENDED TO IMPROVE THE MENTAL MODELS OF RESEARCH MANAGEMENT

Here we set out the arguments for, and provide examples of, simulations that complement rather than replace managerial judgment, making best use of whatever factual information is available to help managers make the necessary choices between possible futures. Such simulations are most needed in support of decisions where even experienced research leaders have "blind spots" in their judgment.

The Sections 11.8 and 11.9 cover:

1. Common errors in research management, indicating the most likely needs for simulations to provide practice in decision making and give feedback on a range of possible outcomes
2. Recent applications of visualization and simulation to support performance improvement in drug discovery

11.8 COMMON ERRORS IN RESEARCH MANAGEMENT

The hardest aspect of management decision making in R&D is the unforgiving, one-off nature of many decisions, not just on disease and target portfolio, but also in the conduct of R&D. Choosing the best business process is especially difficult in drug discovery, which may be 10 to 20 years from peak sales of the resulting product. Especially for the longer-term decisions on resourcing, technologies, and ways of working, managers require sound ways of analyzing and understanding how their choices may impact the downstream pipeline and ultimate sales. This analysis must be based on a underlying model of R&D processes that is capable of convincing both business and technical audiences.

A number of known and consistent biases in human judgment and decision making, particularly severe in estimation and reasoning about probability, are reflected in some common problems experienced or reported by research leaders, for example, undue attention to recent events, neglecting the lessons of the past, failure to balance effort efficiently across resolution of different areas of uncertainty, and systematic blindness to negative findings relative to any hopeful signs that indicate the project may, after all, succeed. The evidence from psychological research is that overcoming such biases is not possible just by knowing their nature but instead requires practice in the solution of problems of relevant structure, with feedback on how well the problem was solved. This suggests that improvement in decision making about R&D process improvement might best be addressed by simulation approaches such as those that we describe in Section 11.9.

11.9 APPLICATIONS OF VISUALIZATION AND SIMULATION TO RESEARCH PLANNING AND PROCESS IMPROVEMENT

The visual display of quantitative information can overcome many barriers to understanding [18]. The most powerful of these pictures are interactive ones, in which the user can explore their assumptions and achieve direct feedback.

The following sections therefore review both pictures and numerical approaches that can help to communicate how value can best be created by R&D, despite uncertainty. Because of all the uncertainties involved in predicting the future, and predicting what might be learned from different kinds of research, all effective research performance models must explicitly incorporate assumptions about sources and levels of uncertainty. We believe that this is the single most important area for improvement in research simulations.

Simulations can help management refine its thinking in four main areas:

1. Identifying the *sources of value* and the "levers that must be pulled" to change performance (we call these "R&D value drivers").
2. Assessing *throughput* and bottlenecks, for a given pattern of attrition, to help longer-term decisions on resourcing and technology investment and to study means of accelerating processes and decision making cycles.
3. Managing *risk*—project managers planning research tasks need to identify the most important outstanding sources of uncertainty and work out which most need resolution at any given point in the R&D process.
4. Making the right *strategic trade-offs* between quality and throughput when working out how to enrich or filter the forward pipeline and how

to resource these processes of "option enrichment" (e.g., library purchase, lead series extension) or "option filtering" (predictive computational and assay methods).

11.9.1 R&D Value Drivers

Ultimately, all of R&D can be seen as some kind of investment. No actual income is obtained until the point at which the new drug is sold, other than through out-licensing, which is not considered further here.

Within drug development, financial valuations are routinely used to assess projects and entire portfolios. For drug discovery groups less familiar with financial methods, who are a long way from the processes of marketing and sales, financial measures of process performance are unfamiliar and may generate resistance. This can sometimes lead to a focus, within R&D improvement initiatives, on improving what can easily be understood through initiatives such as cost cutting or development time compression. Such focus can take attention away from the root causes of good or poor performance, such as the quality profile of leads and candidates and the consequent chances of failing in development or of obtaining the desired high value in the market.

An example is a view given to us by a discovery manager that if a drug candidate could not reach a successful market launch, the next best thing for a discovery team would be to have their compound progress to late stages of development before failure, because this implies that any problem was hard to predict, for example, a rare event. Yet this is exactly the most expensive kind of failure.

Value driver analysis, a development of financial analysis visualizations first created at DuPont [19], provides an intuitive, graphical way of breaking down the sources of value (Fig. 11.4) and, in conjunction with stochastic models of the project process, can be used to quantify the likely contribution of different kind of change.

Graphical representations of complex interactions can aid understanding and show the need for integrated decision making. For the selection of optimum strategies, managers can also visualize and simulate pipeline volume and quality. The two are inextricably linked, and one cannot be changed independently of considering the other if optimum value is to be derived.

Costs in R&D are a mix of short-run cost, dominated by the cost of clinical trials, and long-run cost, dominated by the fixed assets and specialized expertise of discovery and preclinical organizations. Therefore, when seeking to maximize the value of output relative to input, development teams need to be concerned with external spending and the length of tasks, whereas research teams need to look at their investments in capacity and the way they use fixed capacity.

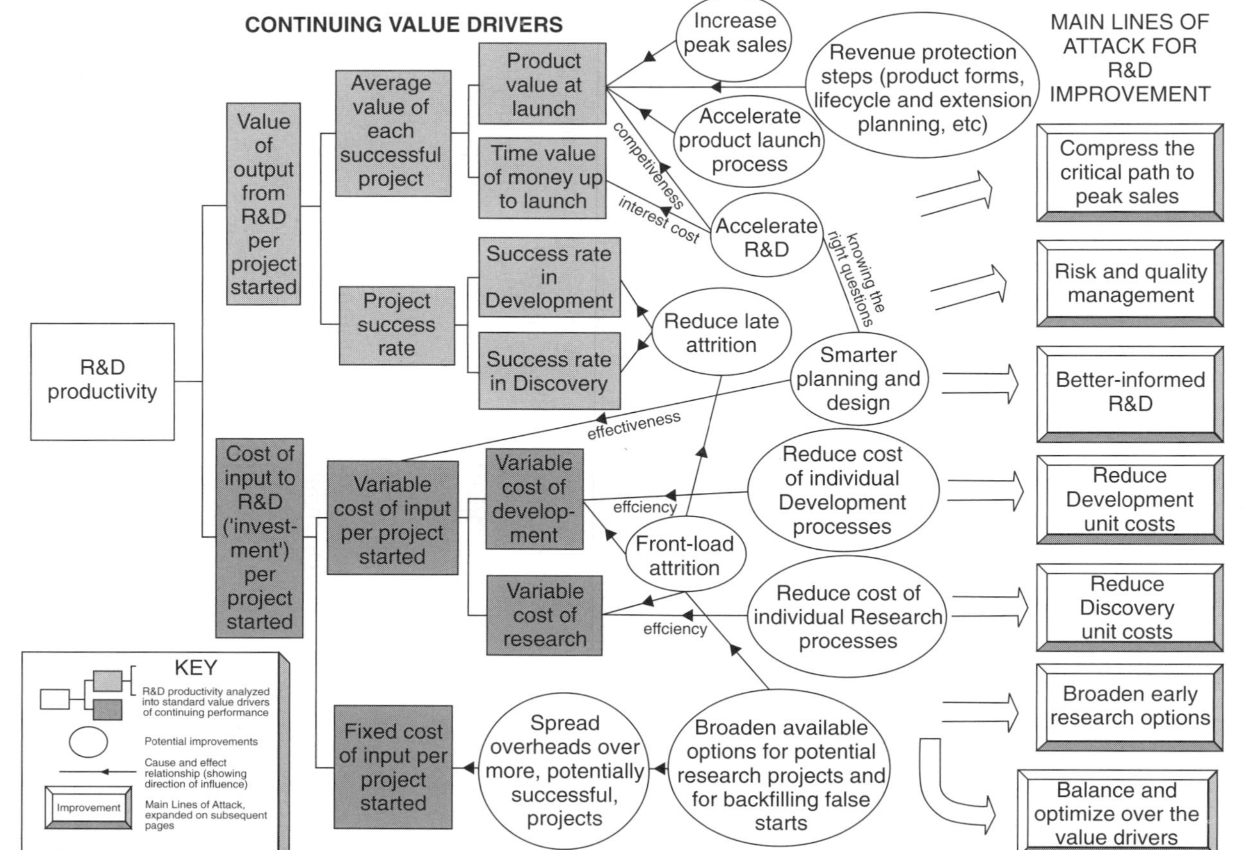

Figure 11.4 Analyzing R&D value generation into drivers such as throughput, compound value ("quality"), time elapsed, and process costs shows how improvement initiatives can best complement each other.

11.9.2 Assessing Throughput and Bottlenecks

The industrialization of drug discovery brings with it the need to build facilities that are dimensioned according to the business objectives. Increasingly, "Big Pharma" has been adopting techniques from the manufacturing world to help guide decisions on facility sizing, staffing, and scheduling. Discrete event simulation (DES) is a long-established technique within the operations research (OR) field, in which a computer version of a proposed or existing system can be built and then used to conduct studies to understand the impacts of changes to the system. Typical situations that are best suited to study with DES models would be those where randomness, variability, prioritization rules, breakdowns, and interprocess dependences are strong factors [20]. These simulation models typically employ animation as a means of illustrating the process flow and bottlenecks and also provide quantitative analysis. Figure 11.5 shows a typical high-level model for R&D project progression, set up in the business modeling environment Corporate Modeler (CASEwise Corporation). Other toolsets such as Promodel or Arena offer finer control over simulation variables and scheduling prioritization rules.

Our colleagues have applied DES in four different pharma companies to help optimize high-throughput screening (HTS) so as to "debottleneck" a process. The simulation must represent the type of compound storage and retrieval equipment, screening platforms, and staff needed to support screening a given annual number of targets against a given compound library. The simulation model helps to answer tactical questions around the impact of different work patterns (24/2 vs. 3 daily shifts, 5-day vs. 7-day working) and also, at a more strategic level, identifying which new investments in technology would best increase total throughput. DES approaches are also well suited to simulation of processes such as adverse event handling.

New combinations of simulation and optimization allow a much wider set of R&D decision making processes to be optimized, at least approximately, than in the past. This exciting new approach has been developed to solve many problems thought to be impossible to solve with classic options analysis. The idea is to trade off the exactness of the optimization for the ability to look at more complex situations [21].

This approach retains the capability to deal with contingent decisions but uses approximations to the value of a project, rather than exact calculations. Decisions are improved iteratively, first improving the approximation to use by simulating the evolution of the project under a given set of policies for decision making and then improving the policies for decision making by optimizing the (approximate) value at each point in time of the simulation.

Blau et al. [22] have applied probabilistic network models to model resource needs and success probabilities in pharmaceutical and agrochemical development, through Monte Carlo analysis. This requires solving the problem of scheduling a portfolio of projects under uncertainty about progression. This approach is tractable for drug development. However, "the inherent complex-

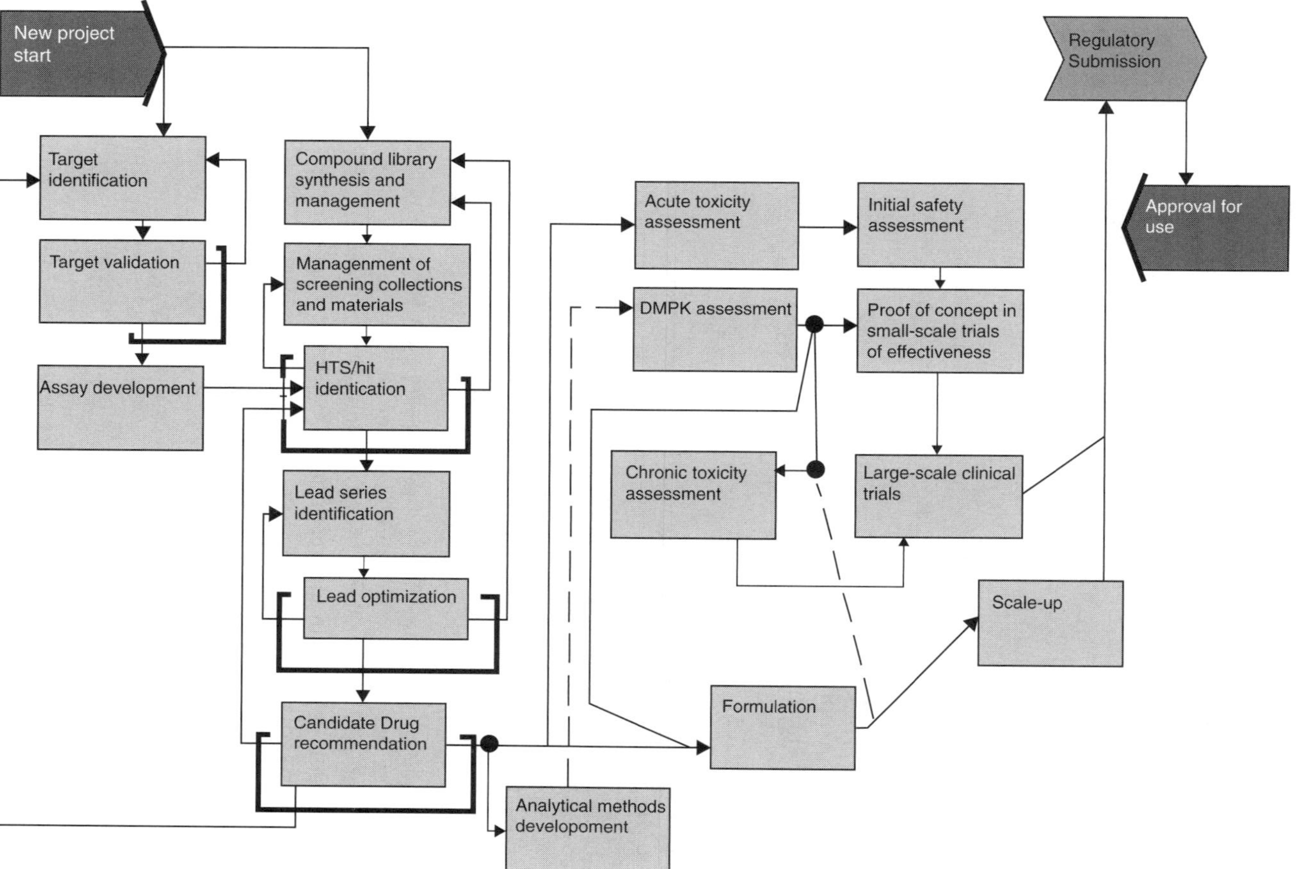

Figure 11.5 A high-level attrition model must represent the success probabilities and time taken at each stage of work, the return loops where rework is necessary, and the criteria for abandoning a project entirely.

ity and creativity of discovery . . . makes it difficult to capture all the activities" within such models applied to pharmaceutical research.

Many companies therefore take a multiproject view of the resources needed at different stages of drug discovery. On the view that where one project fails, another takes over, the drug discovery process can be seen as a continuum of hit generation and confirmation, lead identification, lead optimization, and candidate selection, where the resources needed are proportional to the number of compounds being screened, worked on, made, or optimized at any point in time. This type of "flow" or "throughput" model can give a very clear, intuitive, "five-box" view of the likely demands on resource. Such a view may help to locate a potential bottleneck that, as the input rate of work into the pipeline increases, may limit downstream flow and cause work upstream to back up. It appears that for many large pharma companies this limiting resource has been synthetic chemistry, because this discipline has benefited less from automation than has biological screening. In future, with offshoring of synthetic chemistry, limitations further downstream on pharmacology and biology skills and resources and experience of interdisciplinary working may start to limit R&D productivity.

When the most likely bottleneck stage and limiting resource have been identified, choosing the best management action may well then require lower-level DES that acts behind the scenes to calculate maximum throughput at each relevant step within the bottlenecked research stage. Such a two-step process of analysis is much more efficient than a bottom-up attempt to map the R&D universe before asking critical questions about constraints.

Clearly, however, the "flow" simplification would be invalid on a small site with episodic projects, or in contexts with significant downtime due to change-over and setup activities for project-specific assays. Such simulation problems covering multiple projects and multiple assays, with use of a mix of shared and dedicated resources, can rapidly become intractable, and an early, commonsense selection of the focus area for simulation is essential.

A "time-and-motion" modeling mind-set can easily blinker analysis of how best to improve the value created by research. Truly useful simulations of drug discovery must go beyond simplistic assumptions about yields at stage gates and address the causes of failure, starting to quantify the common concept of pipeline "quality."

Supporting excerpts from R&D management interviews were:

> The danger of a metric-driven approach is to push through quantity instead of quality.
>
> Many improvement attempts have knock-on consequences . . . more compounds delivered faster, not necessarily better, and this leads to bottlenecks.

11.9.3 Managing Risk and Uncertainty

Managing risk and uncertainty was increasingly seen as a priority in recent conferences, reflected in these comments from R&D management interviews:

> The issue of risk lies at the heart of the industry and, broadly speaking, scientists do not understand it well.
>
> The highest priority is to improve our ability to predict.

Uncertainty from the viewpoint of the discovery researcher consists both of controllable and uncontrollable risks [23].

- "Epistemic uncertainty"—missing knowledge—is due to a lack of information that through R&D you could "buy" directly or estimate through proxy methods, if you so chose. These are controllable risks, although in practice they may be unduly expensive to control relative to the risk exposure (threat × likelihood).
- "Aleatory uncertainty"—the roll of the die—describes risks that cannot practicably be predicted within the research process, for example, new failure modes, or modes that can only be detected in late stages of work, for example, humans. An example of aleatory uncertainty is the withdrawal in the UK of Bextra on the basis of two serious adverse events out of 40,000 patients; this could only be discovered after launch [2]. This, without hindsight, was an "uncontrollable risk."

Spending effort on research to attempt to reduce what is really aleatory uncertainty is a waste of time. Accepting some unmanageable risks is simply part of the price of entry to the pharmaceutical industry. Once the limits of possible knowledge are accepted, research people can concentrate on discovering what is genuinely knowable.

We take a Bayesian approach to research process modeling, which encourages explicit statements about the prior degree of uncertainty, expressed as a probability distribution over possible outcomes. Simulation that builds in such uncertainty will be of a "what-if" nature, helping managers to explore different scenarios, to understand problem structure, and to see where the future is likely to be most sensitive to current choices, or indeed where outcomes are relatively indifferent to such choices. This determines where better information could best help improve decisions and how much to invest in internal research (research about process performance, and in particular, prediction reliability) that yields such information.

Such Bayesian models could be couched in terms of parametric distributions, but the mathematics for real problems becomes intractable, so discrete distributions, estimated with the aid of computers, are used instead. The calculation of probability of outcomes from assumptions (inference) can be performed through exhaustive multiplication of conditional probabilities, or with large problems estimates can be obtained through stochastic methods (Monte Carlo techniques) that sample over possible futures.

The main challenge to overcome is obtaining the necessary numbers to input to such models. There is a natural distrust of "rubbish in," "rubbish out," and the teams used to working with "hard data" may be reluctant to express their underlying assumptions about goals, trade-offs, and business processes in terms of numbers: For example, where do the project and stage success rates come from? How far are they adjustable? Are they independent of the therapy area?

Therefore we increasingly take the view that rather than fully simulating the business context, which may seem like a "black box" approach, it is better to have decision makers interact with more selective simulations. These help develop their intuitions and hone their judgment and reasoning ability in focused areas, especially in the area of probability, applied statistics, and decision theory, which is nonintuitive without such practice.

The visualization of trade-offs involving risk and uncertainty is clearly one such powerful aid to insight. Questions frequently encountered are: Where should *in silico* and other predictive technologies best be applied within the R&D process? What workflows involving such technologies add most value? What should be the approach to selecting "cutoffs"?

An application of simple statistical analysis (receiver operating characteristic) combined with a decision analytic valuation of false positives and false negatives may be useful in such cases. The fundamental concept here is one of the method "buying information" that can avoid unnecessary future work but must be reliable enough to avoid wasting valuable opportunities. In many cases there may need even be no need to estimate the cost and effort implications of using the proposed *in silico* method, as it can be proved that a method of less than a critical predictive reliability would destroy value even if it were available for free, owing to the rate of lost opportunities (false negatives).

A further insight is that the best workflow depends on a combination of factors that can in many cases be expressed in closed mathematical form, allowing very rapid graphical feedback to users of what then becomes a visualization rather than a stochastic simulation tool. This particular approach is effective for simple binary comparisons of methods (e.g., use of in vitro alone vs. *in silico* as prefilter to in vitro). It can also be extended to evaluation of conditional sequencing for groups of compounds, using an extension of the "sentinel" approach [24].

Such "sentinel" workflow uses a prediction to select compounds for a more expensive screen that can confirm predicted hazards (liabilities, such as toxicity). It is, provably, the best workflow in contexts where a low prevalence of the hazard is anticipated, and where there is a backstop means further downstream (e.g., preclinical toxicity testing) for detecting hazards before humans are exposed. This workflow then allows the compounds predicted as safe to bypass the expensive hazards screen, without unacceptable risk, and can add significant value in terms of external screening costs or avoiding use of what may be a bottleneck resource.

Our simulation work has identified a value-adding extension of this approach where if there are two alternative liabilities A and B, a prediction of the presence of A or B can select compounds for relatively early screening against either risk factor, leaving the other to be assessed later. For certain combinations of the ratios of costs of screening and prevalence for A and B, a prediction of reliability only just above chance can add some value. The underlying reason is that all compounds will eventually be screened for both liabilities, so there is no downside impact of the predictive method due to false negatives.

There are two key limitations of the use of ROC methods and decision analytic valuations in such applications, each of which gives rise to an opportunity for improving the reach of R&D management simulations:

- ROC analysis, used frequently for assessment of diagnostic methods of all kinds, requires comparison of a "prediction" with an assumed truth or "gold standard." Methods based on Bayesian or belief networks, which can model conditional probability relationships between many possible proxy (surrogate) measures of a given state of nature, have much greater power to model multivariate problems, for example, in comparing a single-factor *in silico* prediction of diffusion rate with a multifactor ADME in vitro measurement that includes the additional factor of solubility.
- The decision theory is valid for variable costs but does not consider the problem of capacity allocation. In many contexts, screening capacity is a sunk cost, and there is a need to consider the "straw that broke the camel's back," the first compound that exceeds capacity. There is no need to ration resources that are not scarce and have trivial variable costs relative to the potential value that their use can create. This reasoning leads naturally back to use of easily understood, intuitive flow and capacity visualizations for the relevant simulations.

There is therefore an as-yet unmet need for helping management intuitions about the best way to invest and use R&D capacity to optimize value added, under conditions of uncertainty.

11.9.4 Making the Right Strategic Trade-Offs About Reducing Uncertainty

There is a vital three-way trade-off between investment (or in general, resourcing), throughput, and quality. Throughput and quality are inextricably linked; when biological and chemical options are limited, more output does not mean better quality. The right balance is not always obvious and may be counterintuitive, which makes the choice of the right investment an even harder problem. For example, if there is an expected bottleneck in the multistage process, is the right thing to invest to elevate this constraint, or to make a more stringent selection of compounds upstream, with potential lost opportunity?

We have developed an approach termed "ARBITER" (Architecture for Reliable Business Improvement and Technology Evaluation in Research) [25], with associated simulation and visualization capability, that combines

Bayesian networks for multivariate reasoning about cause and effect within R&D with a flow bottleneck model (Fig. 11.6) to help combine scientific and economic aspects of decision making. This model can, where research process decisions affect potential candidate value, further incorporate simple estimation of how the candidate value varies based on the target product profile. Factors such as ease of dosing in this profile can then be causally linked to the relevant predictors within the research process (e.g., bioavailability), to model the value of the predictive methods that might be used and to perform sensitivity analysis of how R&D process choices affect the expected added

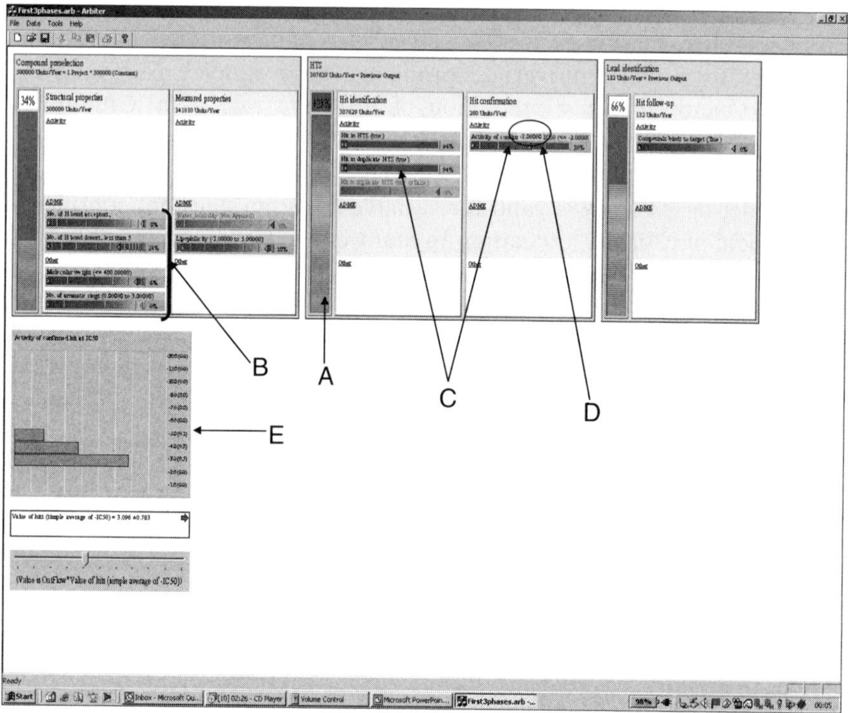

Figure 11.6 ARBITER provides a simulation of R&D throughput, stage success rates, and resource capacity loading (A) as a function of the methods used, the sequence of use (including parallel use), which is based on prior estimates of compound library quality, prevalence of different compound characteristics (B), prediction reliability (C), and user-selectable cutoff levels (D higlighted circle). The combination of throughput and candidate expected value (based on variations around the target product profile and the factors influencing development success rates) gives a direct estimate of the rate at which a particular selection of R&D process can be expected to contribute value. An average yield of successful projects (which may be a fraction) can be converted through use of distribution over a measure of pipeline quality (E), including the chance of having no successes in any given year. See color plate.

value of a given R&D process and pattern of investment in resources. Varying the model structure by "leaving out a step" gives, through the difference in estimated value-add, a financial valuation of a research technology use that includes both throughput and quality impacts.

One challenge in applying this approach, which relies on prior estimates of method prediction reliability, is how to deal with differences between future compounds to be tested and the "universe" of all compounds on which the collected experience of R&D process effectiveness has been based. If new active compounds fall within the "space" previously sampled, then knowledge of chemical properties is just another kind of conditioning within a Bayesian network; if they fall outside this space, then the initial model of both outcomes and predictions has an unpredictable error. The use of sampling theory and models of diversity [16] are therefore promising extensions of the above approach.

The Bayesian network technology embedded in the ARBITER tool is also well suited for learning both probability relationships (e.g., method reliability estimates) and the essential structure of cause and effect, from data sets where predictions and outcomes can be compared. Colleagues have already applied this capability on a large scale for risk management (selection of potentially suspect claims for further inspection and examination) in the insurance industry.

11.10 CONCLUSIONS

How can pharma R&D managers ensure that the future for process and performance improvement is not just like the past, where the long-term trend appears to be decreased, not increased, economic effectiveness?

Perhaps the most relevant interview quotation here is:

> I'm not sure how good big pharma is at knowing what it knows.

So how, in practice can big pharma become more self-aware and self-critical, and what can IT do to help? There are two opposed views, evidenced by these interview comments:

> Discovery is a very creative process; there is a natural desire not to have constraints on this from business and operational considerations.
>
> For continuous improvement, we need to inform scientists of the bigger picture so that individual judgments can be made against the right background.

Only by actively collecting and using the evidence that enables "double loop learning" (including project success/failure tracking data bases, retrospective failure analysis, and tests of prediction reliability), can R&D management take full advantage of the wide range of simulation support tools now available to them. Without this evidence, they must rely on subjective judgments about performance, and the potential to improve performance, which, as we have seen, are shrouded in many doubts.

> If a man will begin with certainties he shall end in doubts; but if he will be content to begin with doubts, he shall end in certainties.
>
> —Francis Bacon, The Advancement of Learning (1605)
> based on Meditations of Marcus Aurelius

ACKNOWLEDGMENTS

We are grateful to:

Nick Hughes, Head of Global Analytics and Life Sciences Consulting, for sponsoring our original work on quantitative methods in support of pharmaceutical R&D performance improvement, and for reviewing a draft.

Michael Aitkenhead, his industrial supervisor Michaela Hajek of PA, and Michael's anonymous interviewees in three large pharmaceutical companies, for the time and effort on interviews and interview analysis.

Radhesh Nair for contributions on discrete event simulation.

Our clients in R&D groups for stimulating discussions on R&D improvement and for requesting and trialing our recent approaches to the simulations of impact and economic assessment of new ways of working and new technology applications in drug discovery.

REFERENCES

1. Ruffolo R. Re-engineering discovery and development: impact on the pharmaceutical industry of tomorrow. In: *Drug Discovery Technology Europe 2005*, IBC Life Sciences.
2. Schmid EF, Smith DA. Is declining innovation in the pharmaceutical industry a myth? *Drug Discov Today* August 2005;1031–9.
3. DiMasi JA New drug development in the United States from 1963–1999. *Clin Pharmacol Therapeut* May 2001;69:286–96.
4. DiMasi JA, Hansen RW, Grabowski HG The price of innovation: new estimates of drug development costs. *J Health Econ* 2003;22:151–85.
5. Luehrman, TA. What's it worth? A general manager's guide to valuation. *Harvard Business Rev* May–June 1997;132–42.
6. http://www.keyitsolutions.com/asp/rptdetails/report/46/cat/1296/
7. Nichols NA. Scientific management at Merck: an interview with CFO Judy Lewent. *Harvard Business Rev* January–February 1994;89–99.

8. Black F, Scholes M. The pricing of options and corporate liabilities. *J Political Econ* 1973;81:637–54.
9. Black, S. Letter to the Editor of *The Economist* (UK), 4 September 1999.
10. Gittins, J. Quantitative methods in the planning of pharmaceutical research. *Drug Inform J* 1996;30:459–87.
11. Palisade Corporation, Ithaca, NY (www.palisade.com).
12. Syncopation Software, London, UK www.syncopationsoftware.com
13. http://ondecidingbetter.editthispage.com/Tools
14. Burman C-F, Senn S. Examples of option values in drug development. *Pharmaceut Statist* 2003;2:113–25.
15. Schjødt-Eriksen J, Clausen J. Optimization and simulation in drug development—review and analysis http://www.imm.dtu.dk/pubdb/views/edoc_download.php/2834/ps/imm2834.ps
16. Wright T, Gillet VJ, Green DVS, Pickett SD. Optimising the size and configuration of combinatorial libraries. *J Chem Info Comput Sci* 2003;43:381–90.
17. Smith MK, Argyris C. Theories of action, double-loop learning and organizational learning. *The encyclopedia of informal education*, 2003; www.infed.org/thinkers/argyris.htm.
18. Tufte ER. *The visual display of quantitative information*, 2nd Ed. Graphics Press 2001.
19. Krumm FV, Rolle CF. Management and application of decision and risk analysis in DuPont. *Interfaces* 1992;22:84–93.
20. Subramanian D, Pekny JF, Reklaitis. A simulation-optimization framework for research and development pipeline management. *AIChE J* 2001;47(10): 2226.
21. Bertsekas D, Tsitsiklis J. *Neuro-dynamic programming*. Belmont, MA: Athena Scientific, 1996.
22. Blau G et al. Risk management in the development of new products in highly regulated industries. *Comput Chem Eng* 2000;24:659–64.
23. http://www.foresight.gov.uk/Intelligent_Infrastructure_Systems/long_paper.pdf
24. Pearl GM, Livingston-Carr S, Durham SK. Integration of Computations Analysis as a Sentinel Tool in Toxicological Assessments. *Curr Topics in Med Chem* 2001;1:247–55.
25. Chadwick A, Hajek M. Learning to improve the decision-making process in research. *Drug Discov Today* 2004;9(6): 251–7.

PART IV

COMPUTERS IN DRUG DISCOVERY

12

COMPUTERS AND PROTEIN CRYSTALLOGRAPHY

David J. Edwards and Roderick E. Hubbard

Contents

Computer Applications in Pharmaceutical Research and Development, Edited by Sean Ekins.
ISBN 0-471-73779-8

12.1 INTRODUCTION

X-ray crystallography became established over forty years ago as the most powerful method for determining the three-dimensional structure of proteins. Such structures provide a detailed description of the arrangement of atoms in a molecule, providing insights into how proteins perform their chemical function. This understanding allows the mechanism of action of the proteins to be related to their biological function, in particular how the proteins recognize and bind other molecules such as substrates, cofactors, and other proteins or nucleic acids.

This detailed knowledge allows a rational approach to many aspects of drug discovery. It can influence the design and interpretation of biological assays and can rationalize why certain ligands bind specifically to a protein. More powerfully, this detailed picture can be used to design changes in the structure of the ligand, to generate new compounds with improved binding affinity and specificity, or to include in the new compound the chemical features that will improve the performance of the compound as a drug. Recently, it has also been realized that various experimental and computational methods can exploit the structure to screen libraries of compounds to discover new classes of molecules that bind to the protein. The power of these methods has been realized in a number of drug discovery projects, with such success that most medium to large pharmaceutical companies now employ a protein crystallographic group as part of their research discovery operations. In addition, a number of new companies have been started with the central aim of structure-based drug discovery, developing and innovating new methods that are now finding application across the industry.

This chapter consists of four main sections. The first provides an overall description of the process of contemporary protein structure determination by X-ray crystallography and summarizes the current computational requirements. This is followed by a summary and examples of the use of structure-based methods in drug discovery. The third section reviews the key developments in computer hardware and computational methods that have supported the development and application of X-ray crystallography over the past forty or so years. The final section outlines the areas in which improved informatics and computational methods will have an impact on the future contributions that X-ray crystallography can make to the drug discovery process.

12.2 OVERVIEW OF THE CRYSTALLOGRAPHIC PROCESS

Figure 12.1 summarizes the main stages in solving the structure of a protein. The following is a brief discussion of the features and issues for each of the steps, with particular reference to the computing and computational requirements. A more detailed description of protein crystallography can be found in numerous text books. Of particular note are the introductory chapters in the *Methods in Enzymology* issues on crystallography, volumes 114, 115, 368, and 374.

12.2.1 Design Construct

A major requirement for structural studies is the availability of large quantities of pure, functional protein. Essentially all proteins are present in only very small quantities in native cells or tissues, so molecular biology techniques

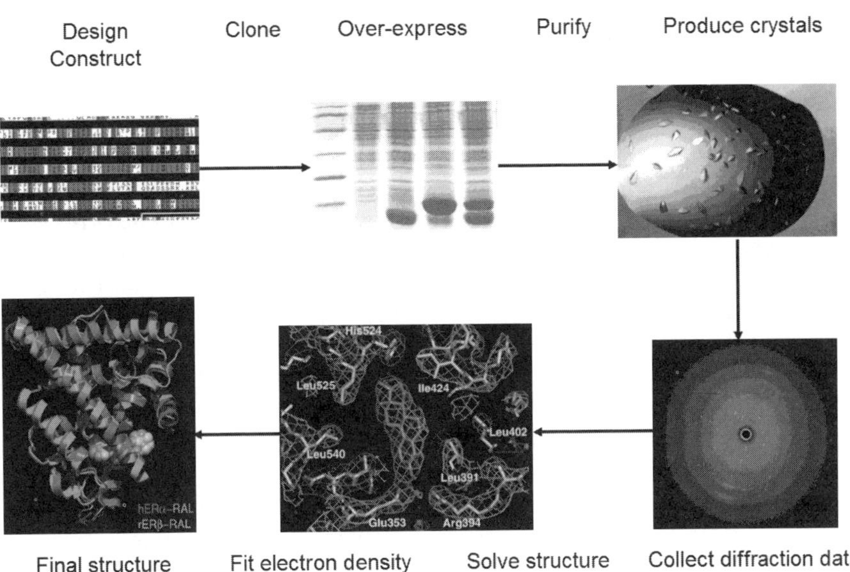

Figure 12.1 The crystallographic pipeline. See color plate.

have been developed to overexpress large quantities of the protein in organisms that can be grown rapidly and in large quantities. To do this requires manipulation of the gene encoding the protein, and an important first step is to select which piece of the DNA is to be used. In many cases, solubility and crystallization of the protein can be problematic, so the gene is often selected just to encode a subpart or domain of the protein that is important for function and that will have an improved chance of folding into a soluble protein that will crystallize.

The design of these constructs draws on experience of working with a particular class of protein and is predominantly informatics—comparing sequences, identifying patterns that indicate domain boundaries, using the structure of related proteins as a guide, if available. The number of constructs designed depends on the protein expression strategy. Where parallel, semiautomated cloning robotics are available, this can involve varying the two ends of the construct (the N and C termini) by, for example, 5, 10, or 15 amino acids and adding a purification tag (often hexa-His, see below) to either N or C terminus.

There are alternative strategies such as expressing the full-length protein and then using mild proteolytic cleavage followed by mass spectroscopy to define the domains. For some targets it is appropriate to attempt the expression of isoforms, homologs, or orthologs of the protein to find a variant that is more amenable to overexpression or crystallization. Some laboratories use mutational strategies (either random or targeted) to improve the properties of the expressed protein, sometimes coupled to other genes that signal when expression has been successful.

12.2.2 Overexpression

Although a variety of different cell systems have been used successfully (including CHO cells for renin, aspergillus for cellulases, yeast for ion channels) the current preferred workhorses for protein expression are bacteria (strains of *Escherichia coli*) transformed to incorporate the gene of interest or insect cells infected with baculovirus containing the gene to be expressed. In both cases there has been extensive optimization of both the cells and the expression construct strategy. Typically, a series of expression trials (different constructs, different expression media and conditions) are assessed for production of protein. The conditions are optimized for a particular clone, and then production is scaled up, either at the liter scale in shaker flasks, or in larger volumes within fermentors of varying levels of sophistication (media/conditions/cell growth control). This step requires no computational support beyond general informatics for tracking and recording results of series of experiments. Some automation is beginning to be used in some laboratories, which is placing an extra requirement on databasing and laboratory information management systems to keep track of all the different samples (see Section 12.6).

12.2.3 Purification

In this step, the cells expressing the protein are broken open and the target protein purified by various forms of chromatography. Most laboratories now engineer the construct for the protein to include a tag (such as histidine residues, so-called His-tag, or a particular peptide or other protein) that binds specifically to a particular column (nickel for His-tag, antibody for most other tags). The join between the tag and the protein is usually designed to have a sequence recognized by a very specific protease, to allow cleavage of the tag after purification. Again, beyond informatics support, this step requires no computational support.

12.2.4 Crystallization

A regularly formed crystal of reasonable size (typically >500 μm in each dimension) is required for X-ray diffraction. Samples of pure protein are screened against a matrix of buffers, additives, or precipitants for conditions under which they form crystals. This can require many thousands of trials and has benefited from increased automation over the past five years. Most large crystallographic laboratories now have robotics systems, and the most sophisticated also automate the visualization of the crystallization experiments, to monitor the appearance of crystalline material. Such developments [e.g., Ref. 1] are adding computer visualization and pattern recognition to the informatics requirements.

In drug discovery, it is usual to determine the structure of a protein in complex with many different small molecules. If the protein crystallizes such that the binding site is open and not occluded by other molecules in the crystal, then there are two options—either to soak crystals with the small molecule or to attempt crystallization of a preformed protein-ligand complex (cocrystallization). For some proteins, the binding of a small molecule either induces a conformational change or changes an important crystal contact. In these cases it may be necessary to screen for different crystallization conditions, often resulting in quite different crystal packing.

12.2.5 Diffraction

When a beam of X rays hits a crystal, the X rays are diffracted by the electrons in the layers of molecules in the crystal to give a pattern of spots of radiation of different intensities. The diffraction pattern is related to the electron density by a Fourier transform. In general terms, the pattern of spots reflects the packing of molecules and the spacing of the spots is related to the dimensions of the asymmetric unit packing in the crystal. The relative intensity of the spots contains information about the distribution of electron density. The number of spots, particularly at higher angles of diffraction, is a function of the quality of the crystal (and the strength of the incident X radiation).

Depending on the size and packing (space group) of the asymmetric unit in the crystal and the resolution available, many tens of thousands of diffraction spots must be recorded to determine a structure.

All crystallographic laboratories have an in-house source of X rays (usually a rotating anode generator) with either an image plate or a CCD camera to record the images. An in-house system is vital for monitoring crystal quality and can be used for collecting a complete set of diffraction data. Synchrotrons have transformed data collection. These large instruments (mostly national facilities) provide high-intensity, tunable sources of radiation. Suitably configured with fast CCD cameras and robotic crystal handling, complete diffraction data sets can be measured for a protein crystal in a few minutes. This generates many gigabytes of images that must be processed to a list of intensities for each of the diffraction spots. Suitably configured multiprocessor PCs can perform this data processing in essentially real time—which can be important for guiding data collection strategies. Another advantage of synchrotrons is that the wavelength of the X rays can be tuned. Collection of diffraction data at a number of wavelengths can be used to solve new structures as discussed in Section 12.2.6.

12.2.6 Initial Structure Solution

When a diffracted X-ray beam hits a data collection device, only the intensity of the reflection is recorded. The other vital piece of information is the phase of the reflected X-ray beam. It is the combination of the intensity and the phase of the reflections that is needed to unravel the contributions made to the diffraction by the electrons in different parts of the molecule in the crystal. This so-called phase problem has been a challenge for theoretical crystallographers for many decades. For practical crystallography, there are four main methods for phasing the data generated from a particular crystal.

Isomorphous replacement is where the phases from a previous sample are used directly for a protein that has crystallized in exactly the same space group as before. This is usually applicable to determining the structure of many protein-ligand complexes or protein mutants.

Molecular replacement is where the phases of a known structure are used to determine the structure of a protein that may be identical but crystallized in a different space group or may adopt essentially the same structure (e.g., a homologous protein). Essentially, the calculations find the rotation and translation of the molecule that work with the phases to produce an interpretable electron density map.

Multiple isomorphous replacement allows the ab initio determination of the phases for a new protein structure. Diffraction data are collected for crystals soaked with different heavy atoms. The scattering from these atoms dominates the diffraction pattern, and a direct calculation of the relative position of the heavy atoms is possible by a direct method known as the Patterson synthesis. If a number of heavy atom derivatives are available, and they are isomorphous, then this combination of data is enough to determine the phases for all reflections.

Multiwavelength methods exploit the tunability of synchrotrons. If data are collected at a number of wavelengths from a crystal that contains an atom that produces anomalous scattering (such as selenium), then this can be sufficient to determine the phases. The selenium is introduced into the protein during protein expression where engineered bacteria can incorporate selenomethionine in place of natural methionine. There have been some recent innovations in anomalous scattering methods, such as bathing the crystal in xenon gas and looking for anomalous signal from sulfur atoms.

The computational requirements of these calculations are relatively modest on modern computers. However, some groups have exploited computer power to design ambitious molecular replacement protocols in which many models are assessed in parallel (see Section 12.6).

12.2.7 Model Building and Refinement

Once the phases are determined, the structure is solved and an electron density map can be generated. The next step is to fit a molecular model of the structure into this map. This can take some time for the very first structure, although there have been some dramatic improvements in semiautomated chain tracing and model building procedures in recent years [2–8]. For molecular replacement or isomorphous replacement solutions, the model will need some rebuilding. Again, this is an area where new software methods are having considerable impact. Finally, any ligands and solvent molecules must be built into the structure. There then follows an iterative process of refinement interspersed with model rebuilding and analysis. Refinement uses computational methods [9, 10] to refine the molecular model into the electron density. This refinement is driven by the so-called R-factor, which is a measure of how well the model fits the density. To avoid overfitting, an additional factor (called the free R-factor [11]) is also tracked, where some of the reflections are left out from calculating the density.

An important step is to validate the structure, that is, to compare features of the structure to features in known protein structures. This includes localized fit to density, hydrogen bonding patterns, divergence from standard geometry, and much more [12]. Such calculations can highlight where the model requires further improvement.

12.3 STRUCTURE AND THE DRUG DISCOVERY PROCESS

There are three main contributions that structural methods are making to the drug discovery process—structural biology, structure-based design, and structure-based discovery.

12.3.1 Structural Biology

The determination of the structure of a protein target, perhaps complexed to partner proteins, lipids, nucleic acid, or substrate, can provide a clear insight into the mechanism of action of a protein, which in turn can often be related to its biological or therapeutic role. It is now possible to generate structures for an increasing number of therapeutically important targets, such as nuclear receptors, kinases, proteases, phosphodiesterases, phosphatases, metabolic enzymes, and key proteins in the life cycle of bacteria or viruses. The two main issues limiting the number of structures are the ability to produce sufficient quantities of pure, soluble, functional, homogeneous protein for crystallization trials and the ability of the protein to form regular crystals suitable for diffraction experiments. This combination of limitations often means that a structure is not available for the whole therapeutic target. However, even the structure of individual domains can be sufficient to make a real impact on a discovery project and provide a context within which to understand the overall function of the protein.

12.3.2 Structure-Based Design

The crystal structure of a ligand bound to a protein provides a detailed insight into the interactions between the protein and the ligand. Such understanding can be used to design changes to the ligand to introduce new interactions to modify the affinity and specificity of the ligand for a particular protein. In addition, the structure can be used to identify where the ligand can be changed to modulate the physicochemical and absorption, distribution, metabolism, excretion, and toxicology properties of the compound, by showing which parts of the compound are important for affinity and which parts can be altered without affecting binding.

This type of analysis is now well established and has been used in many drug discovery projects over the past fifteen years. Examples include HIV protease inhibitors [13], anti-influenza drugs [14], isoform-selective ligands for the estrogen receptor [15], and many more.

12.3.3 Structure-Based Discovery

As the availability of crystal structures increased in the early 1990s, a number of experimental and computational methods were developed to use the structure of the protein target as a route to discover novel hit compounds. The methods include de novo design, virtual screening, and fragment-based discovery. These developments are covered in more detail in the later chapters of this book, but their main features can be summarized as follows.

Virtual screening uses computational docking methods to assess which of a large database of compounds will fit into the unliganded structure of the target protein. Current protocols and methods can, with up to 80% success, predict the binding position and orientation of ligands that are known to bind to a protein. However, identifying which ligands bind into a particular binding site is much less successful, with many more false positive hits being identified. The major challenge remains the quality of the scoring functions—if these were more accurate, then the challenge of predicting conformational change in the protein on binding of ligand would also be more tractable. For a review of current methods, see Reference 16.

De novo design attempts to use the unliganded structure of the protein to generate novel chemical structures that can bind. There are varying algorithms, most of which depend on identifying initial hot spots of interactions that are then grown into complete ligands. As well as the ubiquitous issue of scoring functions, the major challenge facing these methods is generation of chemical structures that are synthetically accessible.

Fragment-based discovery is based on the premise that most ligands that bind strongly to a protein active site can be considered as a number of smaller fragments or functionalities. Fragments are identified by screening a relatively small library of molecules (400–20,000) by X-ray crystallography, NMR spectroscopy, or functional assay. The structures of the fragments binding to the protein can be used to design new ligands by adding functionality to the fragment, by merging together or linking various fragments, or by grafting features of the fragments onto existing ligands. The main issues are designing libraries of sufficient diversity and the synthetic challenges of fragment evolution. Some recent papers on this area are References 17 and 18.

For many proteins, it is possible to generate structures of protein-ligand complexes quite rapidly. It is therefore not uncommon for many hundreds of structures to be determined in support of a drug discovery and optimization project. The major challenge for this level of throughput is informatics support. It is also this type of crystallography that is most in need of semiautomated procedures for structure solution and model building (see Section 12.6).

12.4 HISTORY OF THE DEVELOPMENT OF CRYSTALLOGRAPHIC COMPUTING

It is instructive to look back over the literature of the past fifty years and trace the development of crystallographic computing. The early pioneers in this area (E. J. Dodson, personal communication) do not feel that computing power really limited the development and application of crystallography. There was more of a coevolution of ideas, methods, and experimental data at the same time that computing power was becoming available. However, the computational needs were considerable, and until the early 1990s crystallographic computing both required access to and encouraged some of the major developments in both computing and graphics technology.

The following discussion is necessarily a personal and subjective summary of the major developments in methods and computing. The division into different decades is approximate.

12.4.1 1950s

The 1950s saw the birth of macromolecular crystallography. The first major breakthrough came with the determination of the structure of vitamin B12 by the Hodgkin group in Oxford [19]. This was one of the first documented examples of the use of computers in crystal structure determination, where Ken Trueblood and his team gained access to some of the first analog computers. This also saw the full realization of the methods of multiple isomorphous replacement for phase determination. These developments led to the publication of the first protein structure by the Kendrew group in Cambridge [20].

12.4.2 1960s

This decade saw the establishment of the methods of protein crystallography with a growing number of protein structures from various groups. Examples include the work of Perutz on hemoglobin [21], the first structure of an enzyme (lysozyme) by Phillips et al. [22], and the first structure of a hormone by Hodgkin et al. [23]. These studies established that through structure it was possible to understand the mechanism of action of the proteins and relate this to their biological function. For example, the work on hemoglobin extended to the first attempts to provide a structural understanding of genetic disease, and Perutz and Lehmann [40] mapped the known clinically relevant mutations in hemoglobin to the structure. The major advance in crystallographic methods was the development of molecular replacement techniques by Rossmann and Blow [24].

This decade also saw the first major developments in molecular graphics. The first multiple-access computer was built at MIT (the so-called project MAC), which was a prototype for the development of modern computing. This device included a high-performance oscilloscope on which programs could draw vectors very rapidly and a closely coupled "trackball" with which the user could interact with the representation on the screen. Using this equipment, Levinthal and his team developed the first molecular graphics system, and his article in *Scientific American* [25] remains a classic in the field and laid the foundations for many of the features that characterize modern day molecular graphics systems.

For the most part, however, there was slow development in computers and their availability. The systems were only available at large institutional centers, with limited access, essentially no storage space, and often very long turnaround time on calculations, waiting days for even the smallest calculations to be completed.

12.4.3 1970s

An increasing number of large centers acquired computers dedicated to crystallographic work, and the 1970s saw the emergence of the first laboratory-based computers, such as the PDP series from DEC. These supported important advances in the computational methods. The large centers were particularly important in providing advanced computer graphics systems. This led to the pioneering advances in molecular graphics at laboratories such as those at the University of California-San Francisco and NIH [26, 27] and the first development of interactive graphics systems for fitting molecular models into electron density maps such as skeletonization of electron density maps by Greer [28] and the work by Diamond at the Medical Research Council's Laboratory of Molecular Biology. The most significant advance was by Jones in Munich, who developed the program FRODO [29, 30], reformulated and extended in the program O [31].

The most notable advance in computational crystallography was the availability of methods for refining protein structures by least-squares optimization. This developed in a number of laboratories and was made feasible by the implementation of fast Fourier transform techniques [32]. The most widely used system was PROLSQ from the Hendrickson lab [33].

In terms of crystallographic equipment, the initial synchrotron sources were becoming available, and although most laboratories still relied on diffractometers, some image plate systems were beginning to be developed. Together these advances in methods and equipment led to a steady increase in the number of available protein structures during the 1970s, although the crystallographer was limited to working on naturally abundant proteins. There were sufficient structures, however, for a databank to be required and the Protein Data Bank was established in the late 1970s [34]. The depository was run for many years at Brookhaven National Labs and moved to the Research Collaboratory in Structural Biology during the 1990s (http://www.rcsb.org; Ref. 35).

There were important developments in appreciating how protein structures can be used. A fascinating paper to illustrate this is the description of studies of the enzyme dihydrofolate reductase (DHFR) by Matthews et al. in 1977 [36]. Although the description of the determination of the structure emphasizes just how much the experimental methods of protein crystallography have developed, it does illustrate that many of the ideas of modern structure-based design were well established some thirty years ago. The structure of methotrexate bound to bacterial DHFR allowed quite detailed rationalization of the differences in binding affinity of related ligands and an understanding of why, although there are sequence variations, the ligand bound tightly to all DHFRs known at that time. This type of structural insight led to structure-based design of new inhibitors [37].

12.4.4 1980s

The 1980s saw many important developments in the scientific disciplines that underpin the use of protein crystallography in the pharmaceutical and biotechnology industries. Molecular biology and protein chemistry methods were beginning to dissect many aspects of biological processes, identifying new proteins and, importantly, providing the overexpression methods with which to produce large quantities for structural study. In protein crystallography, synchrotron radiation not only speeded up the data collection process but because of its intensity and focus allowed usable data to be collected from smaller, poorer crystals. In addition, the multiple wavelength methods (MAD [38]) were developed, allowing direct determination of phases from a single crystal. These advances were complemented by developments in methods for refining structures, initially least-squares refinement [33] and later the simulated annealing approach of X-plor [10]. These latter techniques required quite considerable amounts of computer time but did provide real benefit in refining structures with less manual rebuilding.

In computing terms, the 1980s were dominated by laboratory-based, multiaccess computer systems, predominantly the VAX range from DEC. Specialist computer graphics equipment was still required to deliver the performance necessary for interactive display and manipulation of electron density maps and molecular models, and the dominant manufacturer for most of the 1980s was Evans and Sutherland. In the late 1980s, there were two divergent trends. On the one hand there was the emergence of specialist computing equipment such as the Convex and Alliant that used specialized vector hardware to achieve performance. On the other, powerful Unix workstations combined adequate computer power with good graphics, such as the Silicon Graphics 4D range. The pace of development of the RISC-based UNIX workstation was similar to that seen in the Intel PC developments of the past few years. The improvement in price/performance was so rapid for essentially a commodity level of computing that the specialist computers were soon made obsolete.

Whereas at the beginning of the 1980s only a few large groups had access to computing and graphics facilities for protein crystallography, by the end of the decade essentially every crystallographic group was self-sufficient in this regard.

12.4.5 1990s

The major advances in crystallographic methods were both experimental and theoretical. In experimental terms, there was widespread availability of synchrotron data collection resources and the emergence of CCD detectors that dramatically increased the speed at which data could be collected. A particularly important advance was the development of cryocrystallography methods [39] that revolutionized crystallography by making crystals essentially immortal.

This period was dominated computationally by Silicon Graphics, which provided the combination of computational and graphics performance that was accessible to all laboratories. The increased computer power, linked to graphics, led to development of semiautomated fitting of electron density maps. Several automated procedures for model building using de novo density maps have been described in the literature. The majority of these methods are based on either the Greer approach of "skeletonization" of the regions of high electron density to trace the path of the polypeptide chain [5, .28, 41, 42] or on an interpretation of the electron density map in terms of individual atoms, iteratively refined, validated, and interpreted in terms of polypeptide chains [6–8]. These advances were matched by new methods in refinement such as REFMAC from Murshudov [9].

12.4.6 2000s

There are a number of important features of the past five years. The first has been the emergence of the Linux operating system on PC workstations, which has made computing essentially a commodity for most applications. The second is the increasing automation in operation of data collection devices, with new robotic crystal mounting hardware and steady improvements in data processing software and protocols. The third has been the investment in structural genomics methods that has driven the development of new methods and approaches to streamlining the production of protein for structural studies and the determination of structures. There has been considerable investment in the US by government agencies (see for example, http://www.jcsg.org), and a particularly important development for the pharmaceutical industry is the structural genomics consortium (see http://www.sgc.utoronto.ca). This latter initiative aims to solve and make publicly available the structures of 375 therapeutically relevant protein structures over the next three years.

12.5 CURRENT COMPUTING ISSUES

12.5.1 Not Software or Hardware but Informatics and Workflow

As discussed above; the availability of high-performance computing has not been a limiting factor in the advancement of protein structure determination. However, the crystallographic community has consistently been an early adopter of new hardware and software platforms, most recently Linux, in support of structure determination. As these hardware platforms have become available crystallographic methods have "expanded" to consume the available compute power and disk space. For a while now data indexing and reduction have been semiautomated at a minimum, and crystallographers regularly perform these steps on their laptops at the data collection facility as the data are collected with software such as the HKL 2000 suite [43] and X-GEN [44]. Assuming that data collection has been successful, indexing and reduction are normally straightforward steps. The next steps that involve phasing, structure solution, refinement, and model rebuilding then become more of a key focus and bottleneck. The challenge facing the modern crystallographer is now not "what compute resources does he/she bring to bear on the process" but "what methods does he/she bring to bear on the process that most quickly, efficiently, and correctly arrive at a final refined structure."

12.5.2 Toward Semiautomation

What can now be automated is the stage of the crystallographic process that begins with phasing and ends with water fitting and final refinement. A variety of groups (discussed in Section 12.6) have been able to devise ways in which various algorithms can be connected so as to automate the process. The challenge thus becomes less about the connections and more about being able to develop automated protocols for all stages of the structure determination process (from data collection through structure solution, model building, and refinement to analysis) that embody the learned experience of the crystallographer in a rules-based decision making procedure. In a sense the challenge is to reduce the "art" of X-ray crystallography to a science where structure determination "experiments" can be consistently reproduced independent of an individual researcher's personal subjectivity and breadth of expertise. Hence, what is required is systematic investigation and validation of the protocols to be applied, which in turn will drive improvements in the methods. Although great steps have been made toward this goal, the process has not been automated in a way that guarantees success for 100% of cases. Thus a key requirement of a modern-day software package is to be able to "pause" the automated process so that the crystallographer can inspect the results before allowing the process to continue to completion. The ability to direct the process and select which stages should be performed next is also important. Thus the best approach would be to integrate the visual tools required for inspection with the automated structure solution procedure. This is particularly important during protein model building, which is one of the most time-consuming steps in macromolecular structure determination when performed manually, especially when resolution of data is relatively low (2.5 Å or less).

The processing, analysis, and mining of large volumes of data through a user-defined computational protocol is also known as data pipelining in the life sciences industry. Through advances in computer system performance, it is possible for the first time to process whole data collections in real time. And by guiding the flow of data through a network of modular computational components, very fine control over analysis is possible. Data pipelining is a complementary technology to relational database systems—it is not in itself a data management tool. Companies that have developed commercial data pipelining software such as Scitegic (http://www.scitegic.com/) and Inforsense (http://www.inforsense.com/) have shown that data pipelining offers tremendous flexibility advantages for analysis because by processing all the data in real time, it is not constrained by what has been precalculated and stored in a database. An example of a data pipeline in X-ray crystallography could include automated systems for assembling lists of homologous proteins from PDB and alignments to be used as search models for molecular replacement, heuristics for using these proteins in the molecular replacement search, algorithms for building conformationally flexible proteins containing multiple chains and domains, and methods for handling conformations of loops and side chains, coupled with reciprocal space refinement and water fitting.

An additional challenge in the area of automation is to provide an informatics environment that will track the progress of crystallographic projects and provide analysis of results and links to additional important chemical, biological, and experimental data; this challenge is discussed below. This informatics environment must also keep track of exactly what crystallographic methods were brought to bear during the structure procedure. Essentially what is required is an automated electronic laboratory notebook that collects appropriate information as the calculations are performed.

12.6 CURRENT SOFTWARE PROJECTS FOR CRYSTALLOGRAPHY

12.6.1 CCP4

The Collaborative Computational Project Number 4 in Protein Crystallography was set up in 1979 to support collaboration between researchers working on such software in the UK and to assemble a comprehensive collection of software to satisfy the computational requirements of the relevant UK groups. The results of this effort gave rise to the CCP4 program suite [45], which is now distributed to academic and commercial users worldwide (see http://www.ccp4.ac.uk).

Unlike many other packages, particularly for small molecule crystallography, the CCP4 suite is a set of separate programs that communicate via standard data files, rather than all operations being integrated into one huge program. This has some disadvantages in that it is less easy for programs to make decisions about what operation to do next—though it is seldom a problem in practice—and that the programs are less consistent with each other (although much work has been done to improve this). However, the great advantage arising from such loose organization is that it is very easy to add new programs or to modify existing ones without upsetting other parts of the suite. This reflects the approach successfully taken by Unix. Converting a program to use the standard CCP4 file formats is generally straightforward, and the philosophy of the collection has been to be inclusive, so that several programs may be available to do the same task. The components of the whole system are thus a collection of programs using a standard software library to access standard format files (and a set of examples files and documentation) available for most Unix operating systems (including Linux), as well as Windows and Mac OS X. Programs are mostly written in C/C++ and Fortran 77.

12.6.2 PHENIX

A more recently established US consortium is developing a novel software package called PHENIX (Python-based Hierarchical Environment for Integrated Xtallography) to provide tools for automated structure solution. This software is being developed as part of an international collaboration, funded by the National Institute for General Medical Sciences at NIH (http://www.phenix-online.org/). The aim is to provide the necessary algorithms to proceed from reduced-intensity data to a refined molecular model and to facilitate structure solution for both the novice and expert crystallographer. The key is a mechanism to construct networks of crystallographic tasks that represent structure solution strategies (for example, simulated annealing refinement). To minimize the need for human intervention, these task networks encode decisions based on the results of each task, thus enabling different computational paths to be taken. These high-level task networks can be assembled and configured graphically. However, because PHENIX is based on the powerful Python scripting language, all operations can also be controlled at a lower level through text files using Python commands. Similarly, to ensure maximum flexibility the results of running a strategy are presented in a graphical user interface and also in text-based form as lists and tables.

12.6.3 e-HTPX Project

There has been considerable and continuing investment in e-science and Grid-based computing around the world. Of particular interest for protein crystallography is the e-HTPX project funded by the UK research councils (http://www.e-htpx.ac.uk). The aim of e-HTPX is to unify the procedures of protein structure determination into a single all-encompassing interface from which users can initiate, plan, direct, and document their experiment either locally or remotely from a desktop computer.

e-Science is the term used to describe the large-scale science that will increasingly be carried out through distributed global collaborations enabled by the Internet. Typically, a feature of such collaborative scientific enterprises is that they require access to very large data collections and very large-scale computing resources and high-performance visualization is fed back to the individual user scientists. The Grid is an architecture proposed to bring all these issues together and make a reality of such a vision for e-science. Ian Foster and Carl Kesselman, inventors of the Globus approach to the Grid, define the Grid as an enabler for virtual organizations: "an infrastructure that enables flexible, secure, coordinated resource sharing among dynamic collections of individuals, institutions and resources". It is important to recognize that resource in this context includes computational systems and data storage and specialized experimental facilities.

12.6.4 HTC

In June 2000 Accelrys launched Phase I of its High-Throughput Crystallography (HTC) Consortium to advance development and validation of rapid methods for X ray structure determination in structural biology. The consortium provided Accelrys a unique and productive partnership with industrial research and professional software developers and consisted of 18 international members, including Abbott Laboratories, Amgen, Aventis, Bristol-Myers Squibb, Corvas, Exegenics, DeCode, Exelixis, Genencor, Millennium, Pfizer, Procter & Gamble, Schering AG, Tularik, Vertex, and Wyeth. During the consortium Accelrys developed scientific methodology, protocols, and software designed to support high-throughput molecular replacement, automated model building, ligand placement, and structure refinement protocols that represented current best practice in industrial crystallographic laboratories. The first software pipeline developed was HT-XPIPE (Discovery Studio Modeling Environment, Release 1.1, San Diego: Accelrys Inc., 2004), a software pipeline that provides structure determination for protein-ligand complexes with an automated protocol (Fig. 12.2). It was designed for the common scenario in which a user performs structural studies on a series of ligands bound to the same protein target. HT-XPIPE automation takes as input a protein search model and pairs of ligands and structure factor files. It then checks whether the cell defined in the structure factor file varies by a user-defined percentage and performs phasing with a simple molecular replacement protocol if needed. Initial refinement of the protein model in CNX [10] is then performed, followed by a search of the electron density map for density of large enough volume into which the ligand is then placed. Refinement of the protein-ligand complex follows and leads into several iterations of side chain rebuilding and further refinement of the residues in the binding site. Finally, water molecules are placed and then a final refinement of the solvated protein-ligand complex is performed. Some or all of the steps discussed can be performed depending on the point at which the user wishes to initiate the automation. A record is kept of what stages were performed; log file outputs of each individual step for each protein ligand complex are stored and linked in to a final summary report. This allows the user to drill back down into an individual stage of a particular protein-ligand complex in case the overall pipeline does not provide the expected results and manual inspection of models, density maps, and calculations is required.

Out of the work with HT-XPIPE it became clear to the consortium that there was a need to expand the automated molecular replacement protocol embodied in HT-XPIPE to handle scenarios in which either the target was a new project or ligand-binding caused a packing change in the protein that

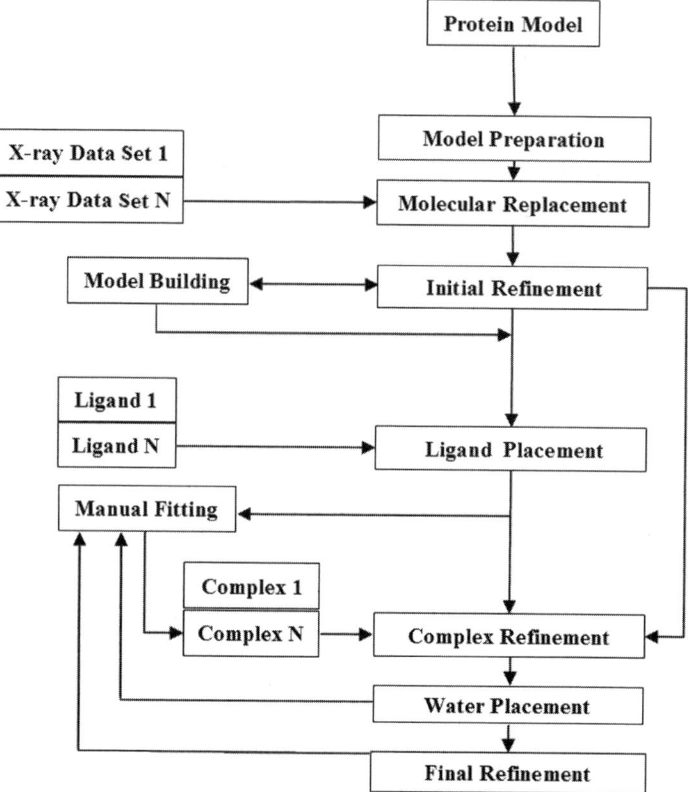

Figure 12.2 Schematic of HT-XPIPE protocol.

gave rise to a different space group. HT-XMR (Fig. 12.3) was developed as a crystallographic software pipeline to meet this need. The automated component of the pipeline requires structural amplitudes from the target crystal, its space group, and unit cell parameters, coordinates for the structural homolog, and sequence alignment between the target protein and the homolog. The user may try alternative space groups, search models, and unit cell packing (for the unit cells with noncrystallographic symmetry). HT-XMR automatically handles the tedious task of preparation of the model(s) for molecular replacement search and model rebuilding. Then, during the search, either the best molecular replacement solution or the first satisfactory solution will be selected for model rebuilding. A decision cascade utilizes a "quick and simple" setting for molecular replacement with the fast molecular replacement program AMoRe [46] (as a first test; if this search fails, a more rigorous search is attempted, using AMoRe or CNX depending on the user's preference. Next

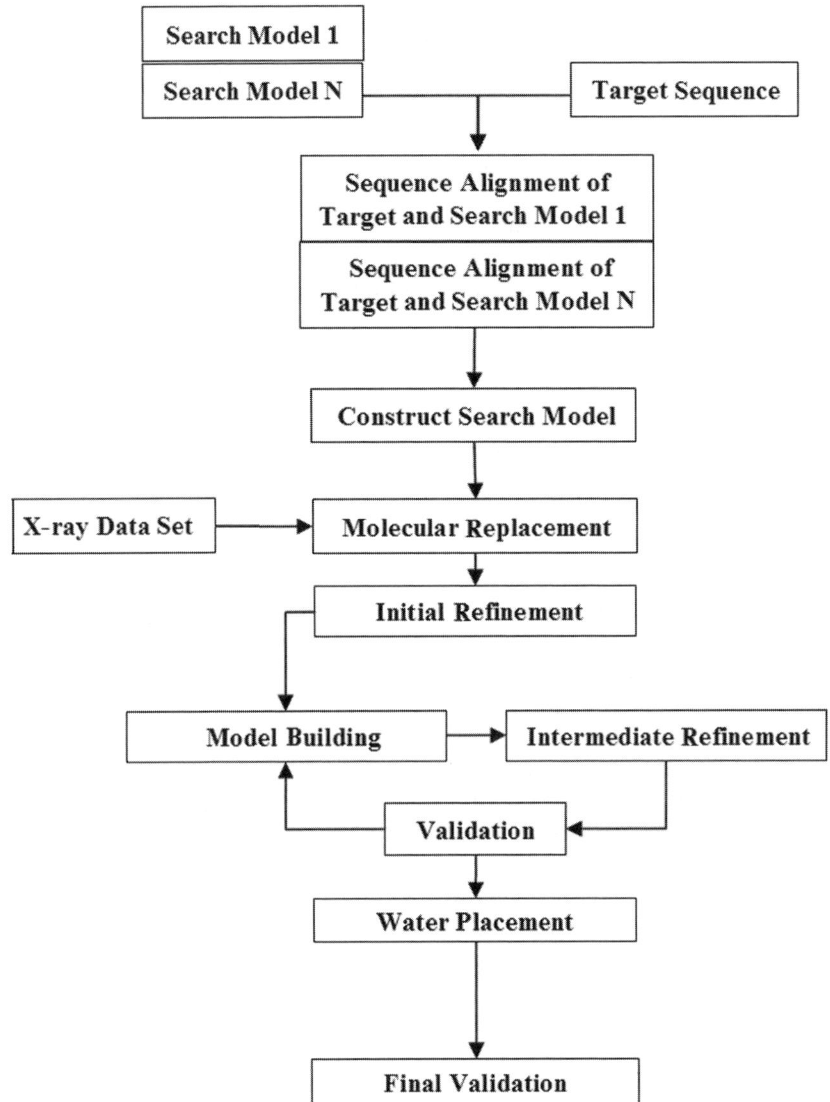

Figure 12.3 Schematic of HT-XMR protocol.

reciprocal space refinement of the initial model is performed, followed by several iterations of model rebuilding, which combines real space and reciprocal space refinements. The pipeline then moves on to perform several iterations of water placement and refinement of a solvated protein model. Finally, the results are validated and a validation report generated that is linked to the final structure complete with a number of electron density maps. Both HT-XPIPE and HT-XMR were validated on a range of systems from the PDB and some consortium members. The HT-XPIPE methods were assessed on their ability to reproduce automatically the position and orientation of the ligand (within 1 Å RMSD) for data sets of resolution 2.5 Å or higher, with ligand density continuous at 3 sigma, and a search model of close to 100% sequence identity. On a set of 34 data sets, 18 data sets passed with default pipeline parameters and an additional 14 data sets passed with nondefault parameter setup. For HT-XMR, the success criteria were set as the ability to correctly rebuild the complete protein with the final model having 90% of the side chains. This was for data sets where the starting model has 51–100% sequence identity from the search model, where no loops longer than seven residues needed rebuilding, and where electron density was continuous at 1 sigma level. HT-XMR successfully completed 9 of 10 test cases with less than 10% of residues in the success cases having mistakes, and the final Rfree factors were similar to those of manually built structures submitted to PDB.

12.7 CONCLUDING REMARKS

Over the past ten years, X-ray crystallography has become established as an important technique to support drug discovery and design for those targets for which structures can be determined. Many companies have invested, or been created, to drive developments in structural methods. As with all new technologies, there has been initial overoptimism and hype as to how the methods will contribute to drug discovery. Perhaps this is necessary to generate the investment and allow the methods to be assessed. However, over time, practitioners have come to recognize which aspects of the methods provide real benefit and how to weave them together to provide the fabric of modern drug discovery research.

Structural methods are beginning to deliver real successes for the drug discovery pipeline. A number of compounds are now on the market for which structural insights have had an important role, and there are many projects across both large and small companies that are progressing into clinical trials. The result is that all large pharmaceutical companies (and many small ones) now have their own crystallographic groups.

This chapter has provided an overview of the main issues for computing and computational methods to support this work. For the past decade or so, the main limitations that have emerged are not in the amount or type of computational hardware that is available. The real issues are in providing a computational environment for informatics support and streamlining of the calculations. It is here that major efforts are still required to ensure effective integration of the methods and data generated into the drug discovery process.

REFERENCES

1. Wilson J, Berry I. The use of gradient direction in pre-processing images from crystallization experiments. *J Applied Cryst* 2005;38:493–500.
2. Oldfield TJ. A number of real-space torsion-angle refinement techniques for proteins, nucleic acids, ligands and solvent. *Acta Cryst* 2001;D57:82–94.
3. Oldfield TJ. X-ligand: an application for the automated addition of flexible ligands into electron density. *Acta Cryst* 2001;D57:696–705.
4. Oldfield TJ. Pattern-recognition methods to identify secondary structure within X-ray crystallographic electron-density maps. *Acta Cryst.* 2002;D58:487–93.
5. Oldfield TJ. Automated tracing of electron-density maps of proteins. *Acta Cryst* 2003;D59:483–91.
6. Lamzin VS, Wilson KS. Automated refinement of protein models. *Acta Cryst* 1993;D49:129–47.
7. Morris RJ, Perrakis A, Lamzin VS. ARP/wARP's model-building algorithms. I. The main chain. *Acta Cryst* 2002;D58:968–75.
8. Perrakis A, Morris R, Lamzin VS. Automated protein model building combined with iterative structure refinement. *Nat Struct Biol* 1998;6:458–63.
9. Murshudov GN, Vagin AA, Dodson EJ. Refinement of macromolecular structures by the maximum-likelihood method. *Acta Cryst* 1997;D53:240–55.
10. Brunger AT, Kuriyan J, Karplus M. Crystallographic r-factor refinement by molecular dynamics. *Science* 1987;235:458–60
11. Brunger AT. Assessment of phase accuracy by cross validation: the free R value. Methods and applications. *Acta Cryst* 1993;D49:24–36.
12. Wilson KS, Butterworth S, Dauter Z, Lamzin VS, Walsh M, Wodak S et al. Who checks the checkers? Four validation tools applied to eight atomic resolution structures. *J Mol Biol* 1998;276:417–36.
13. Greer J, Erickson JW, Baldwin, JJ, Varney MD. Application of three-dimensional structures of protein target molecules in structure-based drug design. *J Med Chem* 1994;37:1035–54.
14. Von Itzstein M, Wu WY, Kok GB, Pegg MS, Dyason JC, Jin B. et al. Rational design of potent siaidase-based inhibitors of influenza-virus replication. *Nature* 2003;363:418–23.
15. Mewshaw RE, Edsall RJ, Yang C, Manas ES, Xu ZB, Henderson RA. et al. ERbeta ligands. 3. Exploiting two binding orientations of the 2-phenylnaphthalene scaffold to achieve ERbeta selectivity. *J Med Chem* 2005;48:3953–79.
16. Barril X, Hubbard RE, Morley SD. Virtual screening in structure-based drug discovery. *Mini Rev Med Chem.* 2004;4:779–91.
17. Zartier ER, Shapiro MJ. Fragonomics: fragment-based drug discovery. *Curr Opin Chem Biol* 2005;9:366–70.
18. Hartshorn MJ, Murray CW, Cleasby A, Frederickson M, Tickle IJ, Jhoti H. Fragment based lead discovery using x-ray crystallography, *J Med Chem* 2005;48:403–13.
19. Hodgkin DC, Kamper J, Mackay M, Pickworth J, Trueblood KN, White JG. Structure of Vitamin B12. *Nature* 1956;178:64–6.

20. Kendrew JC, Bodo G, Dintzis HM, Parrish RG, Wyckoff H, Phillips DC. A three-dimensional model of the myoglobin molecule obtained by x-ray analysis. *Nature* 1958;181:662–6.
21. Perutz MF, Mazzarella H. A preliminary x-ray analysis of haemoglobin H. *Nature* 1963;199:633–8.
22. Blake CC, Koeniz DF, Mair GA, North AC, Phillips DC, Sarma VR. Structure of hen egg-white lysozyme. A three-dimensional Fourier synthesis at 2 Angstrom resolution. *Nature* 1965;206:757–61.
23. Adams MJ, Blundell TL, Dodson EJ, Dodson GG, Vijayan M, Baker EN et al. Structure of rhombohedral 2 zinc insulin crystals. *Nature* 1969;224:491–5.
24. Rossmann MG, Blow DM. Detection of sub-units within crystallographic asymmetric unit. *Acta Cryst* 1962;15:24–31.
25. Levinthal C. Molecular model building by computer. *Sci Am* 1966;214:42–9.
26. Langridge R, Ferrin TE, Kuntz ID, Connolly ML. Real time color graphics in studies of molecular interactions. *Science* 1981;211:661.
27. Feldmann, RJ, Bing DH, Furie BC, Furie B. Interactive computer surface graphics approach to study of the active site of bovine trypsin. *Proc Natl Acad Sci USA* 1978;75:5409–12.
28. Greer J. Three dimensional pattern recognition: an approach to automated interpretation of electron density maps of proteins. *J Mol Biol* 1974;82:279–301.
29. Jones TA. A graphics model building and refinement system for macromolecules. *J Appl Cryst* 1978;11:268.
30. Jones TA. Diffraction methods for biological macromolecules. Interactive computer graphics: FRODO. *Methods Enzymol* 1985;115:157–71.
31. Jones TA, Zou JY, Cowan SW, Kjeldegaard M. Improved methods for building protein models in electron-density maps and the location of errors in these models. *Acta Cryst* 1991;A47:110–9
32. Teneyck LF. Crystallographic fast fourier-transforms. *Acta Cryst* 1973; A29:183–91.
33. Hendrickson WA. Stereochemically restrained refinement of macromolecular structures. *Methods Enzymol* 1985;115:252–70.
34. Bernstein FC, Koetzle TF, Williams GJ, Meyer EE, Brice MD, Rodgers JR. et al. Protein Data Bank—computer-based archival file for macromolecular structures, *J Mol Biol* 1977;112:535–42.
35. Berman HM, Westbrook J, Feng Z, Gilliland G, Bhat TN, Weissig H. et al. The protein data bank. *Nucl Acid Res* 2000;28:235–42.
36. Matthews DA, Alden RA, Bolin JT, Freer ST, Hamlin R, Xuong N et al. Dihydrofolate reductase: X-ray structure of the binary complex with methotrexate. *Science* 1977;197:452–5.
37. Kuyper LF, Roth B, Baccanari DP, Ferone R, Beddell CR, Champness JN et al. Receptor-based design of dihydrofolate reductase inhibitors: comparison of crystallographically determined enzyme binding with enzyme affinity in a series of carboxy-substituted trimethoprim analogues. *J Med Chem* 1982;25:1120–2
38. Hendrickson WA, Smith JL, Sheriff S. Direct phase determination based on anomalous scattering. *Methods Enzymol* 1985;115:44–55.
39. Rodgers DW. Cryocrystallography. *Structure* 1994;2:1135–40.

40. Perutz MF, Lehmann J. Molecular pathology of human haemoglobin. *Nature* 1968;219:902–9.
41. Terwilliger TC. Automated main-chain model building by template matching and iterative fragment extension. *Acta Cryst* 2003;D59:38–44.
42. Terwilliger TC. Automated side-chain model building and sequence assignment by template matching. *Acta Cryst* 2003;D59:45–9.
43. Otwinowski Z, Minor W. Processing of X-ray diffraction data collected in oscillation mode. *Methods Enzymol* 1997;276:307–26.
44. Howard AJ. Data processing in macromolecular crystallography. In: Bourne PE and Watenpaugh KD, editors. *Crystallographic Computing 7: Proceedings from the Macromolecular Crystallographic Computing School, 1996.* Oxford: Oxford University Press, 2000.
45. Collaborative computational project, number 4. The CCP4 Suite: programs for protein crystallography. *Acta Cryst* 1994;D50:760–3.
46. Navaza J. AMORE—an automated package for molecular replacement. *Acta Cryst.* 1994;A50:157–63.

13

COMPUTERS, CHEMINFORMATICS, AND THE MEDICINAL CHEMIST

WEIFAN ZHENG AND MICHAEL JONES

Contents

13.1 INTRODUCTION

Computers have been widely used in the daily practice of the medicinal chemist to search the literature of research articles and patents for competitive intelligence. They have also been extensively used for structure-based

Computer Applications in Pharmaceutical Research and Development, Edited by Sean Ekins.
ISBN 0-471-73779-8

reagent/reaction searches, enumerating virtual libraries for combinatorial chemistry, registration of compounds, and tracking and management of compound inventories. On the science front, the medicinal chemist uses computers to analyze the structure-activity relationship (SAR) data and visualize the three-dimensional (3D) structures of ligand-protein complexes from X-ray crystallographic experiments or computational docking experiments to gain insights into the underlying interaction patterns between a ligand and its target. Such information is often helpful in rationalizing SAR trends and designing new compounds and compound libraries.

In this chapter, we briefly review various aspects of the chemical information systems used by the chemist for literature and patent searches; the field of computer-aided drug design technologies, cheminformatics, as well as other applications. We place special emphases on the ligand-based techniques and only briefly mention the structure-based design technologies.

13.2 COMPUTERIZED CHEMICAL INFORMATION SYSTEMS

During the typical research cycles of drug design–synthesis–biological testing (Fig. 13.1), the medicinal chemist uses the computer to effectively monitor the competitive intelligence from the patent and scientific research literature. He/she designs cost-effective reactions by searching the synthetic chemistry literature and available reagent databases. After obtaining the compounds, he registers and manages them in computerized registration systems and then uses specialized software tools to store, retrieve, and analyze the biological testing data. Today, the medicinal chemist enjoys dramatically improved software tools compared to only ten to fifteen years ago!

Several of the software tools used most frequently today include Beilstein Crossfire (information at www.mdli.com) and SciFinder from the Chemical Abstracts Service (www.cas.org/scifinder/) for structure-based reaction searches. Reagent availability information is often searched with MDL's ACD and CAS's SciFinder. Special compound collections and contract services offered by new companies such as ChemNavigator (www.chemnavigator.com)

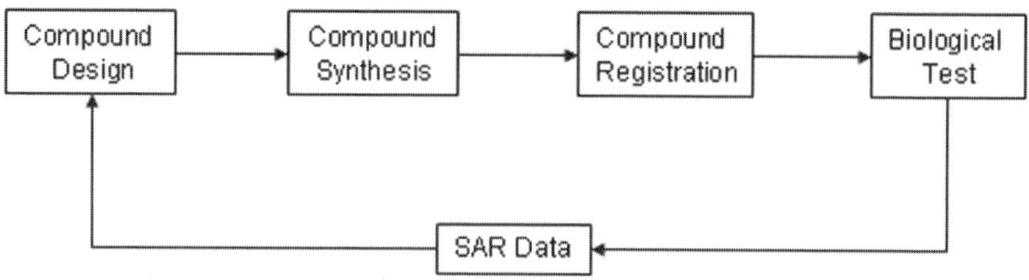

Figure 13.1 The cycle of drug design, synthesis, and biological testing.

allow access to sets of compounds that are highly relevant for groups with specific bioscreening needs. Both IDBS (www.idbs.com) and CambridgeSoft (www.cambridgesoft.com) have developed highly improved compound registration and management systems that have made much easier the daily professional life of the medicinal chemist. Systems for the storage and retrieval of biological data such as *ActivityBase* from IDBS and *BioAssay/BioSAR* from CambridgeSoft are now indispensable tools for the medicinal chemist. Thus informative decisions can be made as to what compounds should be made next to improve biological activity and physical properties. In the following, we will take a look at various aspects where computers have helped tremendously in the work of the medicinal chemist.

13.2.1 Electronic Search for the Patent and Scientific Research Literature

We should not minimize the effects that electronic searching of patents has had on the business of research. In 1990, CAS introduced MARPAT, which is a database of Markush (generic) structures found in patent documents [1]. This database provided a valuable tool for patent searching in a more comprehensive way than had been available previously. In 1995, CAS launched SciFinder, which provided access to the patent literature for chemists on their desktops. Using the SciFinder interface, one may search for research topics, authors, companies, or structures/reactions. From a practical viewpoint, SciFinder did more to enhance the searching capabilities of the medicinal chemist than any other tool. Even today, SciFinder continues to provide a "first pass" through the patent literature when chemists want to include patents in their searching. Indeed, when a search is performed, patent references are included in the answer set. Only very recently have there been additional tools to search the patent literature that have found widespread use.

Searching journal information continues to be the primary use of SciFinder for the medicinal chemist. One finds it especially useful for searching various topics, for instance, "anti-inflammatory treatments." When performing structure/reaction-based searches, many chemists also use Beilstein CrossFire in conjunction with SciFinder. The reaction information from these systems is often complementary, and it is quite useful to have both SciFinder and CrossFire in a medicinal chemistry group. However, companies with restricted budget may have to choose one or the other.

13.2.2 Electronic Search for Clinical and Preclinical Data

Other useful software tools have been directed toward keeping up with clinical trial data via structure searching as well as text-based searching. Software packages such as Pharma Projects [2], Prous Science *Integrity* [3], and of course, Internet search engines such as Google and Yahoo have all contributed to tracking of clinical data and research trends. Some resources such as

Pharma Projects predate the structure-based search tools available today. Twenty years ago, a person would look through three-ring binders of Pharma Projects pages, and now we can more thoroughly find what is needed in a fraction of the time. Access to these types of databases can greatly help the research team that is just beginning to approach a new field of interest. One can quickly find molecules relevant to his/her topic of interest. For example, a quick search on "anti-inflammatory" brings back molecules that are in clinical trials as well as late-stage preclinical development with corresponding journal references. Combining the information related to these compounds in development with the more current molecular modifications can be quite useful for generating new ideas to help in discovery programs.

Prous Science's *Integrity* offers the medicinal chemist structure-searchable access to clinical and preclinical data. The database is searchable by text and sequence as well. This is one way the medicinal chemist can quickly get up to speed on the research programs of interest in terms of what "active" compounds have been reported. This tool "levels the playing field" for small start-up companies. From this database, one may find information related to drug discovery, pharmacodynamics, pharmacokinetics, as well as pathology. In addition to quickly finding molecular structures of interest, one may be updated on a daily or weekly basis with all new information being added to the database in the chosen area. The medicinal chemist will appreciate the synthetic schemes for drugs currently on the market or in development. Through the "Weekly Insights" section of the system, one may find a selection of new molecular entities and biologics ready to enter the research and development arena, as well as descriptions of new therapeutic targets. In addition, changes in the status of drugs under active development are also reported. Furthermore, there are gateways to patents as well as clinical trial data that cover the most recent literature.

13.2.3 The World Wide Web and Chemical Information

It is worth noting that the past few years have witnessed tremendous development of web-based information resources. Notably, the PubMed search tool [4] has made the investigation of any life sciences topic much easier. It offers keyword and author (as well as structure and sequence) searches and covers a wide range of medicinal chemistry-related journals. This resource, coupled with e-journals, affords the medicinal chemist the tools to keep up with any research topics of interest. Because of the public nature of the Web, now a chemist can sometimes find critical journal articles on the Web that do not show up until much later in traditional literature sources. It is not uncommon that scientific meeting presentations can be found on the Web. Indeed, the Internet tools we have all become familiar with also have made the professional life of the medicinal chemist much easier.

It is also worth mentioning the future development of the Web for chemical information purposes. The emergence of the Semantic Web [5] in general and the Chemical Semantic Web [6] in particular would further the roles of the

Web in the life of the medicinal chemist. One may see the development of alerting services for the primary medicinal chemistry journals. The Web-based information search process could be replaced by a much more structured one based on metadata, derived by automated processing of the original full-text article. To discover new and potentially interesting articles, the user subscribes to the RSS feeds of relevant publishers and can simply search the latest items that appear automatically for keywords of interest. The article download is still necessary, but it may be possible for the client software to automatically invoke bibliographic tools to store the found references. Another application of the Chemical Semantic Web may be as alerting services for new additions to chemical databases where users get alerts for the new additions of structures or reactions.

13.2.4 Electronic Searches for Available Reagents

MDL's ACD was among the earliest chemical sourcing databases available. It has been around for over 20 years and has been the de facto standard in the pharmaceutical and biotechnology industries. With MDL's ACD, the medicinal chemist can identify and locate commercially available chemicals and make side-by-side comparisons of reagent purity, quantity, and price information; it readily compiles lists of chemicals of interest along with supplier ordering information. With substructure searching, it is also a valuable research tool for identifying analogs of interest. Most recent development includes the DiscoveryGate platform from MDL. Using the Web browser, the medicinal chemist can execute chemically intelligent structure searches, as well as text-based searches on chemical name, molecular formula, MDL number, and supplier. Similar tools are also available from CambridgeSoft and ChemNavigator.

13.2.5 Electronic Registration Systems for the Medicinal Chemist

As one of the indispensable software tools, the compound registration system provides a mechanism for the medicinal chemist to capture chemical structure information as well as analytical and other data in a database. We mention two of the systems below.

CambridgeSoft's registration system keeps track of newly synthesized or acquired compounds and their physical properties and assigns unique compound identifiers. This system is a Web-based application for storing and searching over a proprietary chemical registry. The registry can contain pure compounds and batches while managing salts, automatic duplicate checking, and unique ID assignments. New compounds are entered through a Web form. When the compound is registered, it is compared for uniqueness via a configurable duplicate check and assigned a registry number. All information about the compound, including its test data, is tracked by the registry number. Names for compounds can also be automatically generated. It also allows batch compound registration based on user-supplied SD files.

IDBS's registration system *ActivityBase* offers the chemist compound registration and compound searching. It fully integrates chemical and biological data. For chemists, *ActivityBase* allows them to register, search, and display complete chemical information alongside the associated analytical data. Key features include advanced structure searching (substructure, exact match, and similarity), as well as stereochemistry representation. *ActivityBase* also offers integration to third-party structure drawing packages and can import and export data to standard file formats such as SD files. It has compound novelty checking, automatic ID generation, calculation of average molecular mass and molecular formula, automatic "salt stripping," and other functionalities.

13.2.6 Electronic Database Systems for Biological Data

It is critically important to capture biological assay data and allow the medicinal chemist to access the information for SAR analysis. Many software systems have been developed for this purpose, and we briefly describe two of them below.

CambridgeSoft's *BioAssay* module has been designed to provide an easy-to-use method to upload assay data from multiple sources to a central, secure location. Once the data have been captured, users can perform various calculations, using the program's built-in calculation and curve-fitting abilities. The validated data can then be published to the larger research group with *BioSAR Enterprise*, which provides storage, retrieval, and analysis of the biological data. In *BioSAR Enterprise*, users define form and report layouts to combine biological and chemical data. It links the registration system to the *BioAssay* module to create customized structure-activity relationship reports. The results can be exported to a MS Excel spreadsheet. The fields exported are defined by the form definition, which allows the medicinal chemist to view both traditional numeric and textual data alongside structure data in the spreadsheet.

IDBS's popular system *ActivityBase* is a comprehensive data management system for both biological and chemical data. For biologists, *ActivityBase* allows them to capture, manipulate, and analyze biological data along with associated chemical information. It has flexible experiment protocol definition and affords reliable data acquisition with the ability to define a company's own standards; it provides automated calculations and curve fitting. It displays biological information for a compound in one simple searchable form; with integrated biological and chemical data one can drill down into and retrieve details about the SAR information.

13.3 COMPUTER-AIDED DRUG DESIGN AND CHEMINFORMATICS

Since the late 1980s, computer-aided drug design (CADD) techniques have found wide application in the pharmaceutical and biotech industries. In the

1990s, the rapid development of small molecule combinatorial chemistry/parallel synthesis and the high-throughput screening (HTS) technologies spurred renewed interests in the quantitative structure-activity relationship (QSAR) technique (see Section 13.3.3) and the development of new tools for library design (see Section 13.3.4). This development produced a new discipline of research called cheminformatics [7]. The applicability of these techniques in a particular project highly depends on the available data and knowledge about the target at hand. Generally, ligand-based techniques are often used when no X-ray structure of the target is available; otherwise, structure-based docking technologies are also employed. Here, we briefly review a few ligand-based techniques including similarity search, pharmacophore perception, and the QSAR technique. We only briefly mention the structure-based design technology because it is covered by other chapters in this book.

13.3.1 Similarity Search and Structure-Based Drug Design

One early step in the workflow of the medicinal chemist is to computationally search for similar compounds to known actives that are either available in internal inventory or commercially available somewhere in the world, that is, to perform similarity and substructure searches on the worldwide databases of available compounds. It is in the interest of all drug discovery programs to develop a formal process to search for such compounds and place them into the bioassays for both lead generation and analog-based lead optimization. To this end, various similarity search algorithms (both 2D and 3D) should be implemented and delivered directly to the medicinal chemist. These algorithms often prove complementary to each other in terms of the chemical diversity of the resulted compounds [8].

Structure-based technology is very helpful for the medicinal chemist when X-ray structures are available. Specifically, visualization of the ligand-receptor interaction is an extremely useful exercise for the medicinal chemist in rationally designing compounds. Experience has indicated that it often makes a huge difference for medicinal chemists to have user-friendly tools at their fingertips so that they can just "play around" with the tools to help the design process. This has been made possible by the availability of desktop tools such as the Weblab Viewer (Accelrys, www.accelrys.com) However, as helpful as these types of visualization tools are, further analysis is still performed by collaboration between the medicinal chemist and the computational chemist (modeler), who accesses more sophisticated software tools such as those from Tripos (www.tripos.com). The successful collaboration can quickly explore modifications of a small molecule and evaluate numerous "if-then" scenarios within the protein structure if available. The quality of the ideas for new modifications is often governed by the creativity of the medicinal chemist as well as the skills and creativity of the modeler. The "modeling" chemist must be able to quickly test new molecules and their placements in the active site of the protein, and the medicinal chemist must be able to quickly give feedback to the modeler in regards to the synthetic feasibility and other chemical properties of the design. Thus, to succeed, there must be a culture and an infrastructure that facilitate rapid communications between the medicinal chemist and the modelers. For more information on structure-based design technologies, the readers are referred to a recent review [9].

13.3.2 Pharmacophore—Concept, Methods, and Applications

The pharmacophore concept has now been widely accepted and used in the medicinal chemistry community as well as the field of computational molecular modeling. Two closely related definitions of pharmacophore have been employed by both the medicinal chemist and molecular modelers, and the root of this concept can be traced back to more than hundred years ago.

The Definition of a Pharmacophore. The very first definition of a pharmacophore was offered by Paul Ehrlich in the early 1900s, which states that a pharmacophore is "a molecular framework that carries the essential features responsible for a drug's biological activity" [10]. This definition is still used today, mostly by medicinal chemists. For example, a chemist may refer to a series of compounds derived from the benzodiazepine scaffold as derivatives of *benzodiazepine pharmacophore* and a COX inhibitor derived from the indoprofen scaffold as a derivative of *indoprofen pharmacophore*. The software tool *LeadScope* (www.leadscope.com) capitalizes on this and attempts to automate the perception of molecular frameworks by comparing sets of structures to a predefined set of some 27,000 chemical substructures in the system, thus categorizing any set of chemical structures into many pharmacophore series. Similarly, *BioReason*'s *ClassPharmer* software (www.bioreason.com) categorizes a set of compounds into clusters and identifies the maximum common substructure (MCS) in each cluster. These MCSs are potential pharmacophores according to this definition. The automated categorization allows the medicinal chemist to analyze large sets of screening data and hunt for interesting chemical series for the follow-up work. However, Ehrlich's definition does not consider the fact that different series of molecules may share important chemical features in 3D space and therefore present similar biological activities, although they may belong to different molecular frameworks.

In 1977, Peter Gund defined a pharmacophore as "a set of structural features in a molecule that is recognized at a receptor site and is responsible for that molecule's biological activity" [11]. This definition is subtly different from Ehrlich's definition in that it implies the 3D nature of the pharmacophore concept, and it is more consistent with the present-day knowledge of the ligand-receptor interaction revealed by X-ray structures of ligand-receptor complexes. By this definition, a pharmacophore can be a set of disconnected features in 3D space that are required and recognized by the receptor and could be held together by different molecular frameworks. Thus this concept provides a platform for an important activity in the medicinal chemistry practice today, that is, the *scaffold hopping* between different chemical series. It was this definition that laid the foundation for many of the state-of-the-art pharmacophore perception algorithms that automate the identification of chemical features shared by molecules.

The Automated Construction of Pharmacophore Models. Manual identification of common 3D pharmacophore features from a set of molecules is a tedious, if not impossible, process, especially when the number of molecules increases. Therefore a computerized system that automates the feature perception process and leaves more time for the medicinal chemist to judiciously collect relevant data sets and critically analyze the results is highly desirable. Since Gund's definition of pharmacophore and their first publication on a computer program for pharmacophore research, [11] several pharmacophore perception algorithms have been developed in the past 20 years: the AAA method (Active Analogue Approach) by Marshall's group [12], DISCO (DIStance Comparison) by Martin et al. [13], the commercial package Catalyst distributed by Accelrys [14], and GASP developed by Willett's group [15] and available from Tripos, just to name a few. These tools have made computerized pharmacophore modeling a standard practice in modern rational drug design in the pharmaceutical industry.

There are two broad categories of pharmacophore construction techniques depending on what initial information is used. The first is the *active analog-based approach*, where no receptor information is employed and only a set of relevant active molecules are provided. These active molecules are believed to act at the same receptor site. In this case, computer algorithms have been developed to perceive the common features shared by the set of molecules. The second approach is the *receptor structure-based approach*, where the target structure is known and employed to derive the pharmacophore features. Various approaches have been developed to derive critical features from the target structure or the structure of a ligand-receptor complex. Catalyst and GASP belong to the first category, whereas the alpha-shape technique in MOE (www.chemcomp.com) belongs to the second category.

Catalyst has two related techniques for pharmacophore analysis: HipHop and HypoGen. The former identifies feature-based alignments for a collection of molecules without considering activity values, and the latter generates 3D pharmacophore hypotheses that can explain the variations of the activity with the chemical structures. In *Catalyst*, a pharmacophore consists of a 3D arrangement of chemical functions surrounded by tolerance spheres. Each sphere defines a space occupied by a particular chemical feature. The commonly seen features include hydrophobic features, hydrogen bond acceptors and donors, aromatic features, charged groups, and so on. During the analysis, the training set molecules are examined for the types of features they have and the ability to adopt a conformation that allows the features to superimpose on a common conformation. *Catalyst* handles conformational analysis in a unique way so that the conformations generated for each training molecule cover as much energetically favorable space as possible. This is important because no prior knowledge of active conformations for each molecule is available. One example of a *Catalyst*-generated pharmacophore is shown in Figure 13.2, and the details of the algorithm can be found in Reference 14.

The GASP software was developed by Jones and Willett [15]. Using the Genetic Algorithm (GA), GASP automatically allows for conformational flexibility and maps features among the training set molecules to determine the correspondence between the features in different molecules. It also automatically aligns the potential pharmacophore groups in a common geometry. In contrast to Catalyst, GASP does not pregenerate conformers; rather it identifies rotatable bonds and pharmacophore features on the fly. The quality of the alignment is determined on the basis of three factors: the quality of the pharmacophore similarity, the common volume of all the molecules in the training set, and the internal energy of each molecule. Recently, a comparative study on Catalyst, DISCO, and GASP was published, and it found that GASP and Catalyst were equally effective in reproducing the known pharmacophores for most of the five data sets tested [16].

As an example of the receptor-based pharmacophore technique, MOE's binding site detection function is an interesting tool. It is based on a robust computational geometry method called alpha-shape analysis. The red and white dots shown in Figure 13.3 were detected by the algorithm, and they coincided well with the known ligand points. When this analysis is combined with the visual pharmacophore definition capability in MOE, one can create 3D pharmacophore features by using the site points as the reference. Inclusion and exclusion volumes can also be added to generate comprehensive receptor-based pharmacophore queries, which can then be used to search 3D conformer databases for potential matches.

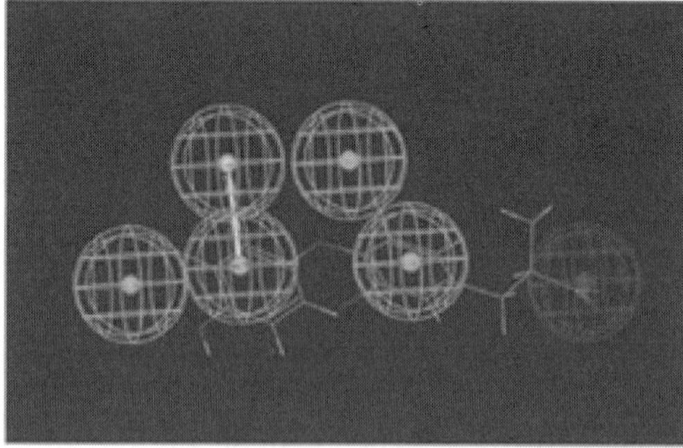

Figure 13.2 A typical Catalyst pharmacophore, where different colors indicate different chemical features and the spheres define tolerance spaces that each chemical feature would be allowed to occupy. See color plate.

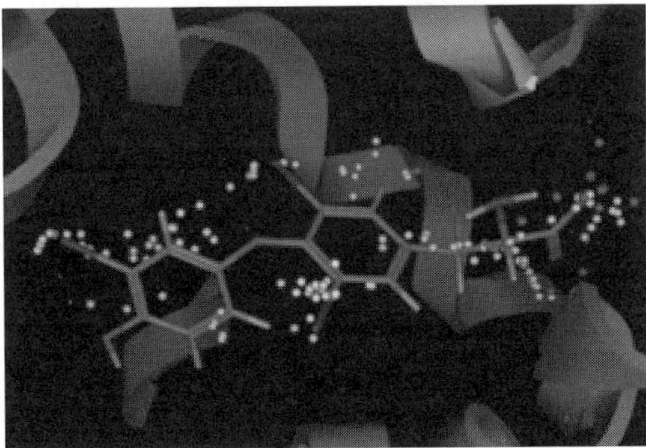

Figure 13.3 Potential pharmacophore points can be generated with MOE's site detection algorithm. The white and red dots are the automatically generated site points, and the ligand structure comes from the X-ray structure of the complex. See color plate.

Nontraditional Pharmacophore Techniques. In the past decade, we have also seen the development of nonclassic pharmacophore methods such as the pharmacophore key technique implemented in Chem-X [17] and subsequently developed and made popular by Mason et al. Mason applied this technique extensively to diversity assessment, similarity searching, and combinatorial library design [18]. Other groups have applied the *recursive partitioning* (RP) technique to discover critical features that distinguish the active molecules from the inactive ones. For example, Chen and Young applied RP to analyze the MAO data set to discover atom pair features as the critical pharmacophores for the MAO inhibitors [19]. Using the *K*-near neighbor principle, Zheng and Tropsha developed a variable selection kNN QSAR technique [20] and applied it to multiple data sets to derive the so-called "descriptor pharmacophores." These descriptor pharmacophores were subsequently used to mine molecular databases for bioactive compounds [21].

These pharmacophore techniques are different in format from the traditional pharmacophore definitions. They can not be easily visualized and mapped to the molecular structures; rather, they are encoded as "keys" or topological/topographical descriptors. Nonetheless, they capture the same idea as the classic pharmacophore concept. Furthermore, this formalism is quite useful in building quantitative predictive models that can be used to classify and predict biological activities.

13.3.3 The Quantitative Structure-Activity Relationship Technique

The Basic Concept of the QSAR Technique. The QSAR technique has been widely employed in modeling biological activities as well as ADME/Tox (absorption, distribution, metabolism, excretion, toxicity) properties. This approach was first introduced by Hansch et al. in 1963, on the basis of linear free-energy relationships (LFER) in general and the Hammett equation in particular. It is based on the assumption that the difference in structural properties accounts for the differences in biological activities of compounds. According to this approach, the structural changes that affect the biological activities of a set of structures are of three major types: electronic, steric, and hydrophobic factors. These structural properties are often described by Hammett electronic constants, Verloop STERIMOL parameters, and hydrophobic constants. The quantitative relationship between the biological activity and these structural parameters can be conventionally obtained with multiple linear regression (MLR) analysis. The fundamentals and applications of this method in chemistry and biology have been summarized by Hansch and Leo [22].

Many different approaches to QSAR have been developed since Hansch's seminal work. These include both 2D and 3D QSAR methods. The differences among these methods can be reviewed in terms of the two fundamental components of the QSAR approach: (1) the structural parameters that are used to characterize molecular structures and (2) the mathematical procedure that is employed to obtain the quantitative relationship between the biological activity and the structural parameters.

A Brief Review of the QSAR Technique. Most of the 2D QSAR methods employ graph theoretic indices to characterize molecular structures, which have been extensively studied by Radic, Kier, and Hall [see 23]. Although these structural indices represent different aspects of the molecular structures, their physicochemical meaning is unclear. The successful applications of these topological indices combined with MLR analysis have been summarized recently. Similarly, the ADAPT system employs topological indices as well as other structural parameters (e.g., steric and quantum mechanical parameters) coupled with MLR method for QSAR analysis [24]. It has been extensively applied to QSAR/QSPR studies in analytical chemistry, toxicity analysis, and other biological activity prediction. On the other hand, parameters derived from various experiments through chemometric methods have also been used in the study of peptide QSAR, where partial least-squares (PLS) analysis has been employed [25].

With the development of accurate computational methods for generating 3D conformations of chemical structures, QSAR approaches that employ 3D descriptors have been developed to address the problems of 2D QSAR techniques, that is, their inability to distinguish stereoisomers. Examples of 3D QSAR include molecular shape analysis (MSA) [26], distance geometry, and Voronoi techniques [27]. The MSA method utilizes shape descriptors and MLR analysis, whereas the other two approaches apply atomic refractivity as structural descriptor and the solution of mathematical inequalities to obtain the quantitative relationships. These methods have been applied to study structure-activity relationships of many data sets by Hopfinger and Crippen, respectively. Perhaps the most popular example of the 3D QSAR is the comparative molecular field analysis (CoMFA) developed by Cramer et al., which has elegantly combined the power of molecular graphics and PLS technique and has found wide application in medicinal chemistry [28].

More recent development in both 2D and 3D QSAR studies have focused on the development of optimal QSAR models through variable selection. This implies that only a subset of available descriptors of chemical structures, which are most meaningful and statistically significant in terms of correlation with the biological activity, is selected. The optimum selection of variables is achieved by combining stochastic search methods with correlation methods such as MLR, PLS analysis, or artificial neural networks (ANN). More specifically, these methods employ either generalized simulated annealing [29] or genetic algorithms [30] as the stochastic optimization tool. Because the effectiveness and convergence of these algorithms are strongly affected by the choice of a fitting function, several such functions have been applied to improve the performance of the algorithms. It has since been demonstrated that these algorithms, combined with various chemometric tools, have effectively improved the QSAR models compared to those without variable selection.

The variable selection methods have been also adopted for region selection in the area of 3D QSAR. For example, GOLPE [31] was developed with chemometric principles and q2-GRS [32] was developed based on independent CoMFA analyses of small areas of near-molecular space to address the issue of optimal region selection in CoMFA analysis. Both of these methods have been shown to improve the QSAR models compared to original CoMFA technique.

Many QSAR techniques (both 2D and 3D) assume the existence of a linear relationship between a biological activity and molecular descriptors, which may be an adequate assumption for relatively small data sets (dozens of compounds). However, the fast collection of structural and biological data, owing to recent development of parallel synthesis and high-throughput screening technologies, has challenged traditional QSAR techniques. First, 3D methods may be computationally too expensive for the analysis of a large volume of data, and in some cases, an automated and unambiguous alignment of molecular structures is not achievable. Second, although existing 2D techniques are computationally efficient, the assumption of linearity in the SAR may not be true, especially when a large number of structurally diverse molecules are included in the analysis.

Several nonlinear QSAR methods have been proposed in recent years. Most of these methods are based on either ANN or machine learning techniques. Both back-propagation (BP-ANN) and counterpropagation (CP-ANN) neural networks [33] were used in these studies. Because optimization of many parameters is involved in these techniques, the speed of the analysis is relatively slow. More recently, Hirst reported a simple and fast nonlinear QSAR method in which the activity surface was generated from the activities of training set compounds based on some predefined mathematical functions [34].

(RP [19], support vector machine (SVM) [35] methods, Bayesian techniques [36] and random forests [37] have all been applied to QSAR studies. Because of the variable performance of all these methods, groups have realized the importance of rigorous model validation that goes beyond the training set and internal cross-validation [38, 39]. Carefully designed external validation sets must be used to supplement the q-square indicator and to select predictive model(s). Consensus modeling has been successfully applied in various problems of drug discovery and ADMET model development [40].

A Simple Example of the QSAR Technique—the kNN QSAR. For illustrative purposes, we describe here the kNN QSAR method, which is conceptually simple and quite effective in a variety of applications. Formally, the kNN QSAR technique implements the active analog principle that is used widely by the medicinal chemist.

In the original kNN method, an unknown object (molecule) is classified according to the majority of the class memberships of its *K* nearest neighbors in the training set (Fig. 13.4). The nearness is measured by an appropriate distance metric (a molecular similarity measure as applied to the classification of molecular structures). It is implemented simply as follows:

1. Calculate distances between the unknown object (*u*) and all the objects in the training set.
2. Select *K* objects from the training set most similar to object *u*, according to the calculated distances (*K* is usually an odd number).

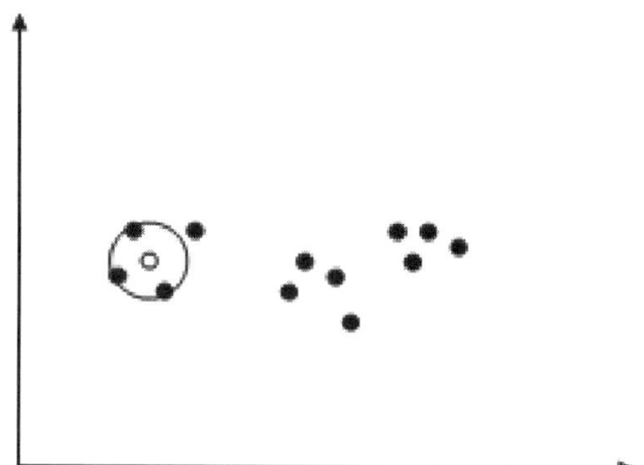

Figure 13.4 The basics of the kNN principle: An unknown object *u* (open circle) is classified into the group to which most of *u*'s *K* near neighbors belong. For QSAR purposes, the activity of molecule *u* is calculated as the average of the activities of its *K* near neighbors in the training set. More sophisticated estimation functions can be applied as well.

3. Classify object u with the group to which a majority of the K objects belongs.

When applied to QSAR studies, the activity of molecule u is calculated simply as the average activity of the K nearest neighbors of molecule u. An optimal K value is selected by the optimization through the classification of a test set of samples or by the leave-one-out cross-validation. Many variations of the kNN method have been proposed in the past, and new and fast algorithms have continued to appear in recent years. The automated variable selection kNN QSAR technique optimizes the selection of descriptors to obtain the best models [20].

Recently, this technique has been applied successfully to the development of rigorously validated QSAR models and virtual screening of large databases for anticonvulsant agents [21]. The model validation was based on several critical statistical criteria, including the randomization of the target property, independent assessment of the predictive power with external test sets, and the establishment of the models' applicability domain. All successful models were employed in database mining concurrently. When these models were applied to search databases containing around 250,000 compounds, 22 compounds were selected as consensus hits. Nine compounds were synthesized and tested (of these 9, 4 were exact database hits and 5 were derived from the hits by minor chemical modifications). Seven of these nine compounds were confirmed to be active, indicating an exceptionally high hit rate.

13.3.4 Cheminformatics and Compound Library Design

Because of space limitations, we cannot cover extensively the applications of the aforementioned tools in both lead generation and lead optimization programs. However, it is worth saying a few words about their applications in the design of chemical libraries for biological screening purposes. The cheminformatics technologies, including similarity/diversity assessment, pharmacophore modeling, the QSAR technique, ADMET/Tox modeling, as well as the structure-based docking tools, have all found wide application in the past several years in the design of compound collections. They have been integrated into various library design tools for diversity, focused libraries, as well as target family-oriented libraries. As the understanding of the requirements for successful drug candidates grows, there is a need to combine activity predictions and drug likeness criteria into one design package so that multiple parameters can be optimized simultaneously. Such tools have been developed in the past; examples include, notably, SELECT [41], HarPick [42], and PICCOLO [43]. In the future, we shall see more systematic applications of such multiobjective optimization tools in lead generation and optimization efforts, especially when they are deployed to the chemist's desktop and become a part of the toolkit for the medicinal chemist.

13.4 CONCLUDING REMARKS

In this chapter, we have presented how computers have had an impact on the life of the medicinal chemist in the past several decades. The topics ranged from computerized chemical information systems to computer-assisted drug design and cheminformatics technologies. The former topic covered scientific literature and patent searches on research topics, reactions, and structures. It also covered computer systems for the management of compound collections and the storage/retrieval of biological data. The impact of Web technologies on the medicinal chemist was also noted, especially in the area of using the Web to keep up with competitive intelligence information. Online search systems include PubMed and the more general search engines (Yahoo, Google). On the science side, we covered the development of CADD and cheminformatics technologies, especially the ligand-based technologies, such as the pharmacophore perception methods (Catalyst, GASP, pharmacophore keys). We also explained the concept and history of the QSAR technique over the past 30 years. Finally, we briefly covered the application of these tools in the area of compound library and screening collection design, where all relevant computational tools should be considered in a comprehensive and balanced manner.

As science and technology continue to progress in the field of structural genomics and chemical genomics [44], more X-ray structures of ligand-receptor complexes will become available, and more structure-activity relationship data will be delivered to the medicinal chemist [45]. Such information will no doubt propel further development and rigorous validation of more accurate structure-based and ligand-based cheminformatics technologies.

As software technologies continue to improve, we shall see these more advanced computational tools delivered to the fingertips of the medicinal chemist. For example, workflow technologies such as Pipeline Pilot [46] will enable the deployment of more specialized computational tools and validated models to the chemist's desktop. The chemist will have an integrated work environment where he/she can access relevant information and predictive cheminformatics tools. Such an environment is not going to replace the chemist's creative thinking but will enhance it via computing and information gathering. Only when this vision is realized will computers and cheminformatics truly become a part of the life of the medicinal chemist and have a greater impact on the delivery of twenty-first century medicines to patients.

REFERENCES

1. http://www.cas.org/ONLINE/DBSS/marpatss.html.
2. http://www.pjbpubs.com/pharmaprojects/index.htm.
3. http://www.prous.com/
4. http://www.ncbi.nlm.nih.gov/entrez

5. Berners-Lee T, Hendler J. Publishing on the semantic web. *Nature* 2001;410(6832): 1023–4.
6. Gkoutos GV, Murray-Rust P, Rzepa HS, Wright M. Chemical markup, XML, and the World-Wide Web. 3. Toward a signed semantic chemical web of trust. *J Chem Inf Comput Sci* 2001;41(5):1124–30.
7. Brown F. Chemoinformatics: What is it and how does it impact drug discovery? *Annu Rep Medicinal Chem* 1998;33:375–84.
8. Sheridan RP, Kearsley SK. Why do we need so many chemical similarity search methods? *Drug Discov Today* 2002;7(17):903–11.
9. Kitchen DB, Decornez H, Furr JR, Bajorath J. Docking and scoring in virtual screening for drug discovery: methods and applications. *Nat Rev Drug Discov* 2004;3(11):935–49.
10. Guner OF. Preface. In: Guner OF, editor, *Pharmacophore perception, development, and use in drug design.* La Jolla: International University Line, 2000.
11. Gund P. Three-dimensional pharmacophore pattern searching. In: Hahn FE, editor, *Progress in molecular and subcellular biology.* Berlin: Springer-Verlag, 1977. p.117–43.
12. Marshall GR, Barry CD, Bosshard HE, Dammkoehler RA, Dunn DA. The conformational parameter in drug design: the active analogue approach. In: Olson EC, Christoffersen RE, editors, *Computer-assisted drug design.* Washington, DC: American Chemical Society, 1979. p.205–26.
13. Martin YC. Distance comparison (DISCO): A new strategy for examining 3D structure-activity relationships. In: Hansch C, Fujita T, editors, *Classical and 3D QSAR in agrochemistry.* Washington, DC: American Chemical Society, 1995. p.318–29.
14. Barnum D, Greene J, Smellie A, Sprague, P. Identification of common functional configurations among molecules. *J Chem Inf Comput Sci* 1996;36(3):563–71.
15. Jones G, Willett P, Glen RC. A genetic algorithm for flexible molecular overlay and pharmacophore elucidation. *J Comput Aided Mol Des* 1995;9(6):532–49.
16. Patel Y, Gillet VJ, Bravi G, Leach AR. A comparison of the pharmacophore identification programs: Catalyst, DISCO and GASP. *J Comput Aided Mol Des* 2002;16(8–9):653–81.
17. Murrall NW, Davies EK. Conformational freedom in 3-D databases. 1. Techniques. *J Chem Inf Comput Sci* 1990;30(3):312–16.
18. Beno BR, Mason JS. The design of combinatorial libraries using properties and 3D pharmacophore fingerprints. *Drug Discov Today* 2001;6(5):251–8.
19. Chen X, Rusinko A, Tropsha A,Young SS. Automated pharmacophore identification for large chemical data sets. *J Chem Inf Comput Sci* 1999;39(5):887–96.
20. Zheng W, Tropsha A. Novel variable selection quantitative structure-property relationship approach based on the k-nearest-neighbor principle. *J Chem Inf Comput Sci* 2000;40(1):185–94.
21. Shen M, Beguin C, Golbraikh A, Stables JP, Kohn H, Tropsha A. Application of predictive QSAR models to database mining: identification and experimental validation of novel anticonvulsant compounds. *J Med Chem* 2004;47(9): 2356–64.

22. Hansch C, Leo A. In Heller SR., editor, *Exploring QSAR. fundamentals and applications in chemistry and biology.* Washington, DC: American Chemical Society, 1995.
23. Kier LB, Hall LH. *Molecular connectivity in chemistry and drug research.* New York: Academic Press, 1976.
24. Jurs PC, Ball JW, Anker LS. Carbon-13 nuclear magnetic resonance spectrum simulation. *J Chem Inf Comput Sci* 1992;32(4):272–8.
25. Wold S, Ruhe A, Wold H, Dunn WJ. The collinearity problem in linear regression. The partial least squares (PLS) approach to generalized inverses. *SIAM J Sci Stat Comput* 1984;5:735–43.
26. Hopfinger AJ. A QSAR investigation of dihydrofolate reductase inhibition by Baker triazines based upon molecular shape analysis. *J Am Chem Soc* 1980;102:7196–206.
27. Crippen GM. Distance geometry approach to rationalizing binding data. *J Med Chem* 1979;22(8):988–97.
28. Cramer RD, Patterson DE, Bunce JD. Comparative molecular field analysis (CoMFA). 1. Effect of shape on binding of steroids to carrier proteins. *J Am Chem Soc* 1988;110:5959–67.
29. Sutter JM, Dixon SL, Jurs PC. Automated descriptor selection for quantitative structure-activity relationships using generalized simulated annealing. *J Chem Inf Comput Sci* 1995;35(1):77–84.
30. Rogers D, Hopfinger AJ. Application of genetic function approximation to quantitative structure-activity relationships and quantitative structure-property relationships. *J Chem Inf Comput Sci* 1994;34(4):854–66.
31. Baroni M, Costantino G, Cruciani G, Riganelli D, Valigi R, Clementi S. Generating optimal linear PLS estimations (GOLPE): an advanced chemometric tool for handling 3D-QSAR problems. *Quant Struct-Act Relat* 1993;12:9–20.
32. Cho SJ, Tropsha A. Cross-validated R2-Guided region selection for comparative molecular field analysis: a simple method to achieve consistent results. *J Med Chem* 1995;38(7):1060–6.
33. Andrea TA, Kalayeh H. Applications of neural networks in quantitative structure-activity relationships of dihydrofolate reductase inhibitors. *J Med Chem* 1991;34:2824–36.
34. Hirst JD. Nonlinear quantitative structure-activity relationship for the inhibition of dihydrofolate reductase by pyrimidines. *J Med Chem* 1996;39(18):3526–32.
35. Zernov VV, Balakin KV, Ivaschenko AA, Savchuk NP, Pletnev IV. Drug discovery using support vector machines. The case studies of drug-likeness, agrochemical-likeness, and enzyme inhibition predictions. *J Chem Inf Comput Sci* 2003;43(6):2048–56.
36. McDowell RM, Jaworska JS. Bayesian analysis and inference from QSAR predictive model results. *SAR QSAR Environ Res* 2002;13(1):111–25.
37. Svetnik V, Liaw A, Tong C, Culberson JC, Sheridan RP, Feuston BP. Random forest: a classification and regression tool for compound classification and QSAR modeling. *J Chem Inf Comput Sci* 2003;43(6):1947–58.
38. Golbraikh A, Tropsha A. Beware of q2! *J Mol Graph Model* 2002; 20(4):269–76.

39. Doweyko AM. 3D-QSAR illusions. *J Comput Aided Mol Des* 2004;18(7–9):587–96.

40. Kovatcheva A, Golbraikh A, Oloff S, Feng J, Zheng W, Tropsha A. QSAR modeling of datasets with enantioselective compounds using chirality sensitive molecular descriptors. *SAR QSAR Environ Re.* 2005;16(1–2):93–102.

41. Gillet VJ, Willett P, Fleming PJ, Green DV. Designing focused libraries using MoSELECT. *J Mol Graph Model* 2002;20(6):491–8.

42. Good AC, Lewis RA. New methodology for profiling combinatorial libraries and screening sets: cleaning up the design process with HARPick. *J Med Chem* 1997;40(24):3926–36.

43. Zheng W, Hung ST, Saunders JT, Seibel GL. PICCOLO: a tool for combinatorial library design via multicriterion optimization. *Pac Symp Biocomput* 2000;588–99.

44. Austin CP, Brady LS, Insel TR, Collins FS. NIH Molecular Libraries Initiative. *Science* 2004;306(5699):1138–9.

45. http://pubchem.ncbi.nlm.nih.gov/

46. http://www.scitegic.com

14

THE CHALLENGES OF MAKING USEFUL PROTEIN-LIGAND FREE ENERGY PREDICTIONS FOR DRUG DISCOVERY

JUN SHIMADA

Contents

Computer Applications in Pharmaceutical Research and Development, Edited by Sean Ekins.
ISBN 0-471-73779-8

14.1 INTRODUCTION

Over the past decade, pressures to improve the efficiency of pharmaceutical research and development (R&D) have steadily increased [1, 2]. At the risk of simplification, the rising costs of R&D can be attributed to a combination of higher regulatory hurdles and increased scientific challenges. Time spent on clinical development has gone up from an average of 7.9 years in the 1960s to 12.8 years in the 1990s [2], largely as a result of increased FDA requirements on safety. Furthermore, the average cost of developing a drug has skyrocketed. Although opinions around this vary considerably, one fairly conservative and frequently cited estimate from 2002 pegs the average cost of developing a drug at $802 million and rising at an annual rate of 7.4% above inflation [3]. To maximize reward in light of this high investment, companies have traditionally pursued the development of blockbuster drugs (annual sales >$1 billion) that can be sold at premium prices to a large patient base. Although many of the past blockbusters were not first-in-class drugs [4], it is clear that today's safety and efficacy hurdles are much higher, because many of the previous generation's well-established therapies have lost patent exclusivity and are available in the form of cheaper generics. In this environment, a pharmaceutical company often has a hard time charging a lofty premium for new drugs that may not be sufficiently differentiated, because insurers can relegate them to lower reimbursement tiers to discourage physician prescription of the new drugs over older generics. Through the dedicated work of many scientists, we now know that, for nearly all indications, maximizing safety and efficacy implies selective targeting of a protein in a complex biological network [see e.g., 5]. It remains a significant intellectual challenge to anticipate the physiological consequences of functionally disrupting a protein (such as COX-2), as it is likely to play significant roles in more than one network. Serendipity combined with the medicinal chemist's intuition have been successful at finding past drugs [6]. However, as our knowledge of human physiology becomes more complex, modern drug discovery requires unprecedented cooperation between scientists of all fields [7]. Modern pressures to improve scientific productivity under even higher safety and efficacy hurdles seem to suggest integrated, parallel approaches [8] to improve the efficiency of drug discovery.

A critical component of modern drug discovery is computational chemistry [7], which should in theory lower R&D costs by improving the outcome of in vitro and in vivo experiments. Because computational chemistry allows any idea from the space of possible compounds to be evaluated before going to the bench, the risk-adjusted costs of discovery are expected to go down. This is particularly important given today's high rates of clinical attrition that result in the vast majority of compounds failing some time during development. One study reported in 2001 showed that 30.8% of compounds entering Phase I failed during the phase, 58.8% for Phase II, and 21.5% for Phase III [9]. When it is noted that these figures do not even include preclinical and registration-stage attrition and failure, it becomes clear how a technology that could potentially improve the probability of success during drug development would be a very significant achievement. However, although the potential of computational methods was stated many years ago [see e.g., 10], it has been a challenge to realize this potential because of the limited accuracy of computational predictions and the difficulty of producing synthesized compounds from *in silico* predictions [11]. My present goal is to suggest some reasons behind the difficulty, and to present some ideas on how computational methods can be effectively utilized in a drug discovery effort. Although it is arguable whether there are clear examples of computational *de novo*-designed drugs currently on the market, it is beyond doubt that computational methods currently play important roles in drug discovery [12]. As this statement suggests, the relevance of computational methods hinges critically on whether they can meaningfully contribute to drug discovery efforts.

In this chapter, I begin by identifying the expectations placed on computational methods when used in the context of drug discovery. I hope to show that there is a fundamental tension underlying the development of computational methods: The need to be commercially relevant for drug discovery is in direct competition with the scientific quest for more accurate, theoretically sound computational methods. Next, I identify several important principles for guiding the development of commercially relevant and scientifically rigorous computational methods. Finally, I demonstrate how these ideas have been successfully put into commercial practice. To focus the discussion, I look specifically at the basic task of predicting protein-ligand *in vitro* binding free energies (or activities; see Appendix) and ask how such predictions can play a practically useful role in drug discovery.

14.2 THE IMPORTANCE OF SPEED, TRANSFERABILITY, ACCURACY, AND INTERPRETABILITY

To maximize safety and therapeutic efficacy, potential drugs are required to be highly specific for their protein target and orally bioavailable. In addition, for a drug candidate to reach the market, it must be patentably novel. A computational approach therefore needs to find novel compounds with well-defined pharmacological properties from the vast space of possible organic compounds ("chemical space").

A back-of-the-envelope calculation [see 13 and Box 4 in 14] demonstrates the magnitude of this task: If we are looking for a handful of 4 residue compounds in a combinatorial chemical space defined by a library of 100 fragments, a random search would have a hit rate of 10^{-8}. Although a more intelligent search may improve this by several orders of magnitude, the computational method would still need to evaluate ~100–1000 compounds. Note that for each compound, we will have to find the global minimum conformation in the target binding site. We now arrive at a critical question: How quickly does a computational method need to finish this task?

In an academic setting where prediction accuracy is the single most important criterion, there is no strict limitation on time. However, timing is a critical aspect in an industrial setting. A fundamental limitation of computational methods is that they have no commercial utility unless predictions lead to synthesized compounds. They must therefore be synergistic to the workflow of synthetic chemists. In general, chemical synthesis is a time-consuming and expensive task that requires considerable planning, from ordering materials to the execution of synthetic routes [7]. Maximal commercial utility would be achieved by a computational method if it could influence the allocation of chemistry resources. This would involve influencing the overall class of reactions and scaffolds to be explored. A more modest scenario is for computational methods to influence the go/no-go decision on specific reactions that alter a particular scaffold. Synthetic work followed by biological characterization typically takes anywhere from a day to several weeks to complete.

During lead optimization, we can imagine that a typical scenario might be for a chemist to approach the computational chemist and say, "We just synthesized and assayed these compounds. Can you (1) rationalize these results, (2) model the following 10 variations, and (3) identify the ones that are worth making?" To be of maximal utility to the drug discovery effort and to maintain the engagement with the chemistry group, we would probably like to return an accurate answer in no more than a day or two. For high-risk tasks such as finding a *de novo* scaffold, we may want to be able to evaluate ~100–1000 compounds in no more than a month. In either scenario, we will be required to evaluate no less than ~10 compounds per day, so the conformational search for one compound needs to average on the order of 1–2 CPU hours.

Novelty requires that computational methods have transferable accuracy. That is, they must be able to make good predictions on protein-ligand complexes that are different from those found in their training set. A modest goal would be for a method to generalize to all classes of compounds (e.g., peptidic and nonpeptidic) for a particular enzyme (e.g., HIV protease) or enzyme class (e.g., aspartic proteases). A more extensive notion of transferability is to generalize across enzyme classes, which is considerably more difficult. Many studies in the past have emphasized transferability as the most important property characterizing computational methods [see e.g., 15, 16], because transferability suggests that the method may be capturing general physical properties of protein-ligand binding.

Synthetic constraints—such as difficulty, yield, management of starting materials, and intermediates—will naturally restrict the diversity of compounds that are made [7]. *In silico* designs with scaffolds that utilize similar synthetic steps will naturally be favored over those that are not. These pressures to make a small number of compounds with limited scaffold variability require computational methods to make exquisitely accurate predictions: The number of *in silico* designs that are predicted to be good binders but turn out not to be upon synthesis (i.e., false positives) must be minimized. False positives are particularly disheartening during the lead discovery phase of drug development, as shifting synthetic efforts towards a different lead scaffold design can result in critical delays.

For the purpose of identifying hits or potential leads, a filter that can reliably distinguish good from bad binders [13] will be sufficient. However, once leads are found, such classification abilities alone will be insufficient to drive optimization. Lead optimization involves small chemical modifications on a fundamental scaffold, and a computational tool must be able to reliably rank order these ideas to help prioritize which of them to pursue [14]. At this stage in discovery, the costs associated with false positives are often less than in lead discovery. Because one good idea may help eliminate a pharmacokinetic problem and thereby save months or years of drug discovery effort, an emerging priority is to reduce the number of false negatives.

Even as the computational prediction error rate is reduced to acceptable levels, many cases will be encountered in which the predictions are indistinguishable to within error. In a scenario in which several different *in silico* designs are given equivalent but favorable activity predictions, the end user's medicinal experience may help decide which to promote to synthesis. The quality of that decision at this point will be strongly influenced by how easy it is to understand the different contributions to the computational predictions. Interpretability is thus critical for synergistically utilizing the experience of the end user.

14.3 CHALLENGES FACING EXISTING METHODS

Are existing methods able to meet the four criteria of speed, accuracy, transferability, and interpretability? The following is meant to be an illustrative, not exhaustive, brief survey of how some popular methods fall short on one or more of these criteria. For recent, comprehensive overviews of computational methods, references [14] and [17] are recommended.

When computer-aided molecular design first came into prominence two decades ago, a major drawback was that the methods were computationally costly. At the time, it was not unusual for rigorous calculations such as free energy molecular dynamics simulations [18] to take several CPU days. Coupled with the inherently limited accuracy of computational methods, it is not surprising that these methods were very difficult to integrate into the drug discovery process. During the optimization stage, medicinal chemists would be more efficient by making compounds and obtaining direct experimental confirmation of their activity than waiting for computational predictions that might be potentially wrong. Even today, slow computational methods are inappropriate for lead discovery, because identifying *in silico* compounds that are predicted to be active, novel, and synthesizable often requires significant

CPU time. In response to these slow and rigorous calculations, many fast heuristic approaches have been developed that are based on intuitive concepts such as docking [10], matching pharmacophores [19], or linear free energy relationships [20]. A disadvantage of many simple heuristic approaches is their susceptibility to generalization error [17], where accuracy of the predictions is limited to the training data.

If we examine the spectrum of existing computational methods, it is clear that all methods can be categorized somewhere between two extremes. At the one end, we have purely *ab initio* approaches that make minimal assumptions. Because they are based on fundamental physical principles, the accuracy of their predictions are expected to be transferable across a diverse collection of proteins and ligands [17]. *Ab initio* approaches typically have two limitations that undercut their intended rigor. First, they are severely limited by computational resources. Because protein-ligand binding is a complex phenomenon involving thousands of atoms, estimation of binding free energies cannot be done without simplifying the problem at hand [21]. Highly rigorous quantum mechanical approaches often require the use of approximate, semiempirical methods in order to accelerate calculations [22]. As a result of these approximations, numerical errors will be inevitable. Even with such simplifications, conformational sampling and calculation of entropy remain prohibitive for *ab initio* methods. Second, our understanding of the protein-ligand binding phenomenon is incomplete. It is currently not possible to write down a numerically solvable, closed-form expression for the free energy of binding. This requires us to make approximations for certain free energy contributions, which in turn will introduce free parameters that require training on experimental data. For example, all force fields have critical parameters, such as harmonic bond force constants [23], tuned to either quantum mechanical calculations or spectroscopic/calorimetric data where available.

At the other extreme of the spectrum, we find computationally fast methods that are not deeply grounded on physical principles. These methods will inevitably rely on data training for their accuracy, and their accuracy is often not transferable outside of their training set. In addition, these predictions may involve nonphysical concepts that are not directly related to the physical phenomena of protein-ligand binding, thus making them difficult to interpret. For example, many statistical methods generate predictions upon transformation to a subspace (e.g., when Gaussian kernels are used in conjunction with support vector machines [24]). These predictions are now given in terms of a new basis set, which may have no direct interpretive connection to the original input.

14.4 WHY IS DATA TRAINING DIFFICULT?

As noted, biological systems are too complex for deriving an expression for free energies from first principles. Consequently, the common thread through all computational methods is their dependence—regardless of the degree—on experimental data for training their methods for estimating free energies. Accuracy and transferability will therefore be a strong function of the effectiveness of data training. For training and testing free energy functions for protein folding or protein-ligand binding, many researchers have turned to structural databases [17].

14.4.1 Statistics Derived from Structural Databases Are Skewed and Sparse

Despite potential anomalies resulting from crystallization conditions [25], structures solved by X-ray crystallography are the main source of data on molecular interactions involving proteins. For training a protein-ligand binding free energy estimator, a protein-ligand cocrystal with a measured binding affinity would be ideal. However, according to recent efforts [26, 27], such co-crystals that are publicly available total less than 1500. Furthermore, compounds that are co-crystals in public databases are not representative of leads or marketed drugs [28]. Structural data on leads and hotly pursued targets are deeply held secrets of pharmaceutical companies and are therefore not available to the general public. Consequently, the public database is predominantly populated by proteins (e.g., nonhuman enzymes) and ligands (e.g., peptides and peptidomimetics, natural products, and biologically relevant cofactors) that are of low interest to drug development [26].

In order to determine N parameters for a free energy predictor, we would need at least N data points in the best-case scenario when all N data points are uncorrelated. However, because of correlation among the training data, we have empirically observed that between N and N^2 data points are often needed [29]. For example, a force field with 100 parameters would in practice need approximately 10,000 data points. This observation suggests a clear scientific challenge for computational drug design methods. Lead discovery and optimization require a computational method that can give refined free energy predictions, which will necessarily feature a large number of parameters to be trained by data. However, as our experience shows, the amount of readily available high-quality data may be too small for training computational models.

14.4.2 Statistics from the Database Are Difficult to Interpret

Structural databases such as the PDB [30], LPDB [31], and BindingDB [26, 27] clearly contain important information about protein-ligand free energies. However, it is also clear that statistical distributions derived from structural databases are subject to influences not relevant to binding free energies [29], such as crystal packing forces or noise associated with crystallization/solvent conditions [25]. Decoupling such noise from "true" free energetic effects when analyzing database statistics can be very difficult [29].

Furthermore, database statistics are heavily influenced by collective effects, including solvent and multibody interactions. Simple potentials based on pairwise interactions are unable to meaningfully capture such effects. To illustrate this point, let us consider a thought experiment using lattice proteins and ligands. Although the robustness of the so-called knowledge-based approach will be specifically tested here [16], the conclusion we reach should be generally relevant to any method used to train protein-ligand binding potentials.

Each lattice protein is compact and of a single type (i.e., a homopolymer) and features a binding site along one face (Fig. 14.1a). Complementary lattice

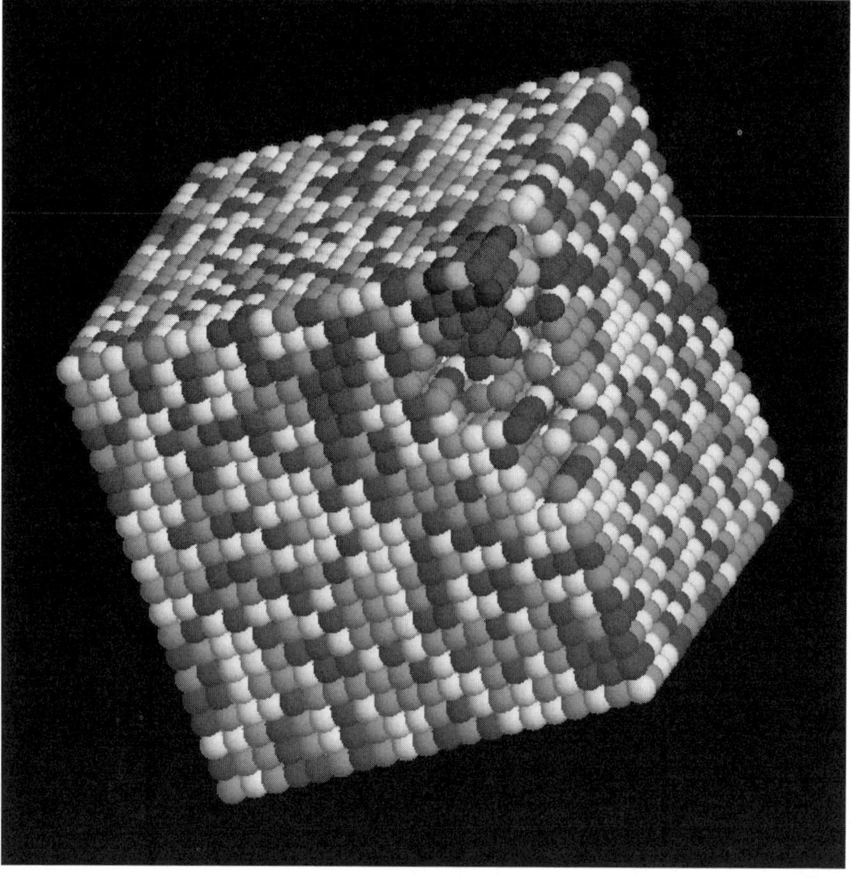

Figure 14.1 (a) A lattice protein-ligand complex. The lattice protein (colored red, yellow, pink, and orange) occupies a 20 × 20 cube, and the binding site is carved out in one corner. In this example, a ligand of 20 atoms was grown into the binding site. The ligand atoms are colored with blues and greens. (b) Effect of the evolutionary temperature on the database composition. The average binding energy of the database members is shown as a function of the temperature at which the ligands in the database were evolved. Clearly, as the temperature is lowered, there is a strong bias in the database towards strong binders. See color plate.

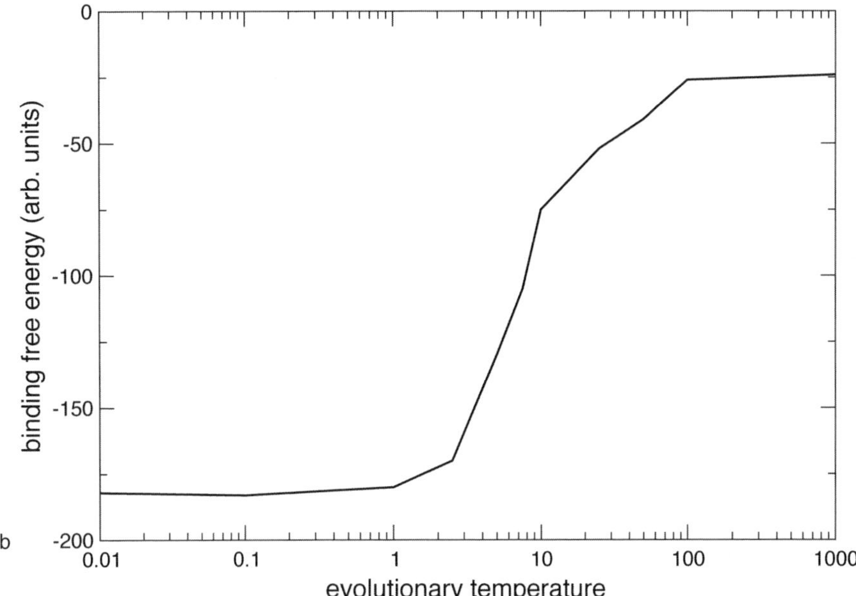

Figure 14.1 *Continued*

ligands are constructed to completely fill the binding site, where the Lth ligand atom is one of four atom types, numbered 0 to 3, denoted by σ_L. The binding free energy is given strictly by the sum of pairwise nearest neighbor interactions. No solvent interactions are assumed. The binding free energy of a protein-ligand complex is therefore simply given by

$$\begin{aligned}\Delta G(L,P) &= G(L,P) - G(L) - G(P)\\ &= \sum_L n_L \varepsilon(\sigma_L)\end{aligned}$$

where $G(L,P)$, $G(L)$, and $G(P)$ are the free energies of the protein-ligand complex, protein, and ligand, respectively, n_L is the number of contacts made by the Lth ligand atom, and $\varepsilon(\sigma_L)$ is the interaction free energy associated with ligand atom L interacting with a protein atom. More precisely, "free energy" refers to an effective free energy, because certain degrees of freedom (e.g., solvent) have been averaged out.

A database of lattice protein-ligand complexes is now constructed with the following steps:

1. Start with a database of randomly chosen N ligands of length M grown in the binding site of protein P.
2. Perform random mutations on each ligand by altering atom types. Mutations do not affect ligand sizes and conformations. During simulated

evolution, mutations that lower the free energy of the ligand are preferentially selected. Namely, mutations are selected according to the Metropolis criterion [32] at an evolutionary temperature $T_{\text{evol}} = 1/\beta_{\text{evol}}$:

$$\text{probability} = \begin{cases} 1 & \Delta\Delta G \leq 1 \\ e^{-\Delta\Delta G/T_{\text{evol}}} & \text{otherwise} \end{cases}$$

where $\Delta\Delta G = \Delta G_{\text{after}} - \Delta G_{\text{before}}$ is the change in the binding free energy upon mutation. Each ligand will be evolved until its free energy stops changing.

Raising β_{evol} plays the role of skewing the database composition toward stronger binders (Fig. 14.1b). In the limit of $\beta_{\text{evol}} \to 0$, the lattice database will consist of randomly selected ligands. It is assumed that a sufficient number of ligands have been added and the evolution process is continued long enough until equilibrium is reached. By this, it is meant that the statistical distributions of contacts in this database are not altered by the inclusion of additional complexes.

It is important to emphasize that this lattice database is highly idealized compared to real databases. Unlike the lattice database, real databases cannot be treated as thermodynamic ensembles of protein-ligand complexes equilibrated at room temperature [33, 34]. Two of the more straightforward reasons are mentioned here. First, real databases are inherently biased toward strong binders ($K_d < 10\ \mu\text{M}$), because weak binders are difficult to crystallize and of lesser interest. Second, as mentioned above, real databases are not composed of a representative selection of proteins and ligands, and their compositions are biased toward peptide and peptidomimetic inhibitors and certain protein superfamilies. In contrast, because only one protein and four ligand types are used, the lattice database should have representative ligand compositions.

With this database in hand, a simple question is asked [29]: How different is a knowledge-based potential derived from this lattice database compared to the actual energy function used to construct the database? If statistical errors are negligible and the knowledge-based method is perfect, the answer is expected to be "They are exactly the same."

The central hypothesis of the knowledge-based approach [16, 17] is that pairwise contacts follow an exponential "Boltzmann-like" distribution [33] according to its interaction energy

$$P_{\text{db}}(\text{contact\_type}) \sim e^{-\beta_{\text{db}} E_{\text{contact}}},$$

with β_{db} being the inverse temperature characterizing the database. Although existing knowledge-based methods differ in how contacts are defined or the reference state [17, 35] is calculated, they all rely on this fundamental assumption to convert observed probabilities to free energy parameters. When the knowledge-based approach is applied to our lattice database, the probability

$P_{db}(\sigma^p, \sigma^l, \beta_{db})$ to observe the (σ^p, σ^l) contact between a protein atom of type σ^p and ligand atom of type σ^l is

$$P_{db}(\sigma^p, \sigma^l, \beta_{db}) = f(\sigma^p, \sigma^l)e^{-\beta_{db}E_{KBP}(\sigma^p, \sigma^l)} \tag{14.1}$$

where $f(\sigma^p, \sigma^l)$ is an energy-independent prefactor and E_{KBP} is the knowledge-based potential. If $\beta_{db} \to 0$, we see that $f(\sigma^p, \sigma^l)$ is equivalent to the infinite temperature probability distribution $P_{db}(\sigma^p, \sigma^l, 0)$, which results from nonenergetic biases that influence the contact distribution. For this thought experiment, the database temperature T_{db} and the functional form of E_{KBP} are assumed to be known. Namely, $T_{db} = T_{evol}$, and E_{KBP} will be a nearest-neighbor contact potential consisting of four free energy parameters, $\varepsilon_{KBP}(\sigma^l)$. Furthermore, because of the idealized nature of the database, we expect statistical errors to be minimized. We are thus testing the knowledge-based approach under idealized circumstances of maximal information (i.e., T_{db} and functional form of E_{KBP}) and minimal statistical error.

If our database is large, standard statistical mechanical theory [32] tells us that the Metropolis algorithm will ensure that our database is a thermodynamic (i.e., canonical) ensemble at inverse temperature β_{evol}. Any ligand atom can have one to six nearest neighbors, and so the free energy contribution of a ligand atom of type σ^l having k homopolymeric protein neighbors is given by $k\varepsilon(\sigma^l)$. Under a canonical ensemble, $P_{db}(\sigma^p, \sigma^l, \beta_{evol})$ is calculated as

$$P_{db}(\sigma^p, \sigma^l, \beta_{evol}) = \sum_{i=1}^{6} k \cdot P_{prot}(k) \cdot e^{-\beta_{evol}k\varepsilon(\sigma^l)} \tag{14.2}$$

where $P_{prot}(k)$ is the fraction of binding site positions with k nearest-neighbor protein atoms. The infinite temperature distribution $P_{db}(\sigma^p, \sigma^l, 0)$ is likewise

$$P_{db}(\sigma^p, \sigma^l, 0) = \sum_{i=1}^{6} k \cdot P_{prot}(k) \tag{14.3}$$

Because $P_{db}(\sigma^p, \sigma^l, \beta_{evol})$ is a higher-order polynomial of the Boltzmann factor, Equation 14.2 cannot have the same structure as Equation 14.1; that is, rewriting Equation 14.2 as

$$P_{db}(\sigma^p, \sigma^l, \beta_{db}) \sim e^{-\beta_{evol}\varepsilon(\sigma^l)} \cdot g(\sigma^p, \sigma^l, \beta_{evol}, \varepsilon(\sigma^l))$$

we see that the prefactor $g(\sigma^p, \sigma^l, \beta_{evol}, \varepsilon(\sigma^l))$ is temperature dependent and not equal to $P_{db}(\sigma^p, \sigma^l, 0)$. This shows that the knowledge-based approach fails our thought experiment. The reason for this failure is that the local density of contacts is not uniform over the ligand.

On the other hand, consider the probability that a particular ligand type is making a certain number of protein contacts. This is given by

$$P_{\mathrm{db}}\left(\sigma^{\mathrm{l}}, k\right) = P_{\mathrm{prot}}\left(k\right) P_{\mathrm{db}}\left(\sigma^{\mathrm{l}} \middle| k\right) = \frac{P_{\mathrm{prot}}\left(k\right) e^{-\beta_{\mathrm{evol}} k \varepsilon\left(\sigma^{\mathrm{l}}\right)}}{\sum_{\sigma^{\mathrm{l}}} e^{-\beta_{\mathrm{evol}} k \varepsilon\left(\sigma^{\mathrm{l}}\right)}},$$

and thus,

$$\varepsilon\left(\sigma^{\mathrm{l}}\right) = -\frac{1}{\beta_{\mathrm{evol}}}\left[\ln \frac{P_{\mathrm{prot}}\left(k-1\right)}{P_{\mathrm{prot}}\left(k\right)} \frac{P_{\mathrm{db}}\left(\sigma^{\mathrm{l}}, k\right)}{P_{\mathrm{db}}\left(\sigma^{\mathrm{l}}, k-1\right)}\right]$$

which yields the correct, exact values of the parameters $\varepsilon(\sigma^{\mathrm{l}})$.

Why was the derivation successful this time around? Interestingly, although the free energies of the database members were based on a pairwise ("two body") contact potential, the contact statistics derived from the database are not distributed accordingly. In fact, the correct application of the knowledge-based formalism requires that the statistics explicitly account for variations in the local density of contacts within the binding pocket. The reason is that when we constructed the canonical ensemble, a ligand atom was favored (or disfavored) according to the total energy contribution it made to the overall binding free energy, which is given by the sum of all the contacts it makes with the protein. In other words, the contacts are distributed according to the energy contribution of the environment in which each ligand atom resides.

Importantly, it is unlikely that we would have derived the correct values of the potential without expert knowledge on how the database was constructed. Critical to success was the knowledge that ligand atoms were mutated so as to form a canonical ensemble. It then made sense to assume that contacts were distributed according to the protein environments they were placed in, even though free energies are given entirely by summing two-body interactions. Clearly, under real-life conditions, it is impossible to know (1) what physical and nonphysical principles were used to construct a database, (2) critical parameters such as T_{db} and the number of atom types, and (3) the correct functional form of the protein-ligand free energy function.

14.5 WHAT STEPS CAN WE TAKE TOWARD A BETTER PROTEIN-LIGAND POTENTIAL?

As stated earlier, a commercially useful computational method must be fast, accurate, transferable, and interpretable. Logical steps one can take towards this goal are now presented. It is important to point out that under current resources, these four criteria cannot be simultaneously optimized. With current computational capabilities, the most complete theoretical description of protein-ligand interactions (which may involve many-body terms) cannot be solved. Hence, any choice we make to improve the speed of a calculation via an approximation will inherently degrade its accuracy. Accuracy will be less sensitive to some approximations, and such approximations are the keys to balancing speed against accuracy.

Likewise, there often is an inverse relationship between transferability and interpretability. Many predictive statistical models are linear or nonlinear functions of descriptors, which may have no direct connection to the property being predicted. One example is the use of 2D descriptors to build models for predicting binding free energies. Such methods often have superior transferability as suggested by cross-validation than many 3D methods. However, 2D methods are difficult to use by a computational chemist when performing critical structure-based modeling tasks. On the other hand, many 3D methods are easy to use in a structure-based setting and allow for the end user's own knowledge and experience to potentially correct the errors of a computational method. Because computational methods can be significantly enhanced by expert human knowledge, it will be important to choose methods with high interpretability even if some transferability is sacrificed.

14.5.1 Using Coarse-Graining to Balance Speed and Accuracy

As we saw with our lattice calculations, for data training to be successful, it is critical to have the correct form of the free energy function. First, the function should capture the components of the free energy that are thermally relevant. Relevant interactions may include van der Waals contacts, hydrogen bonds, electrostatic interactions, solvation effects, and protein and ligand torsional entropies [21]. Second, each free energy contribution should be measured over the appropriate length scales. Hydrogen bonds are short ranged (<3.25 Å) and orientationally specific, in contrast to electrostatic interactions, which decay as $1/r$ when not screened [36]. Third, each component should have the correct scaling behavior with respect to spatial dimensions or contacts. For example, experiments have shown that solvation effects at large length scales are best treated as surface tensions: that is, the free energy scales as the size of the solvent interface ($\sim R^2$) [37]. On the other hand, short-ranged interactions, such as van der Waals interactions, should scale as the number of contacts [38].

When choosing the correct scaling behavior, we are implicitly choosing the time and length scales over which the phenomena of interest are relevant. Stated differently, the fast and short length scale fluctuations of the protein-ligand system are averaged out, or *coarse-grained* [39], without eliminating the important physics of the system. For example, many researchers have noted the importance of solvation effects in protein-ligand binding events, with a key favorable contribution coming from the free energy change associated with desolvating hydrophobic groups and burying them in the interior of proteins [40]. A widely accepted understanding of this hydrophobic effect is that it ought to be treated as a surface tension [21]. Although this empirical observation has held true for large molecules such as polymers and large organics, it did not agree with experimental data for small changes. Recent theory [41] has shown that the hydrophobic effect behaves differently depending on the size of the molecule. For molecules with surface area <100 $Å^2$, the solvation free energy scales as its volume, whereas for larger molecules, the solvation free energy is a surface tension as thought earlier. This sudden transition from volume to surface area scaling is properly modeled by a field-theoretic treatment of liquids. A key step in this treatment is coarse-graining, whereby the microscopic fluctuations of water density are averaged out so that larger length scale effects can be captured. Sudden transitions, such as the drying transition between two hydrophobic surfaces, involve collective effects between molecules separated by distances much longer than typical molecular distances. An important conclusion is that to accurately capture the hydrophobic effect it is not necessary to simulate every water molecule, thereby greatly reducing computational demands.

Coarse-graining correctly is the key to balancing speed and accuracy. Accuracy requires identifying the most important contributions and the correct scaling behavior for those contributions. When deciding what to coarse grain, the question to ask is: If I average out X, do I retain the physics important for prediction? In the case of protein-ligand binding, many length scales are relevant for describing the protein-ligand binding event. It is extremely unlikely that accurate prediction of commercial value can be provided by a single length scale description. A "one size fits all" approach using a single length scale to calculate the number of contacts will likely have limited accuracy, particularly during the lead optimization phase, where subtle chemical modifications must be accurately scored. For example, although useful for elucidating general principles, lattice models are useless for deciding whether a ligand fits a given binding site. For this reason, it does not make sense to coarse grain the protein into a "beads-on-a-string" model.

More generally, solvent can be coarse-grained at large scales, as the hydrophobic effect is best captured with a surface tension model for cavities of sufficient size (>100 $Å^2$). However, for smaller scales (~3–4 Å), all energetic contributions made by a particular atom—including hydrogen bonding, electrostatic and van der Waals interactions with the protein and solvent—may be important. It is also a good assumption that the most relevant effects for noncovalent protein-ligand binding occur at time scales no faster than torsional rotations and distance no shorter than 0.25 Å. More specifically, electron transfer, solvent reorganization, and bond length and angle fluctuations occur at time scales that are faster than the protein-ligand binding event. Electron density (or charges) and bond length/angle geometries can likely be modeled as static entities. Furthermore, steric effects need to be modeled with good precision, as subtle differences in geometric fit could strongly influence their energetic contribution.

14.5.2 Efficient Use of Data Can Improve Accuracy

Typically, many structure-based training algorithms take into account only the X-ray structure, which leads to a practical problem. Each synthesized compound is always put through basic in vitro assays to quickly assess whether it has sufficient potency to be considered worthwhile. If interesting potency is confirmed, further experimental characterization—beginning with X-ray studies or in vivo assays—might be pursued. Thus most assayed data do not lead to structural data, and consequently only a small fraction of synthesized compounds are useful for structure-based training. This results in an inefficient training method: Low trainable information content is obtained per synthesized molecule.

An important capability of computational methods is that alternative conformations of a protein-ligand complex can also be generated. This leads to a natural method for enriching the information content of each experimentally derived data point, regardless of whether X-ray structures are present. For example, take an X-ray structure for which the activity has been measured. We can use any computational method to derive an unlimited number of conformations for this structure. These virtual data are very meaningful, as they provide negative examples to the training procedure. For example, suppose a special salt bridge interaction provides most of the stabilization for an X-ray structure. The computationally generated conformations may not have this salt bridge, but it can feature other types of favorable interactions such as hydrogen bonds. If a training procedure was presented only with the X-ray structure, it might learn that the special salt bridge is a very strong interaction but nothing about its strength relative to other interactions. The information provided by the other conformations can help with the latter. The training procedure will be required to assign higher free energies to the non-X-ray conformations, and in the process, may assign a more refined interaction energy value to the special salt bridge.

This approach can be generalized to all possible types of experimental data that may be generated. All chemical structures available in public databases or internal to a company typically feature at least the in vitro binding assay data and additionally, the three-dimensional structure of the protein and/or bound ligand. A chemical compound C will therefore be:

- Active with a measured binding activity K_C^{exp} or inactive
- Stereochemically pure or racemic
- With or without structural data

For inactive compounds, there will be a lower bound on the activity K_C^{limit}. This limit corresponds to either the point at which the measurements were halted because of lack of interest or the detection limit of the assay. For compounds with X-ray data, there will be an experimentally verified conformation γ_C^{exp}.

Let $\Lambda = \{\gamma_{C,i}\}$, $1 \le i \le N_C$, be conformations generated for C using a computational method. Because the global free energy minimum conformation is expected to statistically dominate the thermodynamic ensemble, the predicted binding activity for C is determined by $F_{\min}(C) \equiv \min_{1 \le i \le N} F(\gamma_{C,i}) = F(\gamma_C^*)$. where the predicted conformation is denoted as γ_C^*. Given this data, the end product of training should be a free energy estimator F that meets the following constraints:

1. Active stereochemically pure compounds with structural data
The minimum energy conformation γ_C^* if it exists in Λ should be the X-ray conformation $\gamma_C^{\exp}$. Because the ground state is given by the X-ray conformation, the calculated free energy of all non-X-ray conformations should be higher than that of $\gamma_C^{\exp}$. In other words:

$$F\left(\gamma_C^{\exp}\right) = -RT \ln K_C^{\exp} \tag{14.4a}$$

and

$$F\left(\gamma_C^{\exp}\right) \le F_{\min}(C) \le F\left(\gamma_{C,i}\right). \tag{14.4b}$$

2. Active stereochemically pure compounds with no structural data
If our conformational and free energy predictions were correct, we expect $F_{\min}(C) = -RT\ln K_C^{\exp}$. Otherwise, the most we could expect is:

$$-RT \ln K_C^{\exp} \le F\left(\gamma_{C,i}\right), \quad \forall i \tag{14.5}$$

3. Inactive stereochemically pure compounds (structural data are not possible)
Because we only have a lower bound on the binding free energy of inactive compounds, we expect:

$$-RT \ln K_C^{\text{limit}} \le F\left(\gamma_{C,i}\right), \quad \forall i. \tag{14.6}$$

4. Active racemic mixture (structural data are not possible)
For a racemic mixture M, the measured binding constant is a sum of the actual binding constants of each species L_i in the mixture weighed by their fraction f_i:

$$K_M^{\exp} = \frac{[\text{bound complex}]}{[\text{free protein}][\text{free ligand}]} = \frac{\sum_{i=1}^{N}[L_i P]}{[P]\sum_{i=1}^{N}[L_i]} = \frac{\sum_{i=1}^{N} K_{L_i}[L_i][P]}{[P]\sum_{i=1}^{N}[L_i]} = \sum_{i=1}^{N} K_{L_i} f_i$$

where $[X]$ denotes the concentration of the species X and $\sum_{i=1}^{N} f_i = 1$. For a given species L_A, we know that:

$$K_{L_A} = \frac{1}{f_A}\left(K_M^{\exp} - \sum_{i \neq A} K_{L_i} f_i\right) \leq \frac{1}{f_A} K_M^{\exp}$$

and

$$K_{L_A} \geq \frac{1}{f_A}\left[K_M^{\exp} - (1 - f_A)\max_{i \neq A}\left\{K_{L_i}\right\}_i\right] \geq \frac{1}{f_A} K_M^{\exp} - \frac{1 - f_A}{f_A} K^{\max}$$

The lower bound is dependent on the worst possible binding affinity $K^{\max}$. Thus, for each isomer L_i with conformations $\{\gamma_{L_i,j}\}$, $1 \leq j \leq N_{L_i}$, we require that:

$$-RT \ln\left[\frac{1}{f_i} K_M^{\exp}\right] \leq F(\gamma_{L_i,j}) \leq -RT \ln\left[\frac{1}{f_i} K_M^{\exp} - \frac{1 - f_i}{f_i} K^{\max}\right], \quad \forall j \quad (14.7)$$

5. Inactive racemic mixture (structural data are not possible)
An inactive racemic mixture M will have an upper bound on its measured binding constant (K_M^{limit}). Following reasoning similar to that leading to the above equation, we require that:

$$-RT \ln\left[\frac{1}{f_i} K_M^{\text{limit}}\right] \leq F(\gamma_{L_i,j}), \quad \forall j \quad (14.8)$$

Any free energy estimate F must satisfy all five constraints in order to be consistent with all data collected during the drug discovery process. These constraints are derived by considering what values F can assume without contradicting experimental data or physical principles. Importantly, biological data obtained for *any synthesized molecule* can be used to generate constraints for training. Training is therefore no longer restricted to structural data or molecules with activity. Furthermore, by generating alternative conformations, one can increase the number of constraints without limitation, although the actual information gained from such constraints may be limited.

14.5.3 Use Algorithms and Physical Ideas to Maximize Transferability

A key problem with constructing accurate computational methods for predicting binding free energy has been overfitting. Many computational methods determine the free energy of the collective protein-ligand interaction by summing together a fairly large number of independent contributions, each of which requires a weight parameter to be determined through training. If the training utilizes only X-ray data, the amount of available training data is sparse, and the risk of overfitting is high. In practice, cross-validation [42] is a useful way to minimize this risk, by empirically determining the relationship between testing error and training set composition.

A more rigorous way to improve transferability is to utilize a data training method that has theoretical guarantees on transferability, such as the support vector machine (SVM) [24]. The SVM was an important advance in machine learning emerging from Vapnik and Chervonenkis (VC) theory [43], which was a general theory for quantifying the complexity of a training problem. VC theory states that the ability of a function to generalize well to data outside of its training set is directly related to its so-called capacity. One measure of capacity is the VC dimension, which is defined as the largest number h of points that can be separated in all possible ways with functions of a given class. If the capacity of a function is known, VC theory can provide bounds on the testing error, depending on the learning task at hand (e.g., regression, classification). For example, for a training data set of m points, a class of pattern recognition functions with a VC dimension of h ($<m$) will have, with a probability of at least $1 - \eta$,

$$\varepsilon_{\text{test}} \leq \varepsilon_{\text{train}} + \sqrt{\frac{h}{m}\left(\log\frac{2m}{h}+1\right)-\frac{1}{m}\log\left(\frac{\eta}{4}\right)}$$

where $\varepsilon_{\text{test}}$ and $\varepsilon_{\text{train}}$ are the test (or generalization) and training errors, respectively. Clearly, both the capacity (h) and the training data size (m) can significantly influence the ability of a data-trained computational model to generalize. Although the utility of bounds depend on how tight they are, they can nonetheless be useful for selecting the model used for making predictions. Vapnik proposed the method of structural risk minimization, whereby models with the smallest value of the upper bound and the lowest VC dimension are chosen. The SVM was one of the first learning procedures for which useful bounds on the VC dimension could be determined, and hence structural risk minimization could be carried out.

Another consideration for improving transferability is to choose models that are grounded in physical principles. Because we are trying to predict a physical quantity (namely, free energy), it is natural to expect a maximally transferable predictor to be based on general physical principles. That is, the less protein-/ligand-/condition-specific the underlying principles are, the more general the predictor will be. To this end, there are several basic properties that models should satisfy. To facilitate the present discussion, consider a free energy predictor of the form $\sum a_i D_i$, which is a linear combination of descriptors, D_i:

1. **Each additive component of the prediction must make physical sense as energies.** That is, each of the components needs to have energy units. A good candidate for a descriptor is the number of hydrogen bonds, because the prefactor a_i will denote the (average) free energy contribution per hydrogen bond, which makes physical sense. However, a poor choice would be the average path length in the bonded structure of a molecule: There is no physically sensible way to relate average path

length to binding free energy. Descriptors that are indirectly related to the free energy can only introduce randomness into the training. This is seen by writing a_iD_i as $a_i D_i^{\text{energetic}} - a_i D_i^{\text{nonenergetic}}$ and observing that the binding data will provide no information on $a_i D_i^{\text{nonenergetic}}$.

2. **Each component should have a physically reasonable scaling behavior.** As stated above, the various contributions to binding free energy have theoretically predicted and/or empirically observed scaling behaviors. If a component is introduced with the incorrect scaling, there will be errors resulting from training. Errors will be introduced, for example, if an energetic quantity with a clear interfacial dependence (solvation for large ligands) is described by a descriptor that scales strictly with distance.
3. **Each component should be nonoverlapping in its energetic contribution.** If a_1D_1 and a_2D_2 make overlapping contributions to the same portion of the free energy, then we can write, using obvious notation, $a_1 D_1^{\text{nonoverlap}} + a_2 D_2^{\text{nonoverlap}} + (a_1 + a_2) D^{\text{overlap}}$. This cannot be optimally trained because the overlapping free energy contribution couples the two variables $a_1 + a_2$.

Although this list clearly is not exhaustive, these properties are challenging for any data-trained model to satisfy. All three argue against including many traditional 2D descriptors. Additionally, the odds of picking a subset of descriptors (typically on the order of 10s) out of a much larger subset (1000s) that satisfies these three properties, particularly property 3, is diminishingly low, which argues against many "feature selection"-based methods. It is stressed that the complete satisfaction of the last two properties is not possible given our current understanding of the protein-ligand binding process. Many difficult questions, such as those related to the role of isolated water molecules, solvent screening in electrostatics, and protein motion, are currently under intense investigation.

14.6 CASE STUDY: TECHNOLOGY PLATFORM AT VITAE PHARMACEUTICALS

Many of the strategies outlined above were implemented into a computational platform at Vitae Pharmaceuticals (formerly Concurrent Pharmaceuticals). When used in the drug discovery effort integrating computational and medicinal chemistry, the platform played a critical role in finding nonpeptidic, high-affinity inhibitors of renin in less than 12 months. This led to a partnership with GlaxoSmithKline, which was announced in June 2005 (see http://www.vitaepharma.com/news/NewsRelease2005Jun20.pdf).

At the heart of the platform was a coarse-grained physical description of the binding free energy, which was trained with a proprietary machine learning algorithm. The coarse-grained physical model used was:

$$\Delta G_{P-L} = F = F_{\text{steric}} + F_{\text{int}} + F_{\text{solv}} + F_{\text{tor}} + F_{\text{strain}}$$

where

- F_{steric} = steric energy
  - This indicates how well the ligand fits in the binding site.
- F_{int} = interaction energy between the protein and ligand
  - This includes hydrogen bonds, electrostatic interactions, and van der Waals contribution.
- F_{solv} = solvation energy
  - This indicates how favorable it is to take the ligand out of solution and into the protein binding pocket.
- F_{tor} = torsional entropy contribution
  - This measures the free energy penalty associated with the freezing of rotatable torsions.
- F_{strain} = strain energy
  - This measures how much the molecule prefers the conformation it adopts in the binding site compared to its conformation in solution.

Note that a fundamental assumption of our physical model is that the binding free energy can be cleanly decomposed in this manner (thus satisfying properties 1–3 in Section 14.5.3).

The training utilized constraints described in Section 14.5 to data consisting of (1) in-house biological assay data, (2) in-house X-ray structures, (3) modeled literature data, and (4) literature X-ray data. Most algorithms used to train an objective function are designed to meet either equality or inequality constraints. Primarily, equality constraints (such as Equation 14.4a) are used to training regression models, whereas inequality constraints (such as Equations 14.4b–14.8) are used for classification models. To meet our unique training requirements, we developed a new algorithm that solves the following optimization problem. Suppose our training set T is the union of three distinct sets: (1) $X=\{(\vec{x}_1, y_1), \ldots, (\vec{x}_n, y_n)\}$, where we want to predict y_i given $\vec{x}_i$; (2) $X_+=\left\{(\vec{x}_1^+, y_1^+), \ldots, (\vec{x}_{n_+}^+, y_{n_+}^+)\right\}$, where the prediction on $\vec{x}_i^+$ must be bounded from above by y_i^+; and (3) $X_-=\left\{(\vec{x}_1^-, y_1^-), \ldots, (\vec{x}_{n_-}^-, y_{n_-}^-)\right\}$, where the prediction on $\vec{x}_i^-$ must be bounded from below by y_i^-. We want to find the predictive function $F(\vec{t}) = b + \vec{w}\cdot\phi(\vec{t})$, where ϕ is the feature space mapping and $\vec{t} \in X \cup X_+ \cup X_-$. In this notation, the data training constraints outlined above that were implemented translate as:

1. Active stereochemically pure compounds with structural data

$$\{(F(\gamma_C^{\text{exp}}), RT \ln K_C^{\text{exp}})\} \in X$$

$$\left\{\left(F\left(\gamma_{C,i}\right), RT \ln K_C^{\exp}\right)\right\} \in X_-$$

2. Active stereochemically pure compounds with no structural data

$$\left\{\left(F\left(\gamma_{C,i}\right), RT \ln K_C^{\exp}\right)\right\} \in X_-$$

3. Inactive stereochemically pure compounds

$$\left\{\left(F\left(\gamma_{C,i}\right), RT \ln K_C^{\text{limit}}\right)\right\} \in X_-$$

The literature/X-ray data was sparse (~1000), so the information content was amplified by generating vast numbers of alternative conformations (~10^6) with a 64-node Linux cluster. Typically, we were able to generate 1 distinct conformation per compound in an average of <1 per minute. At critical points during the drug discovery process, such as when new structural data was obtained, we retrained our free energy model to improve its performance.

14.7 WHAT LESSONS ARE TO BE LEARNED FROM COMPUTATIONAL PROTEIN FOLDING RESEARCH?

It is worthwhile at this point to briefly discuss several problems from the field of protein folding, as they bear a strong similarity to those of computational drug design and have been studied for a longer time. Three fundamental problems underlying most research on protein folding are:

1. Prediction: What is the three-dimensional structure of a given protein?
2. Folding: What is the kinetic mechanism by which the folded state of the protein is reached?
3. Design: Which sequences fold into a given three-dimensional structure?

Presently, a single theory of protein folding that simultaneously solves the three problems does not exist. Separate approaches to each problem have progressed toward separate solutions. Of these, the folding problem is understood best, but the most fruitful approach there can be used neither to predict nor to design real protein structures.

14.7.1 An Important Tool for Understanding Folding: the Lattice Model

Physicists have developed a model that reproduces all of the essential features of protein folding, and in which the three problems have a unified solution. However, the model cannot be used to make specific predictions about real protein sequences because it relies entirely on restricting the polypeptide chain to a cubic lattice—it is therefore only a "toy model." Nevertheless, it is of great importance because it demonstrates that at a coarse-grained level, our basic, physical understanding of proteins is excellent. It is also believed that the principles that were discovered in the toy model are useful for building a high-resolution theory.

The lattice model represents each conformation of the polypeptide chain as a self-avoiding path on a cubic lattice, with consecutive monomers lying on neighboring lattice sites. Each monomer has a sequence identity, which is an integer between 1 and m specifying its amino acid type. The number m is known as the alphabet size of the model. It can be taken to be 20 as in nature, although for a toy representation $m = 3$ (hydrophobic, polar, neutral) is often sufficient. Additionally, the model supplies a function, called the potential energy function, or simply the potential, that assigns an energy to each conformation. Simulation is by Monte Carlo, in which a change of conformation (a move) is made, the resulting energy difference is calculated, and the move is accepted or rejected based on the Metropolis criterion, which allows a fictitious temperature to be specified as a parameter of the simulation.

Different forms of the potential are possible, the simplest being a contact potential in which the energy of a conformation is the sum of all pairwise interaction energies between monomers that are nearest neighbors on the lattice. The energy of each contact is determined by the sequence identities of the two interacting monomers. A contact potential is therefore completely specified by a symmetric $m \times m$ matrix of interaction energies. Given such a potential, the model is capable of reproducing defining features of proteins and can fully address the problems of prediction, folding, and design for toy proteins. That is, for any given sequence, its lowest-energy compact structure is found by simulation (prediction), or, conversely, sequences can be designed to fold into any given compact structure (design). The kinetic mechanism by which this occurs has also been fully explored and elucidated (folding). The signature of proteinlike behavior, namely the cooperative all-or-none transition from unfolded to folded conformations, with a sharp peak in heat capacity at the folding transition temperature, is reproduced in the toy model.

14.7.2 Off-Lattice Models with Coarse-Grained Side Chains

A step closer toward realism is taken by off-lattice models in which the backbone is specified in some detail, while side chains, if they are represented at all, are taken to be single, unified spheres [44–50]. One indication that this approach is too simplistic was given in [51], which proved that for a backbone representation in which only C_{α} carbons were modeled, no contact potential could stabilize the native conformation of a single protein against its nonnative ("decoy") conformations. However, Irback and co-workers were able to fold real protein sequences, albeit short ones, using a detailed backbone representation, with coarse-grained side chains modeled as spheres [49, 52–54].

Although their medium-resolution model was successful for α-helical proteins, folding β-hairpin structures have been difficult. In general, many off-lattice approaches have been tested, and although definitive proof does not exist in most cases, there appears to be a growing consensus that such off-lattice models are not sufficient.

Several reasons exist for the failure of these coarse-grained models. Proteins are stabilized by a variety of forces. Some are largely isotropic, such as the hydrophobic interaction, and are dominated by a term proportional to solvent-exposed surface area. Such interactions might be adequately represented by a backbone model with unified spherical side chains and a contact potential. Other interactions, however, are strongly directional, such as hydrogen bonds and polar interactions. When such interactions occur between two side chains, or between a side chain and the backbone, their strength is highly sensitive to the precise relative orientations. Thus a side chain interaction that appears possible at the coarse-grained level may be entirely unfeasible in reality. As long as some parts of a given protein rely on such side chain-mediated directional interactions for stability, coarse graining side chains is likely to fail.

A single example, given in [55], illustrates why an explicit atomic description may be necessary to discriminate properly between alternative protein conformations. In this example, the side chain carboxyl group of Glu46 and the backbone oxygen of Phe100 in the protein ribonuclease F1 are in contact. Such a contact, the authors note, is highly unfavorable unless the carboxyl is protonated. A coarse-grained protein representation cannot distinguish between these possibilities and will likely designate any glutamine side chain interacting with a backbone oxygen as unfavorable. In this particular case, a favorable long-range interaction will be discounted and the native topology destabilized somewhat. On the other hand, this example shows that even the all-atom description must be handled delicately. The pH of the solution must be considered, and the pK_a values of residues taken into account, either explicitly by including hydrogen atoms or implicitly by modifying the interaction energetics accordingly.

14.7.3 High-Resolution Atomic Models: a Necessary Complexity

Within models that used an all-atom description, major progress has been made on all three of the basic problems. This might be taken as further support for the necessity of high-resolution models. The folding problem has been addressed with the Gōpotential energy function, which utilizes topological information from the native state to strongly bias folding. The Gōpotential cannot be used to fold sequences where the native structure is unknown. Using a Metropolis Monte Carlo simulation, the folding thermodynamics and kinetics of several proteins were studied, starting from completely unfolded conformations and reaching the native state at various fixed temperatures, without simulated annealing, parallel tempering, or other nonphysical computational tricks [56, 57]. It was found that if the energetic scale is properly adjusted to match experimentally measured stabilities of isolated parts of proteins, this method can be used to reproduce faithfully the folding kinetics of a protein. Other groups have used different simulation methodologies of the Gō model with similar success, demonstrating that progress in protein folding theory is not limited by the power of computers to simulate. Rather, it is limited by our knowledge of energetics.

Presently, only the molecular dynamics approach suffers from a computational bottleneck [58–60]. This stems from the inclusion of thousands of solvent molecules in simulation. By using implicit solvation potentials, in which solvent degrees of freedom are averaged out, the computational problem is eliminated. It is presently an open question whether a potential without explicit solvent can approximate the true potential sufficiently well to qualify as a sound protein folding theory [61]. A toy model study claims that it cannot [62], but like many other negative results, it is of relatively little use as it is based on numerous assumptions, none of which are true in all-atom representations.

Significant progress has been made in both the prediction and design problems with all-atom models [63–71]. It is noted, however, that in the most successful approaches, many nonphysical ingredients enter into the models. This does not detract from their power to address the specific problems they have been designed to solve. It only means that they do not qualify as a physical protein folding theory but instead are generating expertise and intuition about protein chemistry that hopefully may be translated into useful knowledge of protein energetics.

Most noteworthy among these approaches are the design [67, 68] and prediction [65, 69] methods developed by Baker and co-workers. Over the last decade, this group has developed an all-atom approach that uses a potential consisting of a weighted sum of different models, each tailored for particular types of interactions. The model uses a special move set, which appears to be crucial to its success. A backbone move consists of simultaneously changing all torsional angles of 3 or 9 consecutive amino acids to angles of a similar 3- or 9-amino acid sequence found within a protein structure in the protein structure database. This clever procedure practically guarantees that locally the resulting conformations will be physically reasonable. Predictions using this approach require some human input but nevertheless consistently perform at or near the top of the class.

A method for protein design with this potential has been used to design a novel protein fold [67] that when synthesized and crystallized had a root-mean-square deviation of 1.2 Å from the target structure. One key to this outstanding success, it was noted, was the addition of backbone moves of the type described above to the design methodology. Traditional protein design methods allow only side chain rotamers and amino acid identities to change during sequence design, while the protein backbone is held fixed. This allowed backbone changes to accommodate bulkier side chains in tight spaces.

Other protein design methods have demonstrated comparable successes [64, 66, 70].

As stated above, the most important missing piece in protein folding theory is an accurate all-atom potential. Recently there has been much effort in this direction, and much more is needed [48, 55, 72–77]. The existence of a potential satisfying minimal criteria such as folding and stability for a single protein was demonstrated in [73]. It is not a realistic potential by any means, but its existence validates the all-atom, implicit solvent, Monte Carlo approach as a serious candidate for theory. The method used to derive this potential was ad hoc, and has recently been compared with other standard methods in a rigorous and illuminating study [77].

Generally, potentials should be derived by an optimization procedure that accounts in some way for the energies of decoys [78]. Explicit decoy methods use an iterative scheme, in which a potential is optimized to give lowest energy to a native structure, folding is initiated with this potential, new true decoys are discovered, and the native energy is reoptimized against these new decoys [50, 79]. Such methods are extremely computationally intensive. As shown in References 77 and 78, decoys can also be included implicitly, without resorting to folding simulations, by taking into account the statistics of atom-atom contacts. There is always some danger in such approaches, however, that the contact statistics are not properly modeled, and more work is presently needed to address this issue. If a good implicit model of decoy contact statistics is found, this will greatly facilitate the process of potential derivation.

14.7.4 Parallels in Computational Drug Design

The most successful protein prediction and design methods employ high-resolution structural models with coarse-grained potentials that contain a combination of physical and nonphysical terms. These models have been tuned for over a decade with rounds of prediction, experimental tests, and retraining. Although the models are still far from perfect, they are now making useful and often accurate predictions, particularly in the fields of protein structure prediction and design. It is clear that drug design will profit greatly from a similar sustained training effort on a huge number of examples, as discussed above.

Another key to success in protein computation has been to try to restrict the search space to proteinlike conformations. This was done, as described above, by using fragments from known crystal structures to build the predictions. Such fragments, when used with the model potential, presumably retain some memory of the true protein energetics and thus might provide some correction of errors. If this is as crucial an innovation as it appears to be, could an analogous principle work in computational drug design?

Indeed it might, but much experimental data would first need to be collected. The general idea would be to bias the test conformations of a ligand inside a binding site to be as near as possible to known X-ray crystal structures of similar ligand-binding site pairs. Because the chemical space we want to explore is large, it would be necessary to have structural information on ligands with all the different chemical moieties that we wish to employ, in diverse binding sites. Supposing that such data become available, it may then be possible to generate ligand conformations based on structural homology with known ligand-binding site pairs. Trained energetics would then be used to evaluate the fit, and make minor adjustments, but the conformations sampled would be strongly biased toward realistic conformations that have been observed for the given chemical moieties and protein environment.

It is altogether unsatisfying from a strictly physical perspective to rely on such hybrid approaches. Nevertheless, problems that are too complex to admit a purely physical solution have been solved brilliantly by engineering. In the case of proteins, it appears that restricting the geometry to locally proteinlike conformations is one way to introduce some part of the true energetics into the model. Analogous approaches for drug design might therefore greatly improve the results of computation, supposing that the true potential is not available. In both cases, discovery of a physical, computationally tractable potential, with sufficient complexity to reliably model the true interactions would render hybrid approaches obsolete, and thus purely physical approaches should continue to be pursued.

14.8 CONCLUSIONS

In the context of drug discovery, computational methods do not add value unless they can achieve practical results. Results must be produced quickly enough so that they can influence decision making in chemical synthesis. Most importantly, computational methods must be accurate enough to maintain the trust of the medicinal chemist. Without this trust, computational predictions will rarely be tested in the laboratory, which will then prevent the generation of critical data useful for improving the original predictions.

Several ideas for balancing speed and accuracy have been presented. Speed can be improved by coarse graining irrelevant degrees of freedom (Section 14.5.1). Because accuracy is ultimately a function of data training, we have presented a way to efficiently use data generated during drug discovery (Section 14.5.2). Another method for improving accuracy is to make rigorous choices with regard to the training algorithm and computational models that improve transferability (Section 14.5.3). Finally, because computational methods will have the computational chemist as the end user, it has been stressed that predictions must be interpretable (Section 14.5.3). Aside from their other merits, purely physical approaches have the distinct advantage of complete interpretability. If predictions are more connected to the basic knowledge base of computational and medicinal chemists, there is a greater likelihood that human judgment can be used to challenge or enhance *in silico* predictions to the betterment of the drug discovery process as a whole.

This final point reminds us that current computational methods are not perfect. We are many years in algorithmic and hardware development away from "touch-button" predictions of binding free energies. Even the task of comparing existing methods has proven challenging. Thus, for computational methods to be an important tool in drug discovery at this moment in time, we must take advantage of the end user's expert knowledge. An important practical challenge for computational methods is to remain commercially relevant for drug discovery. If we ultimately fail to meet this challenge, we will not have the data or experience to improve our methods and will not realize the commercial promise of computational drug discovery.

14.9 APPENDIX: WHAT IS BINDING ACTIVITY?

A necessary condition for a compound to exhibit *in vivo* efficacy is *in vitro* activity. By "activity," we mean that the compound is able to demonstrate binding to the protein target of interest. At constant pressure and temperature, the protein (P) and ligand (L) binding free energy ΔG_{PL} is given by

$$\Delta G_{PL} = G_{PL} - G_P - G_L,$$

where G_{PL}, G_P, and G_L are the Gibbs free energy of the protein-ligand complex, apo-protein, and free ligand, respectively [21, 38]. For drug discovery, we are interested in situations where $\Delta G_{PL} < 0$, which states that the ligand prefers to be bound to the protein. The free energy of binding is logarithmically related to the experimentally measurable equilibrium binding constant (K_b)

$$\Delta G_{PL} = -RT \ln K_b = -2.3RT \log_{10} K_b$$

with $K_b = \dfrac{[PL]}{[P][L]}$, [ ] denoting the concentration of the relevant species, and $2.3RT = 1.35$ kcal/mol at room temperature. This is an important thermodynamic relation, as it relates microscopic physical theories (which serve as the basis for computational models) to experimentally measurable quantities.

ACKNOWLEDGMENTS

I extend enormous thanks to Edo Kussell of The Rockefeller University for his insights and editorial work on this manuscript, particularly with regard to protein folding. Mei Shibata of Clarion Healthcare Consulting, LLC, is also acknowledged for her insights into the business of drug discovery. My former colleagues at Vitae Pharmaceuticals, including Jean-Pierre Wery, Sean Ekins, Eugene Shakhnovich, Suresh Singh, Peter Lindblom, Kam Jim, Carl Elkin, Michael Jastram, Bob Fay, Victor Chubukoff, Maggie Hupcey, Dave Lawson, Alexey Ishchenko, and Guosheng Wu, are thanked for their work on the computational platform.

REFERENCES

1. Mervis J. Productivity counts—But the definition is key. *Science* 2005;309:726–7.
2. Dickson M, Gagnon JP. Key factors in the rising cost of new drug discovery and development. *Nat Rev Drug Discov* 2004;3:417–29.
3. DiMasi JA, Hansen RW, Grabowski HG. The price of innovation: new estimates of drug development costs. *J Health Econ* 2003;22:151–85.
4. Ma P, Zemmel R. Value of novelty? *Nat Rev Drug Discov* 2002;1:571–2.
5. Butcher EC. Can cell systems biology rescue drug discovery? *Nat Rev Drug Discov* 2005;4:461–7.
6. Couzin J. The brains behind blockbusters. *Science* 2005;309:728–30.
7. Lombardino JG, Lowe JA. The role of the medicinal chemist in drug discovery—then and now. *Nat Rev Drug Discov* 2004;3:853–62.
8. Bleicher KH, Bohm HJ, Muller K, Alanine AI. Hit and lead generation: beyond high-throughput screening. *Nat Rev Drug Discov* 2003;2:369–78.
9. DiMasi JA. Risks in new drug development: approval success rates for investigational drugs. *Clin Pharmacol Ther* 2001;69:297–307.
10. Kuntz ID. Structure-based strategies for drug design and discovery. *Science* 1992;257:1078–82.
11. Honma T. Recent advances in de novo design strategy for practical lead identification. *Med Res Rev* 2003;23:606–32.
12. Jorgensen WL. The many roles of computation in drug discovery. *Science* 2004;303:1813–8.
13. Walters WP, Stahl MT, Murcko MA. Virtual screening—an overview. *Drug Discov Today* 1998;3:160–78.
14. Kitchen DB, Decornez H, Furr JR, Bajorath J. Docking and scoring in virtual screening for drug discovery: methods and applications. *Nat Rev Drug Discov* 2004;3:935–49.
15. Ferrara P, Gohlke H, Price DJ, Klebe G, Brooks CL. Assessing scoring functions for protein-ligand interactions. *J Med Chem* 2004;47:3032–47.
16. Grzybowski BA, Ishchenko AV, Shimada J, Shakhnovich EI. From knowledge-based potentials to combinatorial lead design in silico. *Acc Chem Res* 2002;35:261–9.
17. Gohlke H, Klebe G. Approaches to the description and prediction of the binding affinity of small-molecule ligands to macromolecular receptors. *Angew Chem Int Edit* 2002;41:2645–76.
18. Kollman P. Free-energy calculations—applications to chemical and biochemical phenomena. *Chem Rev* 1993;93:2395–417.
19. Ekins S, De Groot MJ, Jones JP. Pharmacophore and three-dimensional quantitative structure activity relationship methods for modeling cytochrome P450 active sites. *Drug Metab Dispos* 2001;29:936–44.
20. Bohm HJ. The development of a simple empirical scoring function to estimate the binding constant for a protein ligand complex of known 3-dimensional structure. *J Comput Aid Mol Des* 1994;8:243–56.

21. Ajay, Murcko MA. Computational methods to predict binding free energy in ligand-receptor complexes. *J Med Chem* 1995;38:4953–67.
22. Raha K, Merz KM. Large-scale validation of a quantum mechanics based scoring function: predicting the binding affinity and the binding mode of a diverse set of protein-ligand complexes. *J Med Chem* 2005;48:4558–75.
23. Brooks CL, Karplus M, Pettitt BM. *Proteins : a theoretical perspective of dynamics, structure, and thermodynamics.* New York: John Wiley & Sons, 1988.
24. Cristianini N, Shawe-Taylor J. *An introduction to support vector machines and other kernel-based learning methods.* Cambridge, UK: Cambridge University Press, 2000.
25. Datta S, Grant DJW. Crystal structures of drugs: advances in determination, prediction and engineering. *Nat Rev Drug Discov* 2004;3:42–57.
26. Wang R, Fang X, Lu Y, Wang S. The PDBbind database: collection of binding affinities for protein-ligand complexes with known three-dimensional structures. *J Med Chem* 2004;47:2977–80.
27. Wang R, Fang X, Lu Y, Yang CY, Wang S. The PDBbind database: methodologies and updates. *J Med Chem* 2005;48:4111–9.
28. Vieth M, Siegel MG, Higgs RE, Watson IA, Robertson DH, Savin KA, et al. Characteristic physical properties and structural fragments of marketed oral drugs. *J Med Chem* 2004;47:224–32.
29. Shimada J, Ishchenko AV, Shakhnovich EI. Analysis of knowledge-based protein-ligand potentials using a self-consistent method. *Protein Sci* 2000;9:765–75.
30. Berman HM, Westbrook J, Feng Z, Gilliland G, Bhat TN, Weissig H, et al. The Protein Data Bank. *Nucleic Acids Res* 2000;28:235–42.
31. Roche O, Kiyama R, Brooks CL 3rd. Ligand-protein database: linking protein-ligand complex structures to binding data. *J Med Chem* 2001;44:3592–8.
32. Newman MEJ, Barkema GT. *Monte Carlo methods in statistical physics.* Oxford: Clarendon Press, 1999.
33. Finkelstein AV, Badretdinov A, Gutin AM. Why do protein architectures have Boltzmann-like statistics? *Proteins* 1995;23:142–50.
34. Finkelstein AV, Gutin AM, Badretdinov AY. Perfect temperature for protein structure prediction and folding. *Proteins* 1995;23:151–62.
35. Godzik A, Kolinski A, Skolnick J. Are proteins ideal mixtures of amino acids? Analysis of energy parameter sets. *Protein Sci* 1995;4:2107–17.
36. Jeffrey GA, Saenger W. *Hydrogen bonding in biological structures.* Berlin: Springer-Verlag, 1991.
37. Tanford C. *The hydrophobic effect : formation of micelles and biological membranes.* New York: John Wiley & Sons, 1980.
38. McQuarrie DA. *Statistical mechanics.* New York: Harper & Row, 1975.
39. Chaikin PM, Lubensky TC. *Principles of condensed matter physics.* Cambridge: Cambridge University Press, 1995.
40. Fersht A. *Structure and mechanism in protein science: a guide to enzyme catalysis and protein folding.* New York: W.H. Freeman, 1999.
41. Chandler D. Interfaces and the driving force of hydrophobic assembly. *Nature* 2005;437:640–7.

42. Hastie T, Tibshirani R, Friedman JH. *The elements of statistical learning: data mining, inference, and prediction*. New York: Springer, 2001.
43. Vapnik VN. *Statistical learning theory*. New York: John Wiley & Sons, 1998.
44. Berriz GF, Shakhnovich EI. Characterization of the folding kinetics of a three-helix bundle protein via a minimalist Langevin model. *J Mol Biol* 2001;310:673–85.
45. Brown S, Fawzi NJ, Head-Gordon T. Coarse-grained sequences for protein folding and design. *Proc Natl Acad Sci USA* 2003;100:10712–7.
46. Clementi C, Nymeyer H, Onuchic JN. Topological and energetic factors: what determines the structural details of the transition state ensemble and "en-route" intermediates for protein folding? An investigation for small globular proteins. *J Mol Biol* 2000;298:937–53.
47. Dokholyan NV, Buldyrev SV, Stanley HE, Shakhnovich EI. Discrete molecular dynamics studies of the folding of a protein-like model. *Fold Des* 1998;3:577–87.
48. Ejtehadi MR, Avall SP, Plotkin SS. Three-body interactions improve the prediction of rate and mechanism in protein folding models. *Proc Natl Acad Sci USA* 2004;101:15088–93.
49. Irback A, Peterson C, Potthast F, Sommelius O. Local interactions and protein folding: A three-dimensional off-lattice approach. *J Chem Phys* 1997;107:273–82.
50. Tobi D, Elber R. Distance-dependent, pair potential for protein folding: results from linear optimization. *Proteins* 2000;41:40–6.
51. Vendruscolo M, Domany E. Pairwise contact potentials are unsuitable for protein folding. *J Chem Phys* 1998;109:11101–8.
52. Favrin G, Irback A, Wallin S. Sequence-based study of two related proteins with different folding behaviors. *Proteins* 2004;54:8–12.
53. Irback A, Sjunnesson F. Folding thermodynamics of three beta-sheet peptides: a model study. *Proteins* 2004;56:110–6.
54. Irback A, Mohanty S. Folding thermodynamics of peptides. *Biophys J* 2005;88:1560–9.
55. Krieger E, Darden T, Nabuurs SB, Finkelstein A, Vriend G. Making optimal use of empirical energy functions: force-field parameterization in crystal space. *Proteins* 2004;57:678–83.
56. Shimada J, Kussell EL, Shakhnovich EI. The folding thermodynamics and kinetics of crambin using an all-atom Monte Carlo simulation. *J Mol Biol* 2001;308:79–95.
57. Shimada J, Shakhnovich EI. The ensemble folding kinetics of protein G from an all-atom Monte Carlo simulation. *Proc Natl Acad Sci USA* 2002;99:11175–80.
58. Gsponer J, Caflisch A. Molecular dynamics simulations of protein folding from the transition state. *Proc Natl Acad Sci USA* 2002;99:6719–24.
59. Beck DAC, Daggett V. Methods for molecular dynamics simulations of protein folding/unfolding in solution. *Methods* 2004;34:112–20.
60. Karplus M, Kuriyan J. Molecular dynamics and protein function. *Proc Natl Acad Sci USA* 2005;102:6679–85.

61. Jaramillo A, Wodak SJ. Computational protein design is a challenge for implicit solvation models. *Biophys J* 2005;88:156–71.
62. Salvi G, De Los Rios P. Effective interactions cannot replace solvent effects in a lattice model of proteins. *Phys Rev Lett* 2003;91.
63. Simons KT, Kooperberg C, Huang E, Baker D. Assembly of protein tertiary structures from fragments with similar local sequences using simulated annealing and Bayesian scoring functions. *J Mol Biol* 1997;268:209–25.
64. Harbury PB, Plecs JJ, Tidor B, Alber T, Kim PS. High-resolution protein design with backbone freedom. *Science* 1998;282:1462–7.
65. Bonneau R, Tsai J, Ruczinski I, Chivian D, Rohl C, Strauss CEM, et al. Rosetta in CASP4: Progress in ab initio protein structure prediction. *Proteins* 2001:119–26.
66. Bolon DN, Mayo SL. Enzyme-like proteins by computational design. *Proc Natl Acad Sci USA* 2001;98:14274–9.
67. Kuhlman B, Dantas G, Ireton GC, Varani G, Stoddard BL, Baker D. Design of a novel globular protein fold with atomic-level accuracy. *Science* 2003;302:1364–8.
68. Dantas G, Kuhlman B, Callender D, Wong M, Baker D. A large scale test of computational protein design: folding and stability of nine completely redesigned globular proteins. *J Mol Biol* 2003;332:449–60.
69. Bradley P, Chivian D, Meiler J, Misura KMS, Rohl CA, Schief WR, et al. Rosetta predictions in CASP5: successes, failures, and prospects for complete automation. *Proteins* 2003;53:457–68.
70. Plecs JJ, Harbury PB, Kim PS, Alber T. Structural test of the parameterized-backbone method for protein design. *J Mol Biol* 2004;342:289–97.
71. Korkegian A, Black ME, Baker D, Stoddard BL. Computational thermostabilization of an enzyme. *Science* 2005;308:857–60.
72. Liu HY, Elstner M, Kaxiras E, Frauenheim T, Hermans J, Yang WT. Quantum mechanics simulation of protein dynamics on long timescale. *Proteins* 2001;44: 484–9.
73. Kussell E, Shimada J, Shakhnovich EI. A structure-based method for derivation of all-atom potentials for protein folding. *Proc Natl Acad Sci USA* 2002;99: 5343–8.
74. Chhajer M, Crippen GM. Toward correct protein folding potentials. *J Biol Phys* 2004;30:171–85.
75. Fujitsuka Y, Takada S, Luthey-Schulten ZA, Wolynes PG. Optimizing physical energy functions for protein folding. *Proteins* 2004;54:88–103.
76. Liang SD, Grishin NV. Effective scoring function for protein sequence design. *Proteins* 2004;54:271–81.
77. Chen WW, Shakhnovich EI. Lessons from the design of a novel atomic potential for protein folding. *Protein Sci* 2005;14:1741–52.
78. Mirny LA, Shakhnovich EI. How to derive a protein folding potential? A new approach to an old problem. *J Mol Biol* 1996;264:1164–79.
79. Vendruscolo M, Najmanovich R, Domany E. Can a pairwise contact potential stabilize native protein folds against decoys obtained by threading? *Proteins* 2000;38:134–48.

15

COMPUTER ALGORITHMS FOR SELECTING MOLECULE LIBRARIES FOR SYNTHESIS

KONSTANTIN V. BALAKIN, NIKOLAY P. SAVCHUK, AND ALEX KISELYOV

Contents

> Designing a combinatorial library is a controversial art that involves a heterogeneous mix of chemistry, mathematics, economics, experience, and intuition.
>
> —D. Agrafiotis

Computer Applications in Pharmaceutical Research and Development, Edited by Sean Ekins.
ISBN 0-471-73779-8

15.1 INTRODUCTION

In the field of drug design, chemists and biologists have always followed some rational guidelines for prioritizing candidate molecules for synthesis, depending on the state of knowledge at the time. The systematic effort in the computational design of chemical libraries was initiated in 1962–1964 by the pioneering works of Corwin Hansch, who laid the foundations of quantitative structure-activity relationship (QSAR) analysis. Further approaches in this discipline were developed in parallel with progress in combinatorial chemistry, molecular modeling, cheminformatics, protein crystallography, and data mining. As it is impossible to cite all the relevant work, the reader is referred to a number of books and reviews that summarize early advances in this area [1–4].

In the new millennium, pharmaceutical drug discovery is undergoing tremendous changes because of the progress in genomic research and the massive impact of combinatorial synthesis and high-throughput biological screening. Although these important modern technologies now provide incredible opportunities to pharmaceutical researchers, there are some serious problems associated with the effect of the combinatorial explosion. The costs of high-throughput screening (HTS) or parallel synthesis per one sample may be very low, but they become fairly expensive when multiplied by millions of compounds. Moreover, several papers report that the large number of compounds synthesized and screened do not necessarily result in an increase in viable drug candidates [5]. Therefore, there is a vital need for the development of novel technologies in order to increase the cost-effectiveness of combinatorial synthesis and library design.

The main objective of a rational library design is the selection of synthetic candidates that possess desirable properties. The "cornerstones" of this process are depicted in Figure 15.1. Initially, research efforts were focused on maximizing diversity [6, 7], sometimes with the introduction of biased pharmacophoric structural motifs. Subsequently, a medicinal chemistry component has been introduced, resulting in drug- and leadlike libraries reflecting the need for soluble molecules with an optimized in vitro PK profile. Further interest in concise screening campaigns yielded biased libraries that are focused on a single biological target or a family of related targets (kinases, G protein-coupled receptors, nuclear receptors, and so forth). Various ligand- and target structure-based design strategies can be implemented in focused library design when a set of known active ligands or the 3D structure of the target is available. Additional design elements include cost, synthetic feasibility, and physicochemical, pharmacokinetic, and toxicity properties. These parameters are taken into account by the knowledge-based approaches when relevant experimental and calculated information empowers the knowledge-oriented process of rational library design. Moreover, modern computational approaches allow for the simultaneous optimization of several variables. These allow a library designer to (1)

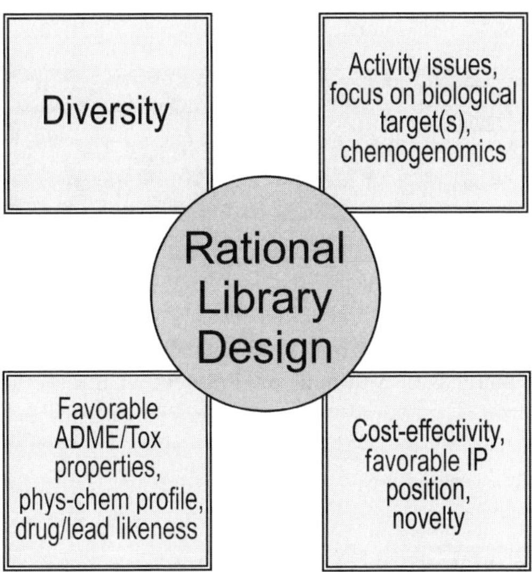

Figure 15.1 "Cornerstones" of rational library design. Modern design strategies require integrative approaches to address many important issues.

control the relative significance of various objectives and (2) intelligently select compounds for synthesis.

In this chapter, we provide an overview of selected advances in computational algorithms for the rational selection of molecule libraries for synthesis. Specifically, the following conceptually and algorithmically diverse topics are addressed:

1. Ligand structure-based design
2. Target structure-based approaches
3. Chemogenomics approaches
4. Design based on special data mining algorithms
5. Optimization of ADME/Tox properties
6. Multiobjective optimization.

15.2 LIGAND STRUCTURE-BASED DESIGN

Historically, ligand structure-based design has been the most widely used approach to the design of target-directed chemical libraries. Methods that start from hits or leads are among the most diverse, ranging from 2D substructure search and similarity-based techniques to analysis of 3D pharmacophores and molecular interaction fields (Fig. 15.2).

Specific structural fragments of biologically active molecules can be used as the core elements for generating targeted libraries. The most straightfor-

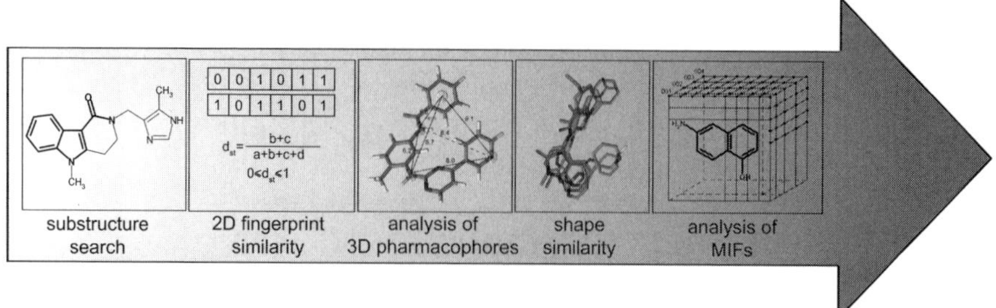

Figure 15.2 Historical progress of ligand structure-based approaches: from substructure search to analysis of 3-dimensional molecular interaction fields.

ward approach is related to 2D substructure search for analogs of known ligands [8]. So called "privileged" substructures [9, 10] have been applied successfully in the framework of the ligand-based strategy. Target-directed libraries based on privileged substructures can be effectively designed without any prior knowledge of the structure of the endogenous ligand, which in turn means that even orphan receptors can be addressed as potential drug targets [11]. Limitations of this approach include the restricted availability of privileged substructures for known target families and related intellectual property issues.

Another group of methods address molecular similarity. A comprehensive review of these is beyond the scope of this paper [12–14]; however, we provide general comments on these useful algorithms. Similarity methods include two independent aspects: representation of the molecules and assessment of their similarity. For example, calculation of similarity of 2D molecular fingerprints represents a relatively simple yet practical library design principle. It is frequently used to select molecules that have diverse structures but similar activities [15]. According to another approach, individual library compounds were represented by Kier–Hall topological descriptors, and molecular similarities between compounds were evaluated quantitatively by modified pairwise euclidean distances in multidimensional descriptor space [16]. This method, called Focus-2D, represents a useful approach to the rational design of targeted combinatorial libraries.

Moving beyond the analysis of 2D structural representations, virtual libraries can be searched with 3D molecular queries [17, 18]. 3D pharmacophore fingerprints detect the presence of predefined pharmacophores in a molecule by a systematic conformational searching method [19, 20]. Researchers at Tripos have developed a topomer-shape similarity searching method, an algorithm that identifies similar compounds by comparing steric interactions between a given query and molecules in a virtual library [21, 22]. This patented technology can effectively generate target-specific libraries around the known ligands used as input queries.

The computational ligand-based strategies are currently progressing toward advanced field fit-based methods. Thus researchers from the University of Florence have set up a novel computational procedure, FIGO (field interaction and geometrical overlap), for the 3D alignment of structures [23]. The alignment of the molecules occurs through the superposition of both the molecular interaction fields (MIFs) for a set of compounds and the heavy atoms (no hydrogens) of their chemical skeleton. The FIGO procedure involves the calculation of MIFs with hydrogen bond acceptor and donor probes as well as factors related to the hydrophobicity and shape of the molecules. This algorithm represents a valid alternative to docking methods in reproducing the orientation of ligands in their binding sites, particularly when the 3D structure of the target is unknown [24].

In general, ligand structure-based methods remain indispensable in those cases when the structure of binding site of the target protein is unknown.

15.3 TARGET STRUCTURE-BASED APPROACHES

Because of the rapidly increasing availability of target protein structures that can be used as templates for virtual screening, combinatorial synthesis and target structure-based design have begun to converge in the process of drug discovery. Many lead generation programs include analysis of X-ray structures of therapeutic biotargets to prioritize compounds for HTS or to establish a tractable collection for lower-throughput assays [25]. A natural trend recognized in the past few years is the application of similar techniques for increasing the likelihood of including active compounds in a focused combinatorial library.

There are many examples from the literature in which combinatorial library synthesis has successfully complemented structure-based design techniques in drug discovery [26]. One novel prospective methodology, in our opinion, perfectly illustrates how the technological advances inherent to the docking approach can be used in the design of biologically diverse and representative chemical libraries. The methodology developed by researchers from MolSoft is based on the new "pocketome" concept [27]. The pocketome is a collection of all currently known "druggable" pocket shapes for a given organism derived from the three-dimensional structures deposited in the Protein Data Bank [28] as well as some validated homology models for known drug targets. The real and hypothetical druggable envelopes are derived with a novel algorithm developed by MolSoft [29]. This algorithm can be used to compile a pocketome, a comprehensive and normalized collection of the unique binding envelopes. Researchers from MolSoft and the Scripps Research Institute have recently completed a large-scale classification of the identified envelopes according to their shape and properties (Totrov M, Abagyan R, personal communication).

In the past few years, we have witnessed a rapid progress in the development of powerful computational technologies that combine elements of structure-based design and combinatorial chemistry [27, 30–34]. Several examples are shown in Table 15.1. Computational programs developed on the basis of these approaches generally start from a synthetically accessible combinatorial template that is complimentary to a target binding site. A database of available building blocks for each point of randomization is then considered. The substituents are selected on the basis of their ability to (1) interact with a specific residue(s) in the active site and (2) couple with the template through accessible synthetic reactions compatible with the combinatorial protocol (synthetic feasibility). The generated list of accessible virtual ligands is then computationally screened against the active site and ranked on the basis of the scoring function available. For example, starting with a combinatorial template positioned in the active site of the target protein, the PRO_SELECT program uses a special scoring function to rank potential substituents at each position on the template [30]. Based on the calculated score, a target-specific library of synthetically accessible molecules is then generated, which may then be prioritized for synthesis and assay.

Alternatively, knowledge of the active site parameters can be used for the generation of pharmacophore hypotheses that are then applied for library design. Thus researchers from DuPont Pharmaceuticals [35] generated active site maps for several protein structures and then enumerated possible pharmacophores as bitstrings via pairwise encoding of the distances between features. The pharmacophores define a design space that can be used to select compounds with an informative library design tool. The method was used in prioritizing molecules biased against a cyclin-dependent kinase target, CDK-2. Researchers at Vernalis developed a set of strategies to address receptor flexibility (CDK-2 and HSP90) in virtual screening experiments using multiple crystallographic structures [36]. Based on their assessment, the combination of a flexible receptor docking algorithm and a robust scoring scheme for hits resulted in a significant improvement of binding affinities.

Customized algorithms, which combine combinatorial library design tools with structure-based design techniques, are viewed by both scientific and business communities as a serious competitive advantage. Despite this fact, there are several key questions about these products. What are the performance and limitations of the approaches? Is the method properly validated? Is the user interface convenient? Are the programs compatible with other industry-standard chemoinformatics platforms? Questions such as these must be taken into consideration when implementing these programs for target-directed research. It should also be noted that most of these technologies are still in their infancy, and future practical work will validate their role in contemporary drug discovery.

The practical utility of the target-structure-based approach in the design of chemical libraries is still limited because of the requirement of quality crystallographic data, detailed knowledge of the ligand binding mode, and

TABLE 15.1 Specialized Computational Technologies for Target Structure-Based Design of Combinatorial Libraries

Program	Description	Developer	Reference
PRO_SELECT	One of the first reported tools for the virtual screening of libraries for fit into a protein active site	Protherics Molecular Design Ltd. http://www.protherics.com	[30]
DREAM++	A set of programs (ORIENT++, REACT++ and SEARCH++) for docking computationally generated ligands into macromolecular binding sites	University of California	[31]
FlexX^C	An extension of the FlexX docking program which increases the efficiency of the docking of combinatorial libraries	Tripos, Inc. http://www.tripos.com	[32]
OptiDOCK	An extension of the CombiDOCK methodology, which selects a diverse but representative subset of compounds that span the structural space encompassed by the full library	Tripos, Inc. http://www.tripos.com	[33]
CombiGlide	A combinatorial version of the Glide algorithm which can be used for the design of focused libraries	Schrodinger, Inc. http://www.schrodinger.com	[34]
ICM PocketFinder	An advanced approach based on the ICM method of flexible docking and the "pocketome" approach	Molsoft LLC http://www.molsoft.com	[27]

inherent issues concerning scoring functions (see Chapter 14). The stepwise procedure of selection and filtering with simpler ligand-based technologies can reduce the virtual databases to a manageable size. Such a prescreening procedure leaves the high-ranking molecules for further analysis by biostructure-based docking and scoring and thus provides both activity enrichment and structural novelty [37].

15.4 CHEMOGENOMICS APPROACHES

The effective identification of high-quality hits and leads across diverse classes of therapeutic targets can be based on the systematic analysis of structural genomics data [38, 39]. The latest human genome initiatives allow for establishing relationships between ligands and targets and thus offer the potential to use the knowledge obtained in the screening experiments for "target hopping."

Several approaches to link chemogenomics data and the generation of target-directed libraries have been reported. The key element of this knowledge space is the ligand-target matrix [40], which represents a comprehensive data source suitable for effective data mining (Fig. 15.3). The collection of properly annotated ligand-target databases can help aid in the understanding of the mechanism and evaluate the potential target specificity of small molecule ligands. Thus a method was recently reported for testing many biological mechanisms and related biotargets in cellular assays with an annotated compound library [41]. Another annotation scheme was described by Jacoby et al. for the ligands of four major target classes, enzymes, G protein-coupled receptors (GPCRs), nuclear receptors (NRs), and ligand-gated ion channels (LGICs) for *in silico* screening and combinatorial design of targeted libraries [42]. Retrospective *in silico* screening experiments have shown that such reference sets can be useful for the identification of ligands binding to receptors closely related to the reference system. The same group of researchers reported a modified [43] homology-based similarity search based on special molecular representations, Similog keys. A recent report by Mestres et al. described an annotated compound library directed to nuclear receptors [44]. Such a systematic exploration of the ligand-target matrix for selected target families appears to be a promising way to speed up the target-directed drug discovery.

15.5 LIBRARY DESIGN BASED ON SPECIAL DATA MINING ALGORITHMS

Pharmaceutical lead discovery and optimization have historically followed a sequential process in which relatively small sets of individual compounds are

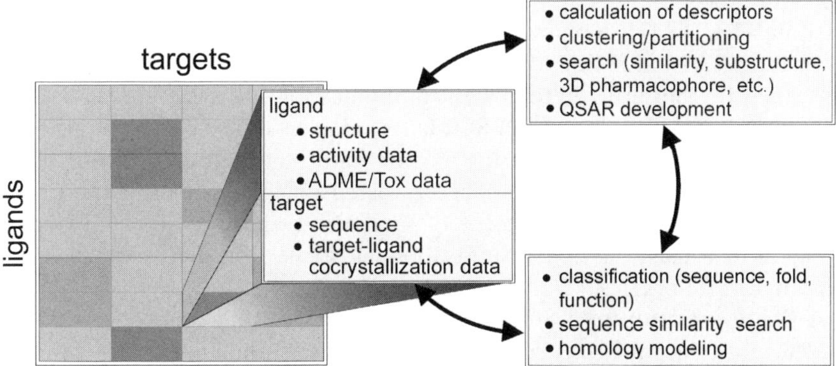

Figure 15.3 Annotated ligand-target knowledge space.

synthesized and tested for bioactivity. The information obtained from such experiments is then used for the selection of further molecules. With the advent of high-throughput synthesis and screening technologies, the fairly simple statistical technique of data analysis has been largely replaced by a massive parallel mode of processing, in which many thousands of molecules are synthesized and tested. As a result, the complete analysis of large sets of diverse molecules and their structural activity patterns has become an emerging problem. Hence, there is considerable interest in novel computational approaches that may be applied to the extraction and utilization of useful information from such data sets. In this section, we review the most frequently employed data mining algorithms that deal with library design based on screening results.

15.5.1 Visualization Techniques

Visual analysis of multivariate data sets has established itself as a powerful means of data mining to detect nonobvious and relevant information for further exploitation. In particular, topology and distance preserving mappings, for example, using the self-organizing feature map (SOM) of Kohonen [45] or the distance preserving nonlinear mapping (NLM) of Sammon [46], are well suited for data visualization and data mining purposes.

The general idea of self-organizing maps or Kohonen networks is to map a set of vectorial samples onto a two-dimensional lattice in a way that preserves the topology of the original space. Kohonen maps have been actively used for the analysis and visualization of large data sets originating from screening campaigns. In particular, Kohonen maps appeared to be effective in the analysis of large databases created and hosted by the National Cancer Institute (NCI) [47]. Kohonen maps were used by Gasteiger et al. for the analysis and visualization of HTS data: The developed structure-activity model was further utilized to design candidates for new sweeteners [48]. The same group of researchers used SOMs for analysis of structure-activity relationships for 5513 compounds from a combinatorial library [49]. Based on the results of these studies, the authors suggested that the self-organizing maps can serve not only as an indicator of structure-activity relationships but as the basis of a classification system allowing for the predictive modeling of combinatorial libraries.

A fine illustration of a SOM-based virtual screening procedure that was used to construct focused combinatorial libraries and to identify products with optimized biological properties against the human A_{2A} purinergic receptor has been reported [50]. A SOM was developed with a 153-member combinatorial library of general **structure 1** (Fig. 15.4). This set was tested to establish a preliminary structure-activity relationship. For SAR modeling by self-organizing networks, all molecules were represented by the CATS pharmacophore descriptor, which is based on a topological correlation of generalized atom types. The secondary combinatorial library design was performed by projecting virtually assembled new molecules onto the SOM. As a result, a small, focused library of 17 selected combinatorial products was synthesized and tested. On average, this small library displayed a 3-fold lower binding constant and 3.5-fold higher selectivity than the initial library. The most selective compound of the product library (Fig. 15.4) has a 121-fold relative selectivity for the A_{2A} receptor.

In contrast to SOMs, nonlinear maps (NLMs) represent relative distances between all pairs of compounds in the descriptor space of a 2D map. The distance between two points on the map directly reflects the similarity of the

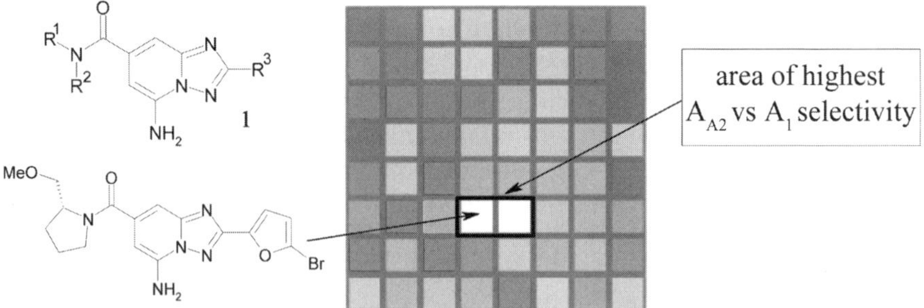

Figure 15.4 Self-organizing maps showing the distribution of selectivity values [K_i (A_1)/K_i (A_{2A})] of the initial 153-member library **1**, and position of the most selective compound from the secondary combinatorial library [50].

compounds [46]. NLMs have previously been used for the visualization of protein sequence relationships in two dimensions, and comparisons between large compound collections, represented by a set of molecular descriptors [51]. However, for large data sets, the NLM computation becomes more and more intractable. In addition, the approach may generate a 2D mapping that poorly approximates the original distances when the number of compounds is large. Several heuristic variants were introduced to alleviate the NLM complexity problem and make it useful for mapping large data sets [52–56]. Usually, a significant speed gain can be achieved by these modified approaches as compared to NLM. At the same time, they provide better distance and topology preservation compared with Kohonen maps.

The described computational tools provide interactive, fast, and flexible data visualizations of chemical data that help and even enhance the human thought processes. However, visualization alone is often inadequate when multiple data points must be considered. A number of data mining methods that seek to identify significant relationships in large multidimensional databases are now being used for library design.

15.5.2 Partitioning Methods

The simplest and fastest techniques for grouping molecules are partitioning methods. Every molecule is represented by a point in an n-dimensional space, the axes of which are defined by the n components of the descriptor vector. The range of values for each component is then subdivided into a set of subranges (or bins). As a result, the entire multidimensional space is partitioned into a number of hypercubes (or cells) of fixed size, and every molecule (represented as a point in this space) falls into one of these cells [57].

Recursive partitioning (RP) has been possibly the most prominent partitioning method for mining bioscreening data and designing libraries. Thus Rusinko, Young, and colleagues established the RP approach for the analysis and mining of large screening data sets [58, 59]. Using RP analysis of the biological activity of a publicly available set of 1650 MAO inhibitors, they designed a screening library, for which a 15-fold improvement in hit rate over random selection was achieved [58]. Another study has demonstrated that it is possible to design targeted libraries by applying RP to large data sets containing thousands of compounds and their associated data [60]. Analysis of a screening data set revealed an approximately four- to fivefold increase in hit rate by application of RP models. The most attractive features of RP are its extreme speed and efficiency, as well as its ability to analyze very large data sets encoded by hundreds of thousands of descriptors and to effectively work with localized and unbalanced data. At the same time, RP has several disadvantages. For example, a single descriptor may not provide adequate information for the splitting process. In addition, single trees are unstable. Often, a minor change in the data can result in a very different tree, with a very distinct series of splits.

To overcome some of the specific problems inherent to this method, the RP approach has been extended through combination with the components of other classification or simulation techniques. Such modifications involved the use of multiple recursion trees (recursion forests) [61], the simulated annealing (SA) algorithm [62], and multiple property recursive partitioning (PUMP-RP) analysis [63]. Significant improvements on the conventional RP method were achieved with the development of a cell-based partitioning algorithm [64], median partitioning [65], and phylogenetic-like trees [66]. It has been demonstrated that these modifications improve the data extraction process and increase the amount of relevant information from screening results.

15.5.3 Classification Methods

Partitioning methods occasionally struggle to provide the accuracy associated with more powerful, albeit less informative techniques such as machine learning and statistical approaches. For this reason, there is a continuing need for the application of more accurate and informative classification techniques to QSAR analysis. The goal of a classifier is to produce a model that can separate new, untested compounds into classes with a training set of already classified compounds.

It is important that QSAR methods are quick, give unambiguous models, do not rely on any subjective decisions about the functional relationships between structure and activity, and are easy to validate. In the past 10–15 years, methods based on artificial neural networks (ANNs) have been shown to overcome some of these problems. For example, they can manage both linear and nonlinear SARs observed in real practice. There are reports that describe the successful application of neural network algorithms to cluster compounds in large data sets with low signal-to-noise values. A recent review [67] on the concepts behind neural networks applied to QSAR analysis, points out problems that may be encountered, suggests ways of avoiding the pitfalls, and introduces several exciting new neural network methods discovered during the last decade.

The support vector machine (SVM) is a relatively recent data mining approach based on the structural risk minimization principle [68] from computational learning theory. SVMs construct a hyperplane that separates classes with a large margin to minimize generalization error. The SVM approach is considered to be at least as powerful and versatile as the ANNs. This algorithm has been customized to specific applications ranging from genomics to face recognition. Recently, the SVM was tested as a classification tool in several drug discovery programs associated with the analysis of experimental biological data [see, for example, 69].

Statistical methods can also be utilized to form probability models or to estimate the likelihood of particular descriptors forming the known classes. Chemical Computing Group Inc. has recently developed a new technology, called QuaSAR-Binary™, which is designed to analyze the results of HTS and make predictions regarding the biological activity of untested compounds. Binary QSAR based on a Bayesian inference technique is an approach for the analysis of bioscreening data by correlation of structural properties of compounds with a "binary" expression of biological activity. It calculates the distribution for active and inactive compounds in a training set [70]. It was demonstrated in several case studies that this method is resistant to experimental errors and exhibits high accuracy. Another approach conceptually similar to binary QSAR—a machine-learning technique known as binary kernel discrimination—has recently been introduced [71]. Two examples described a two- to fourfold enrichment in hit rate when this method was used over a random selection.

15.5.4 Clustering Methods

The goal in clustering a data set is to group similar data together. Clustering forms groups of compounds that maximize internal class similarity while simultaneously minimizing external class similarity. Clustering can be accomplished by either a supervised method, where the number of classes is known, or through unsupervised learning, where the data are not grouped into a fixed set of classes. There are a variety of available clustering algorithms that can be used for analysis of bioscreening data [72]. These include hierarchical and nonhierarchical methods.

A hierarchical clustering (HC) method produces a classification in which smaller clusters of very similar molecules are nested within ever-increasing larger clusters of less closely related molecules. For example, HC analysis has been used for identifying subgroups of compounds related to particular biological targets and for determining the mechanisms of antitumor activity of compounds against the NCI panel of 60 cell lines [73, 74]. A nonhierarchical clustering method generates a classification by partitioning a data set. It further yields a set of generally nonoverlapping groups that have no hierarchical relationships between them. Such methods are less demanding of computational resources than the hierarchical methods. One of the prominent reports of large-scale clustering for compound selection described a system implemented at Pfizer that was based on this method [75]. The system proved to be highly appropriate for the clustering of 240,000 chemical structures represented by 1315 structural fragments.

In general, the described techniques provide an effective, flexible, and relatively fast solution for library design based on analysis of bioscreening data. The quantitative relationships, based on the assessment of contribution values of various molecular descriptors, not only permit the estimation of potential biological activity of candidate compounds before synthesis but also provide information concerning the modification of the structural features necessary for this activity. Usually these techniques are applied in the form of computational filters for constraining the size of virtual combinatorial libraries and selecting the best candidates for synthesis and bioscreening. Modern methods and algorithms of clustering, cell-based partitioning, and other distance-based approaches are reviewed in a recent work [76].

15.6 OPTIMIZATION OF ADME/TOX PROPERTIES

Poor pharmacokinetics and toxicity are important causes of costly late-stage failures in drug development. It is generally recognized that, in addition to optimized potency and specificity, chemical libraries should also possess favorable ADME/Tox and druglike properties [77–80]. Assessment of drug-like character is an attempt to decipher molecular features that are likely to lead to a successful in vivo and, ultimately, clinical candidate [81–83]. Many of these properties can be predicted before molecules are synthesized, purchased, or even tested in order to improve overall lead and library quality.

Considerable research efforts have focused on novel machine learning algorithms that predict ADME/Tox properties of new chemical entities. These calculations can be performed with an extremely large number of molecules and act as a form of multidimensional selection filter. For example, comparative molecular fields analysis (CoMFA) and pharmacophore approaches [for review, see 84, 85] have been used to model binding modes of metabolizing cytochrome P450 (CYP) enzymes as well as transporters such as P-glycoprotein [86], nuclear hormone receptors [87], and ion channels [88] important for drug-drug interactions. Recursive partitioning methods have been used extensively with these large sets of molecules and either continuous or binary data [89, 90]. Kohonen self-organizing maps have only recently been applied to model cytochrome P450-mediated drug metabolism [91], and *k*-nearest neighbors has been used to predict metabolic stability [92].

To date, many of the reported ADME/Tox models have been rule based. For example, some research groups have used relatively simple filters like the rule of 5 [93] and others [94] to limit the types of molecules evaluated with *in silico* methods and to focus libraries for HTS. However, being designed as rapid "computational alert" tools aimed at a single property of interest, they cannot offer a comprehensive picture when it comes to understanding ADME properties.

Multivariate data mining techniques can serve as the basis for advanced ADME filters. Thus we have developed a method for early evaluation of several important pharmacokinetic parameters, including volume of distribution and plasma half-life [95]. These two parameters determine the dose regimen of a drug, and therefore the early prediction of both properties would be of a great benefit. It was demonstrated that such complex properties can be effectively modeled with the nonlinear mapping algorithms based on a preselected set of electronic, topological, spatial, and structural descriptors (Fig. 15.5). Generated models demonstrated good predictive power in the internal and external validation experiments, with up to 80–90% compounds

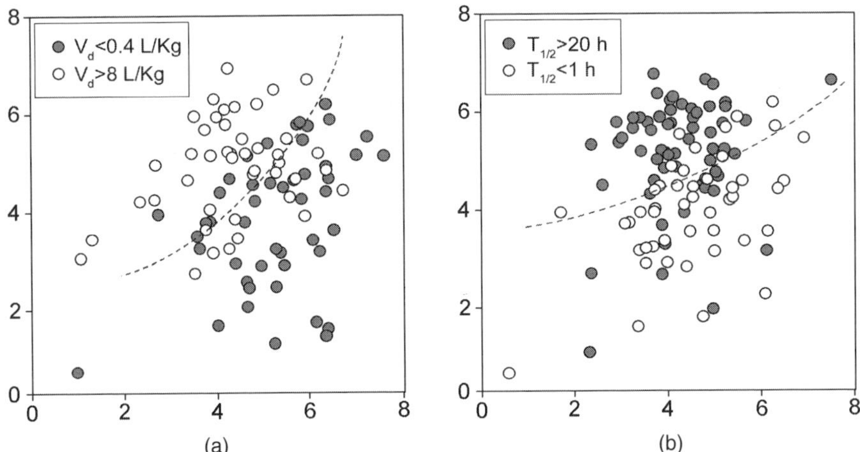

Figure 15.5 Sammon map with SVM classification of drugs based on their volume of distribution (a) and plasma half-life (b) [95].

classified accurately. The accuracy level achieved can be used as a guide in modifying and optimizing these pharmacokinetic properties in chemical libraries before synthesis.

The collection of algorithms for prediction of a number of ADME/Tox-related properties is now integrated in the Smart Mining/ADMET software suite available from ChemDiv. These algorithms were initially validated on human intestinal absorption, blood-brain barrier, plasma half-life, volume of distribution, plasma protein binding [95], CYP450 substrate/nonsubstrate potential [91], as well as cytochrome P450 binding affinity [96] models. These algorithms have been further extended to the evaluation of important physicochemical properties such as DMSO solubility [97] and target-specific activity [98]. Although other software tools for ADME modeling are available [for example, 83, 99], the Smart Mining-based collection of predictive classification tools is both extensive and well validated in multiple library design projects. These methods are particularly suited for the rapid evaluation of both large and medium-sized compound libraries in connection with early ADME/Tox profiling.

15.7 MULTIOBJECTIVE OPTIMIZATION

Knowledge-based data mining algorithms used for correlation of molecular properties with specific activities play an increasingly significant role in modern strategies of chemical library design as relatively inexpensive, yet comprehensive tools. The ability to identify compounds with the desired target-specific activity and to optimize a large number of other molecular parameters (such as ADME/Tox-related properties, lead- and drug-likeness) in a parallel fashion is a characteristic feature of these methods. In the latter case, library design can be considered a multiobjective optimization problem, which has become a topic of growing interest over the last decade in the pharmaceutical industry.

The general idea of multiobjective optimization is to incorporate as much knowledge into the design as possible. Ideally, many factors should be taken into consideration, such as diversity, similarity to known actives, favorable physicochemical and ADME/Tox profile, cost of the library, and many other properties. Several groups have developed computational approaches to allow multiobjective optimization of library design [100, 101]. One method developed by researchers from 3-Dimensional Pharmaceuticals (now Johnson & Johnson) employs an objective function that encodes all of the desired selection criteria and then identifies an optimal subset from the vast number of possibilities [101]. The overall architecture of this approach is shown in Figure 15.6. An optimizer (in this case, a serial or parallel implementation of simulated annealing) produces a state (that is, a collection of subsets from one or more chemical libraries), which is evaluated against all of the desired selection criteria. These are combined into a unifying objective function, which measures the overall fitness of that state—that is, its ability to collectively satisfy all of the specified selection criteria. This fitness value is used by the optimizer to produce a new set of compounds (a new state), which is in turn evaluated against the prescribed selection criteria. The process continues until a predefined termination criterion is met, and the best state identified during the course of the simulation is reported. This approach allows for the

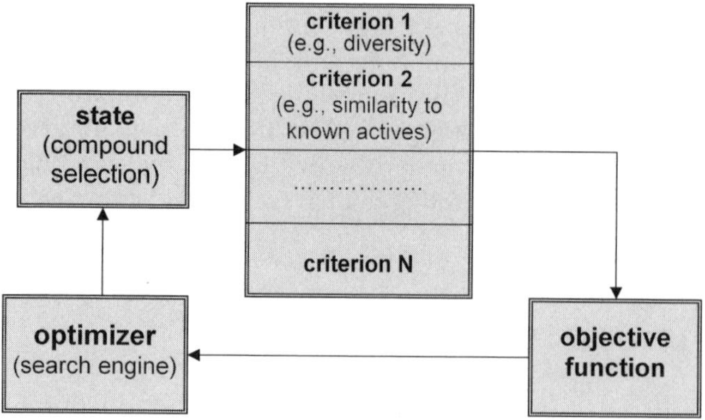

Figure 15.6 Overall architecture of approach used for multiobjective compound selection [101].

simultaneous selection of compounds from multiple libraries and offers the user full control over the relative significance of a number of objectives. These objectives include similarity, diversity, predicted activity, overlap of one set of compounds with another set, property distribution and others. An overview of the general methodology for designing combinatorial and HTS experiments rooted in the principles of multiobjective optimization has been recently presented by Agrafiotis [101].

15.8 CONCLUSIONS

Analysis of information contained within the human genome along with innovations in combinatorial synthesis and biological screening provides new opportunities in the design of novel effective drugs. However, despite the fact that these high-throughput technologies have become common within the modern drug discovery process, their accuracy and efficiency require further improvement. A possible solution is the development and adoption of several novel computational technologies for making combinatorial library design cost-effective.

Over the past few years, various computational concepts and methods have been introduced to extract relevant information from the accumulated knowledge of chemists and biologists and to create a robust basis for rational design of chemical libraries. The obvious trend is that molecular diversity alone cannot be considered to be a sufficient library design criterion. We can also observe a clear shift from the ligand-structure-based methods toward more sophisticated docking algorithms to aid in library design. At the same time, rapid, reliable, and conceptually simple ligand-based strategies are still very useful as prescreening procedures, especially in cases where the structure of a target is unknown. Knowledge-based methods successfully complement the above-mentioned strategies to create information-rich compound collections optimized by consideration of multiple parameters.

Today, the computational community is still in the process of identifying the optimal strategy required for rational library design, and currently there is a trend to combine the existing approaches to achieve better performance. Computational chemistry, bio- and cheminformatics, and chemogenomics all contribute to the development of this strategy. The ultimate goal of the research effort in this field, as with others, is to reduce costs and to accelerate the discovery of novel drugs.

ACKNOWLEDGMENTS

The authors would like to thank Dr. Yan A. Ivanenkov for his assistance in analysis of the literature and preparation of the manuscript.

REFERENCES

1. Kubinyi H. QSAR: Hanch analysis and related approaches. In: Mannhold R, Krogsgaard-Larsen P, Timmerman H, editors, *Methods and principles in medicinal chemistry,* Vol. 1. Weinheim: VCH, 1993.
2. Corey EJ, Long AK, Rubenstein SD. Computer-assisted analysis in organic synthesis. *Science* 1985;228:408–18.
3. Tute MS. History and objectives of quantitative drug design. In: Hansch C, Sammes PG, Taylor JB, editors, *Quantitative drug design (Comprehensive Medicinal Chemistry, Vol. 4).* Oxford: Pergamon Press, 1990. p. 1–31.
4. Purcell WP, Bass GE, Clayton JM. *Strategy of drug design. A molecular guide to biological activity.* New York: John Wiley & Sons, 1973.
5. Oprea TI. Chemical space navigation in lead discovery. *Curr Opin Chem Biol* 2002;6:384–9.
6. Dean PM, Lewis RA. *Molecular diversity in drug design.* Dordrecht: Kluwer Academic Publishers, 1999.
7. Agrafiotis D. Diversity of chemical libraries. In: Allinger NL, Clark T, Gasteiger J, Kollman PA, Schaefer HF III, Schreiner PR, editors, *Encyclopedia of computational chemistry.* Chichester: Wiley, 1998. p. 742–61.
8. Merlot C, Domine D, Cleva C, Church DJ. Chemical substructures in drug discovery. *Drug Discov Today* 2003;8:594–602.
9. Patchett AA, Nargund RP. Privileged structures—an update. *Annu Rep Med Chem* 2000;35:289–98.
10. Muller G. Medicinal chemistry of target family-directed masterkeys. *Drug Discov Today* 2003;8:681–91.
11. Bondensgaard K, Ankersen M, Thogersen H, Hansen BS, Wulff BS, Bywater RP. Recognition of privileged structures by G-protein coupled receptors. *J Med Chem* 2004;47:888–99.
12. Johnson MA, Maggiora GM. *Concepts and applications of molecular similarity.* New York: John Wiley & Sons, 1990.
13. Downs GM, Willett P. Similarity searches in databases of chemical structures. *Rev Comput Chem* 1995;7:1–66.
14. Sheridan RP, Kearsley SK. Why do we need so many chemical similarity search methods? *Drug Disc Today* 2002;7:903–11.
15. Xue L, Stahura FL, Godden JW, Bajorath J. Mini-fingerprints detect similar activity of receptor ligands previously recognized only by three-dimensional pharmacophore-based methods. *J Chem Inf Comp Sci* 2001;41:394–401.
16. Zheng W, Cho SJ, Tropsha A. Rational combinatorial library design 1 Focus-2D: a new approach to the design of targeted combinatorial chemical libraries. *J Chem Inf Comput Sci* 1998;38:251–8.
17. Martin YC. 3D database searching in drug design. *J Med Chem* 1992;35:2145–54.
18. Mason JS, Good AC, Martin EJ. 3D pharmacophores in drug discovery. *Curr Pharm Des* 2001;7:567–97.
19. Mason JS, Morize I, Menard PR, Cheney DL, Hulme C, Labaudiniere RF. New 4-point pharmacophore method for molecular similarity and diversity applica-

tions: overview of the method and applications, including a novel approach to the design of combinatorial libraries containing privileged substructures. *J Med Chem* 1999;42:3251–64.

20. Makara GM. Measuring molecular similarity and diversity: total pharmacophore diversity. *J Med Chem* 2001;44:3563–71.
21. Andrews KM, Cramer RD. Toward general methods of targeted library design: topomer shape similarity searching with diverse structures as queries. *J Med Chem* 2000;43:1723–40.
22. Cramer RD, Jilek RJ, Andrews KM. Dbtop: topomer similarity searching of conventional structure databases. *J Mol Graph Model* 2002;20:447–62.
23. Melani F, Gratteri P, Adamo M, Bonaccini C. Field interaction and geometrical overlap (FIGO): a new simplex/experimental design-based computational procedure for superposing small ligand molecules. *J Med Chem* 2003;46: 1359–71.
24. Gratteri P, Bonaccini C, Melani F. Searching for a reliable orientation of ligands in their binding site: comparison between a structure-based (glide) and a ligand-based (FIGO) approach in the case study of PDE4 inhibitors. *J Med Chem* 2005;48:1657–65.
25. Laird ER, Blake JF. Structure-based generation of viable leads from small combinatorial libraries. *Curr Opin Drug Discov Devel* 2004;7:354–9.
26. Tondi D, Costi MP. Enhancing the drug discovery process by integration of structure-based design and combinatorial synthesis. In: Viswanadhan AK, Ghose VN, editors, *Combinatorial library design and evaluation.* New York: Marcel Dekker, 2001. p. 563–604.
27. An J, Totrov M, Abagyan R. Comprehensive identification of "druggable" protein ligand binding sides. *Genome Informatics* 2004;15:31–41.
28. Berman HM, Westbrook J, Feng Z, Gilliland G, Bhat TN, Weissig H, Shindyalov IN, Bourne PE. The protein data bank. *Nucleic Acids Res* 2000;28:235–42.
29. Cavasotto C, Orry AJW, Abagyan RA. Structure-based identification of binding sites, native ligands and potential inhibitors for G-protein coupled receptors. *Proteins Structure Funct Genet* 2003;51:423–33.
30. Murray CW, Clark DE, Auton TR, Firth MA, Li J, Sykes RA, Waszkowycz B, Westhead DR, Young SC. PRO_SELECT: combining structure-based drug design and combinatorial chemistry for rapid lead discovery. *J Comput Aided Mol Des* 1997;11:193–207.
31. Makino S, Ewing TJ, Kuntz ID. DREAM++: flexible docking program for virtual combinatorial libraries. *J Comput Aided Mol Des* 1999;13:513–32.
32. Rarey M, Lengauer T. A recursive algorithm for efficient combinatorial library docking perspective in drug discovery and design. *Perspect Drug Discov Des* 2000;20:63–81.
33. Sprous DG, Lowis DR, Leonard JM, Heritage T, Burkett SN, Baker DS, Clark RD. OptiDock: virtual HTS of combinatorial libraries by efficient sampling of binding modes in product space. *J Comb Chem* 2004;6:530–9.
34. Friesner RA, Banks JL, Murphy RB, Halgren TA, Klicic JJ, Mainz DT, Repasky MP, Knoll EH, Shelley M, Perry JK, Shaw DE, Francis P, Shenkin PS. Glide: a new approach for rapid, accurate docking and scoring. 1. Method and assessment of docking accuracy. *J Med Chem* 2004;47:1739–49.

35. Eksterowicz JE, Evensen E, Lemmen C, Brady GP, Lanctot JK, Bradley EK, Saiah E, Robinson LA, Grootenhuis PDJ, Blaney JM. Coupling structure-based design with combinatorial chemistry: application of active site derived pharmacophores with informative library design. *J Mol Graph Model* 2002;20:469–77.
36. Barril X, Morley SD. Unveiling the full potential of flexible receptor docking using multiple crystallographic structures. *J Med Chem* 2005;48:4432–43.
37. Gruneberg S, Stubbs MT, Klebe G. Successful virtual screening for novel inhibitors of human carbonic anhydrase: strategy and experimental confirmation. *J Med Chem* 2002;45:3588–602.
38. Bredel M, Jacoby E. Chemogenomics: An emerging strategy for rapid target and drug discovery. *Nat Rev Genet* 2004;5:262–75.
39. Mestres J. Computational chemogenomics approaches to systematic knowledge-based drug discovery. *Curr Opin Drug Discov Dev* 2004;7:304–13.
40. Savchuk NP, Balakin KV, Tkachenko SE. Exploring the chemogenomic knowledge space with annotated chemical libraries. *Curr Opin Chem Biol* 2004;8:412–17.
41. Root DE, Flaherty SP, Kelley BP, Stockwell BR. Biological mechanism profiling using an annotated compound library. *Chem Biol* 2003;10:881–92.
42. Schuffenhauer A, Zimmermann J, Stoop R, van der Vyver JJ, Lecchini S, Jacoby E. An ontology for pharmaceutical ligands and its application for in silico screening and library design. *J Chem Inf Comput Sci* 2002;42:947–55.
43. Schuffenhauer A, Floersheim P, Acklin P, Jacoby E. Similarity metrics for ligands reflecting the similarity of the target proteins. *J Chem Inf Comp Sci* 2003;43:391–405.
44. Cases M, Garcia-Serna R, Hettne K, Weeber M, van der Lei J, Boyer S, Mestres J. Chemical and biological profiling of an annotated compound library directed to the nuclear receptor family. *Curr Top Med Chem* 2005;5:763–72.
45. Kohonen T. *Self-organizing maps,* 3rd edition. New York: Springer Verlag, 2000.
46. Sammon JE. A nonlinear mapping for data structure analysis. *IEEE Trans Comput* 1969; C-18:401–9.
47. Rabow AA, Shoemaker RH, Sausville EA, Covell DG. Mining the National Cancer Institute's tumor-screening database: identification of compounds with similar cellular activities. *J Med Chem* 2002;45:818–40.
48. Polanski J, Jarzembek K, Gasteiger J. Self-organizing neural networks for screening and development of novel artificial sweetener candidates. *Comb Chem High Throughput Screen* 2000;3:481–95.
49. Teckentrup A, Briem H, Gasteiger J. Mining high-throughput screening data of combinatorial libraries: development of a filter to distinguish hits from nonhits. *J Chem Inf Comput Sci* 2004;44:626–34.
50. Schneider G, Nettekoven M. Ligand-based combinatorial design of selective purinergic receptor (A2A) antagonists using self-organizing maps. *J Comb Chem* 2003;5:233–7.
51. Agrafiotis DK, Myslik JC, Salemme FR. Advances in diversity profiling and combinatorial series design. *Mol Div* 1999;4:1–22.

52. Agrafiotis DK, Lobanov VS. Nonlinear mapping networks. *J Chem Inf Comput Sci* 1997;40:1356–62.
53. Xie D, Tropsha A, Schlick T. An efficient projection protocol for chemical databases: singular value decomposition combined with truncated-newton minimization. *J Chem Inf Comput Sci* 2000;40:167–77.
54. Garrido L, Goméz S, Roca J. Improved multidimensional scaling analysis using neural networks with distance-error backpropagation. *Neural Comput* 1999;11:595–600.
55. Pal NR, Eluri VK. Two efficient connectionist schemes for structure preserving dimensionality reduction. *IEEE Trans Neural Networks* 1998;9:1142–54.
56. König A. Interactive visualization and analysis of hierarchical neural projections for data mining. *IEEE Trans Neural Networks* 2000;11:615–24.
57. Mason JS, Pickett SD. Partition-based selection. *Perspect Drug Discov Des* 1997;718:85–114.
58. Rusinko A 3rd, Farmen MW, Lambert CG, Brown PL, Young SS. Analysis of a large structure/biological activity data set using recursive partitioning. *J Chem Inf Comput Sci* 1999;39:1017–26.
59. Chen X, Rusinko A, Young SS. Recursive partitioning analysis of a large structure-activity data set using three-dimensional descriptors. *J Chem Inf Comput Sci* 1998;38:1054–62.
60. Van Rhee AM, Stocker J, Printzenhoff D, Creech C, Wagoner PK, Spear KL. Retrospective analysis of an experimental high-throughput screening data set by recursive partitioning. *J Comb Chem* 2001;3:267–77.
61. Van Rhee AM. Use of recursion forests in the sequential screening process: consensus selection by multiple recursion trees. *J Chem Inf Comput Sci* 2003;43:941–8.
62. Blower P, Fligner M, Verducci J, Bjoraker J. On combining recursive partitioning and simulated annealing to detect groups of biologically active compounds. *J Chem Inf Comput Sci* 2002;42:393–404.
63. Stockfisch TP. Partially unified multiple property recursive partitioning (PUMP-RP): a new method for predicting and understanding drug selectivity. *J Chem Inf Comput Sci* 2003;43:1608–13.
64. Xue L, Stahura FL, Bajorath J. Cell-based partitioning. *Methods Mol Biol* 2004;275:279–90.
65. Godden JW, Xue L, Bajorath J. Classification of biologically active compounds by median partitioning. *J Chem Inf Comput Sci* 2002;42:1263–9.
66. Nicolaou CA, Tamura SY, Kelley BP, Bassett SI, Nutt RF. Analysis of large screening data sets via adaptively grown phylogenetic-like trees. *J Chem Inf Comput Sci* 2002;42:1069–79.
67. Winkler DA. Neural networks as robust tools in drug lead discovery and development. *Mol Biotechnol* 2004;27:139–68.
68. Vapnik V. *Statistical learning theory*. New York: John Wiley & Sons, 1998.
69. Zernov VV, Balakin KV, Ivaschenko AA, Savchuk NP, Pletnev IV. Drug discovery using support vector machines. The case studies of drug-likeness, agrochemical-likeness, and enzyme inhibition predictions. *J Chem Inf Comput Sci* 2003;43:2048–56.

70. Gao H, Williams C, Labute P, Bajorath J. Binary quantitative structure-activity relationship (QSAR) analysis of estrogen receptor ligands. *J Chem Inf Comput Sci* 1999;39:164–8.

71. Harper G, Bradshaw J, Gittins JC, Green DV, Leach AR. Prediction of biological activity for high-throughput screening using binary kernel discrimination. *J Chem Inf Comput Sci* 2001;41:1295–300.

72. Downs GM, Willett P. Clustering of chemical structure databases for compound selection. In: van de Waterbeemd H, editor, *Advanced computer-assisted techniques in drug discovery*. Weinheim: VCH Verlag, 1994. p. 111–30.

73. Shi LM, Fan Y, Lee JK, Waltham M, Andrews DT, Scherf U, Paull KD, Weinstein JN. Mining and visualizing large anticancer drug discovery databases. *J Chem Inf Comput Sci* 2000;40:367–79.

74. Fan Y, Shi LM, Kohn KW, Pommier Y, Weinstein JN. Quantitative structure-antitumor activity relationships of camptothecin analogues: cluster analysis and genetic algorithm-based studies. *J Med Chem* 2001;44:3254–63.

75. Willett P, Winterman V, Bawden DJ. Implementation of non hierarchical cluster-analysis methods in chemical information-systems-selection of compounds for biological testing and clustering of substructure search output. *Chem Inf Comp Sci* 1986;26:109–18.

76. Lam RL, Welch WJ. Comparison of methods based on diversity and similarity for molecule selection and the analysis of drug discovery data. *Methods Mol Biol* 2004;275:301–16.

77. Lipinski CA. Drug-like properties and the causes of poor solubility and poor permeability. *J Pharm Toxicol Methods* 2000;44:235–49.

78. Walters WP, Murcko MA. Prediction of ‚drug-likeness‘. *Adv Drug Del Rev* 2002;54:255–71.

79. Oprea TI. Current trends in lead discovery: are we looking for the appropriate properties? *J Comput Aided Mol Des* 2002;16:325–34.

80. Wenlock MC, Austin RP, Barton P, Davis AM, Leeson PD. A comparison of physiochemical property profiles of development and marketed oral drugs. *J Med Chem* 2003;4:1250–6.

81. Ekins S, Boulanger B, Swaan PW, Hupcey MAZ. Towards a new age of virtual ADME/TOX and multidimensional drug discovery. *J Comput Aided Mol Des* 2002;16:381–401.

82. Ekins S, Rose JP. In silico ADME/Tox: the state of the art. *J Mol Graph* 2002;20:305–9.

83. Van de Waterbeemd H, Gifford E. ADMET in silico modelling: towards prediction paradise? *Nat Rev Drug Discov* 2003;2:192–204.

84. de Groot MJ, Ekins S. Pharmacophore modeling of cytochromes P450. *Adv Drug Del Rev* 2002;54:367–73.

85. Ekins S, de Groot M, Jones JP. Pharmacophore and three-dimensional quantitative structure activity relationship methods for modeling cytochrome P450 active sites. *Drug Metab Dispos* 2001;29:936–44.

86. Ekins S, Kim RB, Leake BF, Dantzig AH, Schuetz E, Lan LB, Yasuda K, Shepard RL, Winter MA, Schuetz JD, Wikel JH, Wrighton SA. Three-

dimensional quantitative structure-activity relationships of inhibitors of P-glycoprotein. *Mol Pharmacol* 2002;61:964–73.

87. Ekins S, Erickson JA. A pharmacophore for human pregnane X-receptor ligands. *Drug Metab Dispos* 2002;30:96–9.
88. Aronov AM, Goldman BB. A model for identifying HERG K+ channel blockers. *Bioorg Med Chem* 2004;12:2307–37.
89. Ekins S, Berbaum J, Harrison RK. Generation and validation of rapid computational filters for Cyp2D6 and Cyp3A4. *Drug Metab Dispos* 2003;31:1077–80.
90. Young SS, Gombar VK, Emptage MR, Cariello NF, Lambert C. Mixture deconvolution and analysis of Ames mutagenicity data. *Chemo Intell Lab Sys* 2002;60:5–22.
91. Korolev D, Balakin KV, Nikolsky Y, Kirillov E, Ivanenkov YA, Savchuk NP, Ivashchenko AA, Nikolskaya T. Modeling of human cytochrome p450-mediated drug metabolism using unsupervised machine learning approach. *J Med Chem* 2003;46:3631–43.
92. Shen M, Xiao Y, Golbraikh A, Gombar VK, Tropsha A. Development and validation of k-nearest-neighbor QSPR models of metabolic stability of drug candidates. *J Med Chem* 2003;46:3013–20.
93. Lipinski CA, Lombardo F, Dominy BW, Feeney PJ. Experimental and computational approaches to estimate solubility and permeability in drug discovery and development settings. *Adv Drug Del Rev* 1997;46:3–25.
94. Veber DF, Johnson SR, Cheng H-Y, Smith BR, Ward KW, Kopple KD. Molecular properties that influence the oral bioavailability of drug candidates. *J Med Chem* 2002;45:2615–23.
95. Balakin KV, Ivanenkov YA, Savchuk NP, Ivashchenko AA, Ekins S. Comprehensive computational assessment of ADME properties using mapping techniques. *Curr Drug Discov Technol* 2005;2:99–113.
96. Balakin KV, Ekins S, Bugrim A, Ivanenkov YA, Korolev D, Nikolsky YV, Skorenko AV, Ivashchenko AA, Savchuk NP, Nikolskaya T. Kohonen maps for prediction of binding to human cytochrome P450 3A4. *Drug Metab Dispos* 2004;32:1183–9.
97. Balakin KV, Ivanenkov YA, Skorenko AV, Nikolsky YV, Savchuk NP, Ivashchenko AA. In silico estimation of DMSO solubility of organic compounds for bioscreening. *J Biomol Scr* 2004;9:22–31.
98. Savchuk NP, Balakin KV. Data mining approaches for enhancement of knowledge-based content of de novo chemical libraries. In: Alvarez H, Shoichet B, editors, *Virtual screening in drug discovery*. New York: CRC Press, 2005. p. 121–49.
99. Davis AM, Riley RJ. Predictive ADMET studies. The challenges and the opportunities. *Curr Opin Chem Biol* 2004;8:378-86.
100. Gillet VJ. Designing combinatorial libraries optimized on multiple objectives. *Methods Mol Biol* 2004;275:335–54.
101. Agrafiotis DK. Multiobjective optimization of combinatorial libraries. *Mol Divers* 2002;5:209–30.

16

SUCCESS STORIES OF COMPUTER-AIDED DESIGN

HUGO KUBINYI

Contents

Computer Applications in Pharmaceutical Research and Development, Edited by Sean Ekins.
ISBN 0-471-73779-8

16.1 INTRODUCTION

Rational approaches have been applied in drug discovery for at least a century. A striking example, with a surprising outcome, was the design of acetylsalicylic acid (ASS). In 1897, Felix Hoffmann synthesized this compound as a more tolerable "prodrug" of salicylic acid. Seventy years later it turned out that ASS has a unique mechanism of action through irreversibly inhibiting the enzyme cyclooxygenase. Many other drugs were developed from natural products and endogenous transmitters, by rational design. Nowadays, the term "rational design" is most often—incorrectly—applied as a synonym for structure-based and computer-aided design, which developed in the early 1970s. With the progress in protein crystallography, Peter Goodford was the first to use protein 3D structures to design ligands that fit a protein binding site [1, 2]. Two successful applications were published by his group.

(1) The 3D structure of the 2,3-diphosphoglycerate (DPG) complex of hemoglobin (Hb) served to derive simple aromatic dialdehydes that mimic the function of DPG as an allosteric modulator of the oxygen affinity of Hb. Some of the resulting compounds were as active and even more active than DPG, the natural ligand [1–3].

(2) Trimethoprim analogs were designed as dihydrofolate reductase (DHFR) inhibitors, starting from the observation that a certain distance from one methoxy group of trimethoprim there is the guanidinium group of an arginine, which can favorably interact with a newly introduced acidic group of the ligand. Analogs with significantly enhanced affinities to bacterial DHFR resulted from this approach [1, 2, 4].

However, in the very end both projects failed with respect to "drug design": The Hb ligands do not permeate the erythrocyte membrane, and the trimethoprim analogs lost the high selectivity for bacterial DHFRs.

The design of the angiotensin-converting enzyme (ACE) inhibitor captopril [5, 6] may be considered as the first real success of structure-based drug design. Long-lasting attempts to derive bioavailable small molecule inhibitors from snake venom peptides were without much success. A breakthrough resulted from the 3D structure of carboxypeptidase A, another zinc protease, in complex with its inhibitor L-2-benzylsuccinic acid. A model of the ACE binding site guided the way to the weakly active ACE inhibitor lead structure *N*-succinoyl-L-proline (IC_{50} = 330 μM). The antihypertensive drug **captopril 1** (IC_{50} = 23 nM; Fig. 16.1) resulted after minor modifications, namely, the introduction of a methyl group (mimicking an alanine side chain) and an exchange of the carboxylate group with a sulfhydryl group [5, 6].

The topically active antiglaucoma agent **dorzolamide 2** (K_i = 0.37 nM; Fig. 16.1), a carbonic anhydrase inhibitor, may be considered as the first drug in the market that originated from the experimentally determined X-ray structure of its target protein. In the very last steps of its design, a favorable conformation of the six-membered ring was stabilized by the shift of a methyl

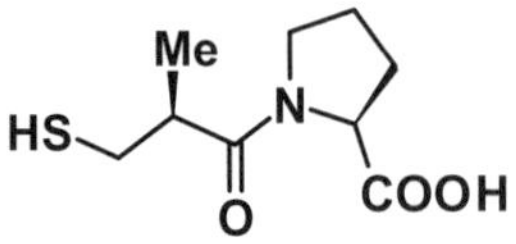

Figure 16.1 Some success stories of structure-based design.

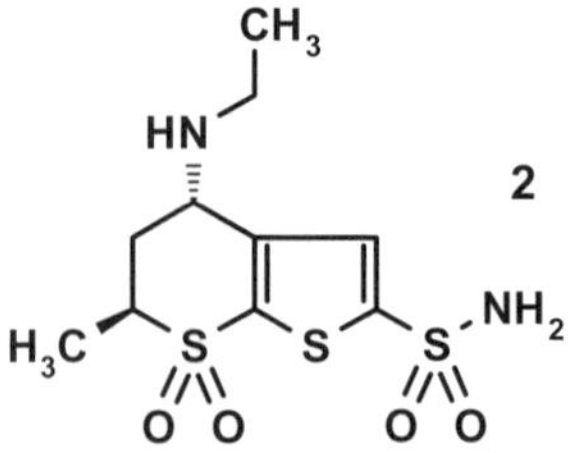

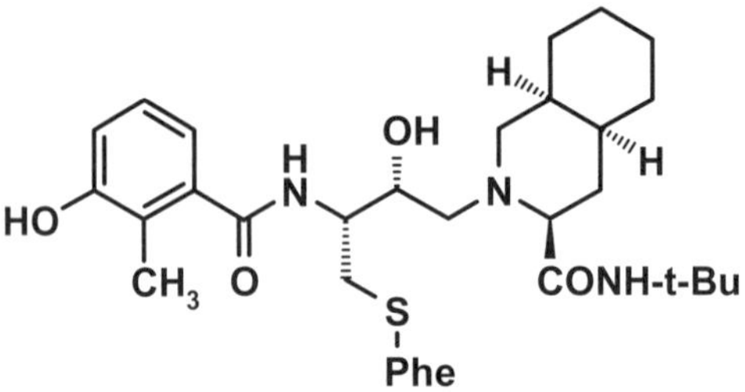

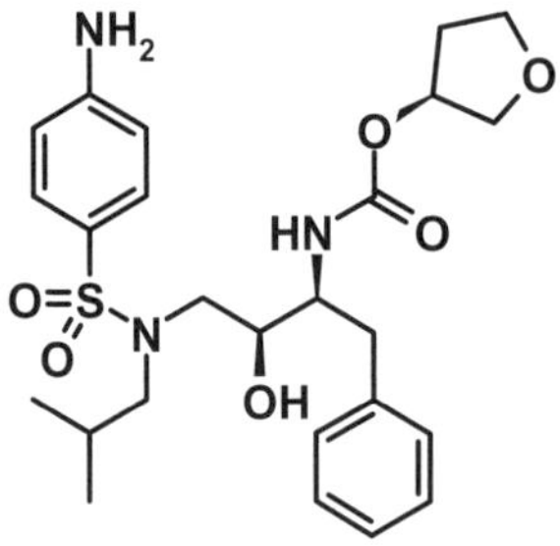

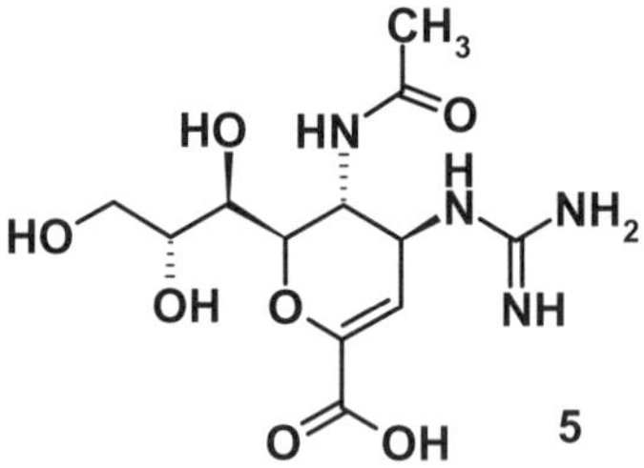

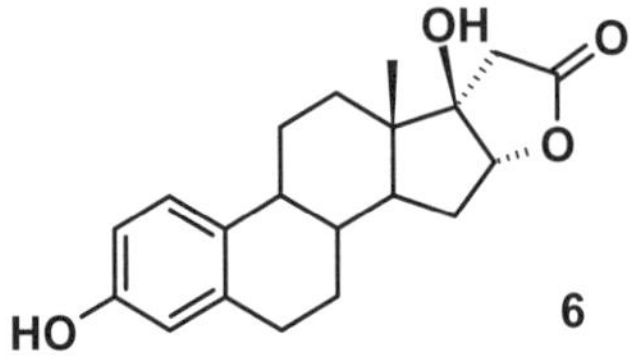

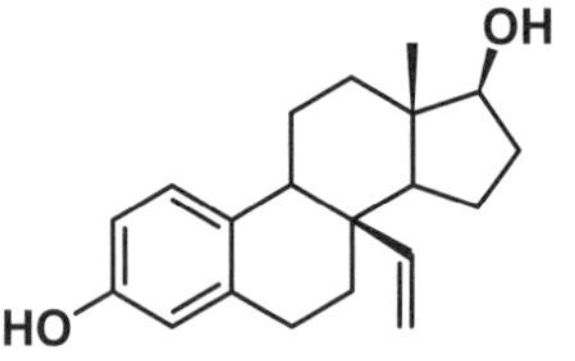

group of an *N*-alkyl substituent to this ring, in this manner enhancing the affinity of the molecule by a factor of two [7].

The very first HIV protease inhibitors in human therapy, saquinavir, indinavir, and ritonavir [8, 9], are often considered as typical examples of structure-based design. However, in reality they resulted from classic medicinal chemistry strategies (as did so many drugs in the decades before), starting from the peptide sequence of the cleavage site of the substrate. The 3D structure of HIV protease, which was available only relatively late, may have helped in understanding the details of the structure-activity relationships, but it did not contribute too much to the design. In the 1980s, several companies started to apply 3D structure-based ligand design as a strategic concept in drug discovery. The two most prominent companies, Agouron Pharmaceuticals and Vertex Pharmaceuticals, were both successful in designing the HIV protease inhibitors **nelfinavir 3** (K_i = 2.0 nM; Fig. 16.1) and **amprenavir 4** (K_i = 0.6 nM; Fig. 16.1), respectively. These drugs resulted from structure-based design, but both also contain some structural elements that were discovered in the design of the first HIV protease inhibitors [8, 9].

An example of a straightforward 3D structure-based design was published by von Itzstein and his group [10]. The enzyme neuraminidase (also called sialidase) is an essential coat protein of the influenza virus. It enables the virus to penetrate into the cell and to leave the cell after reproduction, by cleaving sialic acid from carbohydrate side chains at the cell surface. Correspondingly, the 3D structure of neuraminidase constituted a promising starting point for a structure-based design of anti-influenza drugs. Inspection of the surface of neuraminidase with the computer program GRID [11] indicated a pocket that could accommodate a relatively large positively charged group. Exchange of the –OH group of the weak transition state inhibitor Neu-5Ac-2en ($K_i = 1\,\mu$M) with an ammonium group produced an inhibitor with K_i = 50 nM. If the larger guanidinium group was introduced instead, the strong inhibitor **zanamivir 5** resulted (K_i = 0.1–0.2 nM; Fig. 16.1) [10].

The design of estrogen receptor subtype-selective (ERα and ERβ) ligands is an exciting success story of homology modeling and structure-based design [12–14]. Hillisch et al. investigated the known 3D structure of the human ERα ligand-binding domain (LBD) to derive a homology model of the human ERβ LBD. There are minor but distinct differences in the estradiol binding cavity of the subtypes. Whereas the β side, “above” the steroid ring system, is relatively narrow in ERα, because of a leucine side chain in position 384, there is more space in ERβ, because of a flexible methionine side chain. On the other hand, a methionine in position 421 of ERα is replaced by an isoleucine in ERβ, making the α side of ERβ, “below” the steroid, narrower. Estradiol (E2) analogs were designed to use these structural differences for subtype selectivity, producing the ERα- and ERβ-selective **ligands 6** (40% E2 activity, 300-fold selectivity) and **7** (50% E2 activity, 190-fold selectivity) (Fig. 16.1) [12–14].

There are now many success stories of structure-based design of potent and selective ligands. As these examples have been extensively discussed in books [15–17] and reviews [e.g., 18–24], they are not be repeated here. When combinatorial chemistry and high-throughput screening developed as new approaches to synthesizing and screening thousands, tens of thousands, or even hundreds of thousands of new compounds, it was anticipated that this would generate an unprecedented number of new drugs, marking a milestone in drug discovery. However, the opposite was the case [25, 26]. Most often, screening hits could not be validated or optimized to leads and preclinical candidates. Many such compounds were too large and too lipophilic, too greasy, and they only showed up in the biological tests because of nonspecific binding. It was the merit of Chris Lipinski to take a closer look at the physicochemical properties of biologically active molecules. By an inspection of 2245 drugs and clinical candidates from the World Drug Index he formulated his now famous "rule of five" (Lipinski rule, Pfizer Ro5): To achieve permeability (which is a precondition for oral bioavailability), a molecule should not violate more than one of the following rules: the molecular weight must not be larger than 500, lipophilicity should not be larger than log P = 5, and the molecule should not contain more than 5 hydrogen bond acceptors and not more than 10 N + O atoms (as a rough measure of hydrogen bond acceptors) [27]. However, the rule of five defines only druglike properties, not necessarily druglike character, as expressed by structural features that are typical for drug molecules. This differentiation can be achieved by neural nets that have been trained with drugs (e.g., the World Drug Index or the MDDR) and nondrugs (e.g., the Available Chemicals Directory) [28, 29]. Such neural nets do not allow a discrimination between active and inactive compounds, but they separate druglike structures from mere chemicals, that is, from compounds that contain atypical chemical features, providing about 80% correct assignments to each group.

Molecular modeling plays an important role in all steps of lead discovery and lead optimization. Several computer-aided techniques for automated database searches and docking into protein 3D structures have developed over time. If only ligand structures are available but no 3D structures of the biological target, as until recently was the case for all membrane-embedded proteins, pharmacophore generation and 2D or 3D searches in structural databases are the method of choice [e.g., 30–33]. Starting with the programs DOCK [34] and LUDI [35], the docking of ligands into the binding sites of various proteins, for which 3D structures are available, is now a well-established technique [e.g., 36–45]. A certain problem is the poor reliability of the scoring functions that rank the docking results [e.g., 46–49]. Extensive comparisons of different docking programs and scoring functions [e.g., 50–53], to rediscover known ligands within 3D databases provide evidence that there is no unique solution to the problem. Certain docking and scoring combinations are appropriate for one target, whereas they fail with another target. Consensus scoring, that is, the simultaneous use of several different scoring functions, has been proposed to solve this problem [54, 55]. However, for the most common programs the quality of the obtained results seems to depend more on the experience and skill of the modeler than on the options used. Scoring functions also tend to overestimate the affinity of large molecules [56]. In this context, a posteriori inspection of all docking results is of utmost importance.

By combination of several techniques, from simple filters and pharmacophore searches to docking and scoring, virtual screening developed as a new paradigm in computer-aided ligand design. In contrast to real, "wet" biological screening, virtual screening opens new dimensions: It offers a number of different approaches for the selection of compounds or sublibraries out of huge in-house inventories, compound libraries of commercial suppliers, or virtual libraries, that is, structures that exist only in the computer, not in reality. Such techniques are rule-based or quantitative filters, neural nets, QSAR, 2D and 3D pharmacophore-derived models, and docking and scoring.

Drug research has often been compared with the search for a needle in a haystack. Indeed, this comparison is valid, for two reasons. First, huge numbers of candidates must be investigated in drug research to discover a lead that can be further optimized to a drug candidate. Second, special technologies should be applied to find a needle in a haystack, for example, a magnet; in the very same manner, virtual screening solves the haystack problem of drug discovery by searching for compounds with favorable properties, be it drug-like character, bioavailability, the fit to a pharmacophore, or the complementarity to a binding site. Despite the fact that virtual screening is a relatively young discipline, it has already been reviewed in books [57–59] and in many dedicated publications [60–77].

Retrospective virtual screening studies, in which only known actives are retrieved, are not included in this review, as well as mere enrichment studies and virtual screening, from which some predictions but no experimental confirmation have resulted. Only a few pharmacophore studies without additional filters or docking and scoring are included. To keep this chapter to a reasonable size, no details or references are provided for the individual biological targets and test systems, lead structures, databases, compound collections and libraries, and computer programs that were used in the virtual screening; for all these details the reader is referred to other chapters of this book and to the references of the individual case studies (some references for the most popular computer programs are given in Section 16.6).

Because most often several different techniques of virtual screening are applied in certain combinations, the discussed examples are not ordered by the applied approach but according to the biological targets. Nevertheless, ligand-based approaches and/or homology modeling and docking into a protein 3D model are in the foreground for receptors and ion channels, whereas docking into experimental 3D structures is preferentially applied for enzymes and other soluble proteins.

16.2 RECEPTORS

16.2.1 G Protein-Coupled Receptors (GPCRs)

α_{1A} Adrenergic Receptor. A model of the α_{1A} adrenergic receptor was generated by ligand-supported homology modeling, based on the high-resolution X-ray structure of bovine rhodopsin and also using mutational and ligand SAR data. Virtual screening of the Aventis in-house compound repository was then performed in a stepwise manner. First, compounds with more than nine rotatable bonds and molecular weight >600 were eliminated; then 22,950 compounds were selected, using a α_{1A} receptor ligand pharmacophore hypothesis and the program Catalyst. These compounds were docked into the α_{1A} receptor homology model with the program GOLD and scored with PMF, after calibration of the docking procedure and evaluation of different scoring functions with a data set of 50 α_{1A} receptor antagonists and 990 druglike molecules from the MDDR database. The top-scoring 300 compounds were clustered according to their Unity fingerprint similarity, and a diverse set of 80 compounds was tested in a radioligand displacement assay. Of 37 compounds with K_i <10 μM, the most active hit was **compound 8** (K_i = 1.4 nM; Fig. 16.2) [78].

Dopamine D3 Receptor. The 3D structure of the dopamine 3 (D3) subtype receptor was also modeled from the X-ray structure of rhodopsin, with extensive structural refinement and validation using experimental data. A D3 pharmacophore model was derived from 10 potent and moderately selective known D3 receptor ligands. This pharmacophore model served to search 250,251 compounds from the National Cancer Institute (NCI) 3D database with the program Chem-X. The 6727 resulting hits were docked into four major conformational clusters of the D3 receptor, and ranking of the results was performed with the scoring function of the Cerius2 program. As an independent validation, 20 known D3 ligands were added to the set of 6727 compounds. The hit list of 2478 potential ligands was then filtered for known chemotypes. After removal of all compounds that are structurally similar to known D3 receptor ligands, 1314 candidates remained. Of 60 compounds requested from the NCI, only 20 were available in sufficient quantity. Eight of them had K_i values below 500 nM, for example, **compound 9** (K_i = 11 nM; Fig. 16.2) [79].

Endothelin A Receptor. A common pharmacophore for endothelin A (ET_A) receptor ligands was derived from a cyclic pentapeptide and a triterpene ester. The moderately selective lead structure 2,4-dibenzyloxybenzoic acid (IC_{50} ET_A = 9 μM, ET_B < 20% at 30 μM) was discovered by a 3D pharmacophore search in 60,000 compounds of the Rhone Poulenc Rorer UK corporate database with the ChemDBS-3D system [80]. The highly selective ET_A receptor **ligand 10** (IC_{50} ET_A = 5 nM, IC_{50} ET_B >10 μM; Fig. 16.2) resulted

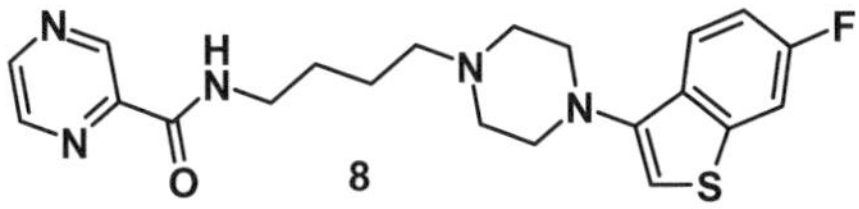

8

α_{1A} adrenergic receptor antagonist, K_i = 1.4 nM

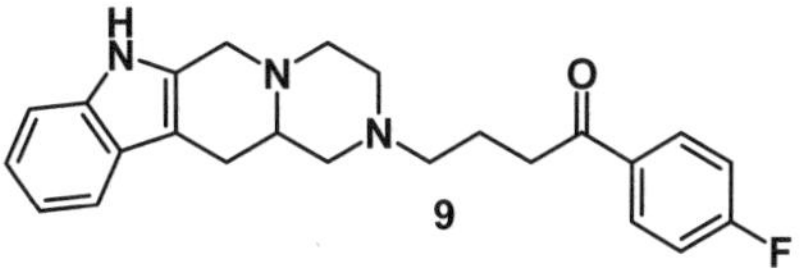

9

Dopamine D3 receptor antagonist, K_i = 11 nM

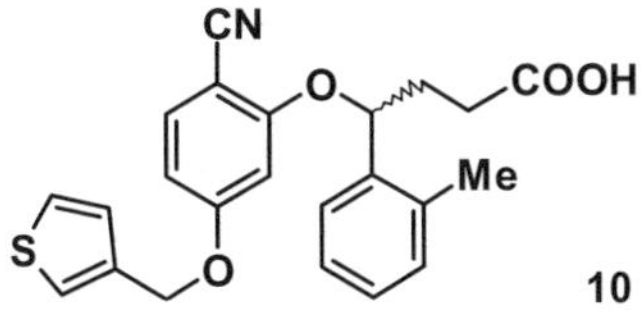

10

Endothelin A (ET_A) receptor antagonist, (R)-isomer, IC_{50} = 5 nM

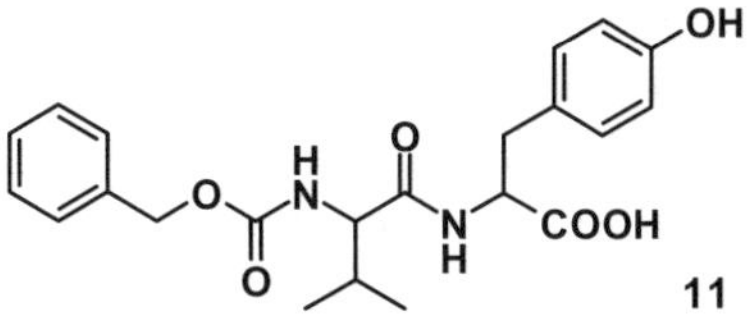

11

Endothelin A (ET_A) receptor antagonist IC_{50} = 220 nM

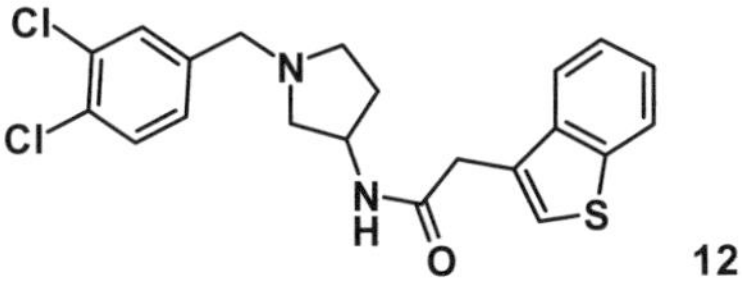

12

MCH-1 receptor ligand, K_i = 360 nM

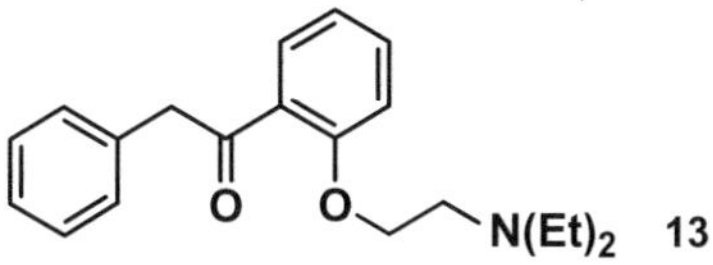

13

Muscarinic M3 receptor antagonist, $[A_{50}]$ M3≈0.2 μM (pA_2 = 6.67)

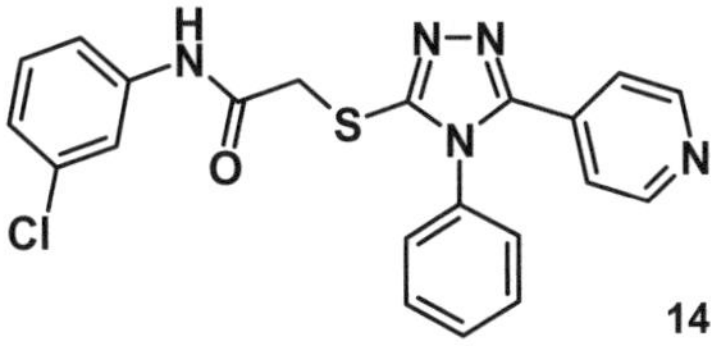

14

Neurokinin NK_1 antagonist, K_i = 251 nM

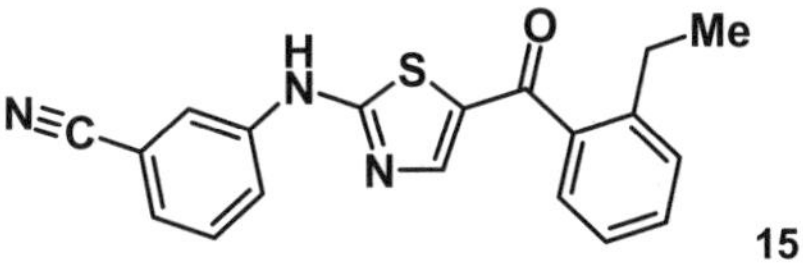

15

Neuropeptide Y (NPY5) receptor antagonist, IC_{50} = 2.8 nM

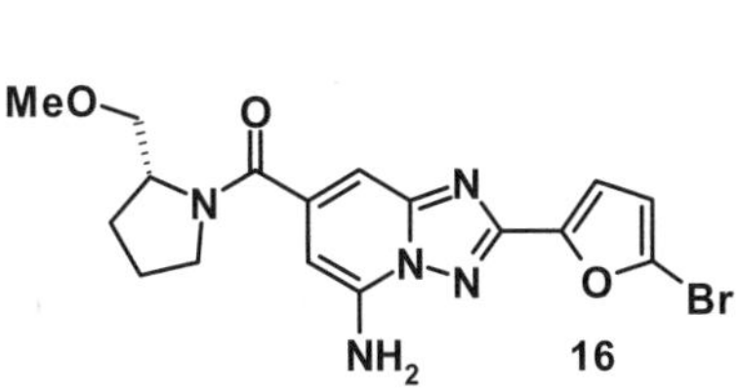

16

Purinergic A_{2A} receptor antagonist, K_i A_{2A} = 2.4 nM, K_i A_1 = 292 nM

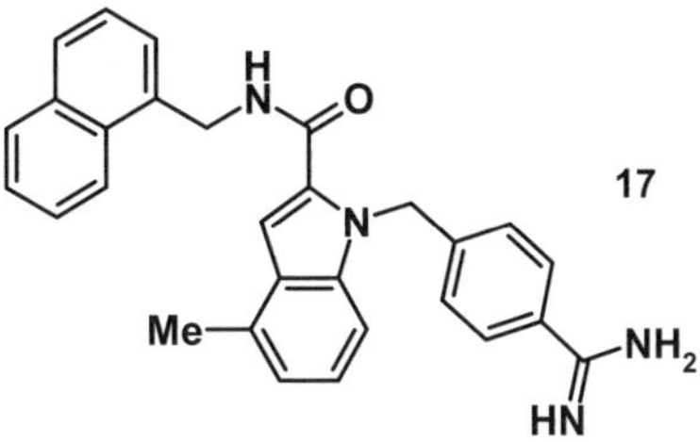

17

Urotensin II receptor antagonist, EC_{50} = 400 nM

Figure 16.2 GPCR ligands from virtual screening.

from a refined pharmacophore hypothesis and further chemical optimization [81, 82].

Another research group generated two pharmacophore models of ET_A-selective receptor antagonists from a training set of 18 ET_A antagonists by using the HypoGen and HipHop options of the program Catalyst. The best HypoGen hypothesis had five pharmacophoric features: two hydrophobic features, one aromatic ring, one acceptor, and one negative ionizable function. The highest-scoring HipHop model had six features: three hydrophobic features, one aromatic ring, one acceptor, and one negative ionizable group. The predictive power of the quantitative models was validated by their ability to extract a test set of 30 known ET_A antagonists from the World Drug Index. A 3D search of 55,000 compounds in the Maybridge database retrieved 498 hits from the HypoGen hypothesis and 5 hits from the HipHop hypothesis. After visual inspection, six hits from both analyses were selected for testing, of which four were biologically active, for example, **compound 11**, Z-Val-Tyr-OH (IC_{50} = 220 nM; Fig. 16.2) [83].

Melanin-Concentrating Hormone Type 1 Receptor. A "drug space" was defined by a BCUT metrics analysis of 81,560 drugs and druglike molecules. The resulting five-dimensional model (hydrogen bond donor and acceptor, two terms for polarizability, and charge) was used to locate the space for peptide G protein-coupled receptor (GPCR) ligands. Analysis of a virtual library of 9 million compounds, constructed from 19 predefined amine templates, yielded 2025 hits. After synthesis and biological testing, potent ligands of the GnRH, galanin, MC4, melanin-concentrating hormone (MCH), orexin, and other peptide GPCRs resulted, with a 4.5-fold (GnRH receptor) to 61-fold (MC4 receptor) enrichment of active analogs, as compared to a random selection of screening compounds from the Neurocrine Biosciences in-house compound repository. Out of several micromolar and submicromolar ligands of the MCH1 receptor, **compound 12** (K_i = 360 nM; Fig. 16.2) had the highest affinity [84].

Muscarinic M3 Receptor. A pharmacophore model was derived from known M3 receptor antagonists, using the program DISCO, and 3D searching was performed by Unity 3D in the Astra Charnwood in-house compound repository and the databases of several commercial suppliers. The 172 compounds that fitted the pharmacophore were screened for their M3-antagonistic potency. Several compounds with micromolar and even submicromolar activities resulted, for example, **compound 13** (A_{50} M3 antagonism ≈ 0.2 μM; pA_2 = 6.67; Fig. 16.2) [85].

Neurokinin-1 Receptor. A homology model of the neurokinin-1 (NK_1) receptor was built from the X-ray structure of rhodopsin, using the MOBILE (modeling binding sites including ligand information explicitly) approach. In this procedure, a preliminary model is generated, which is afterwards refined by docking known ligands into the model. From this model a pharmacophore hypothesis was derived to search eight structural databases for molecules that fit this hypothesis. The workflow shows in an elegant manner how to perform stepwise virtual screening. From the 826,952 compounds of the various databases only 419,747 (51%) molecules passed a filter for molecular weight <450 and less than eight rotatable bonds; 131,967 molecules (16%) had the requested number of hydrophobic, donor, and acceptor properties, and 36,704 molecules (4.4%) fitted the pharmacophore hypothesis in 2D and 3D (database searches with Unity). On the basis of excluded volumes, 11,109 (1.34%) structures remained for docking into the modeled NK_1 receptor binding site, using FlexX-Pharm; the resulting docking poses were ranked with the knowledge-based scoring function DrugScore. The 1000 highest-scoring ligands were force field-minimized in the binding pocket and visually inspected for certain typical receptor-ligand interactions and features: (1) an amino-aromatic interaction between $His197^{5.39}$ and an aromatic ring; (2) a stacking between two aromatic rings; (3) a hydrogen bond between $Gln165^{4.60}$ and an acceptor group of the ligand; (4) similarity to known NK_1 receptor ligands in the β4-hairpin region; and (5) a small number of rotatable bonds. Of seven compounds for biochemical screening, **compound 14** (K_i = 251 nM; Fig. 16.2) showed submicromolar affinity [86, 87]. This result is especially remarkable because **compound 14** does not contain the "magic" 3,5-bis-trifluoromethyl substitution pattern of most highly active NK_1 receptor ligands.

NPY5 Receptor. A pharmacophore hypothesis for NPY5 receptor ligands was derived from three known ligands and used for a Catalyst 3D search in the Hoffmann-La Roche in-house compound repository. Of 632 retrieved molecules, 31 had IC_{50} values <10 μM. The most interesting compound was a substituted aminothiazole (IC_{50} = 40 nM), which after two cycles of chemical optimization resulted in some more nanomolar ligands, for example, **compound 15** (IC_{50} = 2.8 nM; Fig. 16.2) [88].

Purinergic A_{2A} Receptor. The CATS (chemically advanced template search) descriptor compares molecules by the topological pattern of their pharmacophore features [89]. Based on these descriptors, a self-organizing map (SOM) was generated from biologically active molecules, including purinergic receptor antagonists. Virtual libraries were designed from a triazolopyridine carboxylic acid and secondary amines. Projection of the resulting amides onto this map identified several hits with high affinity and selectivity, the most selective A_{2A} antagonist being **compound 16** (K_i A_{2A} = 2.4 nM, K_i A_1 = 292 nM; Fig. 16.2) [90].

Urotensin II Receptor (GPR14). The vasoactive cyclic peptide urotensin II (U-II) is the endogenous ligand of the G protein-coupled orphan receptor GPR14. Structure-activity relationships from 25 peptide analogs, which mobilize intracellular calcium in GPR14-transfected CHO cells, and the

NMR 3D structure of the undecapeptide U-II generated a ligand pharmacophore hypothesis that served as query for the virtual screening of the Aventis in-house compound repository. Active leads from six different chemical classes could be identified by the 3D search, for example, **compound 17** (EC_{50} = 400 nM; Fig. 16.2) [91].

16.2.2 Nuclear Receptors

Retinoic Acid Receptor. A 3D structural model of the inactive conformation of the retinoic acid receptor (RAR) α-subtype (RARα) was developed from the RARγ 3D structure, bound to the agonist all-*trans*-retinoic acid, and the estrogen receptor α-subtype (ERα), bound to an antagonist. After validation of the method with known agonists and antagonists, 153,000 ACD compounds were docked into the RAR binding site with full flexibility of the ligand and the amino acid side chains of the protein, using the Molsoft Internal Coordinates Mechanics (ICM 2.7) program. Two novel RAR antagonists were discovered, for example, **compound 18** (55% inhibition at 20 μM; Fig. 16.3) [92]; comparable results were obtained with all three human isoforms: RARα, RARβ, and RARγ.

In a similar investigation, a model of the active RARα conformation was developed from the agonist-bound RARγ conformation. Docking of the ACD compounds as above but with a refined procedure, considering all atoms of the binding site, resulted in 5364 high-scoring hits. The 300 compounds with the lowest binding energy (i.e., highest predicted affinity) were visually inspected for shape complementarity, hydrogen bonding network, ligand conformations, and possible van der Waals clashes. Finally, 30 compounds were selected for biological testing. Despite the fact that an RARα 3D model was

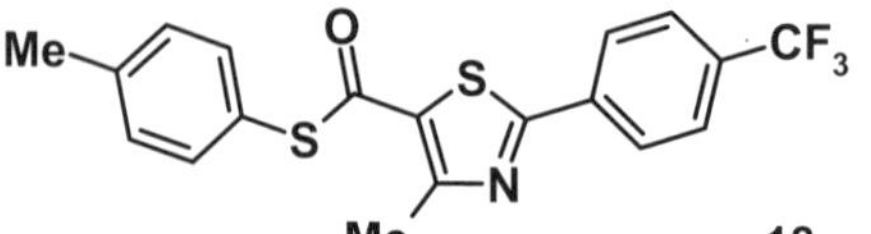

18

Retinoic acid receptor α (RAR α) antagonist, 55% inhibition at 20 μM

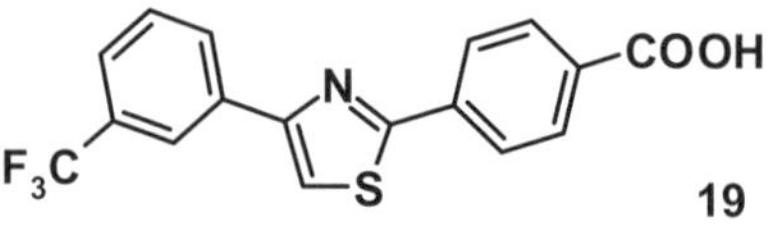

19

Retinoic acid receptor β (RARβ) agonist, EC_{50} RARβ = 200 nM, EC_{50} RARα = 4 μM

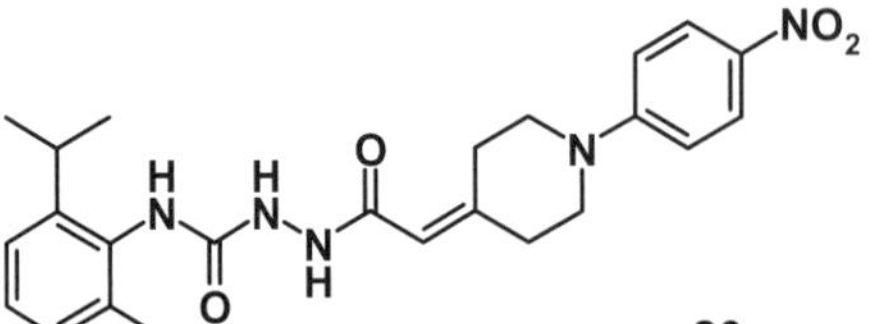

20

Thyroid hormone receptor antagonist, IC_{50} = 0.75 μM

Figure 16.3 Nuclear receptor ligands from virtual screening.

used for the docking, the two most active hits have a higher affinity to RARβ than to RARα, for example, **compound 19** (EC_{50} RARβ = 200 nM, EC_{50} RARα = 4 μM; Fig. 16.3) [93].

Thyroid Hormone Receptor. The 3D structure of the estrogen antagonist raloxifene, bound to the estrogen receptor α-subtype, was used to derive the "antagonist-binding" conformation of the thyroid receptor β-subtype (TRβ) from the 3D structure of an agonist complex of the TRβ ligand binding domain. Five grid potential representations of the binding site were generated by the Molsoft ICM virtual library screening module, accounting for hydrophobicity, van der Waals boundaries, hydrogen bonds, and electrostatic potential of the ligand binding site. The 190,000 rule of five-compatible compounds, out of 250,000 ACD compounds, were docked four times into the receptor grids by the ICM method, and the lowest score (i.e., best fit) of each ligand was retained. The geometry of the top 1000 ligand-protein complexes was refined, and the remaining 300 top-scoring complexes were visually inspected. Of 100 biologically tested compounds, 14 turned out to be TR antagonists. The most active hit (90% inhibition at 20 μM) served as the lead to construct a virtual library of a further 101 analogs. After docking, eight high-scoring compounds were synthesized and tested; all inhibited TR to 10–84% at 5 μM, the most active antagonist being **compound 20** (IC_{50} = 0.75 μM; Fig. 16.3) [94].

16.3 ENZYMES

16.3.1 Kinases

Akt 1 (Protein Kinase Bα, PKBα). The three isoforms of protein kinase B are Akt 1 (PKBα), Akt 2 (PKBβ), and Akt 3 (PKBγ). A 3D structure of the binding site was extracted from the X-ray structure of a ternary complex of Akt1, a nonhydrolyzable ATP analog, and a peptide substrate derived from the binding sequence of glycogen synthase kinase 3β (GSK-3β). About 50,000 ChemBridge compounds were docked into this binding site in a flexible manner, using the program FlexX. The top 2000 compounds were ranked with the consensus scoring function CSORE; the top 100 compounds from the knowledge-based scoring function DrugScore, the top 200 compounds from GoldScore, and the top 200 compounds from ChemScore ranking were biologically tested. Only one hit, **compound 21** (IC_{50} = 4.5 μM, K_i = 3.9 μM; Fig. 16.4) resulted. To improve the result, the 4000 top-ranking compounds from FlexX and DrugScore were ranked according to GoldScore and ChemScore. Two hundred compounds were selected, which showed up within the top 700 rankings of both functions. From this set, 100 compounds were eliminated after visual inspection and 100 compounds were biologically tested. In addition to **compound 21** another low micromolar Akt1 inhibitor, **compound 22** (IC_{50} = 2.6 μM, K_i = 1.1 μM; Fig. 16.4), resulted [95].

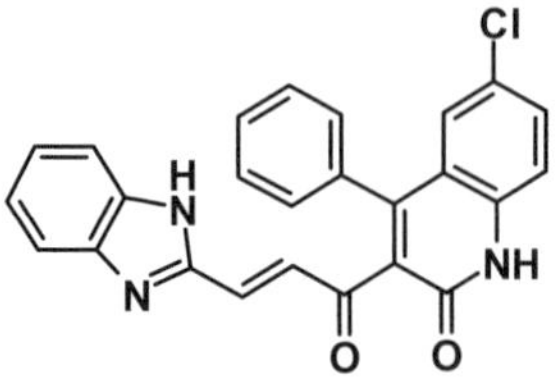

21
Akt 1 (protein kinase Bα, PKBα) inhibitor, IC_{50} = 4.5 μM, K_i = 3.9 μM

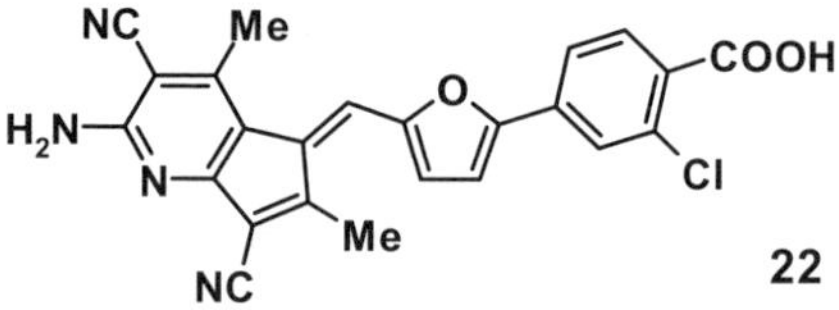

22
Akt 1 (protein kinase Bα, PKBα) inhibitor, IC_{50} = 2.6 μM, K_i = 1.1 μM

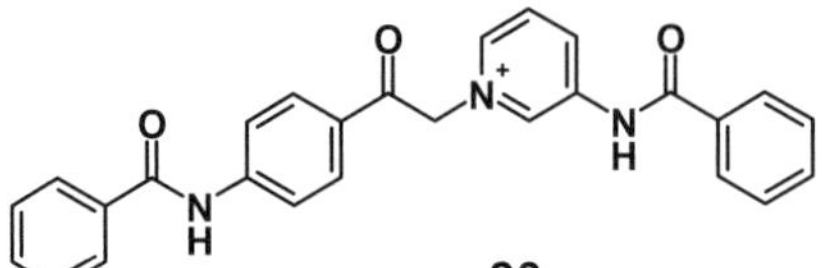

23
Bcr-abl tyrosine kinase inhibitor, IC_{50} = 24 μM

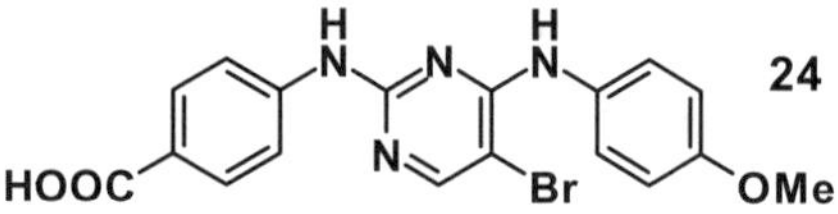

24
Checkpoint kinase 1 (Chk-1) inhibitor, IC_{50} = 450 nM

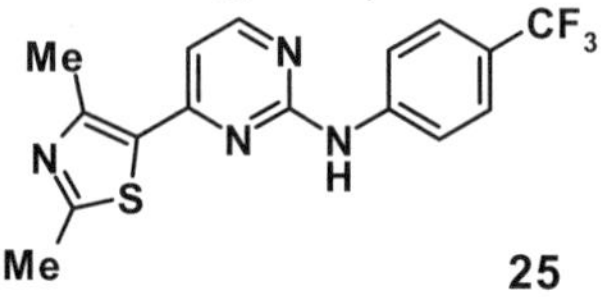

25
Cdk2 inhibitor, K_i Cdk2 = 0.29 μM, K_i Cdk4 > 20 μM

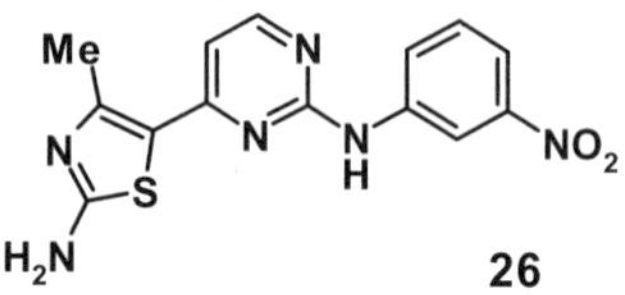

26
Cdk2 inhibitor, K_i Cdk2 = 2 nM, K_i Cdk4 = 53 nM

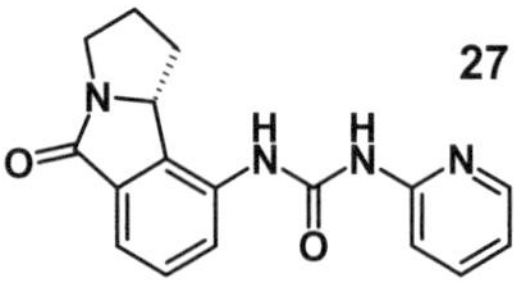

27
Cdk4 inhibitor, IC_{50} = 42 nM

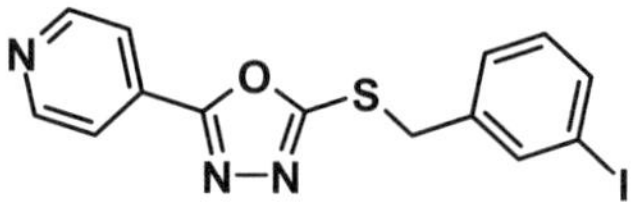

28
Glycogen synthase kinase 3 (GSK-3) inhibitor, IC_{50} = 0.39 μM

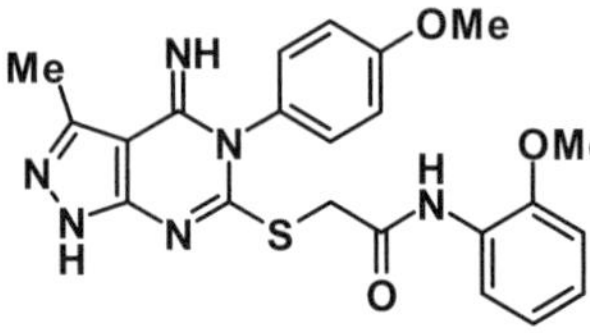

29
p56 lymphoid T cell tyrosine kinase (Lck) inhibitor, ≈75% inhibition of ^{3}H-thymidine uptake at 10 μM

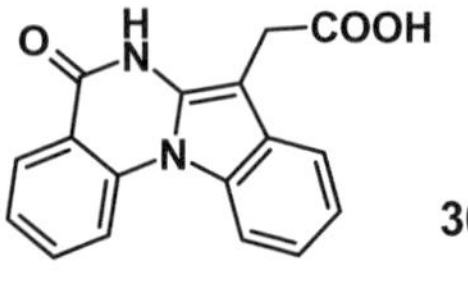

30
Protein kinase CK2 (casein kinase II) inhibitor, IC_{50} = 80 nM

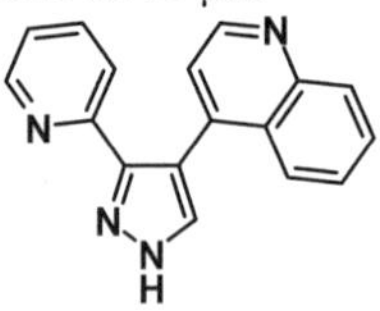

31
TGFβ receptor (TβRI) kinase inhibitor, IC_{50} = 27 nM, K_d = 5 nM

Figure 16.4 Kinase inhibitors from virtual screening.

Bcr-Abl Tyrosine Kinase. A database of 200,000 compounds of the ChemDiv compound collection was converted into 3D format and docked into the binding site of bcr-abl tyrosine kinase, using the program DOCK 4.0.1 for flexible docking. The 1000 top-scoring compounds were clustered by their molecular fingerprints. After filtering by the Lipinski rule of five, 15 compounds from diverse sets were selected for biological testing; eight of these compounds inhibited K562 tumor cell growth with IC_{50} values between 10 and 200 μM, for example, **compound 23** (IC_{50} = 24 μM; Fig. 16.4) [96].

Checkpoint Kinase 1. A subsection of the AstraZeneca in-house compound collection, containing 560,000 compounds, was used for virtual screening for checkpoint kinase 1 (Chk-1) inhibitors. Compounds with molecular weight >600 or with more than 10 rotatable bonds were removed, leaving about 400,000 compounds. Protonation and tautomeric states were corrected with the in-house program Leatherface. Then 3D structures were generated with Corina, with explicit enumeration of stereocenters (generating a maximum of 8 stereoisomers per molecule), and a multiconformer database was produced, using the program Omega. A 3D pharmacophore search was performed with the in-house program Plurality to eliminate compounds that do not have the typical binding motif for the kinase hinge region. The remaining 199,000 compounds (1 conformer per molecule) were flexibly docked into the ATP binding site of Chk-1, using the program FlexX-Pharm, which considers full flexibility of the ligand and demands certain interactions with the binding site, in this case to the backbone NH of Cys 87 and the backbone carbonyl of Glu 85. An enrichment study for known cyclin-dependent kinase 2 (Cdk2) inhibitors served to select the best consensus scoring, resulting in a combination of the FlexX and PMF scoring functions. Visual inspection of the 250 highest-scoring hits for unfavorable interactions with the binding site or compounds with unrealistic conformations resulted in a list of 103 compounds for biological testing. Inhibitory activities of 36 hits were in the range of 110 nM to 68 μM, for example, compound **24** (IC_{50} = 450 nM; Figure 16.4) [97].

Cyclin-Dependent Kinase 2. The flexible docking program LIDAEUS (developed from the program Sandock) was used to dock a database of about 50,000 commercially available compounds into the known 3D structure of the kinase Cdk2, to search for new chemotypes of Cdk inhibitors. Biochemical screening of 200 hits provided moderately active inhibitors. Structure-based modification led to the selective Cdk2 inhibitor **compound 25** (IC_{50} Cdk2/cyclin E = 0.9 μM; IC_{50} Cdk4/cyclin D1 = 5.5 μM [98]; K_i Cdk2 = 0.29 μM, K_i Cdk4 > 20 μM [99]; Fig. 16.4) with antiproliferative activity against tumor cells in vitro and in vivo. Further chemical optimization of **compound 25** produced the moderately selective nanomolar inhibitor **compound 26** (K_i Cdk2 = 2 nM, K_i Cdk4 = 53 nM; Fig. 16.4) [99].

Cyclin-Dependent Kinase 4. A homology model of the cyclin-dependent kinase Cdk4 was constructed from the X-ray structure of activated Cdk2, to perform a structure-based design of Cdk4 inhibitors. For this purpose the de novo design program LEGEND was combined with the program SEEDS (system for evaluation of availability of essential structures generated by de novo ligand design programs). LEGEND constructs ligands within the binding site of a protein on an atom-by-atom basis, and SEEDS extracts relevant scaffolds from the generated ligands to search databases for commercially available or synthetically feasible building blocks or analogs. On searching the ACD, 4884 compounds with molecular weight <350 were retrieved. After visual inspection, 382 compounds were purchased and tested in a cyclin D-Cdk4 complex assay. Eighteen compounds with IC_{50} values <500 μM were identified and clustered into four classes of new scaffolds. A diarylurea class could be further improved in biological activities by a dedicated library design. A docking study confirmed the binding mode of these ligands in the ATP binding pocket of the Cdk4 model. Further modifications led to the Cdk4 inhibitor **compound 27** (IC_{50} = 42 nM; Fig. 16.4) [100].

Glycogen Synthetase Kinase. Inhibitors of glycogen synthase kinase 3 (GSK-3), a serine protein kinase, may play a role in the treatment of diabetes. To search for potential ligands, 32 different virtual libraries with up to about 1.25 million compounds per library were generated. Then 47 hits from GSK-3 inhibitor screening were compared with up to 10,000 compounds from each of these libraries. CATS-2, a modification of the CATS descriptor, which compares molecules by the topological pattern of pharmacophore features assigned to atom pairs [89], was used for similarity search of each of the screening hits against 137,842 molecules that were randomly selected from the different virtual libraries. Whereas a classic 2D fingerprint similarity search did not provide any hits with a Tanimoto index >0.85, the CATS-2 search indicated that one of the virtual libraries had a high similarity to the screening hits. Filtering, library syntheses, and further optimization, including scaffold hopping, led to **compound 28** (IC_{50} = 0.39 μM; Fig. 16.4) [101].

p56 Lymphoid T Cell Tyrosine Kinase. The p56 lymphoid T cell tyrosine kinase (Lck) participates in protein-protein interactions through its Src homology-2 (SH2) domain. Virtual screening was performed, using the X-ray structure of the Lck SH2 domain complex with a pYEEI (pY+3) peptide. A 3D database of 2 million commercially available compounds was built with the 3D generator CORINA and docked into the pY+3 binding site with the program DOCK, using flexible ligands based on the anchored search method. Some further filters selected 25,000 compounds that were more rigorously docked by simultaneous energy minimization of the anchor fragment during the iterative build-up procedure. Two sets of 1000 compounds were selected on the basis of either the total interaction energy or a molecular weight-normalized energy score, to account for the often observed overprediction of large molecules cf. 56]. Similarity clustering was performed for both sets, and compounds from the different clusters were selected according to their physicochemical properties. Thirty-four of 196 selected compounds, without a phosphotyrosine (pY) or a structurally related feature, inhibited Lck. Twenty-four of the active compounds were tested for their modulation of biological function: Thirteen showed inhibitory activity in a lymphocyte culture assay, for example, **compound 29** (~75% inhibition of ^{3}H-thymidine uptake at 10 μM; Fig. 16.4) [102].

Protein Kinase CK2 (Casein Kinase II). A homology model of human protein kinase CK2 (casein kinase II) was generated from the 3D structure of the highly homologous CK2 of *Zea mays*. Docking of 400,000 compounds of the in-house corporate collection of Novartis was performed with the program DOCK. The results were filtered according to the following criteria: Only compounds showing the typical hydrogen bond interaction to the hinge region of the kinase binding site were selected; results were ranked by a second scoring function and visually inspected for unrealistic conformations or unfavorable interactions. Four of twelve biologically tested compounds showed >50% inhibition at 10 μM, the most potent inhibitor being **compound 30** (IC_{50} = 80 nM; Fig. 16.4) [103].

TGFβ Receptor (TβRI) Kinase. TGFβ receptor (TβRI) kinase is activated by its association with the TGFβ type II receptor (TβRII). The activated kinase phosphorylates Smad substrates, which then induce TGFβ-dependent gene expression. The X-ray crystal structure of the unphosphorylated cytoplasmatic region of TβRI in complex with FKBP12, an inhibitor of the TGFβ pathway, served for a structure-based virtual screening to discover novel inhibitors. A starting point of the design was a pharmacophore hypothesis, derived from the experimental X-ray structure of the 2,4,5-triarylimidazole SB 203580 (IC_{50} = 30 μM) in the ATP binding site of TβRI. The pharmacophore search, which also considered shape constraints, identified 87 compounds from a commercially available database of 200,000 molecules, for example, **compound 31** (IC_{50} = 27 nM, K_d = 5 nM; Fig. 16.4) [104].

16.3.2 Proteases

Cathepsin D. The design of inhibitors of the aspartyl protease cathepsin D started from a virtual library of peptide analogs that contained the typical hydroxyethylamine isoster for the cleavable peptide bond. As the availability of starting materials would have generated a library of about 1 billion compounds, virtual screening was applied to reduce this multitude of candidate structures to a reasonable number. The backbone of a peptide analog was docked into the active site of cathepsin D in the same pose as the natural product inhibitor pepstatin. Then fitting side chains for three different pockets of the binding site were selected by the program CombiBuild, which was developed from the program DOCK. A library of 1000 compounds resulted from this procedure, which in the following virtual screening was compared with a diversity-oriented library of peptide analogs. Whereas the directed library produced seven hits with IC_{50} values <100 nM, only one such hit resulted from the diversity-oriented library. In a further step, the best results from the directed library were the starting point for another directed library of 39 compounds. The inhibitor with the highest activity was **compound 32** (K_i = 9 nM, IC_{50} = 14 nM; Fig. 16.5) [105].

Falcipain-2. The 3D structures of the binding pockets of protozoal cysteine proteases are highly conserved. Homology models of the malarial cysteine proteases falcipain-2 and falcipain-3 were used for stepwise virtual screening of 241,000 compounds of the ChemBridge database. First, filters were applied to eliminate metal complexes and counterions, to neutralize charged compounds, and to eliminate compounds with inappropriate ADME properties, poor solubility, and violations of the Lipinski rule of five. 3D structures of the 60,000 compounds of this filtered database were generated and subjected to docking with the program GOLD, using three different protocols that were generated by docking a vinyl sulfone inhibitor into the cysteine protease cruzain. The first two rounds of docking, with 7–8 times and 2 times speed-up as compared to the standard protocol, were performed with the somewhat narrower binding pocket of falcipain-3. The remaining 1500 candidates were docked into both protein binding pockets, using the standard mode settings of GOLD. In both cases 10 known vinyl sulfone inhibitors were included, which showed up in the 20 highest-ranking ligands. The top 200 common hits for both proteins were visually inspected for reasonable geometry of the ligand, proximity of an electrophilic center (if present) to the SH group of the catalytic cysteine, and complementarity of the ligand and the protein. Of 100 selected compounds, 84 were biologically tested to identify 24 diverse inhibitors, of which 12 compounds are dual inhibitors of falcipain-2 and falcipain-3, with IC_{50} values between 1 and 62 μM; although many of these inhibitors are either Schiff bases or hydrazones, some of them have druglike structures, for example, **compound 33** (IC_{50} falcipain-2 = 6.2 μM, IC_{50} falcipain-3 = 12.0 μM; Fig. 16.5) [106]. Five compounds additionally inhibited *Leishmania donovani* cysteine protease, whereas four other, noninhibiting compounds showed strong antileishmanial activity in *L. donovani* promastigotes, obviously by a different mechanism of action.

HIV Protease. Docking of the 3D structures of the Cambridge Structural Database into the HIV protease binding site, by shape and to some extent by chemical complementarity, was performed with an early version of the

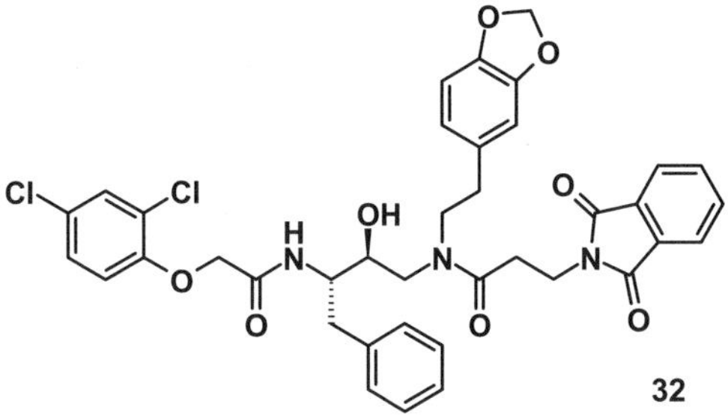

32

Cathepsin D inhibitor,
K_i = 9 nM, IC_{50} = 14 nM

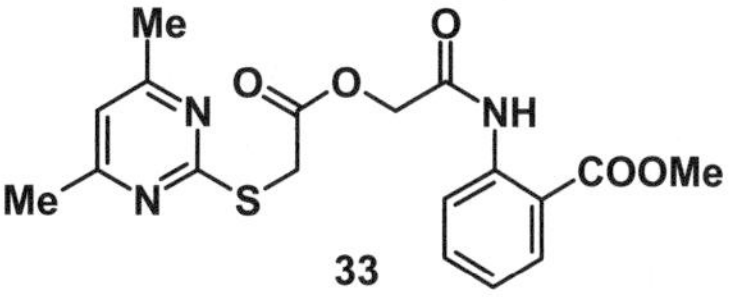

33

Falcipain inhibitor,
IC_{50} falcipain-2 = 6.2 μM,
IC_{50} falcipain-3 = 12.0 μM

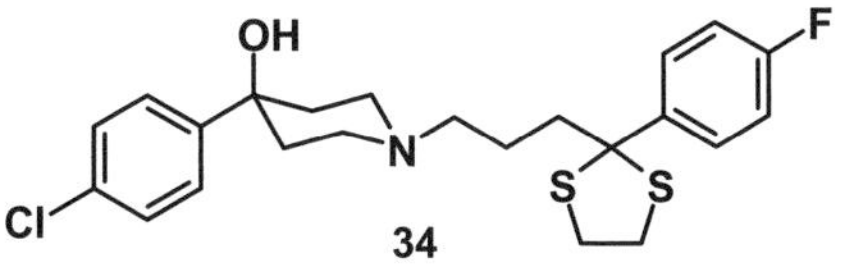

34

HIV protease inhibitor,
K_i HIV-1 protease = 15 μM,
K_i HIV-2 protease = 100 μM

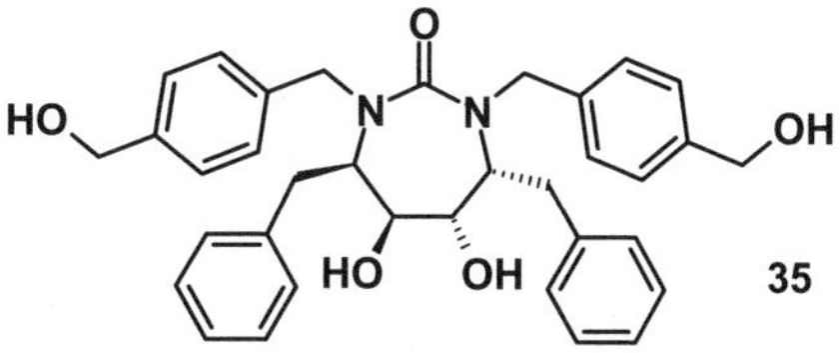

35

HIV protease inhibitor,
K_i = 0.27 nM, IC_{50} = 36 nM

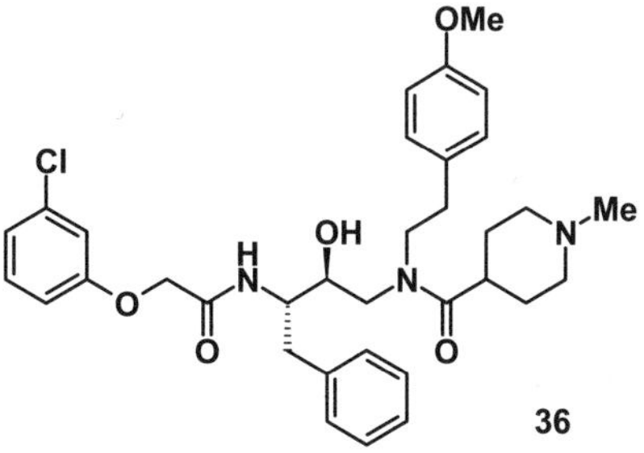

36

Plasmepsin II inhibitor,
K_i plasmepsin II = 2.0 nM,
K_i cathepsin D = 9.8 nM

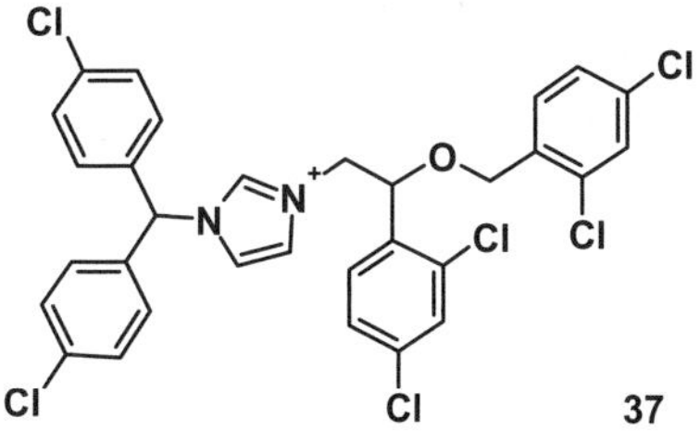

37

SARS CoV 3C-like proteinase inhibitor,
K_i = 61 μM

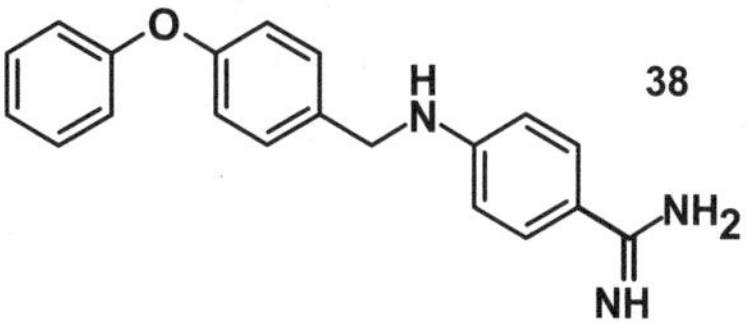

38

Thrombin inhibitor,
K_i thrombin = 95 nM, K_i trypsin = 520 nM

Figure 16.5 Protease inhibitors from virtual screening.

program DOCK. Of the 200 top-scoring hits, 50 were commercially available and 15 were tested for their HIV protease inhibition. The neuroleptic haloperidol had an IC_{50} vs. HIV-1 protease of 100 μM but was toxic at high concentrations [107, 108]. Further chemical optimization resulted in the haloperidol derivative **compound 34** (K_i HIV-1 protease = 15 μM, K_i HIV-2 protease = 100 μM; Fig. 16.5) [108].

A pharmacophore hypothesis for HIV protease inhibitors was derived at Dupont from the X-ray structures of several inhibitor complexes and the modeled binding mode of vicinal diol inhibitors. A 3D database search yielded a substituted terphenyl compound, which suggested as starting point a six- or seven-membered ring, with a carbonyl group to replace a structural water and one or two hydroxy groups to interact with the catalytic aspartates. By extensive structural modification cyclic ureas, for example, **compound 35** (K_i = 0.27 nM, IC_{50} = 36 nM; Fig. 16.5) [109], resulted from which even more active but also poorly soluble inhibitors were derived e.g., [110].

Plasmepsin II. The malarial aspartyl protease plasmepsin II has a significant homology (35%) to cathepsin D. Correspondingly, the very same approach as for the cathepsin D inhibitors (see above) was followed. The best inhibitors have K_i values of 2–10 nM, a molecular weight <650, moderate selectivity vs. cathepsin D, the most closely related human protease, log P values <4.6, and no apparent binding to human serum albumin, for example, **compound 36** (K_i plasmepsin II = 2.0 nM, K_i cathepsin D = 9.8 nM; Fig. 16.5) [111].

SARS CoV 3C-Like Proteinase. For the screening for SARS (severe acute respiratory syndrome) 3C-like proteinase A inhibitors, a "flexible" 3D model was built by homology modeling and molecular dynamics, starting from the known 3D structure of TGEV (transmissible-gastroenteritis virus) coronavirus 3C-like proteinase. Docking of 630,000 compounds from the ACD, MDDR, and NCI 3D databases was performed with the program DOCK 4.01. The docking hits were further ranked by a pharmacophore model, consensus scoring, and "drug-likeness" filters; 40 compounds were biologically tested. Three of these inhibited SARS 3C-like proteinase with K_i values below 200 μM, for example,. the known calmodulin antagonist **calmidazolium 37** (K_i = 61 μM; Fig. 16.5) [112].

Thrombin. New thrombin inhibitors were designed by a two-step procedure at Hoffmann-La Roche. *p*-Amino-benzamidine was the top-scoring ligand from a docking of 5300 commercially available amines into the recognition pocket of the serine protease thrombin. The link mode of the de novo design program LUDI connected this amine with 540 aldehydes by a reductive amination. Ten of the 100 top-scoring candidates were synthesized and tested; five bind with nanomolar affinities, for example, **compound 38** (K_i thrombin = 95 nM, K_i trypsin = 520 nM; Fig. 16.5) [113, 114].

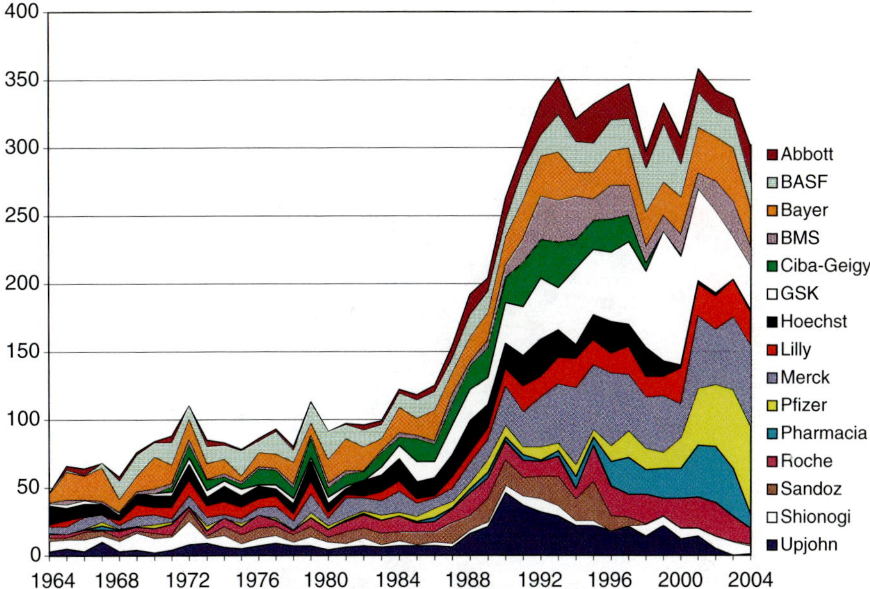

Figure 1.3 Annual number of papers published by researchers at pharmaceutical companies during a 41-year period. For full caption see page 39.

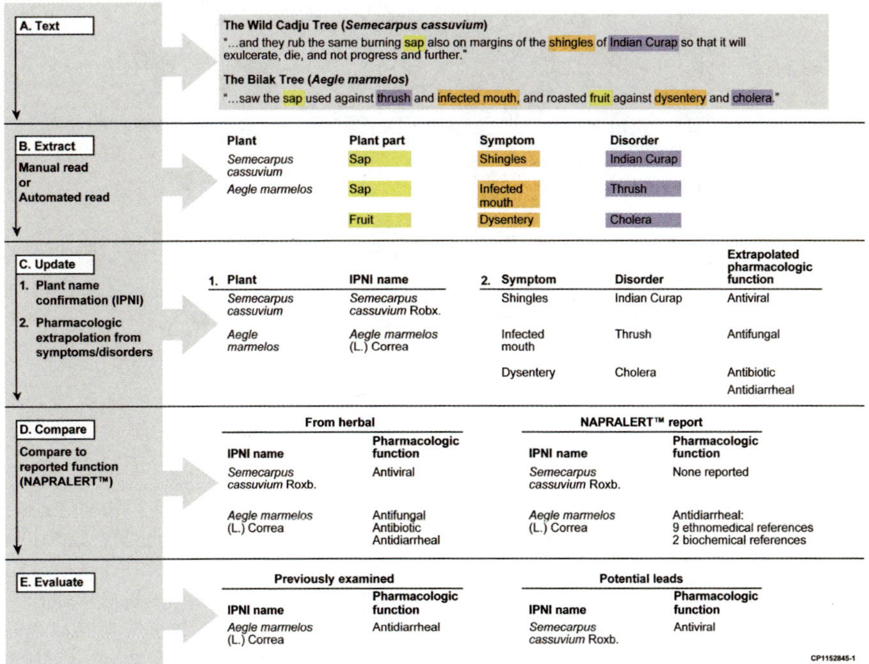

Figure 4.4 The general protocol for information extraction from an herbal text (A–E) is paired with case examples from our work with the *Ambonese Herbal* by Rumphius. For full caption see page 112.

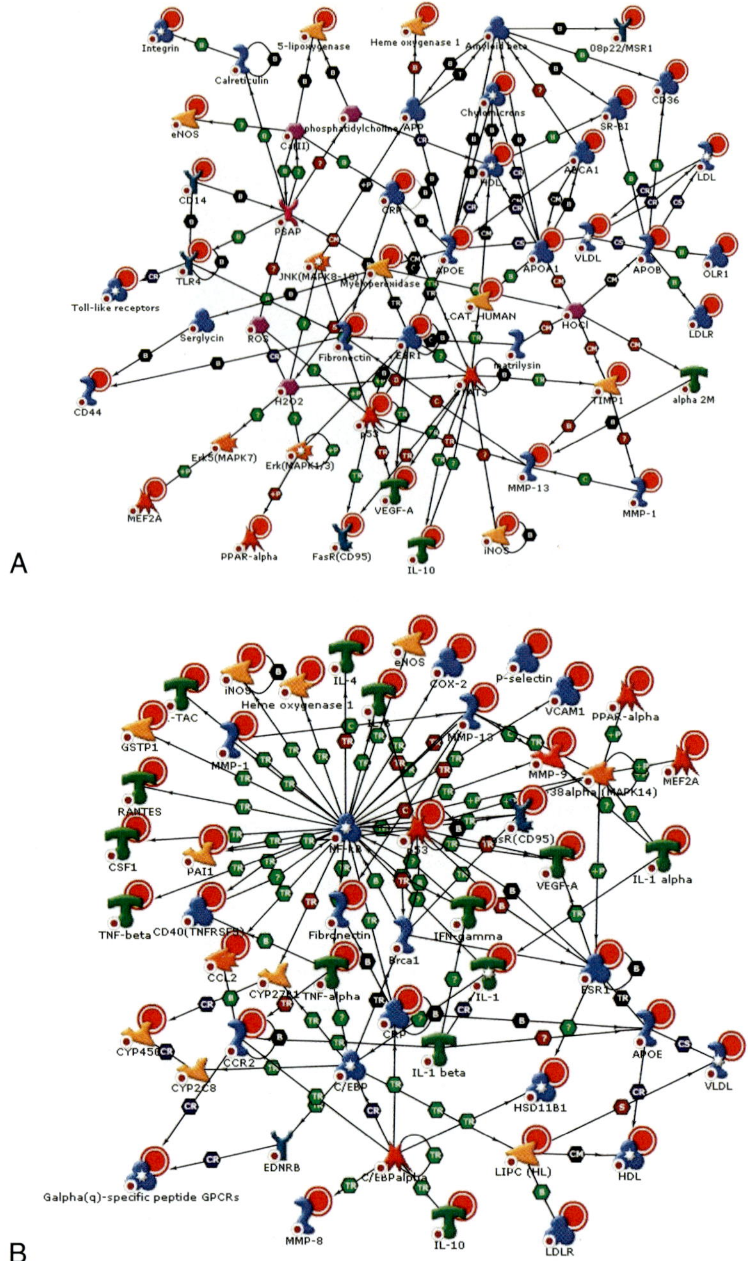

Figure 6.1 Gene interaction networks for atherosclerosis generated with the gene list from Ghazalpour et al. [53] with MetaCore™ (GeneGo, St. Joseph, MI). A. best G-score. B. best p value. The interaction types between nodes are shown as small colored hexagons, e.g., unspecified, allosteric regulation, binding, cleavage, competition, covalent modification, dephosphorylation, phosphorylation, transcription regulation, transformation. When applicable, interactions also have a positive or negative effect and direction. Ligands (purple) linked to other proteins (blue), transfactors (red), enzymes (orange). Genes with red dots represent the members of the original input gene list.

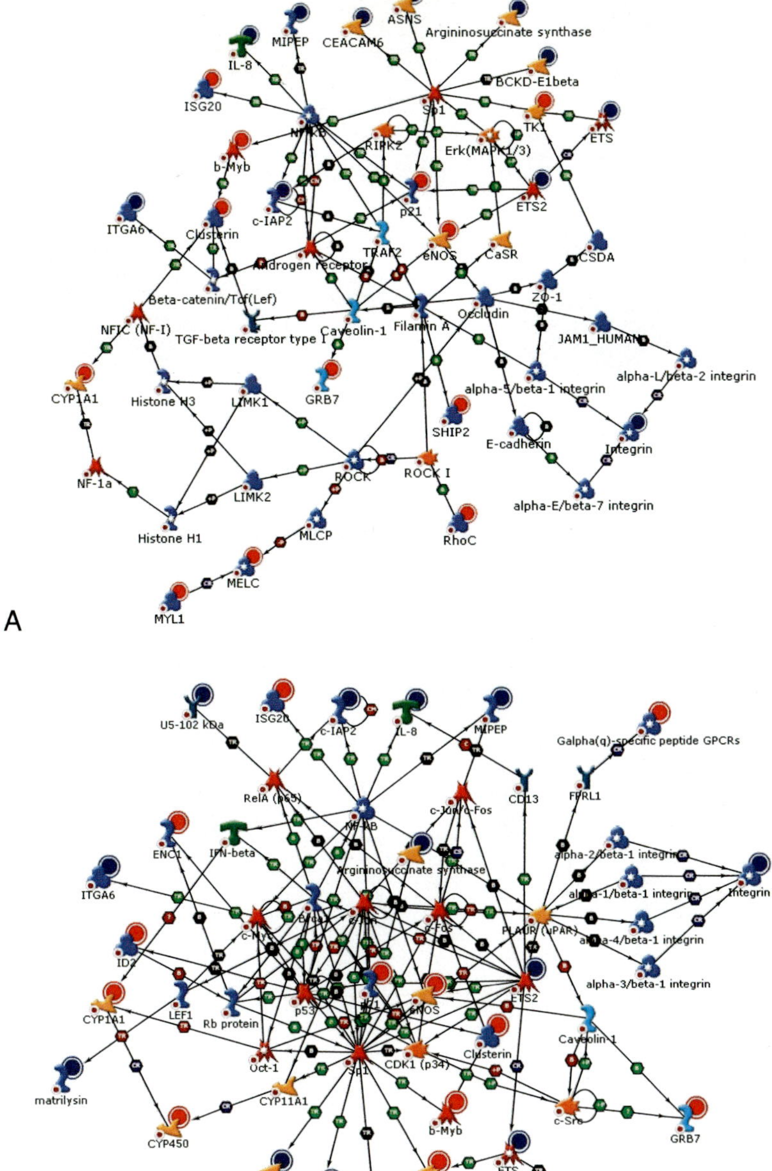

Figure 6.2 Gene interaction networks for tanshinone IIA-treated MCF-7 cells for 72 h [55] were generated with MetaCore™ (GeneGo). A. best G-score. B. best p value. The interaction types between nodes are shown as small colored hexagons, e.g., unspecified, allosteric regulation, binding, cleavage, competition, covalent modification, dephosphorylation, phosphorylation, transcription regulation, transformation. When applicable, interactions also have a positive or negative effect and direction. Ligands (purple) linked to other proteins (blue), transfactors (red), enzymes (orange). Genes with red dots represent the members of the original input gene list that were upregulated, whereas blue dots represent downregulated genes.

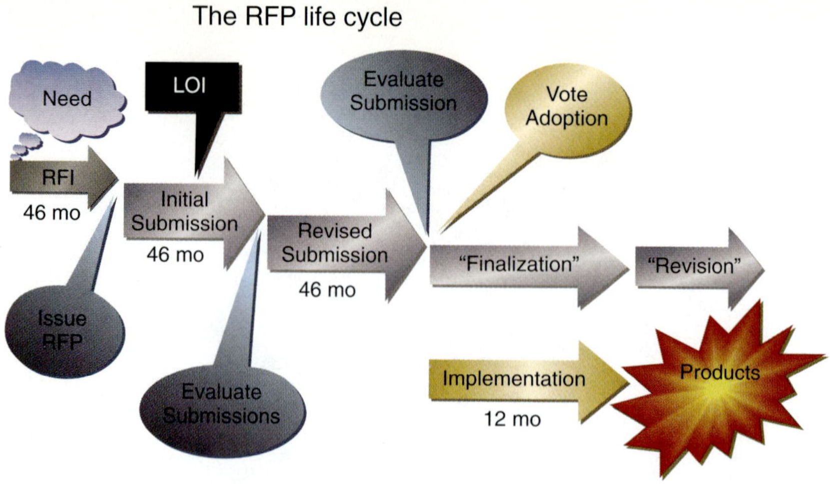

The RFP life cycle

Need
LOI
Evaluate Submission
Vote Adoption
RFI
46 mo
Initial Submission
46 mo
Revised Submission
46 mo
"Finalization"
"Revision"
Issue RFP
Evaluate Submissions
Implementation
12 mo
Products

Figure 7.6 The request for proposals life cycle. Used with kind permission from David Benton, GSK.

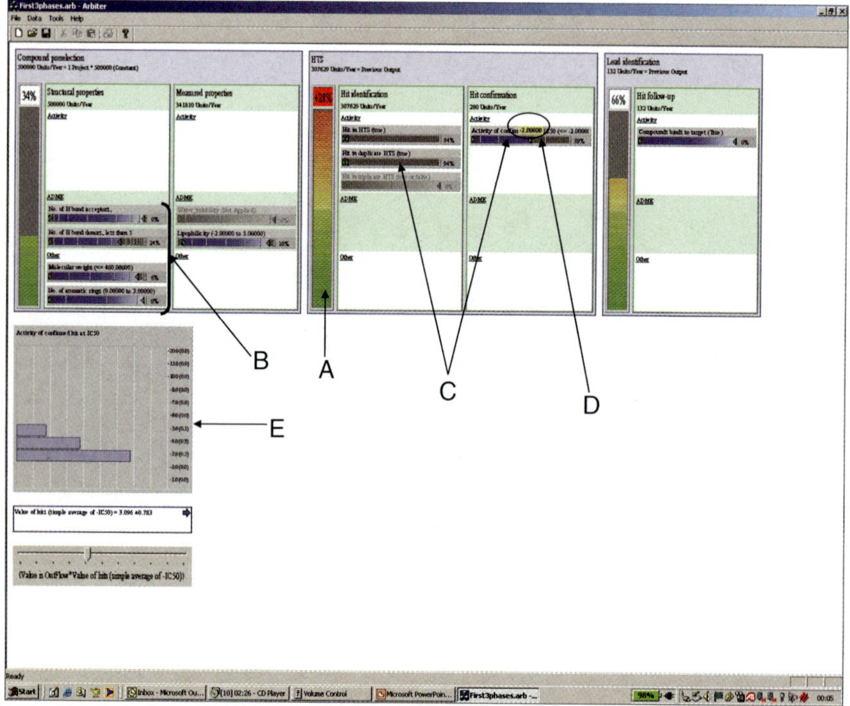

Figure 11.6 ARBITER provides a simulation of R&D throughput, stage success rates, and resource capacity loading (A) as a function of the methods used, the sequence of use (including parallel use), which is based on prior estimates of compound library quality, prevalence of different compound characteristics (B), prediction reliability (C), and user-selectable cutoff levels (D highlighted circle). The combination of throughput and candidate expected value (based on variations around the target product profile and the factors influencing development success rates) gives a direct estimate of the rate at which a particular selection of R&D process can be expected to contribute value. An average yield of successful projects (which may be a fraction) can be converted through use of distribution over a measure of pipeline quality. (E), including the chance of having no successes in any given year.

Determining Protein Structures

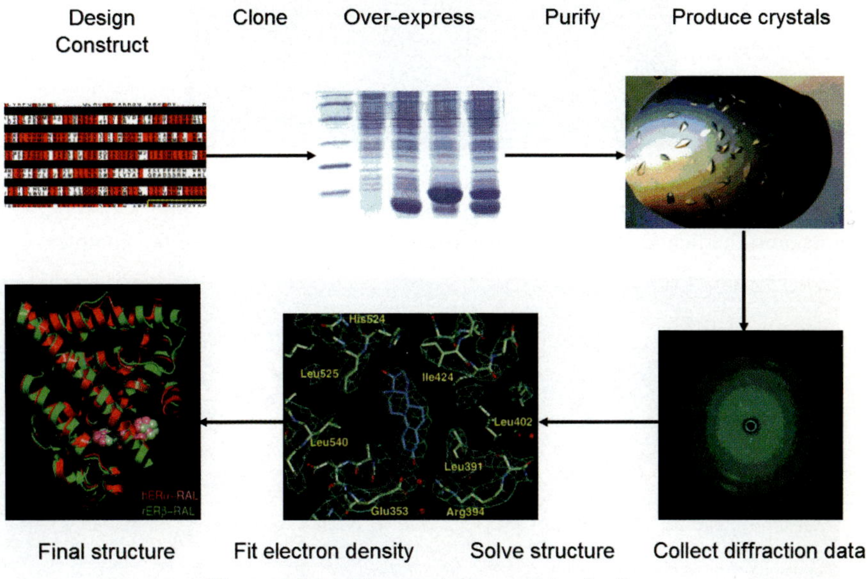

Figure 12.1 The crystallographic pipeline.

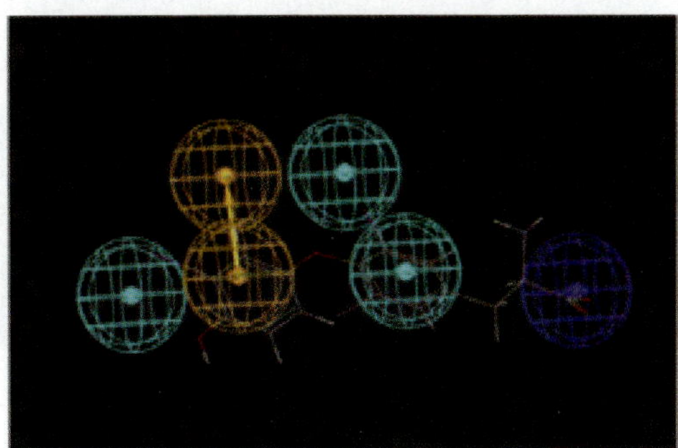

Figure 13.2 A typical Catalyst pharmacophore, where different colors indicate different chemical features and the spheres define tolerance spaces that each chemical feature would be allowed to occupy.

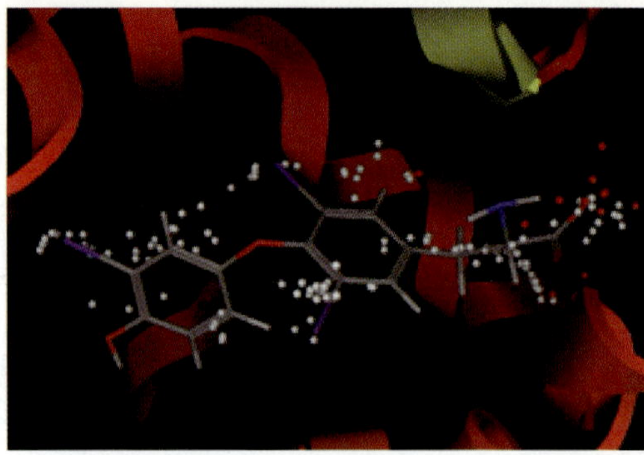

Figure 13.3 Potential pharmacophore points can be generated with MOE's site detection algorithm. The white and red dots are the automatically generated site points, and the ligand structure comes from the X-ray structure of the complex.

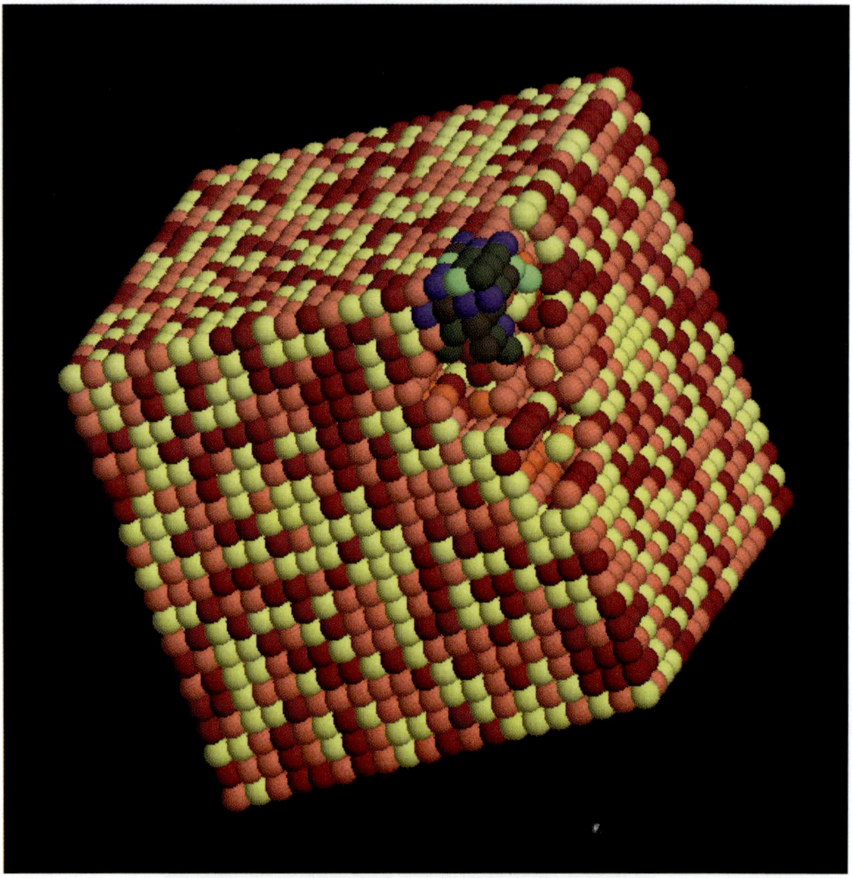

a

Figure 14.1 (a) A lattice protein-ligand complex. The lattice protein (colored red, yellow, pink, and orange) occupies a 20 × 20 cube, and the binding site is carved out in one corner. In this example, a ligand of 20 atoms was grown into the binding site. The ligand atoms are colored with blues and greens. (b) Effect of the evolutionary temperature on the database composition. The average binding energy of the database members is shown as a function of the temperature at which the ligands in the database were evolved. Clearly, as the temperature is lowered, there is a strong bias in the database towards strong binders.

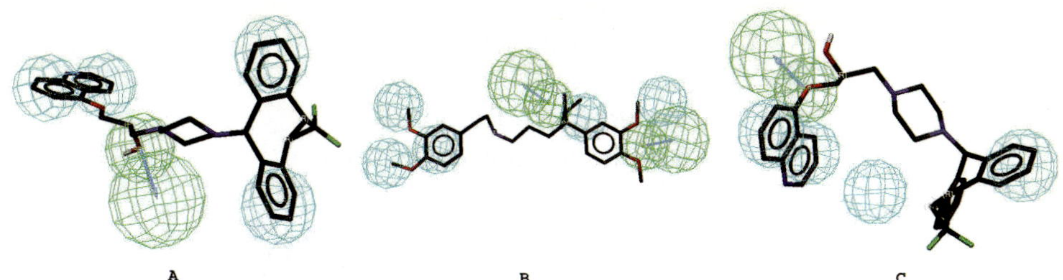

Figure 20.2 Pharmacophore models for P-gp inhibition. A. P-gp inhibition pharmacophore aligned with the potent inhibitor LY335979. B. P-gp substrate pharmacophore aligned with verapamil. C. P-gp inhibition pharmacophore 2 aligned with LY335979. Green indicates H-bond acceptor feature, and cyan indicates H-bond donor feature.

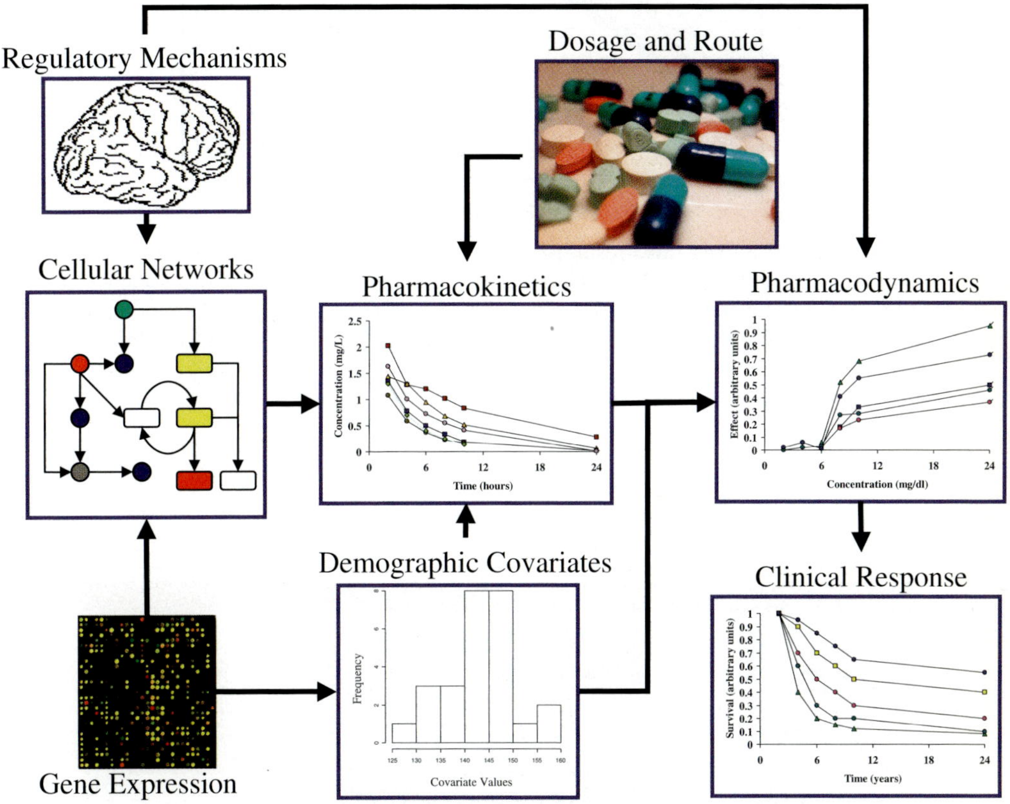

Figure 21.3 Modeling and simulation in the general context of the study of xenobiotics. The network of signals and regulatory pathways, sources of variability, and multistep regulation that are involved in this problem is shown together with its main components. It is important to realize how between-subject and between-event variation must be addressed in a model of the system that is not purely structural, but also statistical. The power of model-based data analysis is to elucidate the (main) subsystems and their putative role in overall regulation, at a variety of life stages, species, and functional (cell to organismal) levels. Images have been selected for illustrative purposes only.

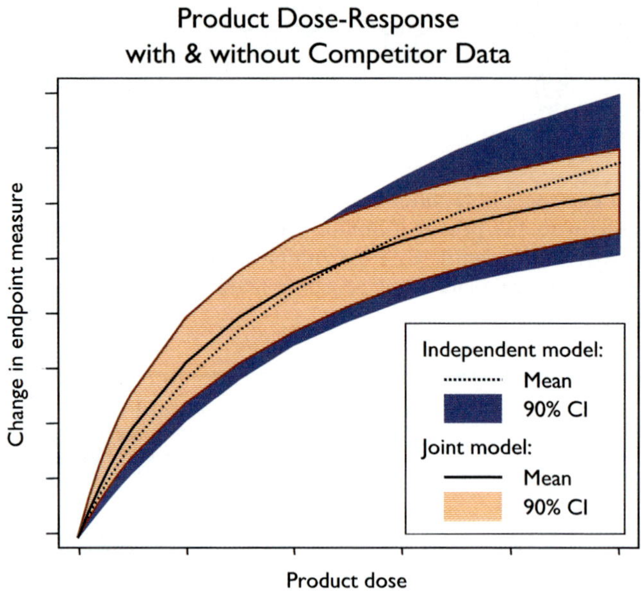

Product Dose-Response
with & without Competitor Data

Change in endpoint measure

Independent model:
Mean
90% CI
Joint model:
Mean
90% CI

Product dose

Figure 22.3 The drug dose-response model was augmented by using data for the comparator drug. Because the mechanism of the drugs was the same, this comprised additional data for the model. This enhanced the predictive power of the model, in a better estimate for central tendency (solid line compared with dotted line) but also in smaller confidence intervals. This is especially pronounced at the higher doses—precisely where data on the drug were sparse.

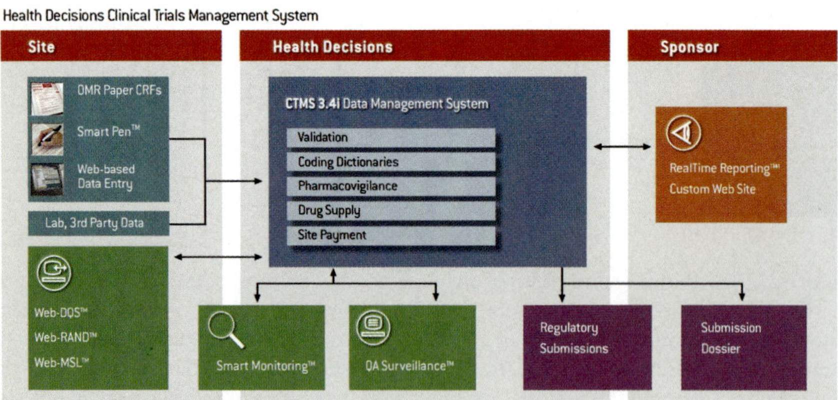

Figure 23.1 Components of the integrated system from the perspective of the clinical site, the data management group, and project management. For full caption see page 564.

Health Decisions WebDQS - Microsoft Internet Explorer

File Edit View Favorites Tools Help

Back Search Favorites History

Queries | Instructions
Reports | Help Desk
Validation Rules | Study List
Study Web Site | Log Out

Health Decisions
INTEGRATED CLINICAL RESEARCH
Sponsor A Protocol A Demo User 10 (Monitor)

Add Request: Step 1
Action: Data Update
Instance: Screening
CRF: Medical History
Continue Request

Step 1 Tips
1. Select an Action.
2. Select an Instance and CRF to indicate which CRF the Request is referring to.
3. Click Continue Request to move to Step 2. From there, you will be able to further define your Request.

Update Required Response Form

Site 60, Subject 200		Query 20055, Outstanding	
CRF:	Screening, Medical History, Log 1	Status:	Not Responded
Description:	Per source documents, the subject's height is 69 inches, but the CRF (MEHI_002) records 68 inches. Please review and reconcile. (Manual Query: Verification)		
Source:	Per Source Documents	Action:	Update Required
Comments:			

Update Requests: Not Submitted / New					
New #:	1			Status:	Not Submitted
Action:	Data Update	CRF:	Screening, Medical History	Log:	Scheduled (Log 1)
Question:	MEHI_002	Old Value:	68	New Value:	69

Remove New Request | Submit Response

Remove All New Requests & Return to Query Details

End document.

Done | Internet

Start 3:13 PM

Figure 23.3 The Data Query System™ is a web-based management tool that sites use to receive and manage queries.

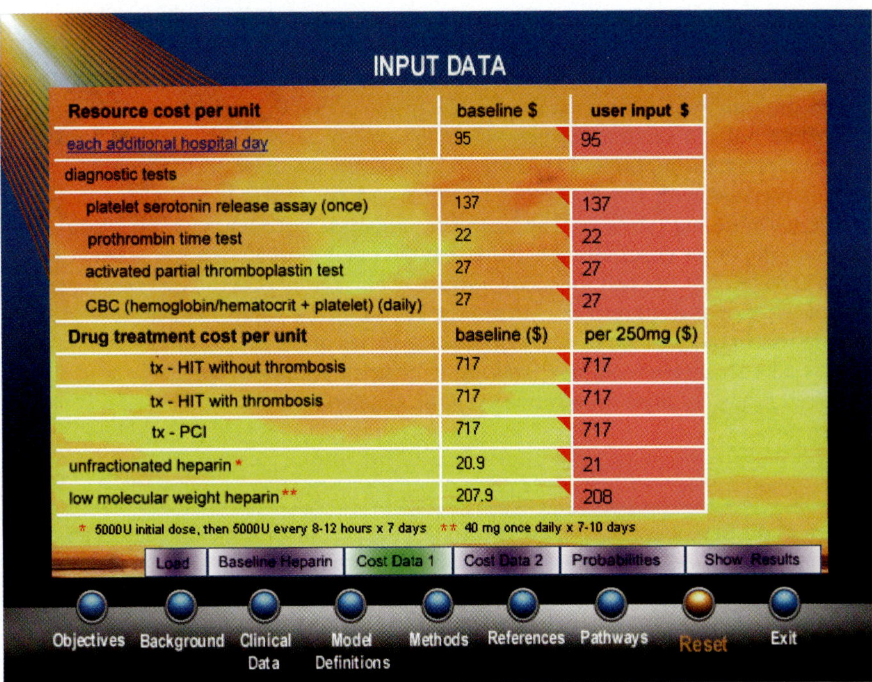

Resource cost per unit	baseline $	user input $
each additional hospital day	95	95
diagnostic tests		
platelet serotonin release assay (once)	137	137
prothrombin time test	22	22
activated partial thromboplastin test	27	27
CBC (hemoglobin/hematocrit + platelet) (daily)	27	27
Drug treatment cost per unit	**baseline ($)**	**per 250mg ($)**
tx - HIT without thrombosis	717	717
tx - HIT with thrombosis	717	717
tx - PCI	717	717
unfractionated heparin *	20.9	21
low molecular weight heparin **	207.9	208

Figure 24.5 Input screen from interactive model.

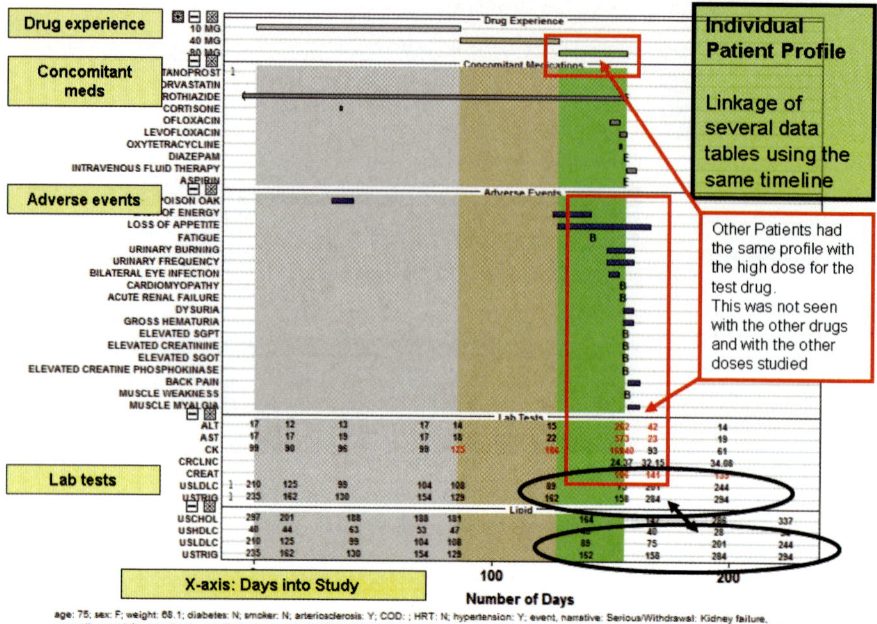

Figure 27.1 An example of New Drug Application (NDA) data graphically displayed for an individual patient in a dose escalation clinical trial. This graph displays and links drug exposure information, clinical adverse events, concomitant medications, clinical laboratory values, demographic information, and narratives. The graph is divided into 4 major sections: The x-axis for all 4 sections depicts time, and the y-axis the labels for each section. The top section displays drug exposure data for the test drug used in various doses (color coded). The second section displays exposure to concomitant medications over time. The third section displays adverse events over time. The bottom sections display when laboratory tests were conducted and the results. Note in the highlighted red squares that clinical and laboratory adverse events were associated with the high dose of the test drug. Other patients had the same profile with the high dose for the test drug. This was not seen with the other drugs and with the other doses studied. Note that the beginning of an adverse event is displayed (B) but not the end for many adverse events. Note that the end of a concomitant medication is displayed (E) but not the beginning for some medications. Observe highlighted in black the areas showing discrepancies in the timing of the same laboratory results in different tables, making it difficult to assess whether these values occurred before or after an adverse event or a concomitant drug.

Figure 27.4 Sector map display of the MGPS data mining profile for each drug, using a dictionary of medical terms. For full caption see page 673.

Cerivastatin

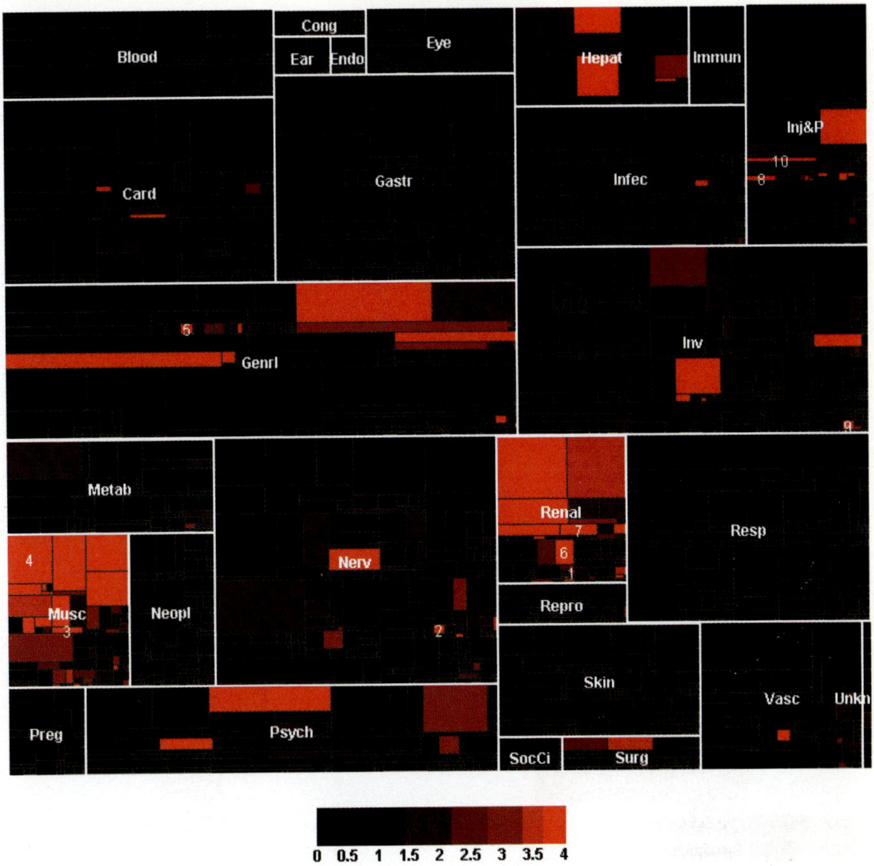

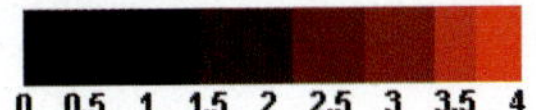

Rank	SOC	Term (PT)	EBGM	AERS cases
1	Renal	Myoglobinuria	15.416	104
2	Nerv	Myasthenic syndrome	12.449	1021
3	Musc	Myositis	12.198	2670
4	Musc	Rhabdomyolysis	11.501	12024
5	Genrl	Organ failure	10.121	685
6	Renal	Chromaturia	9.437	3034
7	Renal	Renal tubular necrosis	9.249	2547
8	Inj&P	Muscle injury	9.025	998
9	Inv	Myoglobin blood increased	8.807	527
10	Inj&P	Polytraumatism	8.497	1105

NOTES: Additional restrictions for graph:

Color controlled by: EBGM.
Size controlled by: relative importance.
Maximum intensity at signal score of 4.0.
Omit rare terms used fewer than 100.0 times
List 10 top scores
Show score indexes.
Group by HLT
Group by HLGT
Group by SOC
Lowest level displayed: PT

Print

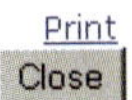

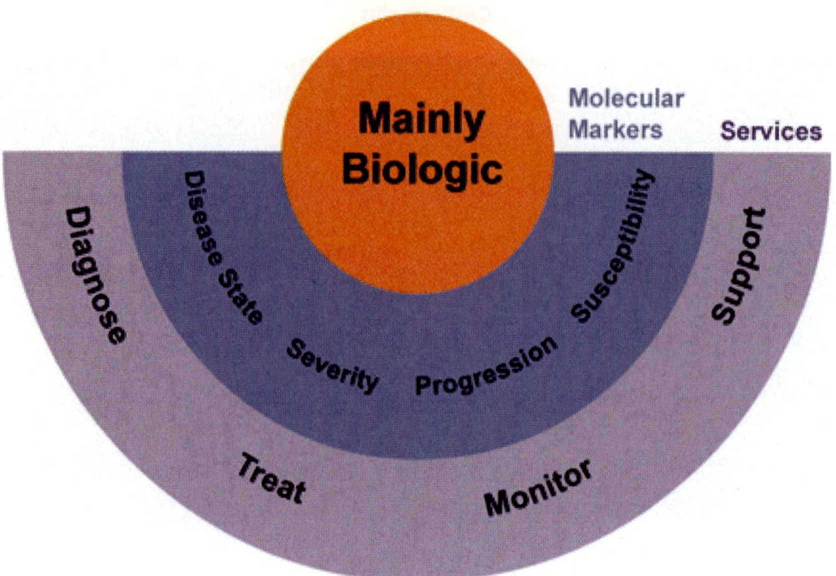

Figure 32.1 Targeted treatment solutions. Reproduced with permission from "Threshold of Innovation" (2005). IBM Business Consulting Services [1].

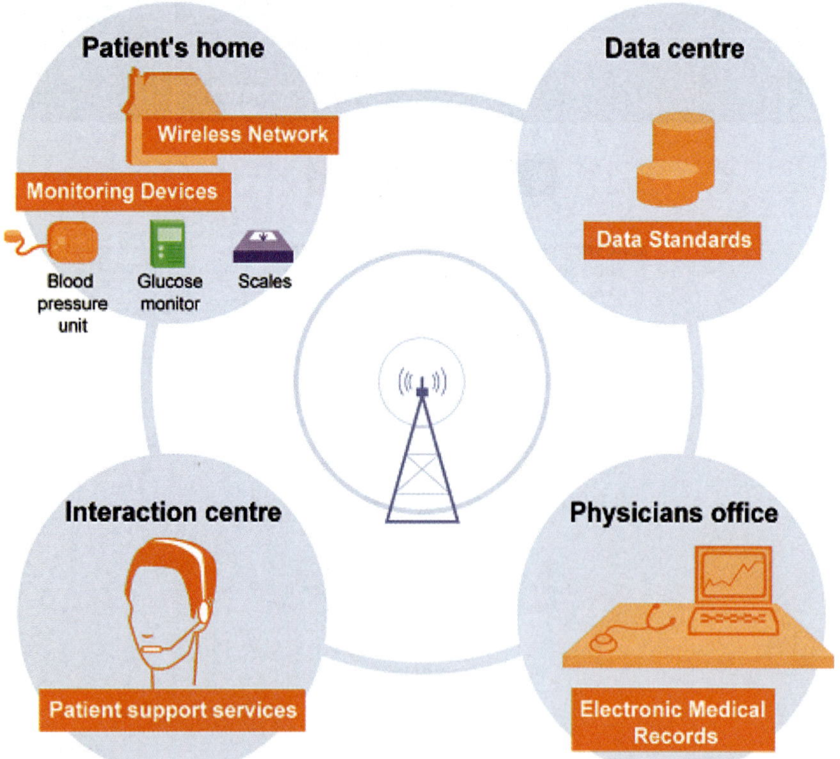

Figure 32.2 Infrastructure required for integrated health care. Reproduced with permission from "Threshold of Innovation" (2005). IBM Business Consulting Services [1].

16.3.3 Other Hydrolases

Acetylcholinesterase. The 3D structure of an acetylcholinesterase (AChE) complex with the natural product galanthamine was used to derive a Catalyst pharmacophore model with the program LigandScout. The pharmacophore, containing one donor, one acceptor, and two hydrophobic features, served to screen a 3D multiconformational database of more than 110,000 natural products. Among the observed hits were the coumarin **scopoletin 39** ($IC_{50} \approx 170\,\mu M$; Fig. 16.6) and its glucoside scopolin. In vivo, both compounds increase the extracellular acetylcholine concentration in rat brain to about 170% and 300% (intracerebrovascular application of 2 μmol compound), which is in the same range as the effect observed from galanthamine [115].

Adenylyl Cyclase (Edema Factor and CyaA). The adenylyl cyclases edema factor (EF) and CyaA are toxins of the pathogenic bacteria *Bacillus anthracis* and *B. pertussis*, which cause anthrax and whooping cough, respectively. The 3D structure of EF served to dock 205,226 ACD compounds into the catalytic site with a university version of the program DOCK. From 24 tested compounds two pyrazoloquinazolines could be identified as selective inhibitors of EF and CyaA, for example, **compound 40** (K_i EF ≈ 20 μM, IC_{50} EF = 90 μM; K_i CyaA ≈ 20 μM, IC_{50} CyaA = 80 μM; Fig. 16.6) [116].

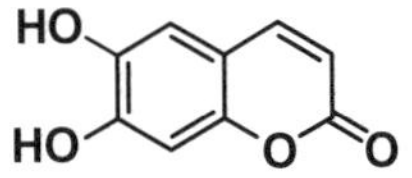

39

AChE inhibitor, $IC_{50} \approx 170\,\mu M$

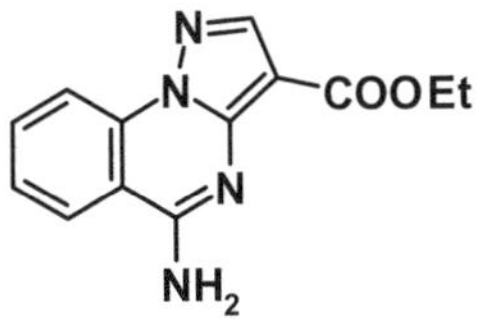

40

Edema factor (EF) adenylyl cyclase inhibitor, K_i EF ≈ 20μM, IC_{50} EF = 90 μM; K_i CyaA ≈ 20μM, IC_{50} CyaA = 80 μM

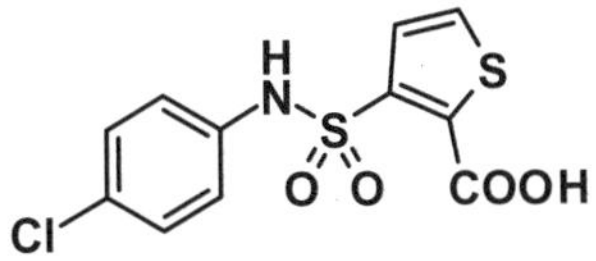

41

AmpC β-Lactamase noncovalent inhibitor, K_i = 26 μM

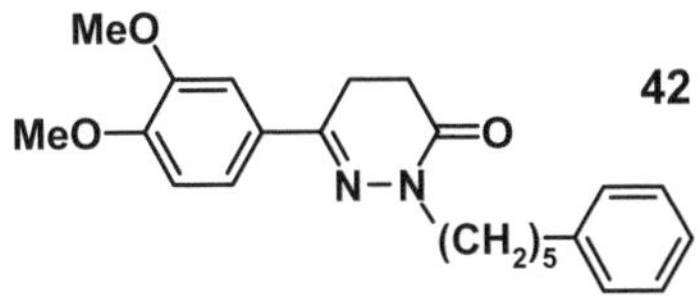

42

Phosphodiesterase 4 inhibitor, IC_{50} = 0.9 nM

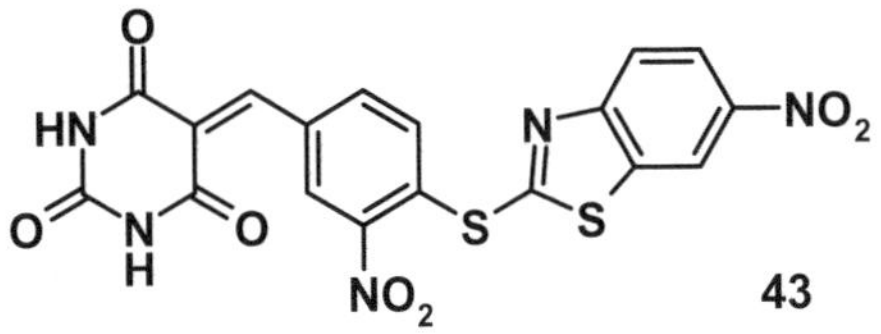

43

Protein tyrosine phosphatase 1B (PTP1B) inhibitor, IC_{50} = 4.1 μM

Figure 16.6 Other hydrolase inhibitors from virtual screening.

AmpC β-Lactamase. A map of "hot spots" was constructed from the X-ray structure of AmpC β-lactamase and a university version of the program DOCK was used to search for noncovalent inhibitors in 229,810 compounds of the ACD database. Of 56 tested compounds three had K_i values <650 μM, for example, **compound 41** (K_i = 26 μM; Fig. 16.6) [117]. The experimental X-ray structure of its complex with AmpC β-lactamase closely resembles the predicted binding mode.

Phosphodiesterase 4. Didier Rognan and his group used a "Scaffold-linker-functional group" (SCF) approach to design a virtual combinatorial library of analogs of the phosphodiesterase 4 (PDE4) inhibitor zardaverine (IC_{50} = 800 nM). All molecules were constructed from the invariable scaffold of zardaverine (with the exception of minor modifications) and a diverse set of variable linkers and building blocks. As the program FlexX produced the best results in the docking of zardaverine itself, this program was also used for the docking of all analogs. Nine molecules, out of 320 candidates, were synthesized and tested. **Compound 42** (IC_{50} = 0.9 nM; Fig. 16.6) was about 900 times more active than the original lead compound zardaverine [118].

Protein Tyrosine Phosphatase 1B. At Pharmacia, the in-house compound collection of 400,000 compounds was screened against protein tyrosine phosphatase 1B (PTP1B), resulting in 85 inhibitors (0.021%) with a validated IC_{50} < 100 μM; the most active compound had an IC_{50} = 4.2 μM. Shoichet and his group compared the efficacy of this high-throughput screening with docking and scoring [119]. Virtual screening was performed with 235,000 commercially available compounds from three different sources. After selection of only molecules with 17–60 nonhydrogen atoms, 165,581 compounds were docked into the 3D structure of PTB1B, using the program DOCK 3.5. Out of 365 high-scoring molecules, 127 (= 34.8%) inhibited PTP1B with an IC_{50} <100 μM, for example, **compound 43** (IC_{50} = 4.1 μM; Fig. 16.6) [74, 119]. The authors claim that the docking hits were more druglike than the screening hits, with respect to their physicochemical properties.

16.3.4 Oxidases/Reductases

Aldose Reductase. The ADAM&EVE docking program was used to screen about 120,000 structures of the ACD 3D database as potential aldose reductase inhibitors. Only one 3D conformation was generated for every molecule, but the ADAM&EVE program performed a systematic conformational search in the docking process, optimizing the conformation by a simplex method. After passing several filters (e.g., MW > 250, at least 1 ring system), total interaction energies were calculated and the resulting hits were visually inspected. An active hit served as a starting point for the dedicated design of analogs, resulting in **compound 44** (IC_{50} = 0.21 μM; Fig. 16.7) as the most potent inhibitor [120].

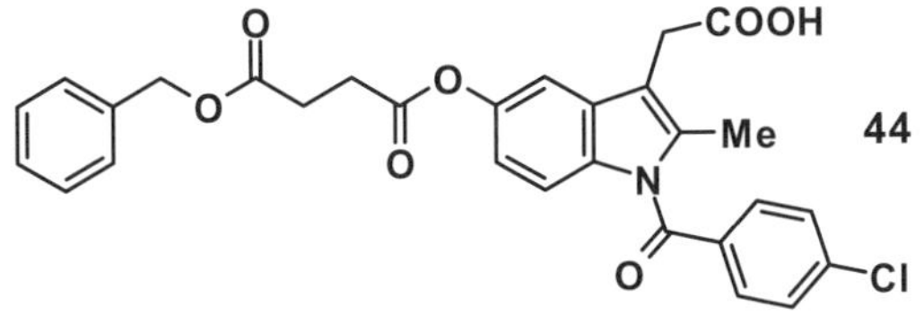

44
Aldose reductase inhibitor, IC_{50} = 0.21 μM

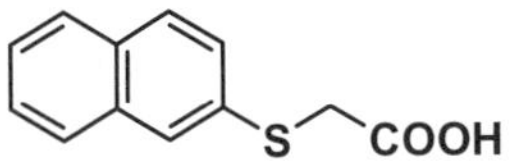

45
Aldose reductase inhibitor, IC_{50} = 28 μM

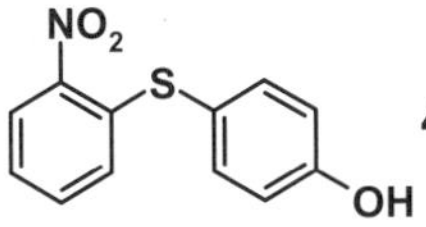

46
Aldose reductase inhibitor, IC_{50} = 4.8 μM

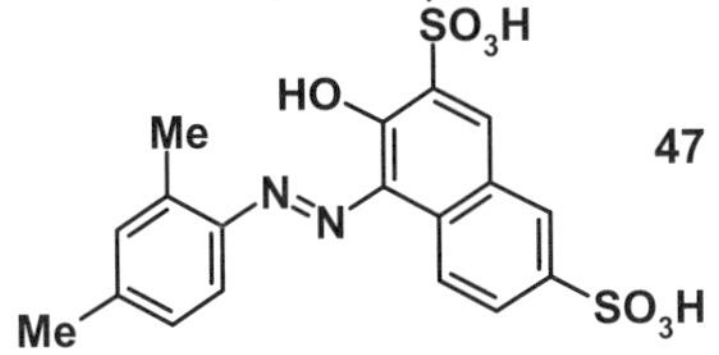

47
Aldose reductase inhibitor, IC_{50} = 0.58 μM

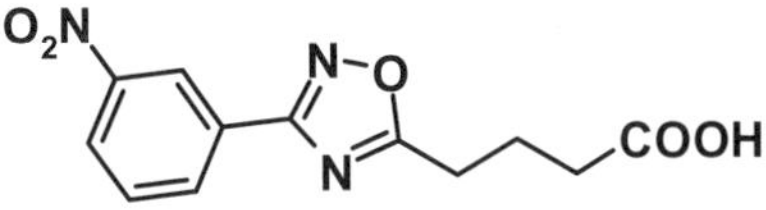

48
Aldose reductase inhibitor, IC_{50} = 2.4 μM

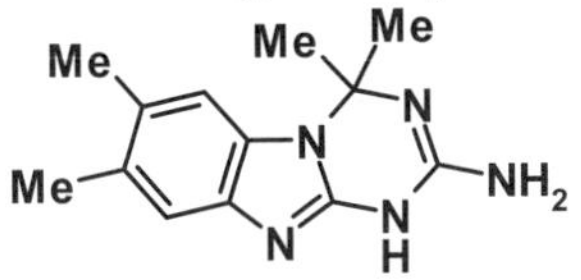

49
Plasmodium falciparum DHFR inhibitor, K_i = 0.54 μM, IC_{50} = 1.4 μM

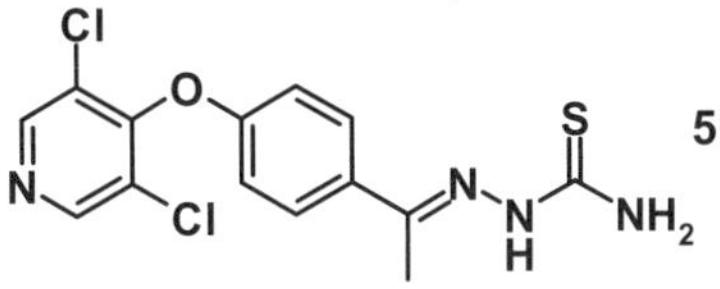

50
Plasmodium falciparum DHFR inhibitor, K_i = 0.9 μM, K_i vs. different resistant strains = 0.6-2.1 μM

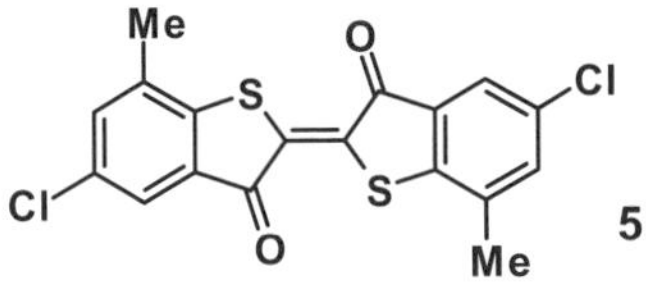

51
Pneumocystis carinii DHFR inhibitor, K_i = 6.9 μM (about 30-fold selectivity vs. human DHFR)

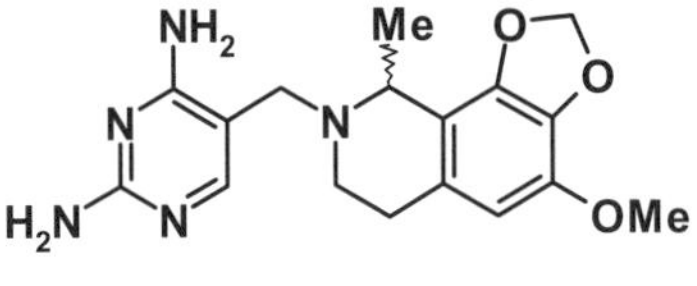

52
Streptococcus pneumoniae DHFR inhibitor, (*R*)-enantiomer, IC_{50} = 9.8 nM (*S. pn*. DHFR), IC_{50} = 2.8 nM (TMP-resistant *S. pn*. DHFR)

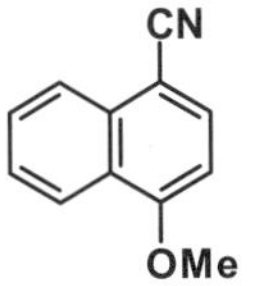

53
Inosine 5′-monophosphate dehydrogenase (IMPDH) inhibitor, IC_{50} = 31 μM

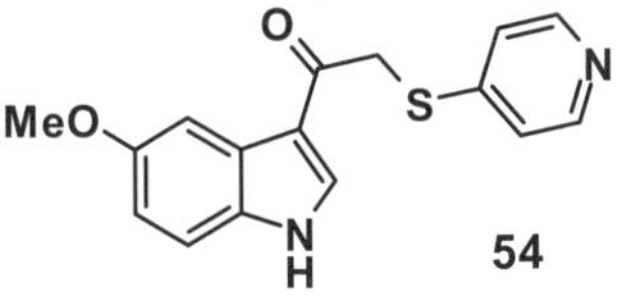

54
Inosine 5′-monophosphate dehydrogenase (IMPDH) inhibitor, IC_{50} = 32 μM

Figure 16.7 Oxidase and reductase inhibitors from virtual screening.

Among different 3D structures of aldose reductase, one with an additional open hydrophobic pocket was selected to search for ligands with additional aromatic rings. Molecular docking of 127,000 molecules of the NCI database into the binding pocket was performed with the program DOCK. The 1270 best-scoring compounds were clustered into chemical families, and a further selection was performed according to the interaction of the ligands with two key amino acids, Tyr48 and His110. Of the original 1270 molecules, 25 were selected; the most similar analogs in the ACD were taken for those that were commercially not available. Micromolar and submicromolar selective inhibitors resulted from biological testing (and chemical optimization of a nitro compound), for example, **compounds 45** (IC_{50} aldose reductase = 28 μM, aldehyde reductase inhibition: 6% at 45 μM; Fig. 16.7), **46** (IC_{50} aldose reductase = 4.8 μM, IC_{50} aldehyde reductase = 48 μM; Fig. 16.7). and **47** (IC_{50} aldose reductase = 0.58 μM, aldehyde reductase: 13% inhibition at 27 μM; Fig. 16.7) [121].

Gerhard Klebe and his group used a high-resolution 3D structure of aldose reductase (0.66 Å resolution) for a stepwise virtual screening for more drug-like inhibitors. First, 259,747 ACD compounds were filtered according to certain properties: presence of a carboxylic group or its isostere and compliance with the Lipinski rule of five (but restricted to MW < 350 and a number of rotatable bonds <9). This resulted in 12,545 candidates that were filtered by a pharmacophore search, using the program Unity and a pharmacophore, which was derived from the aldose reductase binding site with the programs SuperStar and the knowledge-based scoring function DrugScore. The 1261 fitting compounds were flexibly docked with the program FlexX. In the scoring procedure, a correction had to be applied to avoid overprediction of the affinity of large, flexible molecules [cf. 56]. The highest-scoring 216 compounds were clustered and visually inspected for the binding conformation, the surface complementarity of the ligand and the protein, and for unfilled space along the protein-ligand interface. A subset of nine carboxylic acids was selected for acquisition and biological testing. The most active hit was **compound 48** (IC_{50} = 2.4 μM; Fig. 16.7) [122].

Dihydrofolate Reductase. A 3D model of the dihydrofolate reductase (DHFR) domain of the bifunctional DHFR-thymidylate synthase of the malaria parasite *Plasmodium falciparum* was derived from the experimental 3D structures of human, chicken, *Escherichia coli*, and *Lactobacillus casei* DHFRs. Compounds with bifunctional basic groups, like amidines and guanidines, were extracted from the ACD, and the program GREEN was used to dock these compounds into the substrate binding site of the DHFR domain, under the constraint of an interaction of their basic group with Asp54. Among 32 candidates from docking and scoring, 21 were purchased and tested. Two compounds showed significant inhibitory activity, for example, **compound 49** (K_i = 0.54 μM, IC_{50} = 1.4 μM; Fig. 16.7) [123].

In malaria chemotherapy, resistant parasites have significantly reduced the efficiency of classic antifolate drugs. In the search for novel inhibitors of

P. falciparum dihydrofolate reductase (PfDHFR), first 3D pharmacophores and other filters were used to reduce the number of potential candidates in a database of 230,000 ACD compounds to 4061 molecules. Docking of these "focused" compounds was performed with the program DOCK 3.5. Twelve compounds were identified that are structurally unrelated to known antifolates; they inhibit not only wild-type PfDHFR but also different resistant mutants at micromolar concentrations. The most potent inhibitor was **compound 50** (K_i = 0.9 μM, K_i vs. the antifolate-resistant strains A16V, S108T, A16V+S108T, C59R+S108N+I164L, and N51I+C59R+S108N+I164L = 0.6–2.1 μM; Fig. 16.7) [124].

An opportunistic infection with the fungus *Pneumocystis carinii* is the principal cause of mortality in HIV-infected patients. Inhibitors of *P. carinii* DHFR with selectivity against human DHFR were identified by docking 53,328 compounds of the FCD (fine chemicals directory, a precursor of the ACD) into an unpublished 3D structure of the ternary complex of *P. carinii* DHFR with folate and NADPH, using the program DOCK. Of 2700 fitting compounds, 1266 were eliminated by energetic considerations. After two steps of chemical diversity selection the number of candidates was reduced to 89 compounds, of which 40 were ordered for biological testing. The most potent inhibitor was **compound 51** (K_i = 6.9 μM; Fig. 16.7), with about 30-fold selectivity vs. human DHFR [125].

At Hoffmann-La Roche 5-*N*,*N*-disubstituted aminomethyl-2,4-diaminopyrimidines were designed and tested as *Streptococcus pneumoniae* DHFR inhibitors. A virtual library was generated by substituting 2,4-diaminopyrimidine with 9448 secondary amines, and two approaches were followed: (1) a diversity-oriented selection and (1) virtual screening by docking and scoring, using the program FlexX and a homology model that was constructed from the 3D structure of the closely related *S. aureus* DHFR. The FlexX scoring function was modified to penalize hydrogen bonds that are formed at the surface of the protein.

Significantly more hits and more active compounds were obtained from the structure-based library design than from diversity-based design (21% vs. 3% hit rate). In general, the compounds showed high activity against trimethoprim (TMP)-sensitive and TMP-resistant *S. pneumoniae* DHFR. Some compounds were highly selective for the bacterial enzyme, as compared to the inhibition of the human enzyme, for example, the (*R*)-enantiomer of **compound 52** (IC_{50} *S. pn.* DHFR = 9.8 nM, IC_{50} TMP-resistant *S. pn.* DHFR = 2.8 nM, IC_{50} human DHFR = 1.2 μM; Fig. 16.7) [126].

Inosine 5′-Monophosphate Dehydrogenase. A series of 21 known inosine 5′-monophosphate dehydrogenase (IMPDH) inhibitors was used to validate a virtual screening protocol. By application of a molecular weight filter (80 < MW < 400), 3425 compounds were extracted from an in-house reagent inventory system. Docking of these compounds into a substrate-IMPDH complex 3D structure was performed with the program FlexX; three different scoring functions were tested, with and without conserved water molecules in the NAD cofactor binding site. The resulting 74 compounds gave a hit rate of 10% active compounds of diverse chemistry, for example, **compounds 53** (IC_{50} = 31 μM; Fig. 16.7) and **54** (IC_{50} = 32 μM; Fig. 16.7) [127].

16.3.5 Other Enzymes

5-Aminoimidazole-4-Carboxamide Ribonucleotide Transformylase. The NCI diversity library, a set of 1990 compounds with nonredundant pharmacophore profiles, was used for virtual screening of the human 5-aminoimidazole-4-carboxamide ribonucleotide (AICAR) transformylase active site with the program AutoDock. Biological testing of 16 soluble compounds, out of 44 potential inhibitors, revealed eight micromolar inhibitors with novel scaffolds, for example, **compound 55** (IC_{50} = 4.1 μM; Fig. 16.8). Docking of all compounds with similar scaffolds, from the entire NCI 3D database, yielded another 11 inhibitors, for example, **compound 56** (K_i = 154 nM, IC_{50} = 600 nM; Fig. 16.8) [128].

Carbonic Anhydrase II. Carbonic anhydrases are metalloenzymes with a catalytically active Zn^{2+} ion in the catalytic center. Aromatic and other acidic sulfonamides bind as anions that form the warhead group of all carbonic anhydrase inhibitors. The experimental X-ray structure of carbonic anhydrase II was used for virtual screening of potential inhibitors. 3D structures were generated for 98,850 compounds of the Maybridge and LeadQuest compound collections. The binding pocket of carbonic anhydrase was investigated by the computer programs GRID, SuperStar, LUDI, and DrugScore. Hot spots obtained from these programs were converted into a pharmacophore model, and 2D and 3D searches were performed with the program Unity. The resulting 3314 structures were flexibly superimposed on the highly potent inhibitor dorzolamide, using the program FlexS. The best hits were docked as flexible ligands with the program FlexX. Binding affinities to carbonic anhydrase were estimated with the knowledge-based scoring function DrugScore, and the top ranking 13 molecules were biologically tested. Three inhibitors exhibited subnanomolar activity, for example, compounds **57** (IC_{50} = 0.6 nM; Fig. 16.8) and **58** (IC_{50} = 0.8 nM; Fig. 16.8) [129, 130].

A search for even more potent carbonic anhydrase II inhibitors, by a Harvard University group in cooperation with Concurrent Pharmaceuticals (now Vitae Pharmaceuticals), started from the nanomolar inhibitor *p*-$H_2NCO\text{-}C_6H_4\text{-}SO_2NH_2$ (K_d = 120 nM). Derivatives of this base fragment, substituted at the carboxamido nitrogen atom, were generated in the binding site of the protein from 100 different small organic groups. The growth algorithm CombiSMoG (combinatorial small molecule generator) randomly selected fragments from this library and attached them to the growing ligand. The affinity of the generated ligands was estimated by the knowledge-based

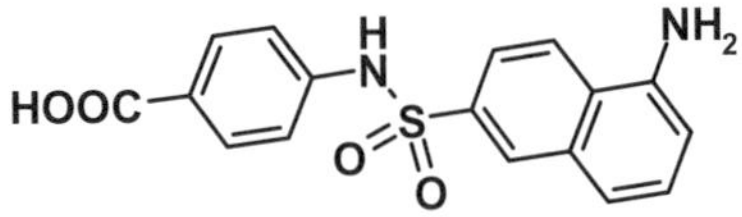

55

5-Aminoimidazole-4-carboxamide ribonucleotide (AICAR) transformylase inhibitor, IC_{50} = 4.1 μM

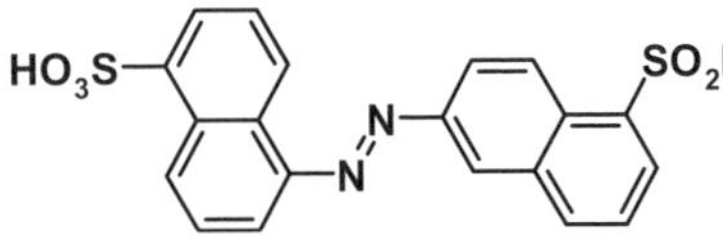

56

5-Aminoimidazole-4-carboxamide ribonucleotide (AICAR) transformylase inhibitor, K_i = 154 nM, IC_{50} = 600 nM

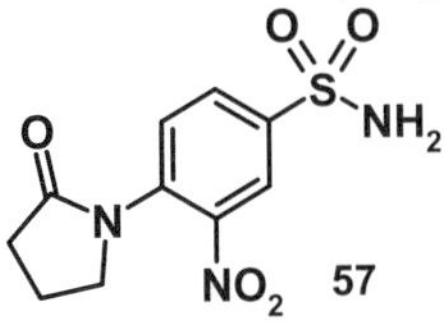

57 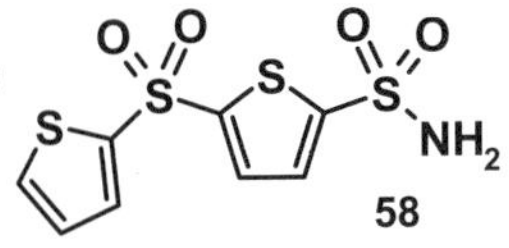 58

Carbonic anhydrase II inhibitors, IC_{50} = 0.6 nM (left) and 0.8 nM (right)

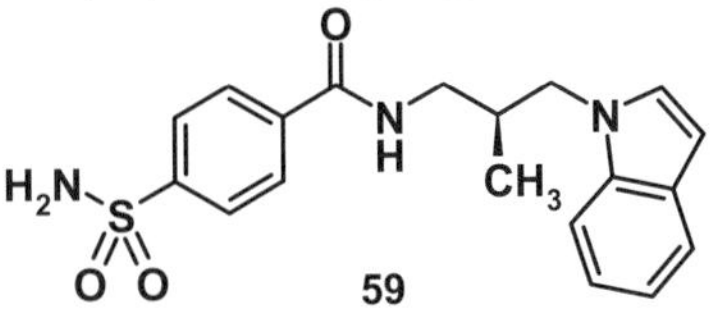

59

Carbonic anhydrase II inhibitor, K_d = 30 pM

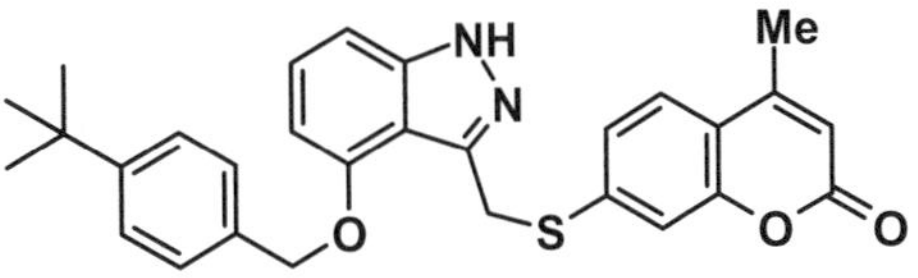

60

DNA gyrase inhibitor MNEC = 0.03 μg/ml

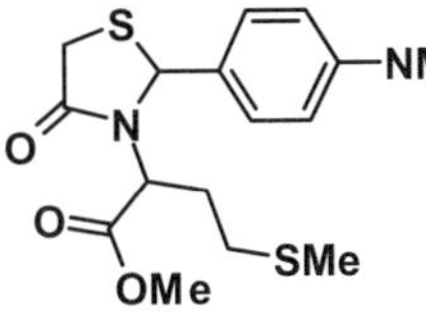

61

dTDP-6-deoxy-D-xylo-4-hexulose 3,5-epimerase (RmlC) inhibitor, 100% inhibition at 20 μM

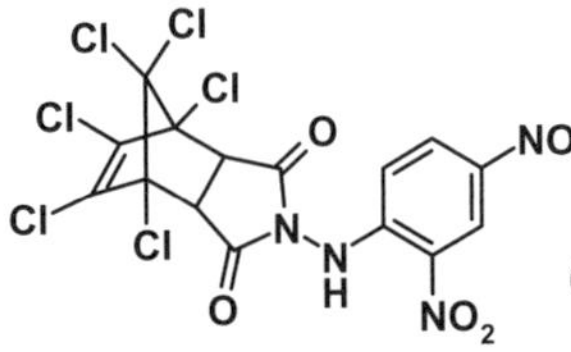

62

Farnesyl transferase inhibitor IC_{50} = 25 μM

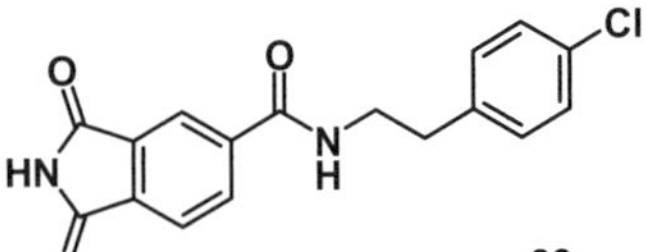

63

Guanine-phosphoribosyl transferase inhibitor, K_i = 23 μM, IC_{50} = 52 μM

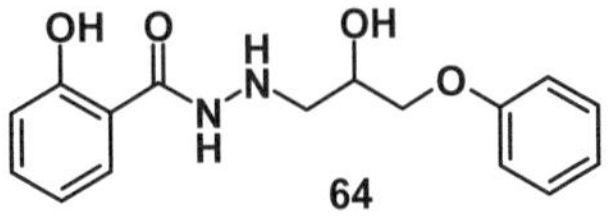

64 and 65 (mixture)

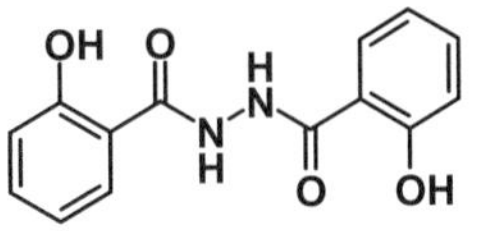

HIV-1 integrase inhibitors, IC_{50} 3′-processing = 0.6 μg/ml, IC_{50} strand transfer = 0.46 μg/ml

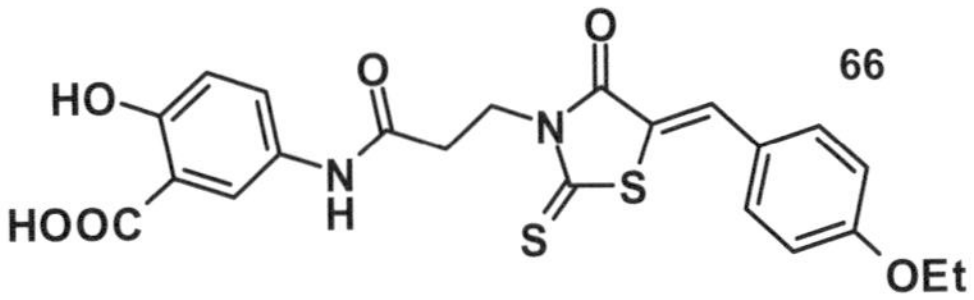

66

HIV-1 integrase inhibitor, IC_{50} 3′-processing = 17 μM, IC_{50} strand transfer = 11 μM

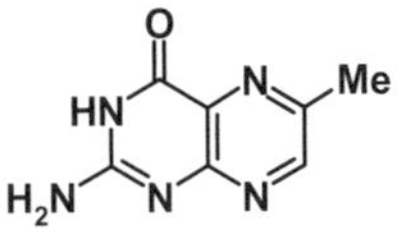

67

tRNA-guanine transglycosylase (TGT) inhibitor, K_i = 0.25 μM

Figure 16.8 Other enzyme inhibitors from virtual screening.

CombiSMoG potential function, which was derived from 1000 protein-ligand complex 3D structures. After inspection of 100,000 candidates, the five best hits were ranked by a force field calculation. The (*R*)-isomer of the indole **compound 59** (K_d = 30 pM; Fig. 16.8) is the highest-scoring compound and has the highest affinity of all synthesized molecules, whereas the (*S*)-isomer has only a K_d = 230 pM [131, 132].

DNA Gyrase. After the failure to find DNA gyrase inhibitors by conventional screening of the Hoffmann-La Roche compound collection, Böhm et al. performed a virtual screening procedure, called "needle screening." First, small "needle-type" molecules were selected from about 350,000 compounds of the ACD and part of the Roche compound inventory and docked into the DNA gyrase active site with the de novo design program LUDI. The resulting hits were then analyzed for their binding site interactions. About 200 compounds were tested for DNA gyrase inhibition, and activities in the range of 5–64 μg/ml were obtained. X-ray structure analysis verified the proposed binding modes of an indazole, an aminotriazine, and a pyrrolopyrimidine lead structure. **Compound 60** [maximal noneffective concentration (MNEC) = 0.03 μg/ml; Fig. 16.8] resulted after 3D structure-guided optimization [133].

dTDP-6-Deoxy-D-Xylo-4-Hexulose3,5-Epimerase (RmlC). dTDP-6-deoxy-D-xylo-4-hexulose 3,5-epimerase (RmlC) has been selected as a new promising target in the fight against tuberculosis. A virtual library of 2,3,5-trisubstituted thiazolidin-4-ones was generated from 24 amino acids, 27 aldehydes, and 2 thioacids with the program CombiLibmaker, and the resulting 3888 structures (containing all possible stereoisomers) were docked into the active site of the enzyme with the program FlexX. After consensus scoring with the CScore module, the top 5% (= 144 compounds) were selected for synthesis and biological tests; 30 of 94 compounds had biological activities >50% at 20 μM, for example, **compound 61** (100% inhibition at 20 μM; Fig. 16.8) [134].

Farnesyl Transferase. A rigid docking of 219,390 ACD compounds into the binding site of farnesyl transferase was performed with the program EUDOC. Of 21 hits, four inhibited the enzyme with IC_{50} values in the range 25–100 μM. The most potent inhibitor, **compound 62** (IC_{50} = 25 μM; Fig. 16.8), inhibited farnesyl transferase also in human lung cancer cells [135a]. A Catalyst 3D pharmacophore search of a Schering-Plough corporate database yielded five compounds with IC_{50} values smaller or equal to 5 μM, representing three different structural classes [135b].

Guanine Phosphoribosyl Transferase. Guanine phosphoribosyl transferase (GPRT) is one of the enzymes of the purine salvage pathway, which is needed by protozoa because they lack the ability to synthesize purine nucleotides.

Two micromolar phthalimide GPRT inhibitors were identified by screening the in-house phthalimide library. On the basis of this result, a virtual library of substituted phthalimides was constructed and docked into the binding sites of six GPRTs from different sources, including *Giardia lamblia*, various trypanosomes, *E. coli*, and human with the program DOCK 4.01. Several micromolar inhibitors resulted, for example, **compound 63** (K_i = 23 µM, IC_{50} = 52 µM; Fig. 16.8) [136].

HIV-1 Integrase. Several 3D pharmacophore models were derived from known HIV-1 integrase inhibitors. These models were validated with a 3D database of 152 compounds with known integrase inhibitory activities. The most probable pharmacophore model was used as query for a 3D search of 206,876 compounds of the NCI 3D database. From 340 hits 29 compounds were selected for biological tests, resulting in 10 novel, structurally diverse HIV-1 integrase inhibitors. Four of these had IC_{50} values <30 µM, for example, a salicylic acid derivative, which later turned out to be a mixture of two salicylic acid hydrazides, **compounds 64** and **65** (IC_{50} 3′-processing ~2.0 µM, IC_{50} strand transfer ~1.5 µM; Fig. 16.8) [137].

A pharmacophore hypothesis for HIV-1 integrase inhibitors was derived from four isosteric β-diketo integrase inhibitors by the HipHop module of Catalyst. A 3D search in a multiconformer Catalyst database of 150,000 ChemBridge compounds yielded 1700 molecules that fitted a four-point pharmacophore. Subsequently, the program GOLD 1.2 was used to dock the structures into the integrase binding site. Afterwards, the 200 top-scoring hits were visually inspected for their ability to chelate a metal ion, for structural novelty, and for compliance with the Lipinski rule of five. Finally, 110 molecules were biologically tested, yielding 48 compounds with IC_{50} values from 7 to 100 µM, for example, **compound 66** (IC_{50} 3′-processing = 17 µM, IC_{50} strand transfer = 11 µM; Fig. 16.8). The most active compounds had a salicylic acid substituent and a 2-thioxo-thiazolidinone (rhodanine) scaffold. On the basis of a 2D substructure search for these moieties, another 22 compounds were selected and tested, resulting in some more micromolar integrase inhibitors [138].

tRNA-Guanine Transglycosylase. In the search for tRNA-guanine transglycosylase (TGT) inhibitors, 800,000 molecules from eight different databases were screened in a stepwise manner, using the programs Selector (to eliminate molecules with more than 7 rotatable bonds and a MW > 450), Unity for 3D pharmacophore search, and FlexX for flexible docking. About 50% of all molecules were eliminated by the Selector procedure. Three different binding site-derived pharmacophore hypotheses were applied to perform 3D pharmacophore searches. This filter reduced the set of compounds to 20% of the original size. In the next step, volume constraints defined the shape of the binding site, producing a hit list of 872 compounds. After flexible docking into two different conformations of the enzyme, some other criteria were applied, to end up with 9 compounds that were biologically tested. All had micromolar to submicromolar activities, for example, **compound 67** ($K_i = 0.25\,\mu M$; Fig. 16.8) [139, 140].

16.4 ION CHANNELS

16.4.1 T-Type Selective Ca^{2+} Channel

The T-type selective channel blocker lead structure mibefradil ($IC_{50} = 1.2\,\mu M$) served as a template for virtual screening of the Hoffmann-La Roche in-house compound collection. Several filters were applied, and the similarity of the candidates to the lead structure was compared by the CATS descriptor [89]. Because only pharmacophoric features and their topological distances describe the molecules, the CATS descriptor enables a "scaffold hopping"; that is, molecules with different scaffolds but comparable biological properties result from this approach. The 12 highest-ranking molecules were biologically tested; nine of them showed T-channel blocking activities in the same range as the lead structure mibefradil. Whereas one highly active compound was the known neuroleptic **clopimozide 68** ($IC_{50} < 1\,\mu M$; Fig. 16.9) [89], several other active hits, for example, **compounds 69** ($IC_{50} = 2.4\,\mu M$; Fig. 16.9) [63,141] and **70** ($IC_{50} = 0.8\,\mu M$; Fig. 16.9) [141], are new chemotypes. Despite the topological pharmacophore similarity, the scaffolds of all compounds are significantly different from mibefradil.

16.4.2 Kv1.5 Potassium Channel

A potent hKv1.5 potassium channel blocker from literature served as template for a TOPAS (topology assigning system) de novo design [142]. The "scaffold hopping" program TOPAS starts from a collection of building blocks that are generated by retrosynthetic fragmentation of the World Drug Index (WDI). By using 11 chemical reactions of the RECAP procedure [143], 24,563 unique building blocks were generated. After assembling new structures from various scaffolds and building blocks, an evolutionary algorithm selects the "fittest" molecules, that is, the ones that are most similar to the original template. Although the "most similar" **compound 71a** (R = OMe, $IC_{50} = 7.34\,\mu M$; Fig. 16.9) is much less active than the template ($IC_{50} = 0.11\,\mu M$), a close analog, **compound 71b** (R = H, $IC_{50} = 0.47\,\mu M$) [142], has about the same order of biological activity (wrong substitution pattern in Scheme 1 of Ref. 142; see Scheme 2).

The same template as for **compound 71** was used by Peukert et al. for a 2D similarity search in the Aventis in-house compound collection [144]. 75 Compounds with a similarity index >0.80 were biologically tested. The moderately active 1-carboxy,8-sulfonamido-naphthalene ($IC_{50} = 9.5\,\mu M$), with insufficient chemical stability, was the starting point for the design of substituted biphenyls, which after further optimization produced **compound 72** (IC_{50} = 0.16 μM; Fig. 16.9) [144].

An improved 3D pharmacophore, considering all results obtained so far, and a new 3D search in the Aventis compound collection with the program

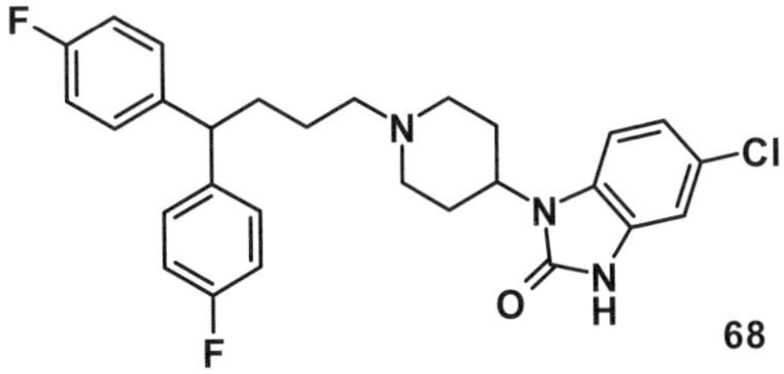

68
Clopimozide, Ca^{2+} antagonist,
IC_{50} < 1 μM

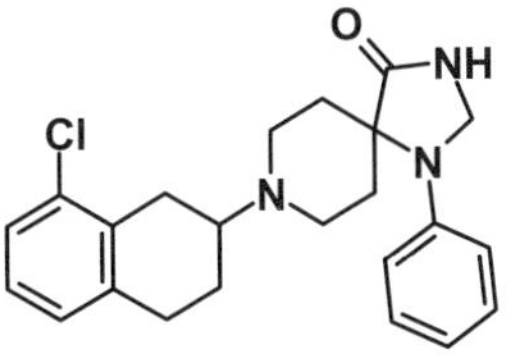

69
Ca^{2+} antagonist (T channel blocker),
IC_{50} = 2.4 μM

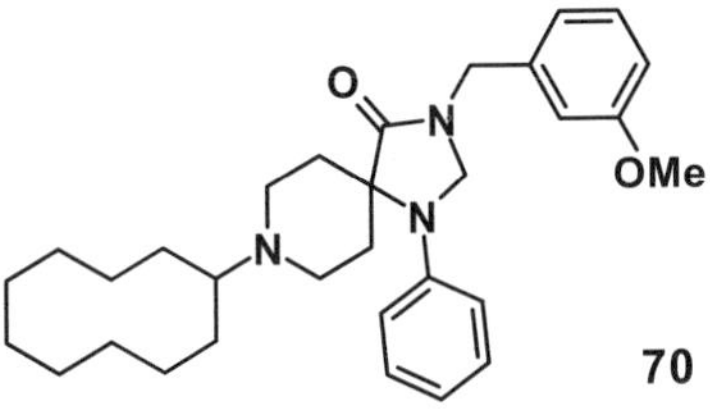

70
Ca^{2+} antagonist (T channel blocker),
IC_{50} = 0.8 μM

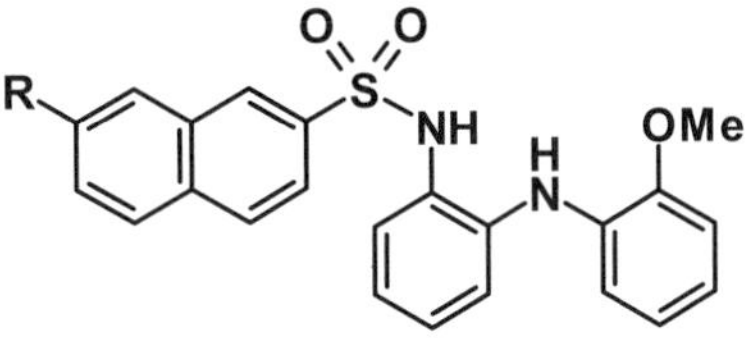

71
hKv1.5 Potassium channel inhibitor,
a R = OMe, IC_{50} = 7.34 μM
b R = H, IC_{50} = 0.47 μM

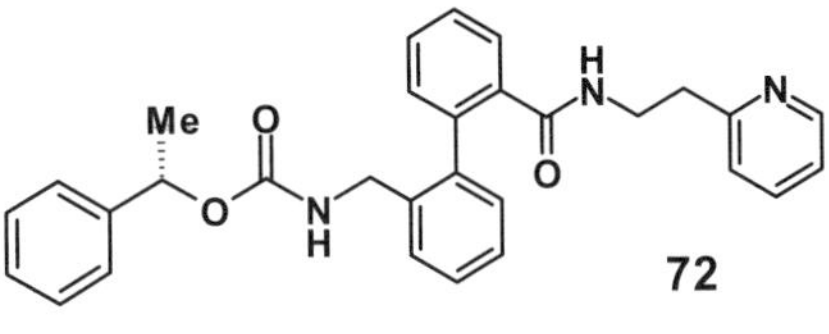

72
hKv1.5 Potassium channel inhibitor,
IC_{50} = 0.16 μM

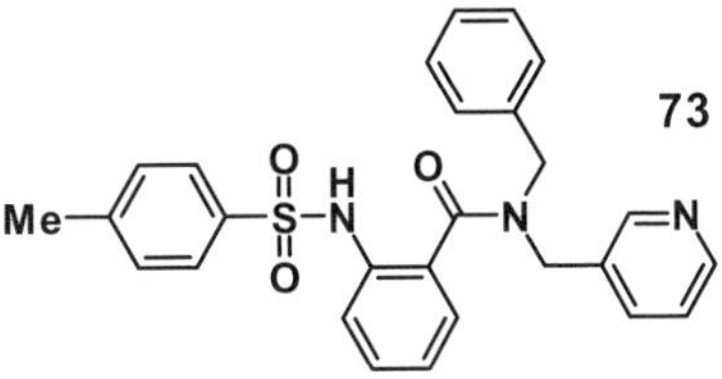

73
hKv1.5 Potassium channel inhibitor,
IC_{50} = 0.7 μM

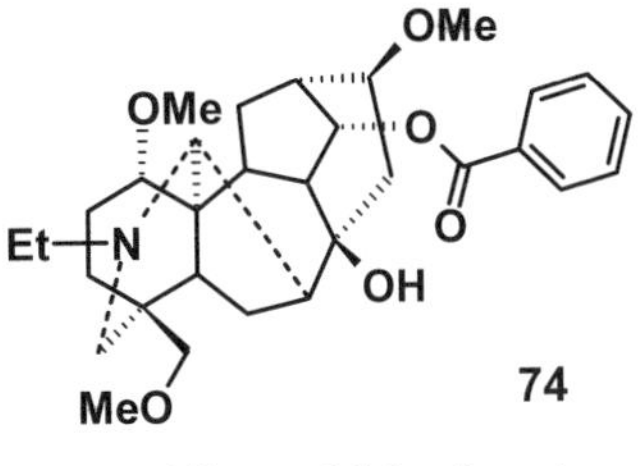

74
Shaker K^+ channel blocker,
IC_{50} = 3.8 μM

Figure 16.9 Ion channel blockers from virtual screening.

Unity resulted in 4234 hits. After application of several filters and clustering of the remaining 1975 molecules, compounds from 18 of the 27 clusters were screened in *Xenopus* oocytes. One compound with an IC_{50} of 5.6 μM belonged to a new class of Kv1.5 blockers and exhibited a favorable pharmacokinetic profile. After further optimization, **compound 73** (IC_{50} = 0.7 μM; Fig. 16.9) resulted, with good oral bioavailability in rats [145].

In a further investigation, the most interesting hits of the prior work were used together with other reference Kv1.5 channel blockers to perform virtual screening for new chemotypes. A protein-based pharmacophore for a 3D search was derived from a homology model of the potassium channel. The five most active hits from the corporate database had IC_{50} values between 0.9 and 7.9 μM (structures not given) [146]. Whereas chemical similarity between these compounds, as measured by pairwise Tanimoto similarity based on Unity fingerprints, was low, feature tree similarity values, which measure pharmacophore similarity across chemically diverse classes, are high.

16.4.3 Shaker K^+ Channel

Although a large number of drugs have their origin in natural products [147], databases of natural products are rarely used for virtual screening. A 3D homology model of the eukaryotic Shaker K^+ channel was built from the known 3D structure of the KcsA potassium channel. The refined 3D model was used to dock more than 50,000 compounds of the China Natural Product Database (Shanghai Institute of Materia Medica, Chinese Academy of Sciences, and Neotrident Technology Ltd.) with the program DOCK 4.0 into the extracellular tetraethylammonium (TEA) binding site. Of 14 hits, only four diterpenoid alkaloids from *Aconitum leucostonum* were accessible. Extracellular application of the four compounds inhibited the delayed rectifier current (I_K) at micromolar concentration, for example, **14-benzoyl-talatisamine 74** (IC_{50} = 3.8 μM; Fig. 16.9) [148].

16.5 OTHER TARGETS; PROTEIN-PROTEIN AND PROTEIN-RNA INTERACTIONS

16.5.1 Bcl-2 Protein-Protein Interaction

Bcl-2 is one of the many factors that control apoptosis, and overexpression of Bcl-2 has been observed in many different cancers. A homology model of Bcl-2 was derived from the NMR 3D structure of the Bcl-XL complex with a Bak BH3 peptide. This model served to search the NCI 3D database of 206,876 organic compounds for potential Bcl-2 inhibitors, which bind to the Bak BH3 binding site of Bcl-2. Full conformational flexibility of the ligands was taken into account in the program DOCK. Thirty-five potential inhibitors were tested, and seven of them had IC_{50} values from 1.6 to 14.0 μM. One of the hits, **compound 75** (Fig. 16.10), had the highest antiproliferative activity (IC_{50} = 10.4 μM) in the human myeloid leukemia cell line HL-60. Whereas **compound 75** induced apoptosis in cancer cells with high Bcl-2 expression, it had only little effect on cancer cells with low or undetectable levels of Bcl-2 [149].

16.5.2 Cyclophilin A

The immunophilins cyclophilin A [CyPA; binds cyclosporin A (CsA)] and FK506-binding protein (FKBP12; binds FK506 and rapamycin) are peptidylprolyl isomerases (PPIases, rotamases). However, it is the interaction of the drug-immunophilin complexes with the calcium/calmodulin-dependent protein phosphatase calcineurin (CsA/CyPA and FK506/FKBP12 complexes) and the serine/threonine kinase FRAP (rapamycin/FKBP12 complex) that is responsible for their immunosuppressive effects. A pharmacophore model for potential cyclophilin ligands was derived from cyclosporin and dipeptides that bind to CyPA. Compounds of the ACD, WDI, and Chapman-Hall Dictionary of Organic Compounds were filtered to remove molecules with MW >700 and reactive compounds. Then 3D structures were generated with the program Concord, and a Unity 3D search was performed, using the cyclophilin ligand 3D pharmacophore. In the resulting hits a lead structure with IC_{50} = 6 μM was identified. It served as the starting point for further chemical optimization, from which several submicromolar CyPA inhibitors resulted, for example, **compound 76** (IC_{50} = 930 nM; Fig. 16.10) [150].

16.5.3 FK 506-Binding Protein (FKBP12)

FK506-binding proteins (FKBP) belong to the family of immunophilins. Together with their ligand FK506 and the serine/threonine phosphatase calcineurin, they form ternary complexes that block signal transduction in T cells. A 3D version of the ACD and the 3D structures of the Cambridge Crystallographic Database (CCD) were docked into the binding pocket of FKBP with the program Sandock. Several hits bound with micromolar affinities, for example, the steroid **compound 77** (K_d = 7 μM) and the spiro **compound 78** (K_d = 11 μM); the dipeptide **Z-L-Pro-L-Pro 79** had even submicromolar affinity (K_d = 0.8 μM) (Fig. 16.10) [151].

16.5.4 HIV-1 RNA Transactivation Response Element

The binding of the HIV-1 transactivating regulatory protein (tat) to the RNA transactivation response element (TAR) is an essential step for HIV-1 replication. The ACD was screened for inhibitors of the tat-TAR protein-RNA interaction. A four-step procedure was used: Rigid docking was followed by three steps of flexible docking, using a stochastic torsional angle modification of the ligands. The procedure was validated by docking ligands of five RNA

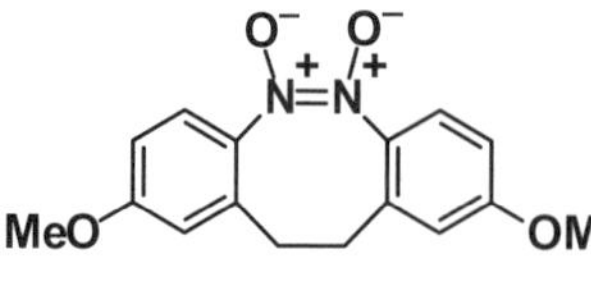

75

Bcl-2 protein-protein interaction inhibition, IC_{50} = 10.4 μM

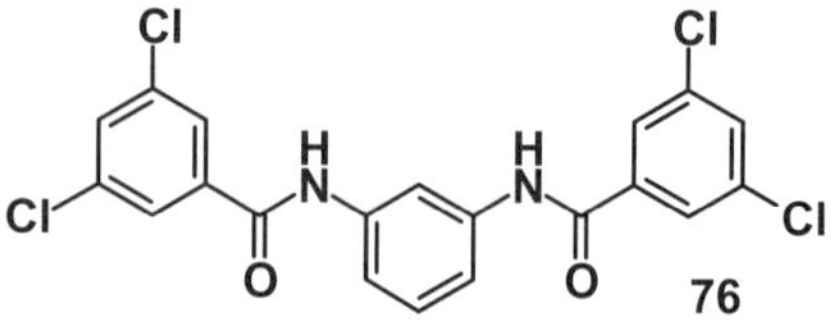

76

Cyclophilin A (CyPA) inhibitor, IC_{50} = 930 nM

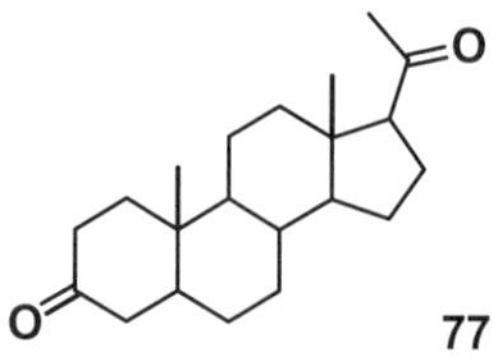

77

FK-506 binding protein (FKBP) ligand, K_d = 7 μM

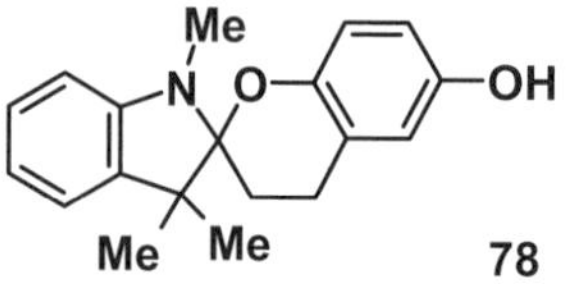

78

FK-506 binding protein (FKBP) ligand, K_d = 11 μM

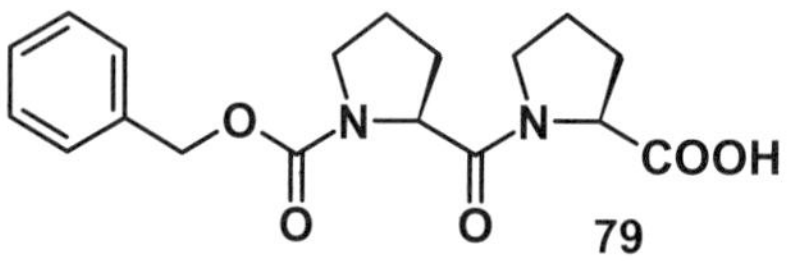

79

FK-506 binding protein (FKBP) ligand, K_d = 0.8 μM

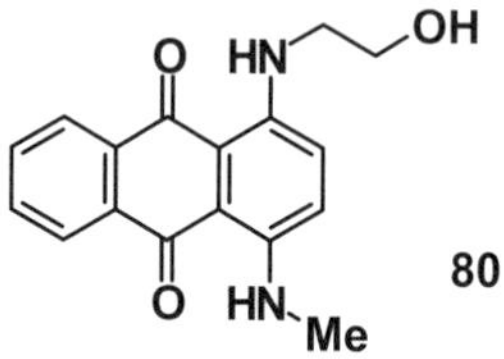

80

HIV-1 RNA Transactivation response element (TAR) inhibitor, $CD_{50} \approx 1$ μM

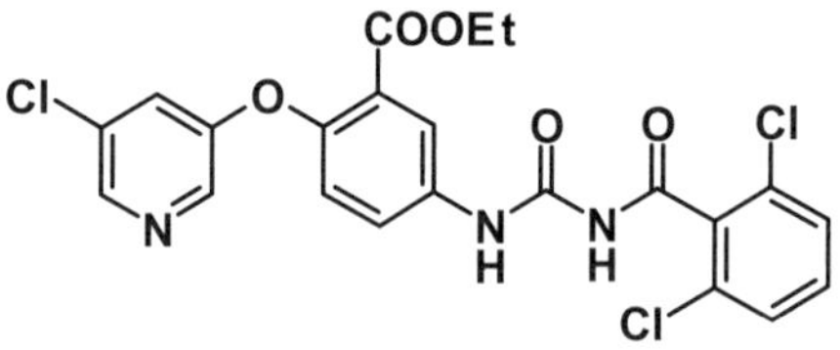

81

Mesangial cell (MC) proliferation inhibitor, 90% inhibition at 100 nM

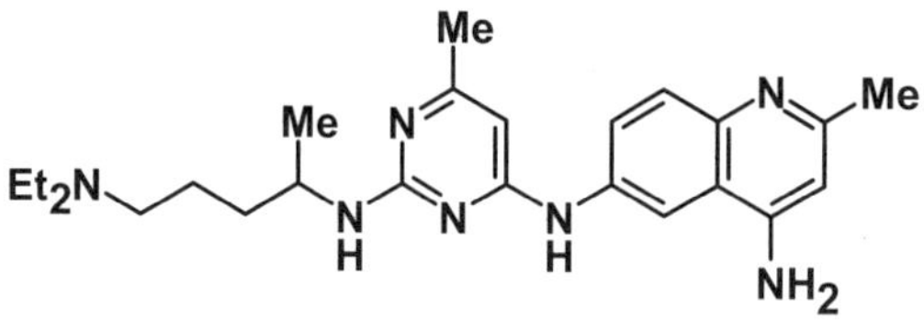

82

Inhibitor of Rac1 protein-protein interaction; $IC_{50} \approx 50$ μM

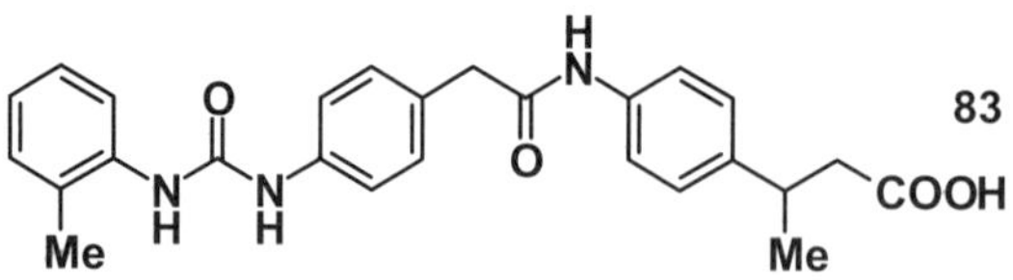

83

VLA-4 (= α4β1 antigen) antagonist, IC_{50} = 1.3 nM

Figure 16.10 Inhibitors of protein-protein and protein-RNA interactions from virtual screening.

complexes of known structure and scoring them by an empirical function, which was derived from ligand-RNA complexes with known structure and affinity, accounting also for solvation and changes in conformational entropy. Screening of about 153,000 ACD compounds yielded high-ranking known TAR ligands, as well as new structures, for example, **compound 80** (CD_{50} $\approx 1\,\mu M$; CD_{50} = competitive dose, concentration of compound required to reduce the binding of the tat protein to TAR to 50%; Fig. 16.10) [152].

16.5.5 Mesangial Cell Proliferation

Mesangial cell (MC) proliferation inhibitors were searched, using the HipHop module of the Catalyst software. A 3D pharmacophore model, consisting of two hydrophobic regions, two hydrophobic aromatic regions, and three hydrogen bond acceptors, was generated from a training set of heterocyclic phosphonic acid diethyl esters, using the Catalyst HipHop option. This model served as a 3D query to search 47,045 compounds of the Maybridge 3D database. Among 41 structurally novel inhibitors with >50% inhibitory activity at 100 nM, the most potent hit was **compound 81** (90 % MC proliferation inhibition at 100 nM; Fig. 16.10) [153].

16.5.6 Rac1 Protein-Protein Interaction

Rac GTPase is involved in one of several signaling pathways mediated by Rho family GTPases. The 3D structure of a Rac1-Tiam1 complex was used to specify the binding pocket for inhibitors, and a flexible 3D search was performed in 140,000 compounds of the NCI database with the program Unity. The hits of this search were flexibly docked with the program FlexX and ranked by the consensus scoring function CScore. By visual inspection, 58 of the 100 highest-scoring hits were eliminated because they did not show an interaction of the ligand with Trp56. Considering solubility and availability of the remaining compounds, finally 15 compounds were tested for their ability to inhibit the Rac1-binding interaction with its guanine nucleotide exchange factor (GEF) TrioN. **Compound 82** ($IC_{50} \approx 50\,\mu M$; Fig. 16.10) was the only active and selective compound, significantly inhibiting TrioN binding to Rac1 but not interfering with Cdc42 binding to Intersectin. Also in cells it effectively inhibited Rac1 binding and activation, and in human prostate cancer PC-3 cells it inhibited proliferation [154].

16.5.7 VLA-4 ($\alpha 4\beta 1$ Antigen)

A 3D model of the fibrinogen-derived (very late antigen-4, VLA-4) inhibitor 4-[N′-(2-methylphenyl)ureido]phenylacetyl-Leu-Asp-Val was derived from the X-ray structure of the related integrin-binding region of the vascular cell adhesion molecule-1 (VCAM-1). A 3D pharmacophore was generated with the program Catalyst, and a 3D search was performed in 8624 molecules from the ACD, containing either a free amino or a nitro group and a carboxyl group, in order to replace the tripeptide part of the inhibitor. All 12 selected molecules that passed additional filters inhibited the association of the $\alpha4\beta1$ antigen with VCAM-1. The most potent analog, **compound 83,** had an IC_{50} = 1.3 nM (Fig. 16.10) [155].

16.6 SUMMARY AND CONCLUSIONS

Virtual screening comprises several computational techniques that have already shown their efficiency in delivering interesting lead structures. In the most effective application, cascades of different steps serve to reduce very rapidly the number of potential candidates from hundreds of thousands or even millions of structures to a manageable size, for example, by first applying simple filters (molecular weight, polar surface area, number of rotatable bonds, Lipinski rule of five, lead-likeness rules, drug-likeness neural nets), followed by pharmacophore generation and pharmacophore searches. The number of potential candidates can be reduced by a filter that checks the presence of all necessary pharmacophoric features. The generation of a pharmacophore hypothesis can be ligand based or may be derived from the protein 3D structure (if available) by a hot spot analysis (programs GRID [11, 156], LUDI [35], DrugScore [49, 157, 158]). Ligand-based pharmacophore generation is most often performed with the HipHop and HypoGen options of the program Catalyst [159–163]. LigandScout is a new program for the automated generation of pharmacophore hypotheses from 3D structures of protein-ligand complexes [164]. Finally, a 2D (topological) or 3D pharmacophore search is performed. The CATS descriptor [89] and the feature trees [165, 166] are extremely fast and effective search tools for pharmacophore similarity, very often producing active hits with new scaffolds. For 3D searches the programs Catalyst [e.g., 78, 81, 82, 88, 91, 104, 115, 138, 153, 155] and Unity [e.g., 78, 122, 139, 140, 145, 146, 150, 154, 167] are most often used.

If a 3D structure of the target is available from protein crystallography or NMR studies, or can be modeled by homology, the last step, using flexible docking and scoring, is more time demanding. For docking, the programs most commonly used in the success stories described in this review are DOCK [34, 168], in several different versions [96, 102, 103, 107, 112, 116, 117, 119, 121, 124, 125, 136, 148, 149], and FlexX and FlexX-Pharm [86, 87, 95, 97, 118, 122, 126, 127, 129, 130, 134, 139, 140, 154, 169–171]. Stepwise virtual screening protocols have been applied in several examples described in this review [e.g., 78, 86, 87, 95, 97, 106, 122, 124, 129, 130, 139, 140]. A surprisingly large number of successful docking studies used a homology model of the respective protein [78, 79, 86, 87, 92–94, 100, 103, 106, 112, 123, 148, 149].

As discussed in the introduction, scoring functions still pose problems (see also Chapter 14). Some of these problems arise from insufficient consideration of details of favorable and unfavorable protein-ligand interactions, whereas others are more systematic in their nature, for example, the overprediction of the affinity of large molecules [56, 102, 122] and the overprediction of the affinity contribution of hydrogen bonds at the solvent-accessible surface of the protein [126]. Thus a visual inspection of the docking results [e.g., 93–95, 97, 100, 103, 106, 120, 122, 138, 154] is of utmost importance, to check for unfavorable geometry of the docked ligand, geometric complementarity, for example, space filling of hydrophobic pockets, key interactions with the protein (which is the key option of the program FlexX-Pharm), and unfavorable electrostatic interactions, for example, oxygen-oxygen repulsion. Of course, synthetic accessibility or commercial availability and certain physicochemical properties, such as solubility, are also critically important for the selection of candidates for biological screening.

Although some virtual screening hits described in this review, do not look very druglike, for example, **compounds 47, 50, 51** (Fig. 16.7), **56, 62** (Fig. 16.8), and **75** (Fig. 16.10), several other compounds have already been optimized to interesting candidates for further development. It must be kept in mind that ligand-based and 3D structure-based approaches enable only ligand design, not drug design. In the future, computer programs for virtual screening not only should aim at the further improvement of the scoring functions but should consider also synthetic accessibility and allow the construction of ligands with chemically reasonable fragment-based approaches.

REFERENCES

1. Goodford PJ. Drug design by the method of receptor fit. *J Med Chem* 1984;27:557–64.
2. Beddell CR, editor. *The design of drugs to macromolecular targets.* Chichester: John Wiley & Sons, 1992.
3. Beddell CR, Goodford PJ, Norrington FE, Wilkinson S, Wootton R. Compounds designed to fit a site of known structure in human haemoglobin. *Br J Pharmacol* 1976;57:201–9.
4. Kuyper LF, Roth B, Baccanari DP, Farone R, Beddell CR, Champness JN, Stammers DK, Dann JG, Norrington FEA, Baker D, Goodford PJ. Receptor-based design of dihydrofolate reductase inhibitors: comparison of crystallographically determined enzyme binding with enzyme affinity in a series of carboxy-substituted trimethoprim analogues. *J Med Chem* 1982;25:1120–2.
5. Cushman DW, Cheung HS, Sabo EF, Ondetti MA. Design of potent competitive inhibitors of angiotensin-converting enzyme. Carboxyalkanoyl and mercaptoalkanoyl amino acids. *Biochemistry* 1977;16:5484–91.
6. Redshaw S. Angiotensin-converting enzyme (ACE) inhibitors and the design of captopril. In: Ganellin CR, Roberts SM, editors, *Medicinal chemistry. The role of organic chemistry in drug research*, 2nd edition. London: Academic Press, 1993. p. 163–85.
7. Baldwin JJ, Ponticello GS, Anderson PS, Christy ME, Murcko MA, Randall WC, Schwam H, Sugrue MF, Springer JP, Gautheron P, Grove J, Mallorga P,

Viader MP, McKeever BM, Navia MA. Thienothiopyran-2-sulfonamides: novel topically active carbonic anhydrase inhibitors for the treatment of glaucoma. *J Med Chem* 1989;32:2510–13.

8. Vacca JP. Clinically effective HIV-1 protease inhibitors. *Drug Discov Today* 1997;2:261–72.
9. Wlodaver A, Vondrasek J. Inhibitors of HIV-1 protease—a major success of structure-assisted drug design. *Annu Rev Biophys Biomol Struct* 1998; 27:249–84.
10. von Itzstein M, Wu WY, Kok GB, Pegg MS, Dyason JC, Jin B, Phan TV, Smythe ML, White HF, Oliver SW, Colman PM, Varghese JN, Ryan DM, Woods JM, Bethell RC, Hotham VJ, Cameron JM, Penn CR. Rational design of potent sialidase-based inhibitors of influenza virus replication. *Nature* 1993;363: 418–23.
11. Goodford PJ. A computational procedure for determining energetically favourable binding sites on biologically important molecules. *J Med Chem* 1985; 28:849–57.
12. Hillisch A, Pineda LF, Hilgenfeld R. Utility of homology models in the drug discovery process. *Drug Discov Today* 2004;9:659–69.
13. Hillisch A, Peters O, Kosemund D, Müller G, Walter A, Schneider B, Reddersen G, Elger W, Fritzemeier KH. Dissecting physiological roles of estrogen receptor α and β with potent selective ligands from structure-based design. *Mol Endocrinol* 2004;18:1599–609.
14. Hillisch A, Peters O, Kosemund D, Müller G, Walter A, Elger W, Fritzemeier KH. Protein structure-based design, synthesis strategy and in vitro pharmacological characterization of estrogen receptor α and β selective compounds. *Ernst Schering Res Found Workshop* 2004;46:47–62.
15. Veerapandian P, editor. *Structure-based drug design*. New York: Marcel Dekker, 1997.
16. Gubernator K, Böhm HJ, editors. *Structure-based ligand design* (Vol. 6 of: Mannhold R, Kubinyi H, Timmerman H, editors, *Methods and Principles in Medicinal Chemistry*). Weinheim: Wiley-VCH, 1998.
17. Babine RE, Abdel-Meguid SS. *Protein crystallography in drug discovery* (Vol. 20 of: Mannhold R, Kubinyi H, Folkers G, editors, *Methods and Principles in Medicinal Chemistry*). Weinheim: Wiley-VCH, 2004.
18. Bohacek RS, McMartin C, Guida WC. The art and practice of structure-based drug design: a molecular modeling perspective. *Med Res Rev* 1996;16:3–50.
19. Böhm HJ, Klebe G. What can we learn from molecular recognition in protein-ligand complexes for the design of new drugs? *Angew Chem Int Ed Engl* 1996;35:2589–614.
20. Babine RE, Bender SL. Molecular recognition of protein-ligand complexes: applications to drug design. *Chem Rev* 1997;97:1359–472.
21. Kubinyi H. Structure-based design of enzyme inhibitors and receptor ligands. *Curr Opin Drug Discov Dev* 1998;1:4–15.
22. Kubinyi H. Combinatorial and computational approaches in structure-based drug design. *Curr Opin Drug Discov Dev* 1998;1:16–27.

23. Davis AM, Teague SJ, Kleywegt GJ. Application and limitations of X-ray crystallographic data in structure-based ligand and drug design. *Angew Chem Int Ed Engl* 2003;42:2718–2736; *Angew Chem* 2003;115:2822–41.
24. Congreve M, Murray CW, Blundell TL. Structural biology and drug discovery. *Drug Discov Today* 2005;13:895–907.
25. Lahana R. How many leads from HTS? *Drug Discov Today* 1999;4:447–8.
26. Ramesha CS. Comment: How many leads from HTS? *Drug Discov Today* 2000;5:43–4.
27. Lipinski CA, Lombardo F, Dominy BW, Feeney PJ. Experimental and computational approaches to estimate solubility and permeability in drug discovery and development settings. *Adv Drug Deliv Rev* 1997;46:3–26.
28. Ajay A, Walters WP, Murcko MA. Can we learn to distinguish between "drug-like" and "nondrug-like" molecules? *J Med Chem* 1998;41:3314–24.
29. Sadowski J, Kubinyi H. A scoring scheme for discriminating between drugs and non-drugs. *J Med Chem* 1998;41:3325–9 (1998).
30. Güner OF, editor. *Pharmacophore perception, development and use in drug design*. La Jolla: International University Line, 2000.
31. Mason JS, Good AC, Martin EJ. 3-D pharmacophores in drug discovery. *Curr Pharm Des* 2001;7:567–97.
32. van Drie J. Pharmacophore discovery: a critical review. In: Tollenaere J, de Winter H, Langenaeker W, Bultinck P, editors, *Computational medicinal chemistry and drug discovery*. New York: Marcel Dekker, 2004. p. 437–60.
33. Langer T, Hoffmann R. *Pharmacophores and pharmacophore searches* (Vol. 32 of Mannhold R, Kubinyi H, Folkers G, editors, *Methods and Principles in Medicinal Chemistry*). Weinheim: Wiley-VCH, 2006.
34. Meng EC, Shoichet B, Kuntz ID. Automated docking with grid-based energy evaluation. *J Comput Chem* 1992;13:505–24.
35. Böhm HJ. The computer program LUDI: a new method for the de novo design of enzyme inhibitors. *J Comput Aided Mol Design* 1992;6:61–78.
36. Lengauer T, Rarey M. Computational methods for biomolecular docking. *Curr Opin Struct Biol* 1996;6:402–6.
37. Dixon JS. Evaluation of the CASP2 docking section. *Proteins Struct Funct Genet* 1997;Suppl 1:198–204.
38. Abagyan R. Totrov M. High-throughput docking for lead generation. *Curr Opin Chem Biol* 2001;5:375–82.
39. Halperin I, Ma B, Wolfson H, Nussinov R. Principles of docking: an overview of search algorithms and a guide to scoring functions. *Proteins Struct Funct Genet* 2002;47:409–43.
40. Böhm HJ, Schneider G, editors. *Protein-ligand interactions. From molecular recognition to drug design* (Vol. 19 of Mannhold R, Kubinyi H, Folkers G, editors, *Methods and Principles in Medicinal Chemistry*). Weinheim: Wiley-VCH, 2003.
41. Brooijmans N, Kuntz ID. Molecular recognition and docking algorithms. *Annu Rev Biophys Biomol Struct* 2003;32:335–73.

42. Erickson JA, Jalaie M, Robertson DH, Lewis RA, Vieth M. Lessons in molecular recognition: the effects of ligand and protein flexibility on molecular docking accuracy. *J Med Chem* 2004;47:45–55.
43. Alvarez JC. High-throughput docking as a source of novel drug leads. *Curr Opin Chem Biol* 2004;8:365–70.
44. Muegge I, Enyedy I. Docking and scoring. In: Tollenaere J, de Winter H, Langenaeker W, Bultinck P, editors, *Computational medicinal chemistry and drug discovery.* New York: Marcel Dekker. 2004. p. 405–36.
45. Krovat EM, Steindl T, Langer T. Recent advances in docking and scoring. *Curr Comput Aided Drug Des* 2005;1:93–102.
46. Böhm HJ. The development of a simple empirical scoring function to estimate the binding constant for a protein-ligand complex of known three-dimensional structure. *J Comput Aided Mol Des* 1994;8:243–56.
47. Ajay A, Murcko MA. Computational methods to predict binding free energy in ligand-receptor complexes. *J Med Chem* 1995;38:4953–67.
48. Muegge I, Martin YC. A general and fast scoring function for protein-ligand interactions: a simplified potential approach. *J Med Chem* 1999;42:791–804.
49. Gohlke H, Hendlich M, Klebe G. Knowledge-based scoring function to predict protein-ligand interactions. *J Mol Biol* 2000;295:337–56.
50. Bissantz C, Folkers G, Rognan D. Protein-based virtual screening of chemical databases. 1. Evaluation of different docking/scoring combinations. *J Med Chem* 2000;43:4759–67.
51. Stahl M, Rarey M. Detailed analysis of scoring functions for virtual screening. *J Med Chem* 2001;44:1035–42.
52. Schulz-Gasch T, Stahl M. Binding site characteristics in structure-based virtual screening: evaluation of current docking tools. *J Mol Model* 2003;9:47–57.
53. Wang R, Lu Y, Wang S. Comparative evaluation of 11 scoring functions for molecular docking. *J Med Chem* 2003;46:2287–303.
54. Charifson PS, Corkery JJ, Murcko MA, Walters,WP. Consensus scoring: a method for obtaining improved hit rates from docking databases of three-dimensional structures into proteins. *J Med Chem* 1999;42:5100–9.
55. Wang RX, Wang SM. How does consensus scoring work for virtual library screening? An idealized computer experiment. *J Chem Inf Comput Sci* 2001;41:1422–6.
56. Kuntz ID, Chen K, Sharp KA, Kollman PA. The maximal affinity of ligands. *Proc Natl Acad Sci USA* 1999;96:9997–10002.
57. Böhm HJ, Schneider G, editors. *Virtual screening for bioactive molecules* (Vol. 10 of: Mannhold R, Kubinyi H, Timmerman H, editors, *Methods and principles in medicinal chemistry*). Weinheim: Wiley-VCH, 2000.
58. Klebe G, editor. *Virtual screening: an alternative or complement to high throughput screening.* Dordrecht: Kluwer Academic Publishers, 2000; also published in *Persp Drug Discov Design* 2000;20:1–287.
59. Alvarez J, Shoichet B, editors. *Virtual screening in drug discovery.* Boca Raton: CRC Press, Taylor & Francis Group, 2005.
60. Walters WP, Stahl MT, Murcko MA. Virtual screening—an overview. *Drug Discov Today* 1998;3:160–78.

61. Good A. Structure-based virtual screening protocols. *Curr Opin Drug Discov Dev* 2001;4:301–7.
62. Langer T, Hoffmann RD. Virtual screening: an effective tool for lead structure discovery? *Curr Pharm Des* 2001;7:509–27.
63. Schneider G, Böhm HJ. Virtual screening and fast automated docking methods. *Drug Discov Today* 2002;7:64–70.
64. Waszkowycz B. Structure-based approaches to drug design and virtual screening. *Curr Opin Drug Discov Dev* 2002;5:407–13.
65. Bajorath, J. Integration of virtual and high throughput screening. *Nat Rev Drug Discov* 2002;1:882–94.
66. Lyne PD. Structure-based virtual screening: an overview. *Drug Discov Today* 2002;7:1047–55.
67. Xu H, Agrafiotis DK: Retrospect and prospect of virtual screening in drug discovery. *Curr Top Med Chem* 2002;2:1305–20.
68. Bissantz C, Bernard P, Hibert M, Rognan D. Protein-based virtual screening of chemical databases. II. Are homology models of G-protein coupled receptors suitable targets? *Proteins Struct Funct Genet* 2003;50:5–25.
69. Bleicher KH, Böhm HJ, Müller K, Alanine AI. Hit and lead generation: beyond high-throughput screening. *Nature Rev Drug Discov* 2003;2:369–78.
70. Shen J, Xu X, Cheng F, Liu H, Luo X, Shen J, Chen K, Zhao W, Shen X, Jiang H. Virtual screening on natural products for discovering active compounds and target information. *Curr Med Chem* 2003;10:1241–53.
71. Lengauer T, Lemmen C, Rarey M, Zimmermann M. Novel technologies for virtual screening. *Drug Discov Today* 2004;9:27–34.
72. Klebe G. Lead identification in post-genomics: computers as a complementary alternative. *Drug Discov Today Technol* 2004;1:225–30.
73. Oprea TI, Matter H. Integrating virtual screening in lead discovery. *Curr Opin Chem Biol* 2004;8:349–358.
74. Shoichet BK. Virtual screening of chemical libraries. *Nature* 2004;432:862–5.
75. Langer T, Wolber G. Virtual combinatorial chemistry and *in silico* screening: efficient tools for lead structure discovery? *Pure Appl Chem* 2004;76:991–6.
76. Rarey M, Lemmen C, Matter H. Algorithmic engines in virtual screening. In: Oprea TI, editor, *Chemoinformatics in drug discovery* (Vol. 23 of Mannhold R, Kubinyi H, Folkers G, editors, *Methods and Principles in Medicinal Chemistry*). Weinheim: Wiley-VCH, 2005. p. 59–115.
77. Anderson AC, Wright DL. The design and docking of virtual compound libraries to structures of drug targets. *Curr Comp Aided Drug Des* 2005;1:103–27.
78. Evers A, Klabunde T. Structure-based drug discovery using GPCR homology modeling: successful virtual screening for antagonists of the alpha1A adrenergic receptor. *J Med Chem* 2005;48:1088–97.
79. Varady J, Wu X, Fang X, Min J, Hu Z, Levant B, Wang S. Molecular modeling of the three-dimensional structure of dopamine 3 (D3) subtype receptor: discovery of novel and potent D3 ligands through a hybrid pharmacophore- and structure-based database searching approach. *J Med Chem* 2003;46:4377–92.

80. Astles PC, Brown TJ, Handscombe CM, Harper MF, Harris NV, Lewis RA, Lockey PM, McCarthy C, McLay IM, Porter B, Roach AG, Smith C, Walsh RJA. Selective endothelin A receptor antagonists. 1. Discovery and structure-activity of 2,4-disubstituted benzoic acid derivatives. *Eur J Med Chem* 1997;32:409–23.

81. Astles PC, Brown TJ, Harper MF, Harris NV, McCarthy C, Porter B, Smith C, Walsh RJA. Selective endothelin A receptor antagonists. 2. Discovery and structure-activity of 5-ketopentanoic acid derivatives. *Eur J Med Chem* 1997; 32:515–22.

82. Astles PC, Brealey C, Brown TJ, Facchini V, Handscombe C, Harris NV, McCarthy C, McLay IM, Porter B, Roach AG, Sargent C, Smith C, Walsh RJA. Selective endothelin A receptor antagonists. 3. Discovery and structure-activity relationships of a series of 4-phenoxybutanoic acid derivatives. *J Med Chem* 1998;41:2732–44.

83. Funk OF, Kettmann V, Drimal J, Langer T. Chemical function based pharmacophore generation of endothelin-A selective receptor antagonists. *J Med Chem* 2004;47:2750–60.

84. Lavrador K, Murphy B, Saunders J, Struthers S, Wang X, Williams J. A screening library for peptide activated G-protein coupled receptors. 1. The test set. *J Med Chem* 2004;47:6864–74.

85. Marriott DP, Dougall IG, Meghani P, Liu YJ, Flower DR. Lead generation using pharmacophore mapping and three-dimensional database searching: application to muscarinic M3 receptor antagonists. *J Med Chem* 1999;42:3210–16.

86. Evers A, Klebe G. Ligand-supported homology modelling of G-protein coupled receptor sites: models sufficient for successful virtual screening. *Angew Chem Int Ed* 2004;43:248–251; *Angew Chem* 2004;116:250–3.

87. Evers A, Klebe G. Successful virtual screening for a submicromolar antagonist of the neurokinin-1 receptor based on a ligand-supported homology model. *J Med Chem* 2004;47:5381–92.

88. Guba W, Neidhart W, Nettekoven M. Novel and potent NPY5 receptor antagonists derived from virtual screening and iterative parallel chemistry design. *Bioorg Med Chem* Lett 2005;15:1599–603.

89. Schneider G, Neidhart W, Giller T, Schmidt G. "Scaffold-hopping" by topological pharmacophore search: a contribution to virtual screening. *Angew Chem Int Ed Engl* 1999;38:2894–2896; *Angew Chem* 1999;111:3068–70.

90. Schneider G, Nettekoven M. Ligand-based combinatorial design of selective purinergic receptor (A_{2A}) antagonists using self-organizing maps. *J Comb Chem* 2003;5:233–7.

91. Flohr S, Kurz M, Kostenis E, Brkovich A, Fournier A, Klabunde T. Identification of nonpeptidic urotensin II receptor antagonists by virtual screening based on a pharmacophore model derived from structure-activity relationships and nuclear magnetic resonance studies on urotensin II. *J Med Chem* 2002;45:1799–805.

92. Schapira M, Raaka BM, Samuels HH, Abagyan R. Rational discovery of novel nuclear hormone receptor antagonists. *Proc Natl Acad Sci USA* 2000; 97:1008–13.

93. Schapira M, Raaka BM, Samuels HH, Abagyan R. *In silico* discovery of novel retinoic acid receptor agonist structures. *BMC Struct Biol* 2001;1:1 (7 pages, www.biomedcentral.com/1472-6807/1/1).
94. Schapira M, Raaka BM, Das S, Fan L, Totrov M, Zhou ZU, Wilson SR, Abagyan R, Samuels HH. Discovery of diverse thyroid hormone receptor antagonists by high-throughput docking. *Proc Natl Acad Sci USA* 2003;100:7354–9.
95. Forino M, Jung D, Easton JB, Houghton PJ, Pellecchia M. Virtual docking approaches to protein kinase B inhibition. *J Med Chem* 2005;48:2278–81.
96. Peng H, Huang N, Qi J, Xie P, Xu C, Wang J, Yang C. Identification of novel inhibitors of BCR-ABL tyrosine kinase via virtual screening. *Bioorg Med Chem Lett* 2003;13:3693–9.
97. Lyne PD, Kenny PW, Cosgrove DA, Deng C, Zabludoff S, Wendoloski JJ, Ashwell S. Identification of compounds with nanomolar binding affinity for checkpoint kinase-1 using knowledge-based virtual screening. *J Med Chem* 2004;47:1962–8.
98. Wu SY, McNae I, Kontopidis G, McClue SJ, McInnes C, Stewart KJ, Wang SD, Zheleva DI, Marriage H, Lane DP, Taylor P, Fischer PM, Walkinshaw MD. Discovery of a novel family of CDK inhibitors with the program LIDAEUS: structural basis for ligand-induced disordering of the activation loop. *Structure* 2003;11:399–410.
99. Wang SD, Meades C, Wood G, Osnowski A, Anderson S, Yuill R, Thomas M, Mezna M, Jackson W, Midgley C, Griffiths G, Fleming I, Green S, McNae I, Wu SY, McInnes C, Zheleva D, Walkinshaw MD, Fischer PM. 2-Anilino-4-(thiazol-5-yl)pyrimidine CDK inhibitors: synthesis, SAR analysis, X-ray crystallography, and biological activity. *J Med Chem* 2004;47:1662–75.
100. Honma T, Hayashi K, Aoyama T, Hashimoto N, Machida T, Fukasawa K, Iwama T, Ikeura C, Ikuta M, Suzuki-Takahashi I, Iwasawa Y, Hayama T, Nishimura S, Morishima H. Structure-based generation of a new class of potent Cdk4 inhibitors: new de novo design strategy and library design. *J Med Chem* 2001; 44:4615–27.
101. Nærum L, Nørskov-Lauritsen L, Olesen PH. Scaffold hopping and optimization towards libraries of glycogen synthase kinase-3 inhibitors. *Bioorg Med Chem Lett* 2002;12:1525–8.
102. Huang N, Nagarsekar A, Xia GJ, Hayashi J, MacKerell AD Jr. Identification of non-phosphate-containing small molecular weight inhibitors of the tyrosine kinase p56 Lck SH2 domain via *in silico* screening against the pY+3 binding site. *J Med Chem* 2004;47:3502–11.
103. Vangrevelinghe E, Zimmermann K, Schoepfer J, Portmann R, Fabbro D, Furet P. Discovery of a potent and selective protein kinase CK2 inhibitor by high-throughput docking. *J Med Chem* 2003;46:2656–62.
104. Singh J, Chuaqui CE, Boriack-Sjodin PA, Wen-Cherng Lee, Pontz T, Corbley MJ, Cheung HK, Arduini RM, Mead JN, Newman MN, Papadatos JL, Bowes S, Josiah S, Ling LE. Successful shape-based virtual screening: the discovery of a potent inhibitor of the Type I TGFβreceptor kinase (TβRI). *Bioorg Med Chem Lett* 2003;13:4355–4359; Corrigendum *Bioorg Med Chem Lett* 2004;14:2991.
105. Kick EK, Roe DC, Skillman G, Liu AG, Ewing TJA, Sun Y, Kuntz ID, Ellman JA. Structure-based design and combinatorial chemistry yield low nanomolar inhibitors of cathepsin D. *Chem Biol* 1997;4:297–307.

106. Desai PV, Patny A, Sabnis Y, Tekwani B, Gut J, Rosenthal P, Srivastava A, Avery M. Identification of novel parasitic cysteine protease inhibitors using virtual screening. 1. The ChemBridge database. *J Med Chem* 2004;47: 6609–15.

107. DesJarlais RL, Seibel GL, Kuntz ID, Furth PS, Alvarez JC, Ortiz de Montellano PR, DeCamp DL, Babé LM, Craik CS. Structure-based design of nonpeptide inhibitors specific for the human immunodeficiency virus 1 protease. *Proc Natl Acad Sci USA* 1990;87:6644–8.

108. Rutenber E, Fauman EB, Keenan RJ, Ortiz de Montellano PR, Meng E, Kuntz ID, DeCamp DL, Salto R, Rosé JR, Craik CS, Stroud RM. Structure of a non-peptide inhibitor complexed with HIV-1 protease. Developing a cycle of structure-based drug design. *J Biol Chem* 1993;268:15343–6

109. Lam PYS, Jadhav PK, Eyermann CJ, Hodge CN, Ru Y, Bacheler LT, Meek JL, Otto MJ, Rayner MM, Wong YN, Chang CH, Weber PC, Jackson DA, Sharpe TR, Erickson-Viitanen S. Rational design of potent, bioavailable, nonpeptide cyclic ureas as HIV protease inhibitors. *Science* 1994;263:380–4.

110. De Lucca GV, Erickson-Viitanen S, Lam PYS. Cyclic HIV protease inhibitors capable of displacing the active site structural water molecule. *Drug Discov Today* 1997;2:6–18.

111. Haque TS, Skillman AG, Lee CE, Habashita H, Gluzman IY, Ewing TJA, Goldberg DE, Kuntz ID, Ellman JA. Potent, low-molecular-weight non-peptide inhibitors of malarial aspartyl protease plasmepsin II. *J Med Chem* 1999;42: 1428–40.

112. Liu Z, Huang C, Fan K, Wei P, Chen H, Liu S, Pei J, Shi L, Li B, Yang K, Liu Y, Lai L. Virtual screening of novel noncovalent inhibitors for SARS-CoV 3C-like proteinase. *J Chem Inf Model* 2005;45:10–17.

113. Böhm HJ, Banner DW, Weber L. Combinatorial docking and combinatorial chemistry: design of potent non-peptide thrombin inhibitors. *J Comput Aided Mol Design* 1999;13:51–6.

114. Stahl M. Structure-based library design. In: Böhm HJ, Schneider G, editors, Virtual screening for bioactive molecules (Vol. 10 of Mannhold R, Kubinyi H, Timmerman H, editors, *Methods and principles in medicinal chemistry*). Weinheim: Wiley-VCH, 2000, pp. 229–64.

115. Rollinger JM, Hornick A, Langer T, Stuppner H, Prast H. Acetylcholinesterase inhibitory activity of scopolin and scopoletin discovered by virtual screening of natural products. *J Med Chem* 2004;47:6248–54.

116. Soelaiman S, Wei BQ, Bergson P, Lee YS, Shen Y, Mrksich M, Shoichet BK, Tang WJ. Structure-based inhibitor discovery against adenylyl cyclase toxins from pathogenic bacteria that cause anthrax and whooping cough. *J Biol Chem* 2003;278:25990–7.

117. Powers RA, Morandi F, Shoichet BK. Structure-based discovery of a novel, noncovalent inhibitor of AmpC beta-lactamase. *Structure* 2002;10:1013–23.

118. Krier M, de Araújo-Júnior JX, Schmitt M, Duranton J, Justiano-Basaran H, Lugnier C, Bourguignon JJ, Rognan D. Design of small-sized libraries by combinatorial assembly of linkers and functional groups to a given scaffold: application to the structure-based optimization of a phosphodiesterase 4 inhibitor. *J Med Chem* 2005;48:3816–22.

119. Doman TN, McGovern SL, Witherbee BJ, Kasten TP, Kurumbail R, Stallings WC, Connolly DT, Shoichet BK. Molecular docking and high throughput screening for novel inhibitors of protein tyrosine phosphatase 1B. *J Med Chem* 2002;45:2213–21.
120. Iwata Y, Arisawa M, Hamada R, Kita Y, Mizutani MY, Tomioka N, Itai A, Miyamoto S. Discovery of novel aldose reductase inhibitors using a protein structure-based approach: 3D-database search followed by design and synthesis. *J Med Chem* 2001;44:1718–28.
121. Rastelli G, Ferrari AM, Constantino L, Gamberini MC. Discovery of new inhibitors of aldose reductase from molecular docking and database screening. *Bioorg Med Chem* 2002;10:1437–50.
122. Krämer O, Hazemann I, Podjarny AD, Klebe G. Virtual screening for inhibitors of human aldose reductase. *Proteins Struct Funct Genet* 2004;55:814–23.
123. Toyoda T, Brobey RKB, Sano G, Horii T, Tomioka N, Itai Akiko. Lead discovery of inhibitors of the dihydrofolate reductase domain of *Plasmodium falciparum* dihydrofolate reductase-thymidylate synthase. *Biochem Biophys Res Commun* 1997;235:515–19.
124. Rastelli G, Pacchioni S, Sirawaraporn W, Sirawaraporn R, Parenti MD, Ferrari AM. Docking and database screening reveal new classes of *Plasmodium falciparum* dihydrofolate reductase inhibitors. *J Med Chem* 2003;46:2834–45.
125. Gschwend DA, Sirawaraporn W, Santi DV, Kuntz ID. Specificity in structure-based drug design: identification of a novel, selective inhibitor of *Pneumocystis carinii* dihydrofolate reductase. *Proteins Struct Funct Genet* 1997;29:59–67.
126. Wyss PC, Gerber P, Hartman PG, Hubschwerlen C, Locher H, Marty HP, Stahl M. Novel dihydrofolate reductase inhibitors. Structure-based versus diversity-based library design and high-throughput synthesis and screening. *J Med Chem* 2003;46:2304–12.
127. Pickett SD, Sherborne BS, Wilkinson T, Bennett J, Borkakoti N, Broadhurst M, Hurst D, Kilford I, McKinnell M, Jones PS. Discovery of novel low molecular weight inhibitors of IMPDH via virtual needle screening. *Bioorg Med Chem Lett* 2003;13:1691–4.
128. Li C, Xu L, Wolan DW, Wilson IA, Olson AJ. Virtual screening of human 5-aminoimidazole-4-carboxamide ribonucleotide transformylase against the NCI diversity set by use of AutoDock to identify novel nonfolate inhibitors. *J Med Chem* 2004;47:6681–90.
129. Grüneberg S, Stubbs MT, Klebe G. Successful virtual screening for novel inhibitors of human carbonic anhydrase: strategy and experimental confirmation. *J Med Chem* 2002;45:3588–602.
130. Grüneberg S, Wendt B, Klebe G. Subnanomolar inhibitors from computer screening: a model study using human carbonic anhydrase II. *Angew Chem Int Ed Engl* 2001;40:389–393; *Angew Chem* 2001;113:404–8.
131. Grzybowski BA, Ishchenko AV, Kim CY, Topalov G, Chapman R, Christianson DW, Whitesides GM, Shakhnovich EI. Combinatorial computational method gives new picomolar ligands for a known enzyme. *Proc Natl Acad Sci* 2002;99:1270–3.
132. Grzybowski BA, Ishchenko AV, Shimada J, Shakhnovich EI. From knowledge-based potentials to combinatorial lead design *in silico*. *Acc Chem Res* 2002;35:261–9.

133. Boehm HJ, Boehringer M, Bur D, Gmuender H, Huber W, Klaus W, Kostrewa D, Kuehne H, Luebbers T, Meunier-Keller N, Mueller F. Novel inhibitors of DNA gyrase: 3-D structure based biased needle screening. Hit validation by biophysical methods, and 3-D guided optimization. A promising alternative to random screening. *J Med Chem* 2000;43:2664–74.

134. Babaoglu K, Page MA, Jones VC, McNeil MR, Dong C, Naismith JH, Lee RE. Novel inhibitors of an emerging target in *Mycobacterium tuberculosis*; substituted thiazolidinones as inhibitors of dTDP-rhamnose synthesis. *Bioorg Med Chem Lett* 2003;13:3227–30.

135a. Perola E, Xu K, Kollmeyer TM, Kaufmann SH, Prendergast FG, Pang YP. Successful virtual screening of a chemical database for farnesyltransferase inhibitor leads. *J Med Chem* 2000;43:401–8.

135b. Kaminski JJ, Rane DF, Snow ME, Weber L, Rothofsky ML, Anderson SD, Lin SL. Identification of novel farnesyl protein transferase inhibitors using three-dimensional database searching methods. *J Med Chem* 1997;40:4103–12.

136. Aronov AM, Munagala NR, Kuntz ID, Wang CC. Virtual screening of combinatorial libraries across a gene family: in search of inhibitors of *Giardia lamblia* guanine phosphoribosyltransferase. *Antimicr Agents Chemother* 2001;45:2571–6.

137. Hong H, Neamati N, Wang S, Nicklaus MC, Mazumder A, Zhao H, Burke Jr TR, Pommier Y, Milne GWA. Discovery of HIV-1 integrase inhibitors by pharmacophore searching. *J Med Chem* 1997;40:930–6.

138. Dayam R, Sanchez T, Clement O, Shoemaker R, Sei S, Neamati N. β-Diketo acid pharmacophore hypothesis. 1. Discovery of a novel class of HIV-1 integrase inhibitors. *J Med Chem* 2005;48:111–20.

139. Brenk R, Naerum L, Gradler U, Gerber HD, Garcia GA, Reuter K, Stubbs MT, Klebe G. Virtual screening for submicromolar leads of tRNA-guanine transglycosylase based on a new unexpected binding mode detected by crystal structure analysis. *J Med Chem* 2003;46:1133–43.

140. Brenk R, Meyer EA, Reuter K, Stubbs MT, Garcia GA, Diederich F, Klebe G. Crystallographic study of inhibitors of tRNA-guanine transglycosylase suggests a new structure-based pharmacophore for virtual screening. *J Mol Biol* 2004;338:55–75.

141. Schneider G, So SS. *Adaptive Systems in Drug Design* (Biotechnology Intelligence Unit 5). Georgetown: Landes Bioscience 2002. p.45–7.

142. Schneider G, Clément-Chomienne O, Hilfiger L, Schneider P, Kirsch S, Boehm HJ, Neidhart W. Virtual screening for bioactive molecules by evolutionary de novo design. *Angew Chem Int Ed Engl* 2000;39:4130–3; *Angew Chem* 2000;112:4305–9.

143. Lewell XQ, Judd DB, Watson SP, Hann MM. RECAP—retrosynthetic combinatorial analysis procedure: a powerful new technique for identifying privileged molecular fragments with useful applications in combinatorial chemistry. *J Chem Inf Comput Sci* 1998;38:511–22.

144. Peukert S, Brendel J, Pirard B, Brüggemann A, Below P, Kleemann HW, Hemmerle H, Schmidt W. Identification, synthesis, and activity of novel blockers of the voltage-gated potassium channel Kv1.5. *J Med Chem* 2003;46:486–98.

145. Peukert S, Brendel J, Pirard B, Strübing C, Kleemann HW, Böhme T, Hemmerle H. Pharmacophore-based search, synthesis, and biological evaluation of anthranilic amides as novel blockers of the Kv1.5 channel. *Bioorg Med Chem Lett* 2004;14:2823–7.
146. Pirard B, Brendel J, Peukert S. The discovery of Kv1.5 blockers as a case study for the application of virtual screening approaches. *J Chem Inf Model* 2005;45:477–85.
147. Newman DJ, Cragg GM, Snader KM. Natural products as sources of new drugs over the period 1981–2002. *J Nat Prod* 2003;66:1022–37.
148. Liu H, Li Y, Song M, Tan X, Cheng F, Zheng S, Shen J, Luo X, Ji R, Yue J, Hu G, Jiang H, Chen K. Structure-based discovery of potassium channel blockers from natural products: virtual screening and electrophysiological assay testing. *Chem Biol* 2003;10:1103–13.
149. Enyedy IJ, Ling Y, Nacro K, Tomita Y, Wu X, Cao Y, Guo R, Li B, Zhu X, Huang Y, Long YQ, Roller PP, Yang D, Wang S. Discovery of small-molecule inhibitors of Bcl-2 through structure-based computer screening. *J Med Chem* 2001;44:4313–24.
150. Wu YQ, Belyakov S, Chi Choi, Limburg D, Thomas BE IV, Vaal M, Wei L, Wilkinson DE, Holmes A, Fuller M, McCormick J, Connolly M, Moeller T, Steiner J, Hamilton, GS. Synthesis and biological evaluation of non-peptidic cyclophilin ligands. *J Med Chem* 2003;46:1112–15.
151. Burkhard P, Hommell U, Sanner M, Walkinshaw MD. The discovery of steroids and other novel FKBP inhibitors using a molecular docking program. *J Mol Biol* 1999;287:853–8.
152. Filikov AV, Mohan V, Vickers TA, Griffey RH, Cook PD, Abagyan RA, James TL. Identification of ligands for RNA targets via structure-based virtual screening: HIV-1 TAR. *J Comput Aided Mol Design* 2000;14:593–610.
153. Kurogi Y, Miyata K, Okamura T, Hashimoto K, Tsutsumi K, Nasu M, Moriyasu M. Discovery of novel mesangial cell proliferation inhibitors using a three-dimensional database searching method. *J Med Chem* 2001;44:2304–7.
154. Gao Y, Dickerson JB, Guo F, Zheng J, Zheng Y. Rational design and characterization of a Rac GTPase-specific small molecule inhibitor. *Proc Natl Acad Sci USA* 2004;101:7618–23.
155. Singh J, van Vlijmen H, Liao Y, Lee WC, Cornebise M, Harris M, Shu I, Gill A, Cuervo JH, Abraham WM, Adams SP. Identification of potent and novel $\alpha 4\beta 1$ antagonists using *in silico* screening. *J Med Chem* 2002;45:2988–93.
156. Cruciani G, editor. *Molecular interaction fields* (Vol. 27 of Mannhold R, Kubinyi H, Folkers G, editors, *Methods and Principles in Medicinal Chemistry*), Weinheim: Wiley-VCH, 2005.
157. Gohlke H, Hendlich M, Klebe G. Predicting binding modes, binding affinities and 'hot spots' for protein-ligand complexes using a knowledge-based scoring function. In: Klebe G, editor, *Virtual screening: an alternative or complement to high throughput screening.* Dordrecht: Kluwer Academic Publishers, 2000; also published in *Persp Drug Discov Des* 2000;20:115–44.
158. Sotriffer CA, Gohlke H, Klebe G. Docking into knowledge-based potential fields: a comparative evaluation of DrugScore. *J Med Chem* 2002;45:1967–70.

159. Catalyst software. Accelrys Inc, San Diego.
160. Li H, Sutter J, Hoffmann R. HypoGen: an automated system for generating 3D predictive pharmacophore models. In: Güner OF, editor, *Pharmacophore perception, development and use in drug design.*, La Jolla: International University Line, 2000. p. 173–89.
161. Clement OO, Mehl AT. HipHop: pharmacophores based on multiple common-feature alignments. In: Güner OF, editor, *Pharmacophore perception, development and use in drug design.* La Jolla: International University Line, 2000. p. 69–84.
162. Kurogi Y, Güner OF. Pharmacophore modeling and three-dimensional database searching for drug design using Catalyst. *Curr Med Chem* 2001;8:1035–155.
163. Güner O, Clement O, Kurogi Y. Pharmacophore modeling and three dimensional database searching for drug design using Catalyst: recent advances. *Curr Med Chem* 2004;11:763–71.
164. Wolber G, Langer T LigandScout: 3-D pharmacophores derived from protein-bound ligands and their use as virtual screening filters. *J Chem Inf Model* 2005;45:160–9.
165. Rarey M, Dixon JS. Feature trees: a new molecular similarity measure based on tree matching. *J Comput Aided Mol Des* 1998;12:471–90.
166. Rarey M, Stahl M. Similarity searches in large combinatorial chemistry spaces. *J Comput Aided Mol Des* 2001;15:497–520.
167. Unity software. Tripos Associates Inc, St. Louis.
168. Ewing TJ, Makino S, Skillman AG, Kuntz ID. DOCK 4.0: search strategies for automated molecular docking of flexible molecule databases. *J Comput Aided Mol Des* 2001;15:411–28.
169. Rarey M, Kramer B, Lengauer T, Klebe G. A fast flexible docking method using an incremental construction algorithm. *J Mol Biol* 1996;261:470–89.
170. Kramer B, Rarey M, Lengauer T. Evaluation of the FlexX incremental construction algorithm for protein ligand docking. *Proteins Struct Funct Genet* 1999;37:228–41.
171. Hindle SA, Rarey M, Buning C, Lengauer T. Flexible docking under pharmacophore type constraints. *J Comput Aided Mol Des* 2002;16:129–49.

17

PHARMACEUTICAL RESEARCH AND DEVELOPMENT PRODUCTIVITY: CAN SOFTWARE HELP?

CHRISTOPHE G. LAMBERT AND S. STANLEY YOUNG

Contents

17.1 INTRODUCTION

Let's examine the challenge of producing and selling scientific software that produces meaningful business results for pharmaceutical research and development (R&D) productivity. Software is necessary but not sufficient to provide a solution to the apparent drop in R&D productivity. Some potentially disruptive technologies in cheminformatics and pharmacogenetics have the potential to dramatically improve productivity as they mature, assuming the industry makes appropriate policy shifts to take advantage of the technology.

Ultimately, software is bought to accomplish a business result. Therefore, software offerings in pharmaceutical R&D ought to somehow accelerate R&D productivity, or at least give cost savings along the pipeline. Yet the reality is that most scientific software is not sold on the basis of delivering

Computer Applications in Pharmaceutical Research and Development, Edited by Sean Ekins.
ISBN 0-471-73779-8

economic value. Rather, most software is sold based on novel and exciting features, ease of use, or at best solving some current scientific problem that faces the scientist within the context of a massive organization devoted to creating better treatments for diseases.

For scientific knowledge workers, the currency of the new knowledge economy is the transformation of data into useful information. We are inspired by the promise of genetic medicine and unraveling the mysteries of life itself to find breakthrough cures for the diseases that plague humankind. The average scientist in a large pharmaceutical corporation knows that he or she is working toward bringing better medicines to market, but the average scientist would have little idea of how to quantify the economic contribution of his/her work. How then, in turn, can a scientific software provider hope to provide an economic justification for an expenditure of funds? How can a software provider set a fair price for its products? How can a software supplier choose financially viable markets to enter with new products?

The pharmaceutical industry is one of the most difficult in which to answer these questions. This is due to two major factors, one that is industry specific and one that is not.

First, the pharmaceutical pipeline typically spans approximately 14+ years from early-stage discovery to bringing a drug to market, depending on the therapeutic target (sometimes longer). For a pharmaceutical company, the economic reality of today is a largely a function of decisions made over a decade ago. CEOs are praised or blamed for quarterly results that were largely the business decisions of their predecessors. How then can the worker in the trenches hope to have a better picture of the economic consequence of a software purchase? The time horizon of return on investment (ROI) for innovative scientific software expenditures may be more than twice the expected lifetime of the average small software company. The idea of value paid for value received appears to be untenable on these large time horizons. As always, the price is set by what the market will bear, which is usually based on price comparisons with marginally similar packages and with open-source offerings averaged in. In our experience, the total costs of ownership for internal solutions, factoring in salaries, overhead, and time cost of money, are usually significantly underestimated.

Second, despite the fact that we work in a knowledge economy, the business practices in use today largely operate from paradigms set in motion during the Industrial Revolution. In particular, organizational complexity is handled by divide and conquer: Functional units operate semiautonomously, with each suborganization striving to meet metrics that may or may not be good for the organization as a whole. This worked reasonably well in a textile factory, but not in a knowledge industry. For a knowledge worker to make decisions that are good for the organization as a whole, she must have relevant information from many parts of the organization. Software technology has the potential to provide instantaneous information about all relevant aspects of an organization to the individual worker, yet decisions are largely made locally, as was done in the nineteenth century. The pharmaceutical pipeline is basically an assembly line paradigm where the worker/organization from one stage does his job, then passes it on to the next person. Although this has been slowly changing, it remains difficult for the software provider to make a bottom-line value proposition, particularly within the silos that are furthest from bringing product to market. In many situations, it may well be the case that software offerings have small relevance to the bottom line, particularly if they do not address a system constraint, see [22] for an introduction to the Theory of Constraints.

Goldratt has outlined the necessary and sufficient conditions for a technology to confer a benefit [23]. To generate productivity from a new technology he advocates answering a set of questions about the technology. Let's use them in detail to examine software solutions in the pharmaceutical industry. Goldratt's questions are as follows:

1. What is the main power of the technology?
2. What limitation does it diminish?
3. What rules (policies) helped us to accommodate the limitation?
4. What rules (policies) should we use now?

These seemingly simple questions have profound implications because they ask us to examine possibly obsolete policies and behaviors that have become deeply ingrained and unexamined habit patterns. For instance, let us consider the fields of genomics, proteomics, metabolomics, and systems biology as applied to pharmaceutical R&D:

1. In general, the power of these technologies is to profoundly understand cause/effect within biological systems.
2. Without understanding cause/effect sufficiently in biological systems, we have been limited in our ability to change these systems for the better, for example, to treat/cure disease. The process of trial and error in pharmaceutical R&D is tremendously expensive and time consuming, with most diseases going untreated.
3. A number of policies and paradigms currently exist to deal with the limitation of our ability to change biological systems toward beneficial ends. The centuries-old paradigm of disease diagnosis as a pattern recognition exercise in observing similar effects is no longer viable. We now know that there is a many-to-many relationship between causes and effects. Obesity, heart disease, diabetes, Alzheimer disease—all the big diseases that impact millions late in life involve multiple genes, if not hundreds. Furthermore, defects in one genetic mechanism can give rise to many different so-called diseases. Although everybody knows this, consider the policies we use in the US and elsewhere in the world to approve medicines. Currently, drugs are approved based on their ability to treat an indication (a disease). Suppose a drug treats an underlying

cause—a mutation in a single gene, which gives rise to 5% of 20 different diseases. As a whole, this might represent a very large group. However, a pharmaceutical company would have to run one clinical trial for each "disease," likely making it financially prohibitive to bring the drug to market.

Another paradigm is the "one size fits all" paradigm for disease treatment that has been slowly changing over the centuries. Although most people no longer apply leeches or snake oil to cure all our ailments in one fell swoop, the dream of a universal panacea lives with us still. In an old *Superman* comic book story [2], Superman's brain power is magnified 100-fold, he develops an antievil ray to wipe out all evil on earth, and a reformed Lex Luther creates a serum that is an antidote to all sickness on earth (including baldness). The reality is that disease is as complex as our individual genetic variations, various environmental exposures, and the interactions between the two; the paradigms of today are far from treating each patient according to the specific cause-effect pattern of disease that exists within his/her body.

Thankfully, for many diseases, blockbuster drugs at standard dosages are reasonably safe and effective at saving lives and alleviating suffering for large numbers of people. However, many of the best blockbusters (particularly anticancer drugs) work for only 30–50% of a diseased population. Furthermore, the NIH Office of Rare Diseases estimates there are 6000+ rare diseases collectively afflicting about 25 million Americans. These so-called "orphan" diseases, defined as affecting fewer than 200,000 Americans, are currently too "small" to provide ROI for most pharmaceutical companies. Clearly, the blockbuster and the one drug fits all paradigms must be changed to help these people.

Another paradigm is treatment versus cure. If we can understand the genetic causes of the disease, and if in the years to come technologies such as gene therapy allow us to change our genes, the economic model of drug treatment for the rest of our lives may no longer be viable for most diseases.

4. What new paradigms and policies do we need? Most of the major pharmaceutical companies are moving in the direction of developing pharmacogenetic-based drugs. That is individualized medicine—where different subpopulations of patients are prescribed different medicines based on their genetic profiles. To take advantage of the power of genetics to differentiate responders and nonresponders, we need to look at new policies that facilitate drug approvals based on treatment of underlying causes, instead of the effects we term "disease." Alternately, we need to redefine our notion of disease in terms of cause, so that a disease will be specified by the genetic mutation, rather than the observable symptoms. At the present time, it might be useful to define a complex disease, like depression or schizophrenia, by the drug or drug combination that works for the patient.

What does this all mean for the scientific software? If you want to make a difference to pharmaceutical R&D productivity, you need to understand what is limiting productivity today, then you must develop technologies for addressing that limitation, and finally new policies and paradigms must be instituted to take advantage of the power of your software. This concept is aptly illustrated in [3], a business novel that makes the observation that despite its power, Enterprise Resource Planning (ERP) software was bringing limited ROI because of policy holdovers from a previous century. That is, the power of ERP software was to give instantaneous access to relevant data throughout the enterprise for better decision making. Yet the policies of local decision making based on local information were firmly in place, resulting in suboptimal decision making, with most ERP implementations bringing marginal benefits at great expense. To bring true value, software companies have to engineer change at key leverage points within their customers' organizations.

To bring significant economic value to pharma today requires a change in paradigm for the software maker. No longer can software providers just be good at solving a specific scientific problem with a shrink-wrapped package. They must take a holistic view of their industry, market, and customer. Software providers must understand the minutiae of the systems and businesses of their customers as well or better than they do. As silos are collapsing within the pharmaceutical industry, and work teams are being assembled that draw from talents across the R&D pipeline, the software provider needs to follow suit. Increasingly, the average software provider will be ineffective at providing value for the pharmaceutical company because it is generally ignorant of its complex internal workings.

All of the big pharmaceutical companies are currently consolidating their IT resources. Although stand-alone solutions are tolerated on the bleeding edge of technology, once a field matures software applications for that field must fit within an overall IT infrastructure. Increasingly, this infrastructure is being custom built by pharmaceutical companies themselves (often with the help of contract programmers) because no software provider comes close to being able to span the breadth and depth of pharmaceutical R&D complexity. Furthermore, manufacturing, sales and marketing, and supply chain logistics will increasingly need to integrate in a more profound way with the activities of R&D. For instance, in drug development, there is much consternation over the high cost of running large clinical trials. Yet in many cases with large successful clinical trials, the word-of-mouth marketing effect of many patients sharing their success stories has provided an huge unforeseen marketing boost. To capitalize on this in the future, marketing and development silos would need better communication to tune a strategy to optimize the expected bottom-line return. Consider also where genetic results of clinical trials can be fed back to research to help with target identification. If silos don't look at the overall system picture, suboptimal resource allocation decisions end up being made.

We have been developing cutting-edge data analysis tools for the pharmaceutical industry for over a decade, with a particular focus in the fields of cheminformatics and bioinformatics. We now describe how our insights apply to these areas.

Over the past couple of decades pharmaceutical companies have made massive expenditures in scaling up their ability to perform high-throughput screening (HTS) on large numbers of compounds. Large investments in information technology have also been made to support these data collection efforts. Unfortunately, although millions of compounds can be screened per day, there has been a steady decline of new molecular entities (NMEs) coming to market for about a decade now [4]. HTS is definitely a powerful technology, yet the adoption of this technology has not led to improved bottom line results.

Furthermore, for the last 7 years or so, a great deal of investment has been made by pharmaceutical companies and investors in the science of pharmacogenetics. Pharmacogenetics relates directly to delivering the right drug for the right patient at the right dosage based on the patient's genetic differences. There have been some promising success stories of drugs brought to market that target a particular subpopulation, for example, the beneficial effects of BiDil in African Americans [5]. However, there is also great concern that, given the high cost of drug development, pharmacogenetic medicine may only be economically viable for subpopulations of blockbuster-sized diseases.

What are the real problems plaguing the pharmaceutical industry, and why have these promising technologies not been silver bullets as initially hoped? To answer this question we need to take a holistic view of the forces at work in the industry. Surprisingly, it is often easier to deal with organizational complexity by looking at the whole at a sufficient level of abstraction, rather than looking at the parts without that larger context.

Figure 17.1 presents a "current reality tree" showing some of the major problems that afflict the pharmaceutical industry at present. Good sources of background information on the current reality tree approach and other Theory of Constraints "thinking tools" are [6] and [7]. Rounded rectangles represent causes/effects, with connecting arrows pointing from cause to effect. Small, empty ovals represent the "and" operation, where more than one cause is needed to produce the effect. Arrows that start high in the tree and point to lower sections are feedback loops that amplify the problems over time. In the upper part of the tree we see the symptoms of the underlying productivity disease that the pharmaceutical industry is faced with:

- Pharma cannot sustain the double-digit growth demanded by investors.
- When market exclusivity ends, revenues drop by 50–80%.
- Drug prices keep rising for consumers.
- Pharmaceutical company productivity is declining.
- It now costs $1.25 billion+ in R&D to develop a new drug.

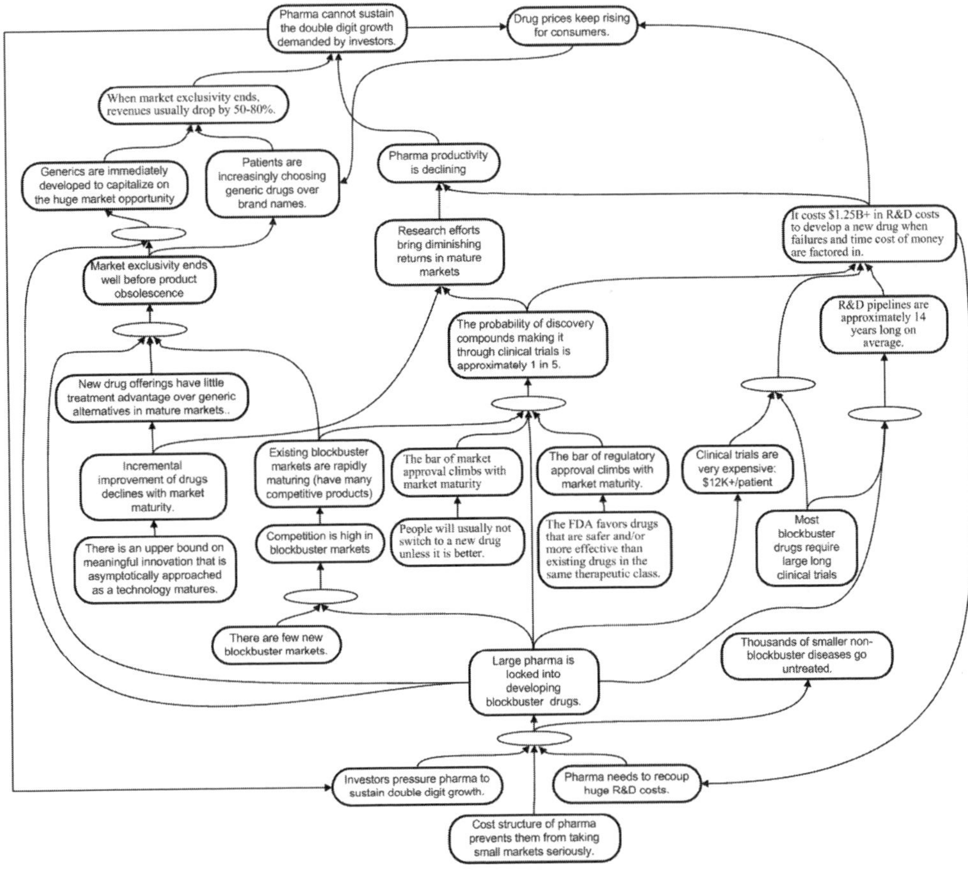

Figure 17.1 Pharmaceutical industry current reality tree.

- The probability of discovery compounds making it through clinical trials is 1 in 5.
- R&D pipelines are approximately 14 years long on average.
- Thousands of smaller nonblockbuster diseases go untreated.

When we look at the detailed cause-effect pattern, we see a fascinating picture emerging. To meet the revenue demands of large pharmaceutical companies, to cover the $1.25 billion+ costs of bringing drugs to market, and to keep investors happy by not losing money, they are locked into developing blockbuster drugs. However, the proportion of diseases that are blockbuster-sized is small, leading to stiff competition in these markets. As a result, the blockbuster markets quickly mature, with the safety and efficacy of drugs in those markets rapidly climbing the innovation "S" curve described by Christensen in *The Innovator's Dilemma* [8]. As the incremental improvement of each new generation of drugs necessarily shrinks, the marginal value that a new drug for a blockbuster disease delivers to the market shrinks as well. Decades ago, the new generation of patent-protected drugs were far superior to their off-patent predecessors, providing less market opportunity for generic companies to copy the off-patent drugs. But as innovation approaches its practical limits, the generic drugs become comparable in value to the latest and greatest patent-protected drugs, increasing the market demand for off-patent drugs as they have converged in quality, safety, and efficacy. Without generics needing to recoup large R&D costs, the new drug that might provide a 5% improvement is competing with a generic drug that is a fraction of the cost to the consumer of the new one. Time to competition is decreasing as the financial incentive for generics is so large. The last phase of technology maturity is competition on price, further bolstering our argument that it is the innovation curve that the pharmaceutical industry is up against. Generics will win in the price war game because of their cost structure, but their growth is capped by the innovation rate of the pharmaceutical industry unless they enter the drug discovery business themselves, something that has already begun to happen. There are other factors related to generics not included in this model such as the impact of the Wax–Hatchman FDA regulatory changes that encouraged generic competition, the increasing success of generics at challenging pharmaceutical patents, or the fact that your local pharmacist has stickers on his wall encouraging the use of generics over brand-name drugs.

Returning to other parts of the current reality tree we see that as drugs improve in safety and efficacy with each generation, the bar of market and FDA approval rises, making the success rate of clinical trials drop. That is, drug quality is a roughly monotonically increasing sequence, and the probability that a random attempt for higher quality exceeds all previous attempts drops inversely with the number of drugs on the market in a given therapeutic area. Technically, a drug only has to beat the placebo. In practice, the FDA is unlikely to approve a drug with a success rate lower than the market leader unless the side effects profile is better.

Currently about 80% of clinical trials fail (which is an astounding number) [9]. As the safety bar goes up, the costs of clinical trials go up as ever larger clinical trials are required to provide the necessary statistical power to demonstrate safety equivalent to or better than the last innovative drug that jumped through all the hoops. Note also that the $1.25 billion+ cost of bringing a drug to market is amortizing clinical failures and time cost of money into the equation.

As a consequence of all the aforementioned issues, the pharmaceutical industry cannot reasonably sustain its historic double-digit growth without some dramatic change in the way it discovers drugs. This further creates more pressure from investors to press forward with ever more efforts and technologies to find mega-blockbusters to somehow sustain profits. These efforts cost money, and drug prices continue to rise for consumers, often leading to public outcry and public policy changes that create negative feedback loops, further impeding the industry's ability to sustain revenue growth. Ironically, many of the consumers who criticize the high cost of medicines are the same ones who expect their pharmaceutical and biotechnology company stocks to deliver double-digit growth! Many pundits say that the pharmaceutical industry is in some kind of innovation slump, but the truth is that the industry has had to be tremendously innovative to jump the ever higher bars of safety and efficacy within these mature markets. The "productivity" challenges we see for the pharmaceutical industry are not due to a drop in innovation; rather, these challenges are a consequence of the properties of the system. The impersonal understanding that deep systems knowledge gives us allows us to fix the problems instead of affixing blame to one party or the other that appears to be the villain from the limited local perspective of where we feel our pain most personally.

At the bottom of the tree is the core problem: The cost structure of the pharmaceutical industry prevents companies from taking small markets seriously. There are plenty of diseases to go around, but only a handful can be lucrative within the limitations of the current system. This brings us to the critical question, Where does a technology company focus its efforts? The answer is, obviously, at the core problem! The pharmaceutical companies need to be able to enter immature small disease markets and produce drugs cost effectively. The software provider must figure out how to help them do that. It is interesting to note that Roche has already made the bold strategic move of targeting smaller markets [see 10].

This leads us to the realm of disruptive technologies. Christensen [8] presents the innovator's dilemma, where the large company focused on meeting current customer demand on a large scale ignores the disruptive opportunity because it looks like too small a market to make a difference on the balance sheet. Further, the opportunity is ignored because it does not fit in the current business model or address the needs of the current customer base.

Two key technologies the authors have specialized in over the last decade are sequential screening [see 1, 27] and pharmacogenetics [see 25]. Both of these complementary technologies have the potential to address the core problem discussed above. However, the current evidence is that most pharmaceutical companies are making the classic mistake Christensen describes of evaluating these potentially disruptive technologies within the limitations of their existing paradigms. (These companies may be destined to fail.)

Sequential screening has been largely applied within the pipeline paradigm. Compounds are optimized for their ability to bind to a target in vitro and then handed off to the next stages of optimization with the hope that this compound with nanomolar potency against the target will be optimizable to one with good absorption, distribution, metabolism, excretion, and toxicity (ADME/Tox) properties and be safe and effective in humans.

Although many companies have advocated "personalized" or "individualized" medicine, with a few exceptions, pharmacogenetics operationally has been seen as a mechanism to salvage a failed blockbuster after the fact, rather than a way to go after small markets from the beginning with a precise focus. The most widely heralded example of a pharmacogenetic drug, Herceptin®, which treats breast cancer for women with a particular genetic variant, is still a blockbuster seller in its own right. The same will probably be true of BiDil®, NitroMed's recently launched medication for the treatment of heart failure in African American patients (described above). Even if it proves to be a limited financial success, the point holds that the drug was originally targeted to the blockbuster-sized market of 5,000,000 Americans who are affected by the disease, not just the 750,000 African Americans the drug was eventually approved for.

We believe the direction to a solution to low-cost drug R&D is therefore a combination of sequential screening and pharmacogenetics-based medicine. We do not claim the solution is here today. Like other disruptive technologies, these technologies will need to mature before significant benefits come. Also, we have to be willing to change our paradigms so that these disruptive technologies can bear fruit. Disruptive forces involve change, and change involves discomfort because we must face the inevitable uncertainty ahead of us. To engineer change we must not only hold out the golden apple of promise but also provide enough security that the proposed change will bring the promised benefits for the industry.

We have worked in the field of cheminformatics for about a decade, and in particular we have developed statistical and computer science technology for sequential screening and advocated a paradigm shift to its adoption within the pharmaceutical and biotechnology industries (see Fig. 17.2).

Briefly, the idea is to take the results of an assay of a relatively small number of compounds along with chemical structure information and use statistical and computer science algorithms and chemistry knowledge to predict what will happen on new compounds that are candidates to be acquired or synthesized and tested. The idea is that if you can predict with some confidence the results of a screen, you can make more effective resource allocation decisions than just screening random available compounds. Moreover, the ability to predict with a computer gives one the ability to search toward an optimum in an automated fashion [see in particular 1, 11, and 12. The ChemTree® package from Golden Helix 13 enables this type of predictive modeling, yet few are taking advantage of the power of this technology throughout the drug discovery pipeline; rather, they are using it and similar commercially available tools in a more limited mode.

Let us examine cheminformatics technologies with our four questions:

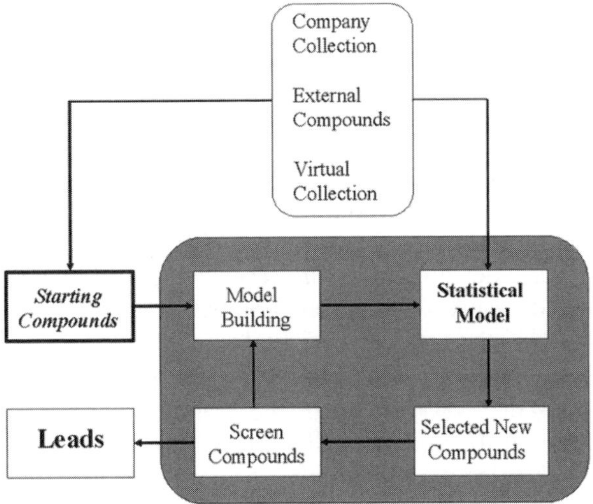

Figure 17.2 The sequential screening process.

1. The power of the technology is to predict what a compound will do in a biological system, reducing or eliminating the need for biological testing.
2. The less we can predict what a compound will do, the more we rely on trial and error with expensive and time-consuming laboratory work.
3. We will focus on two of the many policies we have in place that enabled us to deal with our inability to predict the outcome of an assay. First, although this approach is dying off, many screening groups still use brute force to screen thousands of compounds and skim off the most active, passing them off to medicinal chemists for further optimization. The tremendous information inherent in this data is lost, and the scientist relies on human pattern recognition alone to take compounds forward towards clinical development. Second is the practice of screening many compounds for activity against a target and then asking teams of medicinal chemists to modify the most promising lead series until compounds are found with good ADME/Tox properties. These two paradigms are useful when you count on human beings to do pattern recognition and optimization. However, to use prediction optimally, we need to use all of the data, and not limit our optimization to a one-dimensional perspective. We examine appropriate new approaches in the next section.
4. There are a number of reasons why HTS may not be delivering. Lipinski has argued that compounds coming out of HTS are not druglike [14]. They are too large and too lipophilic. HTS systems by their nature are

isolated systems; the correlation from these systems to intact cells or animal models is often problematic, if indeed there is any correlation at all. It is well known in optimization theory that to optimize multiple criteria, it is much better to simultaneously optimize rather than sequentially optimize one property at a time. Many times highly potent compounds lack other necessary properties or features, and it has not been easy to build these in without losing potency. There is growing awareness of the multiple optimization problem, where focus has recently shifted toward developing *in silico* (i.e., computer) models for the more expensive to assay secondary end points. A much better way to use the power of HTS and sequential virtual screening is to:

a. Set up an assay for the primary target and, simultaneously, set up hundreds of assays for all of the secondary end points that could possibly be affected by a drug treatment: ADME/Tox, selectivity. Although price may be an object now, remember that once a compound is assayed for ADME/Tox properties, that data point can be used predictively in all future drug discovery efforts. In any event, price will come down with economy of scale.
b. Screen thousands of compounds against all these assays with the power of HTS, instead of millions of compounds against just the primary target.
c. Use the predictive power of sequential screening to decide which compounds to build or buy next that most drive in the direction of not only optimizing the primary target, but also having good ADME/Tox and selectivity properties against all of the secondary screens.
d. With those compounds, go back to Step b and repeat until optimization (within desired thresholds) is complete.

As this sequential screening technology matures this procedure should allow automated production of drugs that are safe and effective in humans. All of the technologies necessary to perform this already exist. To our knowledge, they have never been assembled as described, although some companies such as Neurogen have gone far in this direction [15]. What is required is:

1. *Good validated targets.* This is not always easy, but the genomics revolution has opened the way to finding many more targets more cost effectively. Good genetic analysis software is needed to find the association between disease and genetic factors. Furthermore, a deeper understanding must be developed around gene-gene and gene-environment interactions. The authors and co-workers have developed HelixTree® genetics analysis software over the past 7 years with those ends in mind [16].
2. *Good secondary screens for ADME/Tox and selectivity.* It used to be these were too expensive to consider at medium throughput, but this is

changing. Companies such as NovaScreen have a few hundred such screens available on demand, but right now they are mostly used at the end of lead optimization by pharmaceutical companies. Hurel Corp., recently profiled in *Forbes Magazine* [17], has created a chip that purports to enable predictive toxicology and metabolic, absorption and bio-availability studies with compounds. Currently their product appears to be targeted to preclinical studies with the idea of minimizing failed animal studies by incorporating cells from the liver and intestine containing key transporters and enzymes important for limiting a drug's bioavailability. If this or other predictive technologies for ADME/Tox were placed within the predictive feedback loop described above, the revenue possibilities for automated drug discovery could be even more significant.

3. *Good predictive algorithms.* Prediction doesn't have to be perfect; it just has to be better than random. ChemTree® from Golden Helix (www.goldenhelix.com) has been validated in numerous pharmaceutical installations and provides outstanding predictions using recursive partitioning [see 24, 26, 28]. Metadrug™ from GeneGo (www.genego.com) has the extra capability of determining what compounds a given compound may be metabolized to, which in turn can be run through predictive algorithms such as those in ChemTree integrated within this software.
4. *Good automated compound creation* is required in which compounds can be synthesized by robots on demand, driven by predictive software. This is achieved with combinatorial chemistry. In particular, Click Chemistry [18] provides very stable and predictable reactions that would be ideal for this application.
5. *Pharmacogenetics-based assays*, in which different genetic variants of biological systems can be interrogated to develop individualized medicine. Note also that the new specialized medicine paradigm will require rethinking the expensive safety requirements used for general-purpose drugs. For example, long-term rodent tests are too expensive, and they have poor prediction characteristics for humans.
6. Tying all of these competencies together within *an integrated system.*

Thirty years ago, pharma was chemistry driven. Synthetic chemistry was well understood, and the biological mechanism for most drugs was generally poorly understood. More recently, the amount of biological knowledge has exploded, and one can argue that the pharmaceutical industry is becoming increasingly biology driven (leaving marketing out of consideration). We are making the case that chemistry and biology need to be in balance in a very tight molecule design and testing loop with a range of different molecules designed for the different human genotypes. Inside drug companies there will have to be efficient information extraction from data and efficient information flow. Software will obviously be the key to enabling the flow of such huge quantities of information. One aspect of the software is that it should embed or be linked to subject matter knowledge so that desk scientists of ordinary skill can function near the level of world-class experts. There will not be enough experts to go around for the many drug design projects that need to be sustained. Analysis and triage of HTS is a case in point. Evaluation of these large, up to 1 million compound, complex data sets calls for multiple experts in biology, medicinal chemistry, and statistics. Much of the medicinal chemistry is embedded in ChemTree® for smart statistical analysis and PowerMV for linking to annotated chemistry databases. The genetics data sets coming from clinical trials are and will be very complex. There could be hundreds of candidate genes and hundreds of thousands of single nucleotide polymorphism (SNP) markers. Complex correlation structures are implicit in the nature of genetics. The supply of quantitative or statistical genetics experts is quite limited, and therefore software such as HelixTree® puts complex analysis within the reach of clinical trial statisticians.

What might a new vision of drug discovery be? Think of a large feedback loop. We observe disease-gene associations in large clinical trials or prospective population studies. Young, Zaykin, and Ge have outlined many key challenges in the analysis of genetics data previously in [19] and [20]. Multiple genes are likely to be involved. We expect to see interactions between genes. We also expect to see subpopulations that are homogeneous within a heterogeneous named disease. We will therefore need to find one or more drugs to modify the biochemical pathways indicated by the large studies. This process will lead to relatively many, smaller-use drugs. To capture the promise of this vision, we will also need much less expensive safety and efficacy drug testing. As fewer patients will be exposed to these specialized medicines and they are the ones that will directly benefit or suffer side effects, risk/benefit will be more individually focused. It seems clear that safety testing strategies will have to be modified to move to individualized medicine.

Returning to our discussion of the current reality tree in Figure 17.1, the core problem is the cost structure of the pharmaceutical companies that prevents them from taking small markets seriously. We can then construct a future reality tree, to project the consequences of alleviating the core problem (see Fig. 17.3). Rectangular boxes indicate "injections" or additional action steps that need to be taken to get the desired positive outcomes. At the bottom to overcome the core problem, we propose sequential virtual screening, pharmacogenetics, and other technologies to maximize downstream success, such as the novel use of chemistry technologies described earlier.

The authors have developed software, ChemTree and HelixTree, to meet many of the challenges at the core of this problem. Nevertheless, the full value of these software technologies will only be realized through transformation of the policies and paradigms of the pharmaceutical industry. It is the goal of this chapter to spark other change agents toward making this transformation a reality.

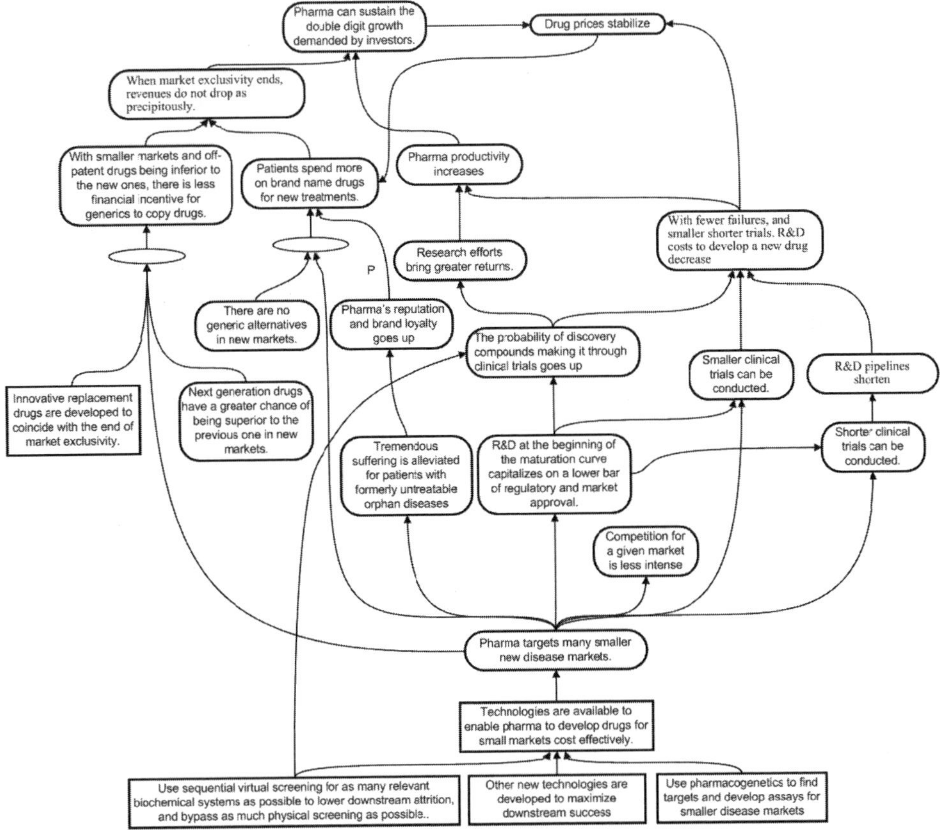

Figure 17.3 Pharmaceutical industry future reality tree.

17.2 CONCLUSIONS

For pharmaceutical companies to get back on track to double-digit growth, they must be able to compress the time and resources it takes to bring a drug to market. To move to personalized medicine, the cost to develop each drug must be dramatically lower. This is possible with current technologies, and we have outlined the software and laboratory components necessary for success. Are these technologies sufficient? Perhaps not currently, but as these disruptive technologies continue to climb the innovative "S" curve, they will surely surpass the laborious expensive and time-consuming techniques we count on today.

The biggest payoff for software vendors and the pharmaceutical industry alike is not likely to come from developing or buying that next exciting new piece of scientific software in isolation. Rather, it is deeply understanding system dynamics [21] and making informed changes of policy in concert with investing in R&D technologies that provide leverage points for change. The role of the niche software provider will be as a piece of a larger business process. It appears that the consultants, in-house visionaries, and change agents will need to play a larger role in moving pharmaceutical companies to personalized medicine. To receive maximum value for their innovative solutions, software providers will either need to become consultants and change agents themselves or add this capacity through strategic alliances or mergers.

REFERENCES

1. Abt M, Lim Y-B, Sacks J, Xie M, Young SS. A sequential approach for identifying lead compounds in large chemical databases. *Stat Sci* 2001;16:154–68.
2. Dorfman L. The amazing story of Superman-Red and Superman-Blue. In: *Superman* #162. DC Comics, 1963.
3. Goldratt EM, Schragenheim E, Ptak CA. *Necessary but not sufficient.* North River Press, 2000.
4. FDA. Innovation or Stagnation? Challenge and Opportunity on the Critical Path to New Medical Products. March 16, 2004. http://www.fda.gov/oc/initiatives/criticalpath/whitepaper.pdf.
5. Taylor AL, Ziesche S, Yancy C, Carson P, D'Agostino R Jr, Ferdinand K, Taylor M, Adams K, Sabolinski M, Worcel M, Cohn JN; African-American Heart Failure Trial Investigators. Combination of isosorbide dinitrate and hydralazine in blacks with heart failure. *N Engl J Med* 2004; Nov 11;351(20):2049–57.
6. Scheinkopf LJ. *Thinking for a change: putting the TOC thinking processes to use.* CRC Press, 1999.
7. Dettmer HW. *Goldratt's theory of constraints: a systems approach to continuous improvement.* ASQ Quality Press, 1997.
8. Christensen CM. *The innovator's dilemma: when new technologies cause great firms to fail.* Harvard Business School Press, 1997.
9. DiMasi JA. *Risks in new drug development: Approval success rates for investigational drugs.* Tufts Center for the Study of Drug Development, Tufts University, Boston, MA, 2001.
10. Whalen J. A big drug maker moves to play down mass-market pills: Roche seeks pricey products in specialties like cancer and rejects megamergers: Pfizer's edge in sales muscle. *Wall Street Journal*, September 20, 2004.
11. Jones-Hertzog DK, Mukhopadhyay P, Keefer CE, Young SS. Use of recursive partitioning in the sequential screening of G-protein-coupled receptors. *J Pharmacol Toxicol* 2000;10:207–15.
12. Engels MFM, Venkatarangan P. Smart screening: Approaches to efficient HTS. *Curr Opin Drug Discov Devel* 2001;4:275–83.

13. Lambert CG. ChemTree® HTS Analysis Software. Golden Helix, Inc. 2005; http://www.goldenhelix.com.
14. Lipinski CA, Lombardo F, Dominy BW, Feeney PJ. Experimental and computational approaches to estimate solubility and permeability in drug discovery and development settings. *Adv Drug Delivery Rev* 1997;23:3–25.
15. Manly CJ, Hamer J, Louise-May S. The impact of informatics and computational chemistry on synthesis and screening. *Drug Discov Today* 2001;6:1101–10.
16. Lambert CG. HelixTree® Genetics Analysis Software. Golden Helix, Inc. 2005; http://www.goldenhelix.com.
17. Schupak A. The Bunny Chip. *Forbes Magazine* 2005; vol. 176 no. 3 pp. 53–4.
18. Kolb HC, Finn MG, Sharpless KB. Click chemistry: diverse chemical function from a few good reactions. *Angew Chemie Intl Ed* 2001; vol. 40 no. 11, pp. 2004–21.
19. Young SS, Ge N. Recursive partitioning analysis of complex disease pharmacogenetics studies. I. Motivation and overview. *Pharmacogenomics* 2005;6(1):65–75.
20. Zaykin DV, Young SS. Large recursive partitioning analysis of complex disease pharmacogenetic studies. II. Statistical considerations. *Pharmacogenomics* 2005;6(1):77–89.
21. Sterman JD. *Business dynamics: systems thinking and modeling for a complex world*. McGraw-Hill/Irwin, 2000.
22. Goldratt EM, Cox J. *The goal: a process of ongoing improvement,* 3rd edition. North River Press. 2004.
23. Goldratt EM. *Necessary & sufficient: CD01 The reason for technology*. CD-ROM video series, 2003.
24. Hawkins DM, Young SS, Rusinko A III. Analysis of a large Structure-activity data set using recursive partitioning. Quantitative Structure-Activity Relationships, 1997;16:296–302.
25. Lambert CG. Compound-selection & pharmacogenetics tools. *Genet Eng News* 2003;23(1):30–2.
26. Rusinko A III, Farmen MW, Lambert CG, Brown PL, Young SS. Analysis of a large structure/biological activity data set using recursive partitioning. *J Chem Inf Comput Sci* 1999;39(6):1017–26.
27. Young SS, Ekins S, Lambert CG. So many targets, so many compounds, but so few resources, *Curr Drug Discov* 2002; December:17–22.
28. Young SS, Gombar VK, Emptage MR, Cariello NF, Lambert CG. Mixture deconvolution and analysis of Ames mutagenicity data. *Chemometrics Intell Lab Syst* 2002;60:5–11.

PART V

COMPUTERS IN PRECLINICAL DEVELOPMENT

18

COMPUTER METHODS FOR PREDICTING DRUG METABOLISM

SEAN EKINS

Contents

18.1 INTRODUCTION

Metabolic transformations of pharmaceuticals occurring in vivo can modify their bioavailability, efficacy, chronic toxicity, and excretion rate and route. Both the parent molecule and the products of such metabolic pathways may also interfere with endogenous metabolism or interfere with other coadministered compounds. For example, the inhibition of metabolizing enzymes can be associated with drug-drug interactions, which can have potentially fatal consequences for the patient. Key issues in drug metabolism include identifying the enzyme(s) involved, the site(s) of metabolism, the resulting metabolite(s), and the rate of metabolism [1]. The majority of drugs as well as other xeno-

Computer Applications in Pharmaceutical Research and Development, Edited by Sean Ekins.
ISBN 0-471-73779-8

biotics undergo phase I metabolism via the cytochrome P450 (P450) enzymes predominantly in liver, although these enzymes are present in other organs such as the intestine. These enzymes are capable of either inactivating or activating both xeno- and endobiotic molecules. Of the approximately 40 human P450 genes cloned and classified according to sequence homology, three P450 families and fewer than a dozen unique enzymes have been shown to play a substantial role in human hepatic metabolism of drugs [2]. In addition, further metabolism may then occur, including glucuronidation, sulfation, or other phase II reactions that can result in important metabolites for some drugs that are widely used clinically [3]. Although these phase II enzymes have not received anywhere near as much attention as the P450s, there is interest in their role in drug metabolism [3]. Therefore, depending on the pharmaceutical molecule structure and the enzymes involved, there could be a range of possible metabolites that may be more or less reactive than the parent. Prediction of these possible metabolites and subsequent disposition is desirable.

Although P450s display high structural homology, they often have distinct roles in xenobiotic metabolism, with active sites that enable broad and overlapping substrate specificity that is complicated by ligand binding promiscuity [4]. The substrate selectivity of human P450s is related to both the substrate structure and the key molecular features of the active sites, namely, the disposition of certain amino acid residues around the heme [5]. In the absence of X-ray crystal structures for many of these enzymes, the prediction of whether a molecule binds to them rests with our limited knowledge for specificity and selectivity of the binding sites derived from in vitro data. The prediction of metabolism via the various phase I and phase II drug-metabolizing enzymes has therefore progressed in a number of directions (Table 18.1) over more than 30 years, and the different types of computational technologies discussed here represent the current state of the art (Table 18.2). The prediction of metabolites is a useful technology before assessment and detection with analytical methods. Metabolism prediction tools would also be of particular use before the generation of combinatorial libraries [6] or purchasing of compounds from external vendors. Because of the combinatorial explosion in the number of possible metabolites for each molecule in such libraries, the prediction methods will need to either produce a simple score as output or identify substructures of key metabolites produced by specific enzymes that may need to be avoided. The various metabolism prediction technologies are described in this chapter.

18.2 STATISTICAL, PHARMACOPHORE, AND HOMOLOGY MODELS AND CRYSTAL STRUCTURES OF DRUG-METABOLIZING ENZYMES

In the 1960s it was discovered that a mathematical model could describe the relationship between simple calculated molecular properties for a series of

TABLE 18.1 Human Enzymes Involved in Drug Metabolism That Have Been Computationally Modeled to Date

Enzyme	Cellular Location	Reaction	Cofactor	Phase	QSAR	Pharmacophore	Homology models	Crystal structures
Cytochrome P450	Microsomal	Oxidation and reaction	NADPH	1	[9–12] [13–18, 36]	[20–33]	[44–54]	[39–43]
Flavin Containing Monooxygenase	Microsomal	Oxidation	NADPH	1	[123]			
Monoamine oxidases	Mitochondrial	Oxidation		1	[124–126]	[127]	[128]	[129–132]
Aromatases	Mitochondrial	Oxidation	FAD	1	[133]	[134]	[135–137]	
Esterases	Microsomal and cytosolic	Hydrolysis		1	[138]			
Epoxide hydrolases	Microsomal and cytosolic	Hydration		1	[139]	[140]	[141]	[142]
UDP-glucuronosyl-transferases	Microsomal	Glucuronidation	UDPGA	2	[68]	[63–65]		
Sulfotransferases	Cytosolic	Sulfation	PAPS	2	[69, 143]			[69, 70, 144–147]
Glutathione S-transferases	Microsomal and cytosolic	Glutathione conjugation	Glutathione	2	[124]			[148–152]

Abbreviations NADPH, b-nicotinamide adenine dinucleotide phosphate reduced from; FAD, flavin adenine dinucleotide; PAPS, 3′-phosphoadenosine 5′-phosphosulfate; UDPGA, uridine diphosphate-glucuronic acid.

TABLE 18.2 Commercially Available Computational Technologies for Drug Metabolism Evaluation and Prediction

Software	Function	Website
MetaDrug™	Metabolism database, Metabolite prediction, Metabolite prioritization, QSAR models for enzymes, transporters and network building algorithms for Systems-ADME/Tox	www.genego.com
Metabolite™	Metabolism content database	www.mdl.com
Metabolism™	Metabolism content database	www.accelrys.com
BioFrontier/P450™	Metabolism content database	www.fqspl.com.pl
PharmGKB	Pharmacogenetics and pharmacogenomics knowledgebase	www.pharmgkb.org
METEOR™	Rule-based Metabolite prediction software Predicts the metabolic fate of chemicals Displays results as a metabolic tree. User can filter results for 'likely' metabolites. Links directly to MetaboLynx™ for analysis of mass spectrometry data	www.lhasalimited.org
META™	Rule-based Metabolite prediction software	www.multicase.com
MetabolExpert™	Rule-based Metabolite prediction software Predicts the most common metabolic pathways in animals, plants or through photodegradation. Results are presented in metabolic tree format. Graphical interface for editing and adding rules	www.compudrug.com
MetaSite™	Site of metabolism prediction for CYP2C9 and CYP3A4 and others	www.moldiscovery.com

molecules and a particular biological property [7, 8]. The application of the quantitative structure-metabolism relationships (QSMR) was pioneered by Hansch and co-workers [9–12], using small homologous sets of molecules and a few molecular descriptors. Following on from this work, Lewis and co-workers [13–18] provided many quantitative structure-activity relationships

(QSAR) studies that enabled them to suggest a simple decision tree for human P450 substrates [14]. Lipophilicity expressed as log P or molecular refractivity was one of the first important molecular properties found to be important for enzyme substrate binding. Steric, electronic, and molecular shape properties are also important for enzyme binding and transformation, whereas metabolite release likely requires the opposite properties to binding [1]. QSMR or QSAR models have since been constructed for each major P450 enzyme. The availability of more complex and graphically intensive software tools in the late 1980s to the 1990s initiated a new era in ligand-based computational modeling or QSAR analysis. QSAR technologies available include Catalyst (Accelrys, San Diego, CA), DISCO, CoMFA, ALMOND (Tripos Associates, St. Louis, MO), and GOLPE (Multivariate Infometric Analysis, S.r.l., Perugia) and have been described in detail elsewhere [19]. CoMFA has been used to describe key molecular features of ligands for human CYP1A2 [20] and CYP2C9 [21].

Computational pharmacophore models could also now be generated that represented the key features present in ligands that were necessary for a biological response. In pharmacophore software the molecular features of ligands are translated into spheres, points, or a mesh onto which molecule structures themselves can be mapped in 3D space [19]. Recent research has described and compared the many pharmacophores that have been generated for P450s [22], providing insight into the important features for interaction of ligands and proteins. The human enzymes CYP1A2, CYP2A6, CYP2B6, CYP2C9, CYP2D6, CYP3A4, CYP3A5, and CYP3A7 [20, 23–33] have received most of the focus of computational pharmacophore approaches to date. The CYP3A enzymes are the most important in terms of human drug metabolism [34], as they have a very broad substrate specificity. Computational pharmacophores for CYP3A4 have therefore been derived for substrates [35] and inhibitors [31, 35, 36], using kinetic constants K_m, $K_{i(apparent)}$, and IC_{50} data [22]. The computational pharmacophore approach has also been used to provide the first example of a model for the important features of molecules that increase their own metabolism (autoactivators) via CYP3A4 [35]. Recently, the pharmacophore approach has also been similarly applied to understanding heteroactivators of CYP3A4 and CYP2C9 metabolism [37, 38]; in such cases a molecule can increase the metabolism of another molecule that is metabolized by the same enzyme.

The 3D structure of the membrane-bound P450s were largely unknown until the relatively recent crystallization of the rabbit and human CYP2C forms [39–41] as well as the human CYP3A4 [42, 43]. Up until this time there were many efforts at homology modeling the various P450s using bacterial P450s as template structures [44–54], and once the rabbit CYP2C enzyme became available this was also utilized for modeling other human P450s [30, 55–58]. The merger of pharmacophore and homology modeling has also been frequently used [30, 59, 60] as a means to both validate and improve the models resulting from each method separately. These 3D structures are now obviously potentially useful for modeling of other enzymes involved in drug metabolism.

Small lipophilic molecules can also undergo glucuronidation, which is a further important route for drug clearance [61]. These membrane-bound enzymes have not been crystallized to date. A recent study described the glucuronidation of simple 4-substituted phenols by the human recombinant UGT1A6 and UGT1A9 enzymes [62]. The use of a genetic algorithm and a range of molecular surface and atomic descriptors enabled one of the first attempts to predict the K_m for these enzymes [62]. Analogous to their use in modeling P450s, pharmacophores have also been applied to various human enzymes involved in glucuronidation with a custom metabolism pharmacophore feature [63–65]. In this way it was possible to derive pharmacophore models for UDPGT 1A4 [64], UDPGT 1A1 [65, 66], and others [67]. More recently, other QSAR algorithm methods such as support vector machines have been used with quantum chemical and 2D descriptors for the same enzymes [68]. At present the data sets from which the models were constructed are still relatively limited in terms of structural diversity compared with the P450 models, but this situation is likely to improve as more data are generated. A further class of conjugating enzymes are the sulfotransferases, which have been crystallized [69, 70], and a QSAR method has also been used to predict substrate affinity to SULT1A3 [69].

More recently other types of QSAR methods have been used to generate predictions for metabolic stability. For example, recursive partitioning is a simple but powerful statistical method that can uncover relationships in large complex data sets involving thresholds, interactions, and nonlinearities to classify objects into categories based on similar activities [71]. A recursive partitioning model containing 875 molecules with human liver microsomal metabolic stability was used to predict and rank the clearance of 41 drugs [72]. A *k*-nearest neighbor statistical model finds a subspace of the original descriptor space where activity of each compound in the data set is most accurately predicted as the averaged activity of its *k* nearest neighbors in this subspace. This approach has been used with metabolic stability data from human S9 homogenate for 631 diverse molecules and was able to adequately classify metabolism of a further set of over 100 molecules [73]. Kohonen maps are a multivariate statistical technique that approximates local geometric relationships of a multidimensional property space on a 2D plot [74]. Kohonen maps have also been useful for differentiating high- and low-affinity CYP3A4 substrates [75]. Neural networks are biologically relevant based on ideas from neuroscience; they include "neurons" that are weighted connecting an input layer, one or more hidden layers, and an output layer [76]. Neural networks have been used to predict *N*-dealkylation rates for CYP3A4 and CYP2D6 substrates [77]. This latter work represents a foundation for a software system to predict metabolites and the enzymes involved from an input molecular structure and has also been applied to the differentiation of P450 substrates from nonsubstrates [78, 79]. A recent technique called MetaSite (Molecular

Discovery, Middlesex, UK) generates GRID field descriptors (used for determining energetically favorable binding sites on molecules of known structure) using crystal structures or homology models for the P450 enzymes, as well as the interaction energy descriptors for the molecules evaluated as substrates [80]. A reactivity component is also considered in the MetaSite calculation, which produces a probability for an atom to be metabolized. To date this approach has been applied with AT receptor antagonists to predict the site of metabolism for the P450s CYP2C9 and CYP3A4 [80].

18.3 ELECTRONIC MODELS FOR METABOLISM PREDICTION

Other molecular models accounting for electronic effects of ligands for P450-mediated metabolism have also been produced [21, 81, 82]. These methods depend on the calculation of ground-state energies and in some cases have also combined aliphatic and aromatic oxidation reactions. In this way predictions have been generated for metabolic regioselectivities of enzymes in general [81, 83] or for specific enzymes such as CYP2E1 [84] and CYP3A4 [82]. In the latter case, a partial least-squares method was trained with AM1 calculated hydrogen abstraction energy data to rapidly speed up the prediction of these values for molecules. The combination of electronic methods with steric and orientation terms has also been described to limit overfitting of the training data and improve predictions [85]. An electronic model has been developed for hydrogen abstraction for a series of steroidal androgens [86]. Electronic methods have to date been less widely applied than QSMR methods, and there have been no comparisons of predictions from electronic models and other QSMR. There is certainly some scope for the further development of these technologies as applied to metabolism prediction.

18.4 DATABASES AND RULE-BASED APPROACHES FOR METABOLISM PREDICTION

There have been very limited efforts to organize ADME/Tox data, exceptions being databases such as PharmaGKB [87], the nuclear receptor database [88], the human membrane transporter database [89], and the ADME-AP database [90]. Commercial drug metabolism databases such as Metabolite™, Metabolism™, and BioFrontier/P450™ represent a broad collection of metabolic data [91]. These databases are useful for calculating probabilities for a given metabolic reaction [92], indicating possible metabolites [93] or the sites of metabolism with a statistical approach [94]. Accumulation of drug metabolism data from the literature has also resulted in the creation of expert systems for metabolism prediction for esters, *O*-, *N*-alkyl derivatives, and aromatic fragments [95] and has resulted in commercial rule-based products such as MetabolExpert™ [96], META™ [97–99], and METEOR™ [100, 101]. These expert systems have been reviewed previously [100], and the reasoning behind metabolite prediction for one of these knowledge-based approaches has been described in some detail [101]. One of the main drawbacks of databases and similar expert systems is combination of data or rules from many different mammalian species. Ideally, the data and rules for each species should be separate. The computer programs using this combined information tend to predict all the metabolic possibilities for a molecule even though the metabolic pathways can be very different even in close mammalian species. Metabolism of the same drug may further vary substantially between individuals depending on the expression level of particular enzymes, polymorphisms, and the presence of particular enzymes in normal and disease states as well as different tissues. Analogous metabolism prediction methods include those developed as part of the University of Minnesota biocatalysis/biodegradation database, merging a database of molecules with metabolite prediction rules [102–104] for small organic molecules. A second example is the tissue metabolism simulator (TIMES), which combines a database with probability of occurrence of metabolites to produce a metabolic map that has to date been tested with 179 molecules, with published rat data reproducing 86% of the documented metabolic pathways [105]. To date these latter approaches have not been applied to human metabolism data.

The sheer complexity of predicting metabolites has prompted some to apply graph theory to the metabolism problem. In this case the overall topology of the resulting reactivity maps based on molecular descriptors describing the site of metabolism of molecules undergoing the same metabolic pathway suggests clusters of structurally similar molecules [106]. This approach has also been applied by the same research group to visualize the biological data, source, and analytical method used as well as other types of information. This method has not been commercialized or widely utilized. As a drug-metabolizing enzyme may produce multiple products from a single substrate, predicting the important metabolites is a challenge. A theoretical model has been used to demonstrate that a single enzyme can create a distributed catalysis network in such cases [107]. In this published example, a substrate produces multiple metabolites with a lower concentration than the initial substrate concentration. Under these conditions the toxicity of a given compound is likely to be minimized. The substrate promiscuity of P450s such as CYP3A4 [4], which can metabolize molecules at multiple positions, complicates the ability to reliably make predictions for metabolite formation. The various methods to predict affinity for enzymes may be required in combination to improve accuracy as a consensus approach.

A new tool for computational ADME/Tox called MetaDrug™ includes a manually annotated Oracle™ database of human drug metabolism information including xenobiotic reactions, enzyme substrates, and enzyme inhibitors with kinetic data. The MetaDrug™ database has been used to predict some of the major metabolic pathways and identify the involvement of P450s [78]. This database has enabled the generation of over 80 key metabolic pathways for predicting likely metabolic reactions. In addition, there are over 40 recursive partitioning QSAR models [36, 108, 109] implemented in MetaDrug, enabling the prediction of affinity and rate of metabolism for numerous enzymes as well as prediction of other ADME/Tox properties. The user can also upload their own QSAR or QSMR data into the software. Structural alerts for likely reactive metabolites [110–112] are also integrated in the MetaDrug™ software. Finally, the molecules can also be visualized as temporary objects with connections on a network diagram (see also Chapter 6) with the various proteins to which they are predicted to bind, representing a valuable method for understanding potential drug-drug interactions graphically. To date this method has been used to show the predicted binding interactions for 4-hydroxytamoxifen derived from QSAR models for P-gp and CYP3A4 [113].

Machine learning tools that utilize databases of human metabolism information represent methods for calculating more reliable predictions of metabolites from an input structure alone. For each molecule in the database with metabolism information we could calculate a binary string of metabolites that are seen experimentally and that correspond with our large number of metabolite rules (Fig. 18.1). This molecule-metabolite fingerprint can then be used in a multivariate model alongside 2D molecular path length descriptors (or other descriptors) to generate a machine learning model or multiple models for each metabolic reaction. The combination of these models for all reactions would then be used to predict the likely metabolite profile for a new molecule from the input structure. Using this approach with the Kernal-partial least squares (K-PLS) algorithm devised by Rosipal and Trejo [114] and implemented by Dr. Mark Embrechts (Rensselaer Polytechnic Institute) as a component of the Analyze/Stripminer software [115], we have evaluated several classification models for predicting metabolic reactions using over 300 molecules and their metabolites. Not surprisingly, reaction models that are well populated with literature data (*N*-dealkylation, aromatic and aliphatic hydroxylation, and *O*-glucuronidation) perform well when assessed with the receiver operator curve (Fig. 18.2) in these initial experiments. This preliminary work with phase I and II reactions (Fig. 18.2) indicates that such a classification approach may be even more successful with larger databases than the sample of just over 300 molecules and metabolites selected from MetaDrug.

18.5 APPLICATIONS OF METABOLISM PREDICTION

Computational methods including both metabolism databases and predictive metabolism software can be used to aid bioanalytical groups in suggesting all possible potential metabolite masses before identification by mass spectroscopy (MS) [116, 117]. This approach can also combine specialized MS spectra feature prediction software that will use the outputs from databases and prediction software and make comparisons with the molecular masses observed

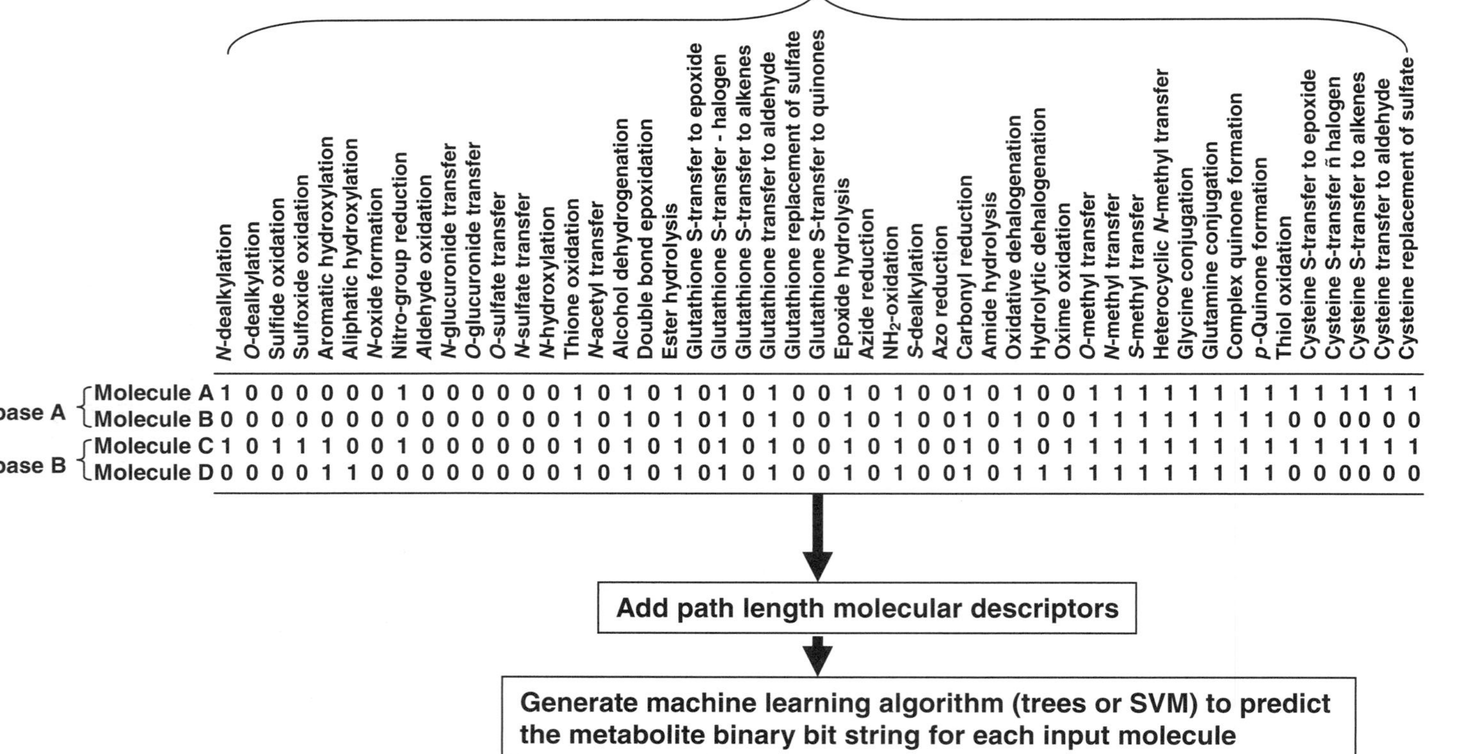

Figure 18.1 Schematic representation for the prediction of the complete metabolic profile of a molecule using databases and a machine learning approach. In this example various metabolite rules are used to illustrate how this method will be implemented. Molecule B could also represent metabolites derived from Molecule A.

(Apex from Sierra Analytics, www.massspec.com). Predicting metabolite fingerprints for libraries of compounds also suggests a role for software in screening large numbers of molecules efficiently [6]. Because of the massive estimated size of synthetically tractable chemistry space, on the order of 10^{20} and 10^{24} molecules [118], it is clear that we have to limit the expectations of QSAR models for metabolism based on small sets of molecules as they are unlikely to be predictive for all available molecules. One method that can be used is a simple Tanimoto similarity score calculated with molecular descriptors both for the molecules in the model training set and for those molecules predicted [119]. In this way molecules with predicted metabolism data that are similar to those in the training set based on the Tanimoto similarity score may be suggested as more reliable than ones that are too dissimilar from the training set. It is also important to update such computational models with new data when available at regular intervals so that they remain relevant over time. This may require constant annotation of literature data or the collation of more proprietary experimental information from a company database. The generation of many more enzyme crystal structures beyond CYP2C9 and CYP3A4 may also aid in understanding the promiscuity of the enzymes, assist in the prediction of metabolites, and direct the improvement of the homology models that have been generated [120]. Many efforts have focused on human metabolism prediction, but there is a considerable amount of metabolism information for mouse and rat that might enable us to better understand differences in metabolism between species. For example, human cytochromes P450 differ from rodent cytochromes P450 in both isoform composition and catalytic activities [121]. Other potential limitations of animal data include sex differences in xenobiotic metabolism, which to date have been most extensively studied in the rat, where they are most pronounced.

The history of methods used for the computational prediction of human drug metabolism includes several different approaches such as databases, QSMR/QSAR, pharmacophores, rule-based approaches, electronic models, homology models, and crystal structures. These techniques have been used individually with different levels of success, although they could ultimately be combined to improve predictions. To date specific P450-substrate/inhibitor recognition interactions have been studied extensively, and several QSAR and pharmacophore models have been built for a limited number of these enzymes. These models have generally shown the importance of hydrophobic, hydrogen bonding, and ionizable features for both substrates based on K_m data and inhibitors based on K_i, IC_{50} and percent inhibition data [22]. Molecular models that account for electronic effects of ligands for P450-mediated metabolism have also been produced [21, 81], and these have combined aliphatic and aromatic oxidation reactions to generate predictions for metabolic regioselectivities. These preceding types of computational technologies represented the current state of the art for ligand-based predictions of binding, inhibition, and metabolism up until the development of newer technologies integrating multiple methods.

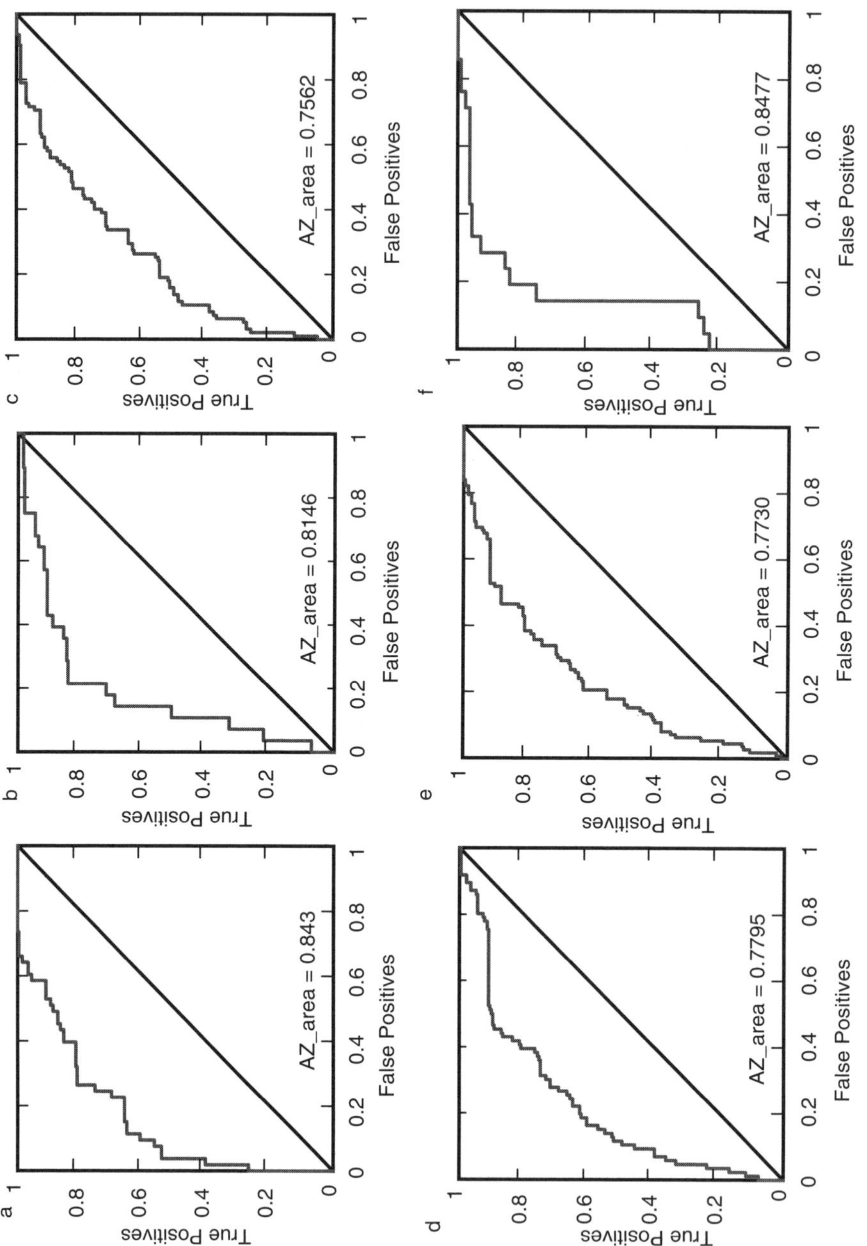
a
b
c
d
e
f
True Positives
False Positives
0
0.2
0.4
0.6
0.8
1
AZ_area = 0.843
AZ_area = 0.8146
AZ_area = 0.7562
AZ_area = 0.7795
AZ_area = 0.7730
AZ_area = 0.8477

Figure 18.2 Representative receiver operator curves to demonstrate the leave *n* out validation of K-PLS classification models (metabolite formed or not formed) derived with approximately 300 molecules and over 60 descriptors. The diagonal line represents random. The horizontal axis represents the percentage of false positives and the vertical axis the percentage of false negatives in each case. a. *N*-dealkylation. b. *O*-dealkylation. c. Aromatic hydroxylation. d. Aliphatic hydroxylation. e. *O*-glucuronidation. f. *O*-sulfation. Data generated in collaboration with Dr. Mark Embrechts (Rensselaer Polytechnic Institute).

Simulation methods have also been developed that include physiologically based pharmacokinetic modeling (PBPK) and methods such as Cloe PK™, QMPRPlus™, GastroPlus™, SimCYP™, and others [122] that are described elsewhere in this book. It is likely that the computational metabolism predictions could be integrated with these to assist in deriving more accurate predictions of human pharmacokinetic parameters.

As the approaches used previously were rather reductionist, it is also important to consider the impact of the global biological complexity of the organism. The field of systems biology is likely to incorporate metabolism information and ADME/Tox data in general as we attempt to reconcile the data available for drug disposition, alongside predictive models to assess metabolism and binding to different proteins by druglike molecules [113]. The networks of interactions between molecules and different enzymes in humans are likely to become more complex as metabolism and drug-drug interaction data continue to be generated. Methods to reliably predict metabolites and their further effects on the complete biological system are certainly needed to aid in the selection of molecules to be synthesized and tested in vivo.

There is an urgent requirement within the pharmaceutical and biotechnology industries, regulatory authorities, and academia to improve the success of molecules selected for clinical trials. Metabolism is just one component contributing to successful drug discovery and development. There is therefore a need for *in silico* methodologies for uncovering the relationships between the structure and metabolic activity of novel molecules. For such computational models to be relevant they should be able to determine the complete xenobiotic biotransformation pathways in the body that define activity, toxicity, and interactions with normal endogenous metabolism. The limitations of virtually all of the computational methods developed thus far are related to the fact that the experimental measurement of metabolism-related parameters is inherently prone to errors. For instance, kinetic constants for the same compound vary substantially between studies, depending on the enzyme source (recombinant P450s, purified enzyme, or human liver microsomes). Additionally in some cases, the reported V_{max} values for the same compound may vary by 2–3 orders of magnitude, which can seriously impact regression-based QSMR or

QSAR modeling. Therefore considerably larger and more consistent data sets for each enzyme will be required in future to increase the predictive scope of such models. The evaluation of any rule-based metabolite software with a diverse array of molecules will indicate that it is possible to generate many more metabolites than have been identified in the literature for the respective molecules to date, which could also reflect the sensitivity of analytical methods at the time of publishing the data. In such cases, efficient machine learning algorithms will be necessary to indicate which of the metabolites are relevant and will be likely to be observed under the given experimental conditions.

18.6 CONCLUSIONS

In conclusion, it is likely that computational approaches for metabolism prediction will continue to be developed and integrated with other algorithms for pharmaceutical research and development, which may in turn ultimately aid in their more widespread use in both industry and academia. Such models may already be having some impact when integrated with bioanalytical approaches to narrow the search for possible metabolites that are experimentally observed. Software that can be updated by the user as new metabolism information becomes available would also be of further potential value. The field of metabolism prediction has therefore advanced rapidly over the past decade, and it will be important to maintain this momentum in the future as the findings from crystal structures for many discrete metabolic enzymes are integrated with the diverse types of computational models already derived.

ACKNOWLEDGMENTS

I gratefully acknowledge the contributions to some of the work described, in particular Dr. Sergey Andreyev (GeneGo, Inc) and Dr. Mark Embrechts (Rensselaer Polytechnic Institute). I appreciate the valuable suggestions in preparing this article from Dr. Maggie A. Z. Hupcey.

REFERENCES

1. Austel V, Kutter E. Absorption, distribution, and metabolism of drugs. In: Topliss, EJ, editor, *Quantitative structure-activity relationships of drugs*. New York: Academic Press, 1983. p. 437–96.
2. Nelson DR. Introductory remarks on human CYPs. *Drug Metab Rev* 2002;34: 1–5.
3. Williams JA, Hyland R, Jones BC, Smith DA, Hurst S, Goosen TC, et al. Drug-drug interactions for UDP-glucuronosyltransferase substrates: a pharmacoki-

netic explanation for typically observed low exposure (auci/auc) ratios. *Drug Metab Dispos* 2004;32:1201–8.

4. Ekins S. Predicting undesirable drug interactions with promiscuous proteins *in silico. Drug Discov Today* 2004;9:276–85.
5. Lewis DFV. *Cytochromes P450.* Bristol, UK: Taylor & Francis, 1996.
6. Kesuru GM, Molnar L. METAPRINT: a metabolic fingerprint. Application to cassette design for high-throughput ADME screening. *J Chem Inf Comput Sci* 2002;42:437–44.
7. Hansch C, Deutsch EW, Smith RN. The use of substituent constants and regression analysis in the study of enzymatic reaction mechanisms. *J Am Chem Soc* 1965;87:2738–42.
8. Hansch C, Steward AR, Iwasa J. The use of substituent constants in the correlation of demethylation rates. *J Med Chem* 1965;8:868–70.
9. Hansch C. Quantitative relationships between lipophilic character and drug metabolism. *Drug Metab Rev* 1972;1:1–14.
10. Hansch C. The QSAR paradigm in the design of less toxic molecules. *Drug Metab Rev* 1984;15:1279–94.
11. Hansch C, Lien EJ, Helmer F. Structure-activity correlations in the metabolism of drugs. *Arch Biochem Biophys* 1968;128:319–30.
12. Hansch C, Zhang L. Quantitative structure-activity relationships of cytochrome P-450. *Drug Metab Rev* 1993;25:1–48.
13. Lewis DFV. Quantitative structure activity relationships in substrates, inducers, and inhibitors of cytochrome P4501 (CYP1). *Drug Metab Rev* 1997;29:589–650.
14. Lewis DFV. On the recognition of mammalian microsomal cytochrome P450 substrates and their characteristics. *Biochem Pharmacol* 2000;60:293–306.
15. Lewis DFV. Structural characteristics of human P450s involved in drug metabolism: QSARs and lipophilicity profiles. *Toxicology* 2000;144:197–203.
16. Lewis DFV, Eddershaw PJ, Dickins M, Tarbit MH, Goldfarb PS. Structural determinants of cytochrome P450 substrate specificity, binding affinity and catalytic rate. *Chem Bio Interact* 1998;115:175–99.
17. Lewis DFV, Eddershaw PJ, Dickins M, Tarbit MH, Goldfarb PS. Erratum to "Structural determinants of cytochrome P450 substrate specificity, binding affinity and catalytic rate". *Chem Biol Interact* 1999;117:187.
18. Lewis DF, Jacobs MN, Dickins M. Compound lipophilicity for substrate binding to human P450s in drug metabolism. *Drug Discov Today* 2004;9:530–7.
19. Ekins S, Swaan PW. Computational models for enzymes, transporters, channels and receptors relevant to ADME/TOX. *Rev Comp Chem* 2004;20:333–415.
20. Fuhr U, Strobl G, Manaut F, Anders E-M, Sorgel F, Lopez-de-brinas E, et al. Quinolone antibacterial agents: relationship between structure and in vitro inhibition of human cytochrome P450 isoform CYP1A2. *Mol Pharmacol* 1993;43:191–9.
21. Jones JP, Korzekwa KR. *Predicting the rates and regioselectivity of reactions mediated by the P450 superfamily.* New York: Academic Press. 1996.
22. Ekins S, de Groot M, Jones JP. Pharmacophore and three dimensional quantitative structure activity relationship methods for modeling cytochrome P450 active sites. *Drug Metab Dispos* 2001;29:936–44.

23. Ekins S, VandenBranden M, Ring BJ, Wrighton SA. Examination of purported probes of human CYP2B6. *Pharmacogenetics* 1997;7:165–79.
24. Ekins S, VandenBranden M, Ring BJ, Gillespie JS, Yang TJ, Gelboin HV, et al. Further characterization of the expression and catalytic activity of human CYP2B6. *J Pharmacol Exp Ther* 1998;286:1253–9.
25. Ekins S, Bravi G, Ring BJ, Gillespie TA, Gillespie JS, VandenBranden M, et al. Three dimensional-quantitative structure activity relationship (3D-QSAR) analyses of substrates for CYP2B6. *J Pharmacol Exp Ther* 1999;288:21–9.
26. Ekins S, Bravi G, Wikel JH, Wrighton SA. Three dimensional quantitative structure activity relationship (3D-QSAR) analysis of CYP3A4 substrates. *J Pharmacol Exp Ther* 1999;291:424–33.
27. Ekins S, Bravi G, Binkley S, Gillespie JS, Ring BJ, Wikel JH, et al. Three and four dimensional-quantitative structure activity relationship (3D/4D-QSAR) analyses of CYP2D6 inhibitors. *Pharmacogenetics* 1999;9:477–89.
28. Ekins S, Bravi G, Binkley S, Gillespie JS, Ring BJ, Wikel JH, et al. Three and four dimensional-quantitative structure activity relationship analyses of CYP3A4 inhibitors. *J Pharmacol Exp Ther* 1999;290:429–38.
29. Ekins S, Bravi G, Binkley S, Gillespie JS, Ring BJ, Wikel JH, et al. Three and four dimensional-quantitative structure activity relationship (3D/4D-QSAR) analyses of CYP2C9 inhibitors. *Drug Metab Dispos* 2000;28:994–1002.
30. Snyder R, Sangar R, Wang J, Ekins S. Three dimensional quantitative structure activity relationship for CYP2D6 substrates. *Quant Struct Act Relationship* 2002;21:357–68.
31. Ekins S, Stresser DM, Williams JA. In vitro and pharmacophore insights into CYP3A enzymes. *Trends Pharmacol Sci* 2003;24:191–6.
32. Ekins S, Wrighton SA. Application of *in silico* approaches to predicting drug-drug interactions: a commentary. *J Pharm Tox Methods* 2001;44:1–5.
33. Asikainen A, Tarhanen J, Poso A, Pasanen M, Alhava E, Juvonen RO. Predictive value of comparative molecular field analysis modelling of naphthalene inhibition of human CYP2A6 and mouse CYP2A5 enzymes. *Toxicol In Vitro* 2003;17:449–55.
34. Wrighton SA, Schuetz EG, Thummel KE, Shen DD, Korzekwa KR, Watkins PB. The human CYP3A subfamily: practical considerations. *Drug Metab Rev* 2000;32:339–61.
35. Ekins S, Wrighton SA. The role of CYP2B6 in human xenobiotic metabolism. *Drug Metab Rev* 1999;31:719–54.
36. Ekins S, Berbaum J, Harrison RK. Generation and validation of rapid computational filters for CYP2D6 and CYP3A4. *Drug Metab Dispos* 2003;31:1077–80.
37. Egnell AC, Houston JB, Boyer CS. Predictive models of CYP3A4 heteroactivation: in vitro—in vivo scaling and pharmacophore modelling. *J Pharmacol Exp Ther* 2005;312:926–37.
38. Egnell AC, Eriksson C, Albertson N, Houston B, Boyer S. Generation and evaluation of a CYP2C9 heteroactivation pharmacophore. *J Pharmacol Exp Ther* 2003;307:878–87.
39. Cosme J, Johnson EF. Engineering microsomal cytochrome P450 2C5 to be a soluble, monomeric enzyme. Mutations that alter aggregation, phospholipid dependence of catalysis, and membrane binding. *J Biol Chem* 2000;275:2545–53.

40. Williams PA, Cosme J, Ward A, Angove HC, Matak Vinkovic D, Jhoti H. Crystal structure of human cytochrome P450 2C9 with bound warfarin. *Nature* 2003;424:464–8.
41. Williams PA, Cosme J, Sridhar V, Johnson EF, McRee DE. Mammalian microsomal cytochrome P450 monooxygenase: structural adaptations for membrane binding and functional diversity. *Mol Cell* 2000;5:121–31.
42. Williams PA, Cosme J, Vinkovic DM, Ward A, Angove HC, Day PJ, et al. Crystal structures of human cytochrome P450 3A4 bound to metyrapone and progesterone. *Science* 2004;305:683–6.
43. Yano JK, Wester MR, Schoch GA, Griffin KJ, Stout CD, Johnson EF. The structure of human microsomal cytochrome P450 3A4 determined by X-ray crystallography to 2.05-Å resolution. *J Biol Chem* 2004;279:38091–4.
44. Koymans LMH, Vermeulen NPE, Baarslag A, Donne-Op den Kelder GM. A preliminary 3D model for cytochrome P450 2D6 constructed by homology model building. *J Comput-Aided Mol Des* 1993;7:281–9.
45. Modi S, Paine MJ, Sutcliffe MJ, Lian L-Y, Primrose WU, Wolf CR, et al. A model for human cytochrome P4502D6 based on homology modeling and NMR studies of substrate binding. *Biochemistry* 1996;35:4540–50.
46. Lewis DFV, Lake BG, Dickins M, Eddershaw PJ, Tarbit MH, Goldfarb PS. Molecular modelling of CYP2B6, the human CYP2B isoform, by homology with the substrate-bound CYP102 crystal structure: evaluation of CYP2B6 substrate characteristics, the cytochrome b5 binding site and comparisons with CYP2B1 and CYP2B4. *Xenobiotica* 1999;29:361–93.
47. Szklarz GD, Halpert JR. Use of homology modeling in conjunction with site-directed mutagenesis for analysis of structure-function relationships of mammalian cytochromes P450. *Life Sci* 1997;61:2507–20.
48. Szklarz GD, Halpert JR. Molecular modeling of cytochrome P4503A4. *J Comput-Aided Mol Des* 1997;11:265–72.
49. Szklarz GD, Graham SE, Paulsen MD. Molecular modeling of mammalian cytochromes P450: application to study enzyme function. *Vitamins Hormones* 2000;58:53–87.
50. Lewis DFV, Eddershaw PJ, Goldfarb PS, Tarbit MH. Molecular modelling of cytochrome P4502D6 (CYP2D6) based on an alignment with CYP102: structural studies on specific CYP2D6 substrate metabolism. *Xenobiotica* 1997;27:319–40.
51. Lewis DFV, Eddershaw PJ, Goldfarb PS, Tarbit MH. Molecular modelling of CYP3A4 from an alignment with CYP102: identification of key interactions between putative active site residues and CYP3A- specific chemicals. *Xenobiotica* 1996;10:1067–86.
52. Lewis DFV, Dickins M, Weaver RJ, Eddershaw PJ, Goldfarb PS, Tarbit MH. Molecular modelling of human CYP2C subfamily enzymes CYP2C9 and CYP2C19: rationalization of substrate specificity and site-directed mutagenesis experiments in the CYP2C subfamily. *Xenobiotica* 1998;28:235–68.
53. Lewis DFV. Three-dimensional models of human and other mammalian microsomal P450s constructed from an alignment with P450102 (P450bm3). *Xenobiotica* 1995;25:333–66.
54. Wiseman H, Lewis DFV. The metabolism of tamoxifen by human cytochromes P450 is rationalized by molecular modelling of the enzyme substrate interac-

tions: potential importance to its proposed anti-carcinogenic/carcinogenic actions. *Carcinogenesis* 1996;17:1357–60.

55. Afzelius L, Zamora I, Ridderstrom M, Andersson TB, Karlen A, Masimirembwa CM. Competitive CYP2C9 inhibitors: enzyme inhibition studies, protein homology modeling, and three dimensional quantitative structure activity relationship analysis. *Mol Pharmacol* 2001;59:909–19.
56. Barhelt C, Schmid RD, Pleiss J. Regioselectivity of CYP2B6: homology modeling, molecular dynamics simulation, docking. *J Mol Model* 2002;8:327–35.
57. Wang Q, Halpert JR. Combined three-dimensional quantitative structure-activity relationship analysis of cytochrome P450 2B6 substrates and protein homology modeling. *Drug Metab Dispos* 2002;30:86–95.
58. de Groot MJ, Alex AA, Jones BC. Development of a combined protein and pharmacophore model for cytochrome P450 2C9. *J Med Chem* 2002;45:1983–93.
59. de Groot MJ, Ackland MJ, Horne VA, Alex AA, Jones BC. Novel approach to predicting P450-mediated drug metabolism: development of a combined protein and pharmacophore model for CYP2D6. *J Med Chem* 1999;42:1515–24.
60. de Groot MJ, Ackland MJ, Horne VA, Alex AA, Jones BC. A novel approach to predicting P450 mediated drug metabolism. CYP2D6 catalyzed *N*-dealkylation reactions and qualitative metabolite predictions using a combined protein and pharmacophore model for CYP2D6. *J Med Chem* 1999;42:4062–70.
61. Tukey RH, Strassburg CP. Human UDP-glucuronosyltransferases: metabolism, expression, and disease. *Annu Rev Pharmacol Toxicol* 2000;40:581–616.
62. Ethell BT, Ekins S, Wang J, Burchell B. Quantitative structure activity relationships for the glucuronidation of simple phenols by expressed human UGT1A6 and UGT1A9. *Drug Metab Dispos* 2002;30:734–8.
63. Smith PA, Sorich M, McKinnon R, Miners JO. QSAR and pharmacophore modelling approaches for the prediction of UDP-glucuronosyltransferase substrate selectivity and binding. *Pharmacologist* 2002;44 supplement.
64. Smith PA, Sorich MJ, McKinnon RA, Miners JO. Pharmacophore and quantitative structure-activity relationship modeling: complementary approaches for the rationalization and prediction of UDP-glucuronosyltransferase 1A4 substrate selectivity. *J Med Chem* 2003;46:1617–26.
65. Sorich M, Smith PA, McKinnon RA, Miners JO. Pharmacophore and quantitative structure activity relationship modelling of UDP-glucuronosyltransferase 1A1 (UGT1A1) substrates. *Pharmacogenetics* 2002;12:635–45.
66. Smith PA, Sorich MJ, McKinnon RA, Miners JO. *In silico* insights: chemical and structural characteristics associated with uridine diphosphate-glucuronosyltransferase substrate selectivity. *Clin Exp Pharmacol Physiol* 2003;30:836–40.
67. Sorich MJ, Miners JO, McKinnon RA, Smith PA. Multiple pharmacophores for the investigation of human UDP-glucuronosyltransferase isoform substrate selectivity. *Mol Pharmacol* 2004;65:301–8.
68. Sorich MJ, McKinnon RA, Miners JO, Winkler DA, Smith PA. Rapid prediction of chemical metabolism by human UDP-glucuronosyltransferase isoforms using quantum chemical descriptors derived with the electronegativity equalization method. *J Med Chem* 2004;47:5311–7.

69. Dajani R, Cleasby A, Neu M, Wonacott AJ, Jhoti H, Hood AM, et al. X-ray crystal structure of human dopamine sulfotransferase, SULT1A3. *J Biol Chem* 1999;53:37862–8.
70. Gamage NU, Duggleby RG, Barnett AC, Tresillian M, Latham CF, Liyou NE, et al. Structure of a human carcinogen-converting enzyme, SULT1A1. *J Biol Chem* 2003;278:7655–62.
71. Rusinko A, 3rd, Farmen MW, Lambert CG, Brown PL, Young SS. Analysis of a large structure/biological activity data set using recursive partitioning. *J Chem Inf Comput Sci* 1999;39:1017–26.
72. Ekins S. *In silico* approaches to predicting metabolism, toxicology and beyond. *Biochem Soc Trans* 2003;31:611–4.
73. Shen M, Xiao Y, Golbraikh A, Gombar VK, Tropsha A. Development and validation of k-nearest neighbour QSPR models of metabolic stability of drug candidates. *J Med Chem* 2003;46:3013–20.
74. Kohonen T. *Self-organisation and associative memory*. Berlin: Springer-Verlag, 1989.
75. Balakin KV, Ekins S, Bugrim A, Ivanenkov YA, Korolev D, Nikolsky Y, et al. Kohonen maps for prediction of binding to human cytochrome P450 3A4. *Drug Metab Dispos* 2004;32:1183–9.
76. Mitchell M. *An introduction to genetic algorithms*. Cambridge, MA: MIT Press, 1996.
77. Balakin KV, Ekins S, Bugrim A, Ivanenkov YA, Korolev D, Nikolsky Y, et al. Quantitative structure-metabolism relationship modeling of the metabolic *N*-dealkylation rates. *Drug Metab Dispos* 2004;32:1111–20.
78. Korolev D, Balakin KV, Nikolsky Y, Kirillov E, Ivanenkov YA, Savchuk NP, et al. Modeling of human cytochrome P450-mediated drug metabolism using unsupervised machine learning approach. *J Med Chem* 2003;46:3631–43.
79. Bugrim A, Nikolskaya T, Nikolsky Y. Early prediction of drug metabolism and toxicity: systems biology approach and modeling. *Drug Discov Today* 2004;9:127–35.
80. Berellini G, Cruciani G, Mannhold R. Pharmacophore, drug metabolism, and pharmacokinetics models on non-peptide AT_1, AT_2, and AT_1/AT_2 angiotensin II receptor antagonists. *J Med Chem* 2005;48:4389–99.
81. Jones JP, Mysinger M, Korzekwa KR. Computational models for cytochrome P450: a predictive electronic model for aromatic oxidation and hydrogen abstraction. *Drug Metab Dispos* 2002;30:7–12.
82. Singh SB, Shen LQ, Walker MJ, Sheridan RP. A model for likely sites of CYP3A4-mediated metabolism on drug-like molecules. *J Med Chem* 2003;46:1330–6.
83. Csanady GA, Laib JG. Metabolic transformation of halogenated and other alkenes- a theoretical approach. Estimation of metabolic reactivities for in vivo conditions. *Toxicology* 1995;75:217–23.
84. Yin H, Anders MW, Korzekwa KR, Higgins L, Thummel KE, Kharasch ED, et al. Designing safer chemicals: predicting the rates of metabolism of halogenated alkanes. *Proc Natl Acad Sci USA* 1995;92:11076–80.
85. Korzekwa K, Ewing TJ, Kocher JP, Carlson TJ. Models for cytochrome P450-mediated metabolism. In: Borchardt RT, Kerns EH, Lipinski CA, Thakker DR,

Wang B, editors, *Pharmaceutical profiling in drug discovery for lead selection*. Arlington, VA: AAPS Press, 2004. p. 69–80.

86. Bursi R, de Gooyer ME, Grootenhuis A, Jacobs PL, van der Louw J, Leysen D. (Q)SAR study on the metabolic stability of steroidal androgens. *J Mol Graph Modelling* 2001;19:552–6.
87. Kliewer SA, Moore JT, Wade L, Staudinger JL, Watson MA, Jones SA, et al. An orphan nuclear receptor activated by pregnanes defines a novel steroid signalling pathway. *Cell* 1998;92:73–82.
88. Nakata K, Yukawa M, Komiyama N, Nakano T, Kaminuma T. A nuclear receptor database that maps pathways to diseases. *Genome Infomatics* 2002;13:515–6.
89. Schapira M, Raaka BM, Samuels HH, Abagyan R. Rational discovery of novel nuclear hormone receptor antagonists. *Proc Natl Acad Sci USA* 2000;97:1008–13.
90. Sun LZ, Ji ZL, Chen X, Wang JF, Chen YZ. ADME-AP: a database of ADME associated proteins. *Bioinformatics* 2002;18:1699–700.
91. Erhardt PW. A human drug metabolism database: potential roles in the quantitative predictions of drug metabolism and metabolism-related drug-drug interactions. *Curr Drug Metab* 2003;4:411–22.
92. Boyer S, Zamora I. New methods in predictive metabolism. *J Comput-Aided Mol Des* 2002;16:403–13.
93. Borodina Y, Sadym A, Filimonov D, Blinova V, Dmitriev A, Poroikov V. Predicting biotransformation potential from molecular structure. *J Chem Inf Comput Sci* 2003;43:1636–46.
94. Borodina Y, Rudik A, Filimonov D, Kharchevnikova N, Dmitriev A, Blinova V, et al. A new statistical approach to predicting aromatic hydroxylation sites. Comparison with model-based approaches. *J Chem Inf Comput Sci* 2004; 44:1998–2009.
95. Smith RV, Erhardt PW, Leslie SW. Microsomal *O*-demethylation, *N*-demethylation and aromatic hydroxylation in the presence of bisulfite and dithiothreitol. *Res Commun Chem Path Pharmacol* 1975;12:181–4.
96. Darvas F, Dorman G, Papp A. Diversity measures for enhancing ADME admissibility of combinatorial libraries. *J Chem Inf Comput Sci* 2000;40:314–22.
97. Klopman G, Dimayuga M, Talafous J. META. 1. A program for the evaluation of metabolic transformations of chemicals. *J Chem Inf Comput Sci* 1994;34: 1320–5.
98. Talafous J, Sayre LM, Mieyal JJ, Klopman G. META. 2. A dictionary model of mammalian xenobiotic metabolism. *J Chem Inf Comput Sci* 1994;34:1326–33.
99. Klopman G, Tu M, Talafous J. META. 3. A genetic algorithm for metabolic transform priorities optimization. *J Chem Inf Comput Sci* 1997;37:329–34.
100. Langowski J, Long A. Computer systems for the prediction of xenobiotic metabolism. *Adv Drug Del Rev* 2002;54:407–15.
101. Button WG, Judson PN, Long A, Vessey JD. Using absolute and relative reasoning in the prediction of the potential metabolism of xenobiotics. *J Chem Inf Comput Sci* 2003;43:1371–7.
102. Hou BK, Ellis LB, Wackett LP. Encoding microbial metabolic logic: predicting biodegradation. *J Ind Microbiol Biotechnol* 2004;31:261–72.

103. Hou BK, Wackett LP, Ellis LB. Microbial pathway prediction: a functional group approach. *J Chem Inf Comput Sci* 2003;43:1051–7.
104. Ellis LB, Hou BK, Kang W, Wackett LP. The University of Minnesota Biocatalysis/Biodegradation Database: post-genomic data mining. *Nucleic Acids Res* 2003;31:262–5.
105. Mekenyan OG, Dimitrov SD, Pavlov TS, Veith GD. A systematic approach to simulating metabolism in computational toxicology. I. The TIMES heuristic modelling framework. *Curr Pharm Des* 2004;10:1273–93.
106. Gifford EM, Johnson MA, Smith DA, Tsai CC. Structure-reactivity maps as a tool for visualizing xenobiotic structure reactivity relationships. http://wwwnetsciorg/Science/Special/feature04html 1996.
107. Cook DL, Atkins WM. Enhanced detoxication due to distributive catalysis and toxic thresholds: a kinetic analysis. *Biochemistry* 1997;36:10802–6.
108. Young SS, Ekins S, Lambert C. So many targets, so many compounds, but so few resources. *Curr Drug Discov* 2002;December:17–22.
109. Young SS, Gombar VK, Emptage MR, Cariello NF, Lambert C. Mixture deconvolution and analysis of Ames mutagenicity data. *Chemo Intell Lab Sys* 2002;60:5–11.
110. Li AP. A review of the common properties of drugs with idiosyncratic hepatotoxicity and the "multiple determinant hypothesis" for the manifestation of idiosyncratic drug toxicity. *Chem Biol Interact* 2002;142:7–23.
111. Williams DP, Park BK. Idiosyncratic toxicity: the role of toxicophores and bioactivation. *Drug Discov Today* 2003;8:1044–50.
112. Uetrecht J. Screening for the potential of a drug candidate to cause idiosyncratic drug reactions. *Drug Discov Today* 2003;8:832–7.
113. Ekins S, Nikolsky Y, Nikolskaya T. Techniques: Application of systems biology to absorption, distribution, metabolism, excretion, and toxicity. *Trends Pharmacol Sci* 2005;26:202–9.
114. Rosipal R, Trejo LJ. Kernel partial least squares regression in reproducing Kernel Hilbert space. *J Machine Learning Res* 2001;2:97–123.
115. Bennett KP, Embrechts MJ. An optimization perspective on kernel partial least squares regression. In: Suykens JAK, Horvath G, Basu S, Micchelli J, Vandewalle J, editors, *Advances in learning theory; methods, models and applications*. Amsterdam: IOS Press, 2003. p. 227–50.
116. Anari MR, Baillie TA. Bridging cheminformatic metabolite prediction and tandem mass spectrometry. *Drug Discov Today* 2005;10:711–7.
117. Anari MR, Sanchez RI, Bakhtiar R, Franklin RB, Baillie TA. Integration of knowledge-based metabolic predictions with liquid chromatography data-dependent tandem mass spectrometry for drug metabolism studies: application to studies on the biotransformation of indinavir. *Anal Chem* 2004;76:823–32.
118. Ertl P, Rohde B, Selzer P. Fast calculation of molecular polar surface area as a sum of fragment-based contributions and its application to the prediction of drug transport properties. *J Med Chem* 2000;43:3714–7.
119. Willet P. Similarity-based approaches to virtual screening. *Biochem Soc Trans* 2003;31:603–6.

120. Kirton SB, Baxter CA, Sutcliffe MJ. Comparative modelling of the cytochromes P450. *Adv Drug Del Rev* 2002;54:385–406.
121. Nedelcheva V, Gut I. P450 in the rat and man: methods of investigation, substrate specificities and relevance to cancer. *Xenobiotica* 1994;24:1151–75.
122. Leahy D. Drug Discovery information integration: virtual humans for pharmacokinetics. DDT: *Biosilico* 2004;2:78–84.
123. Kim YM, Ziegler DM. Size limits of thiocarbamides accepted as substrates by human flavin-containing monooxygenase 1. *Drug Metab Dispos* 2000;28:1003–6.
124. Soffers AEMF, Ploeman JHTM, Moonen MJH, Wobbes T, van Ommen B, Vervoort J, et al. Regioselectivity and quantitative structure-activity relationships for the conjugation of a series of fluoronitrobenzenes by purified glutathione *S*-transferase enzymes from rat and man. *Chem Res Toxicol* 1996;9:638–46.
125. Medvedev AE, Veselovsky AV, Shvedov VI, Tikhonova OV, Moskvitina TA, Fedotova OA, et al. Inhibition of monoamine oxidase by pirlindole analogues: 3D-QSAR and CoMFA analysis. *J Chem Inf Comput Sci* 1998;38:1137–44.
126. Miller JR, Edmondson DE. Structure-activity relationships in the oxidation of *para*-substituted benzylamine analogues by recombinant human liver monoamine oxidase A. *Biochemistry* 1999;38:13670–83.
127. Ekins S, Waller CL, Swaan PW, Cruciani G, Wrighton SA, Wikel JH. Progress in predicting human ADME parameters *in silico*. *J Pharmacol Toxicol Methods* 2000;44:251–72.
128. Reck F, Zhou F, Girardot M, Kern G, Eyermann CJ, Hales NJ, et al. Identification of 4-substituted 1,2,3-triazoles as novel oxazolidinone antibacterial agents with reduced activity against monoamine oxidase A. *J Med Chem* 2005;48:499–506.
129. Edmondson DE, Mattevi A, Binda C, Li M, Hubalek F. Structure and mechanism of monoamine oxidase. *Curr Med Chem* 2004;11:1983–93.
130. Binda C, Hubalek F, Li M, Edmondson DE, Mattevi A. Crystal structure of human monoamine oxidase B, a drug target enzyme monotopically inserted into the mitochondrial outer membrane. *FEBS Lett* 2004;564:225–8.
131. Binda C, Hubalek F, Li M, Herzig Y, Sterling J, Edmondson DE, et al. Crystal structures of monoamine oxidase B in complex with four inhibitors of the *N*-propargylaminoindan class. *J Med Chem* 2004;47:1767–74.
132. Binda C, Li M, Hubalek F, Restelli N, Edmondson DE, Mattevi A. Insights into the mode of inhibition of human mitochondrial monoamine oxidase B from high-resolution crystal structures. *Proc Natl Acad Sci USA* 2003;100:9750–5.
133. Cavalli A, Greco G, Novellino E, Recanatini M. Linking CoMFA and protein homology models of enzyme-inhibitor interactions: an application to nonsteroidal aromatase inhibitors. *Bioorg Med Chem* 2000;8:2771–80.
134. Sonnet P, Dallemagne P, Guillon J, Enguehard C, Stiebing S, Tanguy J, et al. New aromatase inhibitors, synthesis and biological activity of aryl-substituted pyrrolizine and indolizine derivatives. *Bioorganic Med Chem* 2000;8:945–55.
135. Laughton CA, Zvelebil MJ, Neidle S. A detailed molecular model for human aromatase. *J Steroid Biochem Mol Biol* 1993;44:399–407.

136. Lewis DF, Lee-Robichaud P. Molecular modelling of steroidogenic cytochromes P450 from families CYP11, CYP17, CYP19 and CYP21 based on the CYP102 crystal structure. *J Steroid Biochem Mol Biol* 1998;66:217–33.

137. Vanden Bossche H, Koymans L, Moereels H. P450 inhibitors of use in medical treatment: focus on mechanisms of action. *Pharmacol Ther* 1995;67:79–100.

138. Buchwald P. Structure-metabolism relationships: steric effects and the enzymatic hydrolysis of carboxylic esters. *Mini Rev Med Chem* 2001;1:101–11.

139. McElroy NR, Jurs PC, Morisseau C, Hammock BD. QSAR and classification of murine and human epoxide hydrolase inhibition by urea-like compounds. *J Med Chem* 2003;46:1066–80.

140. Kim EJ, Kim KS, Shin WH. Electrophysiological safety of DW-286a, a novel fluoroquinolone antibiotic agent. *Hum Exp Toxicol* 2005;24:19–25.

141. Lewis DF, Lake BG, Bird MG. Molecular modelling of human microsomal epoxide hydrolase (EH) by homology with a fungal (*Aspergillus niger*) EH crystal structure of 1.8 Å resolution: structure-activity relationships in epoxides inhibiting EH activity. *Toxicol In Vitro* 2005;19:517–22.

142. Gomez GA, Morisseau C, Hammock BD, Christianson DW. Structure of human epoxide hydrolase reveals mechanistic inferences on bifunctional catalysis in epoxide and phosphate ester hydrolysis. *Biochemistry* 2004;43:4716–23.

143. Sipila J, Hood AM, Coughtrie MW, Taskinen J. CoMFA modeling of enzyme kinetics: K_m values for sulfation of diverse phenolic substrates by human catecholamine sulfotransferase SULT1A3. *J Chem Inf Comput Sci* 2003;43: 1563–9.

144. Lee KA, Fuda H, Lee YC, Negishi M, Strott CA, Pedersen LC. Crystal structure of human cholesterol sulfotransferase (SULT2B1b) in the presence of pregnenolone and 3′-phosphoadenosine 5′-phosphate. Rationale for specificity differences between prototypical SULT2A1 and the SULT2BG1 isoforms. *J Biol Chem* 2003;278:44593–9.

145. Rehse PH, Zhou M, Lin SX. Crystal structure of human dehydroepiandrosterone sulphotransferase in complex with substrate. *Biochem J* 2002;364: 165–71.

146. King RS, Sharma V, Pedersen LC, Kakuta Y, Negishi M, Duffel MW. Structure-function modeling of the interactions of the *N*-alkyl-*N*-hydroxyanilines with rat hepatic aryl sulfotransferase IV. *Chem Res Toxicol* 2000;13:1251–8.

147. Bidwell LM, McManus ME, Gaedigk A, Kakuta Y, Negishi M, Pedersen L, et al. Crystal structure of human catecholamine sulfotransferase. *J Mol Biol* 1999;293:521–30.

148. Gu Y, Guo J, Pal A, Pan SS, Zimniak P, Singh SV, et al. Crystal structure of human glutathione *S*-transferase A3-3 and mechanistic implications for its high steroid isomerase activity. *Biochemistry* 2004;43:15673–9.

149. Le Trong I, Stenkamp RE, Ibarra C, Atkins WM, Adman ET. 1.3-Å resolution structure of human glutathione *S*-transferase with *S*-hexyl glutathione bound reveals possible extended ligandin binding site. *Proteins* 2002;48:618–27.

150. Oakley AJ, Lo Bello M, Battistoni A, Ricci G, Rossjohn J, Villar HO, et al. The structures of human glutathione transferase P1-1 in complex with glutathione and various inhibitors at high resolution. *J Mol Biol* 1997;274:84–100.

151. Oakley AJ, Lo Bello M, Mazzetti AP, Federici G, Parker MW. The glutathione conjugate of ethacrynic acid can bind to human pi class glutathione transferase P1-1 in two different modes. *FEBS Lett* 1997;419:32–6.

152. Ji X, Tordova M, O'Donnell R, Parsons JF, Hayden JB, Gilliland GL, et al. Structure and function of the xenobiotic substrate-binding site and location of a potential non-substrate-binding site in a class pi glutathione *S*-transferase. *Biochemistry* 1997;36:9690–702.

19

COMPUTERS IN TOXICOLOGY AND RISK ASSESSMENT

JOHN C. DEARDEN

Contents

Computer Applications in Pharmaceutical Research and Development, Edited by Sean Ekins.
ISBN 0-471-73779-8

19.1 INTRODUCTION

The design and development of a new drug entity is a lengthy and costly process; failure can occur for a number of reasons, such as poor pharmacokinetics, lack of efficacy, and toxicity [1], that is, absorption, distribution, metabolism, excretion and toxicology (ADME/Tox) properties. Such failures are disastrous and expensive when they occur late in the development process, and worst of all when they occur during clinical trials or after the drug is put on the market. Kennedy [1] reported in 1997 that 16% of new drug entities failed in animal toxicity testing, and 14% failed because of adverse effects in humans. However, Ekins et al. [2] have commented that the majority of adverse effects are related to measurable ADME/Tox properties that could be predicted in vitro or *in silico*. Hence it should be possible, given the right tools, to design out such adverse effects early in the design/development process and even, with *in silico* tools, before synthesis, although Tute [3] pointed out that because a drug structure has to be optimized for many facets of its action (e.g., solubility, stability, metabolism, transport, receptor binding), a single universal *in silico* prediction covering all of these aspects is not possible. But computer hardware and software have improved immensely in the past decade, and although in 2002 Ekins et al. [2] also pointed out that because a change in molecular structure affects every property of a compound one cannot design out one adverse effect unilaterally, they nevertheless suggested, as a feasible proposition, the development of new computational tools for more rapid and successful drug discovery. This chapter examines the development of *in silico* tools to model and predict one adverse effect, namely, toxicity.

19.1.1 History of Toxicity Prediction

In 1868 two Scottish scientists, Crum Brown and Fraser [4] recognized that "a relation exists between the physiological action of a substance and its chemical composition and constitution." That recognition was in effect the birth of the science that has come to be known as quantitative structure-activity relationship (QSAR) studies; a QSAR is a mathematical equation that relates a biological or other property to structural and/or physicochemical properties of a series of (usually) related compounds. Shortly afterwards, Richardson [5] showed that the narcotic effect of primary aliphatic alcohols varied with their molecular weight, and in 1893 Richet [6] observed that the toxicities of a variety of simple polar chemicals such as alcohols, ethers, and ketones were inversely correlated with their aqueous solubilities. Probably the best known of the very early work in the field was that of Overton [7] and Meyer [8], who found that the narcotic effect of simple chemicals increased with their oil-water partition coefficient and postulated that this reflected the partitioning of a chemical between the aqueous exobiophase and a lipophilic receptor. This, as it turned out, was most prescient, for about 70% of published QSARs contain a term relating to partition coefficient [9].

Despite the work of Overton and Meyer, it was to be many years before structure-activity relationships were explored further. In 1939 Ferguson [10] postulated that the toxic dose of a chemical is a constant fraction of its aqueous solubility; hence toxicity should increase as aqueous solubility decreases. Because aqueous solubility and oil-water partition coefficient are inversely related, it follows that toxicity should increase with partition coefficient. Although this has been found to be true up to a point, it does not continue ad infinitum. Toxicity (and indeed, any biological response) generally increases initially with partition coefficient, but then tends to fall again. This can be explained simply as a reluctance of very hydrophobic chemicals to leave a lipid phase and enter the next aqueous biophase [11]. An example of this is shown by a QSAR that models toxicity of barbiturates to the mouse [12]:

$$\log 1/LD_{50} = 1.02 \log P - 0.27(\log P)^2 + 1.86 \qquad (19.1)$$

$$n = 13 \qquad r^2 = 0.852 \qquad s = 0.113$$

This is an example of a multilinear regression (MLR) QSAR. LD_{50} is the dose required to kill 50% of the animals within a specified time; its reciprocal is used so that higher values represent higher toxicity, and its logarithm is used so that a wide range of values can conveniently be represented, and also because a QSAR is a form of linear free energy relationship (LFER) in which, from the van't Hoff isotherm, a free energy change is proportional to the logarithm of an equilibrium or reaction constant. P is the octanol-water partition coefficient, n is the number of compounds used to develop the QSAR, r^2 is the square of the correlation coefficient and indicates the fraction of the variation of toxicity that is accounted for by the terms on the right-hand side of the equation (in this case 85.2%), and s is the standard error of the estimate.

It was not until 1962 that the first quantitative structure-activity relationship was published by Corwin Hansch and co-workers [13], relating to the herbicidal activity of a series of phenoxyacetic acids:

$$\log 1/C = 4.08\pi - 2.14\pi^2 + 2.78\sigma + 3.36 \qquad (19.2)$$

where C is the concentration inducing a 10% growth in *Avena* coleoptiles in 24h, π is the hydrophobic substituent constant [defined as $\log (P_X/P_H)$], and σ is the Hammett substituent constant, a measure of electron-directing effect. Although no statistics were given for this QSAR, it was nonetheless of immense significance, for several reasons: It was the first example of MLR, showing that a biological end point could be modeled by more than one molecular descriptor; it introduced the hydrophobic substituent constant π, which recognized the essentially additive nature of hydrophobicity; it demonstrated that within a congeneric series of compounds, substituent constants such as π and σ could be used as descriptors to model the variation of biological activity; it introduced the octanol-water partition coefficient as a descriptor of hydrophobicity; and it pioneered the use of the quadratic equation to describe the biphasic variation of biological activity with hydrophobicity.

Since that time thousands of QSARs, covering a wide and diverse range of end points, have been published [9]; most of these have used MLR, but numerous other statistical techniques have also been used, such as partial least squares, principal component analysis, artificial neural networks, decision trees, and discriminant analysis [14].

19.1.2 Uses of QSAR and Basis for Development

A QSAR has two main uses. Its prime use is predictive, to estimate the activity or toxicity of a compound not used to develop the QSAR. However, it is important to note here that predictions must not be made for compounds that are outside the descriptor space of the compounds in the training set. To take a simple example, if the log P values of the training set compounds range from −1 to 5, the QSAR must not be used to predict the activity of a compound with a log P value of 7. Second, the descriptors selected, if they model the biological data well, should be related to the process(es) by which the biological activity is achieved, and thus could throw light on the mechanism(s) of action. It should always be remembered, however, that the existence of a correlation between structure and activity is not proof of causality. Walker et al. [15] have recently published guidelines for developing and using QSARs.

Clearly, there are three basic steps to developing a QSAR:

1. Acquisition of relevant biological data for a series of compounds. The compounds used in developing a QSAR (the training set) should preferably all act by the same mechanism. If this is not the case, the QSAR will be less accurate and there will be outliers, that is, compounds that are not modeled well. Because it is difficult to establish a mechanism, QSAR analysis is usually carried out on congeneric series of compounds, in the expectation (or hope) that this will mean that they have a common mechanism of action. The data should be as accurate as possible and should have been determined with the same protocol—preferably in the same laboratory. They should for best results be in the form of dose or concentration to produce a defined effect (e.g., LD_{50}, the dose required to kill 50% of the organisms) and as such must be reported in mole units (e.g., $mmol{\cdot}kg^{-1}$, $mmol{\cdot}l^{-1}$). The compounds should cover as wide a range of chemical space as is feasible and as wide a range of end point values as possible. The design of series of compounds for QSAR analysis has been reviewed by Pleiss and Unger [16].

Strictly speaking, toxicity values should be given relative to the values for the desired activity, that is as selectivity values, because absolute toxicity values are not particularly meaningful. For example, if a drug is toxic at $1\,\mu mol{\cdot}kg^{-1}$ but the therapeutically effective dose is $0.1\,\mu mol{\cdot}kg^{-1}$, the drug is

probably safe to use; if, on the other hand, the therapeutically effective dose is $10\,\mu mol \cdot kg^{-1}$, the drug is clearly not safe to use.
Some biological data are, of course, reported in a categorical manner, for example, as simply toxic or nontoxic. It is valid to class correlations involving such data as QSARs, because although the biological data are not quantitative (or are at best semiquantitative), the descriptors are.

2. Selection and/or generation of physicochemical and/structural molecular descriptors that will model the biological data. There are essentially two ways to approach the selection of descriptors. The first is to choose only those descriptors that are relevant to a putative mechanism of action. This has the advantage that one is not burdened with a large number of descriptors, but has the disadvantage that if the chosen descriptors are not relevant a good QSAR will not be obtained. The second approach is to generate a large number of descriptors and use an appropriate statistical method to select those that best model the biological activity. The disadvantage here is that the more descriptors one has to choose from, the greater is the risk of chance correlation [17], and the greater the risk that one or more of the descriptors selected will be difficult or impossible of physicochemical interpretation. There is now a vast range of descriptors available—hydrophobic, electronic, steric, quantum chemical, topological, and electrotopological—and there are a number of commercially available software packages, such as Tsar [18], MDL QSAR [19], CODESSA [20], Dragon [21], Cerius^2 [18], HYBOT [22], and MOLCONN-Z [23] that will each generate many descriptors.

3. Application of an appropriate statistical method to develop the best QSAR. As mentioned above, MLR is the most widely used type of correlation in QSAR, although there are several others (*vide ultra*). If one is using a large descriptor library, some means must be found to select the descriptors that will best model the biological data. Livingstone [14, 24] has discussed in detail the various statistical methods (stepwise regression, best subsets, genetic algorithms), with their attendant advantages and disadvantages, that are available to the QSAR practitioner. Checks must also be made for collinearity of descriptors, which can lead to statistical instability and the inability to interpret a QSAR mechanistically; if any pair of descriptors is found to be highly collinear, one of the pair must be deleted from the descriptor pool [25]. Any descriptors for which most values are the same should also be removed from the descriptor pool.

A fourth step, increasingly recognized as crucial, is that of validation [26, 27]. However good the statistics of a correlation, if it is unable to predict the activity of similar compounds that were not included in the training set, it is useless for predictive purposes. One common test for predictivity is the LOO (leave one out) procedure, in which one compound is removed from the training set, the QSAR is regenerated using the remaining compounds, and the activity of the deleted compound is then predicted with the new QSAR. The deleted compound is then reinstated and the procedure repeated until each compound in turn has been left out. A cross-validated r^2 value (q^2) is obtained that is a guide to the predictivity of the QSAR; Walker et al. [15] have proposed that for acceptability, q^2 should not be more than 0.3 lower than the r^2 value for the correlation, whereas Perkins et al. [28] have suggested that a q^2 value of >0.5 is acceptable. However, the LOO procedure has come in for criticism recently [24, 28]. A better procedure, if one has sufficient data, is to leave an appreciable proportion (20–50%) of compounds out of the training set and to use them as an external test set. Finally, whether or not the developed QSAR is a chance correlation can be checked by scrambling the biological response values and trying to build a model using the scrambled data. This procedure is then repeated, say, 100 times and the r^2 values are checked against that for the real QSAR; for a 1% risk that the QSAR is a chance correlation, only one of the r^2 values from the scrambled data should be as high as that from the real QSAR.

Livingstone [24] has given a number of recommendations for successful QSAR modeling:

1. If possible, select chemicals for testing to provide as much physicochemical information as possible.
2. Ensure that the biological response data are appropriate for modeling.
3. If a large number of descriptor variables are utilized, reduce the number by variable elimination before modeling.
4. Use a variable selection technique appropriate to the problem.
5. Use a modeling technique appropriate to the data and data set being modeled. Preference should be given to simple modeling techniques.
6. Models should be assessed not only in terms of their goodness of fit (i.e., statistical quality) but also in terms of their predictive power. The predictive power of a model can be assessed only by estimating the activity of a set of compounds not included in the original model.
7. In all modeling techniques, and neural networks in particular, care must be taken not to overtrain or overfit the model.
8. If possible, models should be interpreted in terms of their mechanistic meaning.

19.1.3 QSARs for Drug Toxicity

What is the status of QSAR in drug toxicology? Published QSAR studies of drug toxicity cover over 30 different end points, from acute toxicity to carcinogenicity to gastric irritancy [29], and most of these studies were made in the period 1970–1990. There is little evidence from *published* work that the pharmaceutical industry is using *in silico* prediction of drug toxicity extensively. For example, of the 208 presentations made at the 2002 European Symposium on QSAR, only five dealt with the prediction of drug toxicity.

However, pharma industries are, understandably, reticent about their work on the design and development of new drug entities, and they are undoubtedly using QSAR and related techniques for toxicity prediction [2]. The advent of combinatorial chemistry and high-throughput screening has meant that vast quantities of data on potential drug compounds are now available, through in vitro testing and the use of expert systems for toxicity prediction such as DEREK [30], CASE/MultiCASE [31], HazardExpert [32], TOPKAT [18], and OncoLogic [33]. Dearden et al [34] have reviewed the performance of such software.

In silico methods are being developed, often by software companies such as Spotfire, Leadscope, Tripos, and Accelrys, to deal with the huge number of data generated in ADME/TOX testing [2]. Because of the importance of optimizing several drug properties together, techniques such as multicriteria decision methods or multiobjective optimization methods are being explored [35, 36].

Nowhere is the generation of huge amounts of data greater than in the field of gene expression [37], so a major challenge for this rapidly emerging and potentially vitally important area is how to handle such data and how to incorporate structure-activity and related techniques to convert the data into knowledge useful for drug design [38, 39].

19.2 STRATEGIES FOR THE USE OF *IN SILICO* TOXICOLOGY IN DRUG DEVELOPMENT

19.2.1 General Screening of Drug Libraries

The tools for *in silico* toxicology are broadly applied in the drug development process. The particular use of the tools is clearly context-dependent, which includes the quality of the prediction and the applicability domain of the model.

At the outset of the drug discovery process *in silico* tools are highly valued to eliminate "obviously" toxic drug candidates. This process has become particularly useful in the screening of large databases of candidate drugs, and techniques such as virtual screening for toxicity have become commonplace. There is a clear role for automated techniques such as the commercial expert systems at this stage.

A number of commercial expert systems have been applied to screen drug libraries. For instance, DEREK, TOPKAT, MultiCASE, and many other systems all have possibilities in this regard. However, it should be noted that for broad screening only compounds with toxicity associated with them can be identified, and hence these are very crude measures of hazard assessment. The use of expert systems to screen libraries is fraught with dangers, not least that no performance statistics are available for these systems being used for such an application. It is also highly probable that the vast majority of predictions will be made for compounds that are well outside of the area of knowledge of the training sets of the original models. Thus predictions for these compounds may be better when there is some form of consensus, that is, when the prediction is made from a number of different models.

Predictions of no, or low, toxicity in a general drug screening approach should be used to indicate a possible absence of toxicity in potential drug candidates. Inevitably this would require further toxicological assessment of potential drugs to ensure safety.

19.2.2 In-Depth Assessment of Candidates

Once candidate molecules have been selected, there is an increased possibility for more in-depth *in silico* studies for toxic effects. These could, for instance, take the form of attempts to "design out" toxicities from a fundamental point of view, or may involve de novo modeling efforts. For instance, just as drug activity is optimized by QSAR, toxicity could also be minimized.

If in-depth toxicological QSAR is to be performed on a series of candidates, it is likely that new data and modeling will be required.

19.2.3 Regulatory Usage

There is increasing use of *in silico* techniques to predict toxicity by regulatory agencies worldwide. There are a number of applications from regulatory agencies that include prioritization of chemicals, filling data gaps, and classification and labeling. Most regulatory applications have been for environmental end points, for instance, as part of the United States Environmental Protection Agency's Pre-Manufactory Notification procedure.

Increasingly *in silico* technologies are being considered with regard to the registration of drugs. The US Food and Drug Administration (FDA) Center for Drug Evaluation and Research (CDER) operates a number of programs and activities in the area of *in silico* toxicology. These include *Database Projects* for creating a FDA knowledge base and institutional memory of the results of clinical and nonclinical studies and of postmarketing clinical adverse events. There are also *Chemical Structure Similarity Searching* tools, for example, developed from the ISIS/Host software program [19], to evaluate the capability to retrieve toxicological and chemical structure information in the database. The *Computational Toxicology Program and ComTox Consulting Service* incorporates information from toxicology databases and applies advances in computer technology and QSAR methods to screen compounds for potential toxicity. There are also applications of computational toxicology to assess clinical adverse drug reactions. Further information on US FDA CDER activities is available from its website [40].

Although there is considerable activity in developing computational toxicology for regulatory applications, the reality for the foreseeable future is that QSARs and related techniques are not yet sophisticated enough to replace whole animal testing.

19.3 TECHNIQUES FOR THE DEVELOPMENT OF QSARs TO PREDICT TOXICITY

A large variety of techniques are available to develop predictive models for toxicity. These range from relatively simple techniques to relate quantitative levels of potency with one or more descriptors to more multivariate techniques and ultimately the so-called expert systems that lead the user directly from an input of structure to a prediction. These are outlined briefly below.

19.3.1 Multiple Linear Regression

MLR is the most widely used of the QSAR modeling techniques. Walker et al. [15] have published guidelines for the development and use of MLR-based QSARs, and Cronin and Schultz [41] have discussed their potential pitfalls.

Their advantages are that they are simple to use and are transparent; that is, the descriptors that best model the biological activity can be seen and—hopefully—understood. Their disadvantages are that they work best when restricted to congeneric series of compounds, they assume that the biological activity is a rectilinear function of each descriptor, and they can suffer from a high risk of chance correlations, especially when a large pool of descriptors is used.

Concerning the last point, Topliss and Costello [42] proposed that, to minimize the risk of chance correlations, a QSAR developed with MLR should utilize at least five data points (compounds) for each descriptor included in the equation. Later work [17] showed that it was necessary to take into account not only the number of descriptors in the QSAR (usually several) but also the whole of the descriptor pool (often several hundred) from which the "best" descriptors were selected.

The descriptors used should not be highly collinear with each other, for two reasons. First, this can lead to statistical instability and overprediction, and second, collinearity makes mechanistic interpretation difficult. For example, Cronin and Schultz [41] have pointed out that although a good correlation could be obtained between the skin sensitization potential and the hydrophobicity of a series of bromoalkanes, a correlation between skin sensitization potential and molecular weight had exactly the same statistics, because hydrophobicity and molecular weight are very highly correlated in homologous series.

An example of a valid, easily interpretable QSAR is that relating to P-glycoprotein-regulated multidrug resistance reversal (MDRR) by phenothiazines [43]:

$$\log \mathrm{MDRR} = 0.195\ {}^{5}\chi_{\mathrm{p}} + 0.147\ E_{\mathrm{SsssN}} + 0.00597\ \mathrm{PSA} - 0.00240\ \mathrm{TSA} - 0.255N_{5\text{-AR}} + 0.094 \tag{19.3}$$

$$n = 38 \qquad r^2 = 0.864 \qquad q^2 = 0.820 \qquad s = 0.168 \qquad F = 40.6$$

where ${}^5\chi_p$ is fifth-order path molecular connectivity [44], E_{SsssN} is the sum of electrotopological state indices for singly-bonded nitrogen [45], PSA is polar surface area, TSA is total surface area, and $N_{5\text{-AR}}$ is the number of five-membered aliphatic rings. There is no collinearity among descriptors, and each descriptor is significant at the 5% level (i.e., there is <5% risk that each descriptor has been selected by chance). The data set is too small to be split into separate training and test sets, but the internal cross-validated q^2 value is high, indicating that the QSAR has good predictivity.

On the other hand, it is all too easy to find QSARs that fail one or other of the statistical criteria, or have other faults. An early example, involving the tumor-promoting ability of aniline mustard drugs, was [46]:

$$\log 1/C = -1.17\,\sigma + 3.30\,\sigma^2 - 1.70\,I_4 + 5.03 \tag{19.4}$$

$$n = 11 \qquad r^2 = 0.819 \qquad s = 0.482 \qquad F = 10.6$$

where C is the concentration to produce tumors above the background level, σ is the Hammett substituent constant, I_4 is an indicator variable for the presence of a 4-substituent, and F is the Fisher statistic, a measure of the probability that the correlation has not occurred by chance. This QSAR fails the Topliss–Costello rule [42] and also is not validated. Furthermore, no indication of the statistical significance of individual descriptors is given. This is usually done by including in brackets, after the coefficient for each descriptor, the standard error; if the standard error approaches the value of the coefficient, the significance of that descriptor is low, and it should strictly not be included in the QSAR.

A QSAR for which the standard error of each descriptor is given concerns the bradycardic effect of a series of tetraalkylbispidines [47]. The QSAR models the selectivity between the desired bradycardic effect and the adverse contractile effect. It is important, in assessing and modeling drug toxicity, that the toxic effect is assessed relative to the desired effect as described above. The QSAR developed for the selectivity of the tetraalkylbispidines was:

$$\log(\text{selectivity}) = 0.37(\pm 0.33)\,\text{MR}_1 - 0.010(\pm 0.007)\,(\text{MR}_1)^2 + 0.17(\pm 0.10)\,\text{MR}_{3,4} - 0.0043(\pm 0.002)\,(\text{MR}_{3,4})^2 + 0.43(\pm 0.40)\,I_2 - 3.03 \tag{19.5}$$

$$n = 16 \qquad r^2 = 0.950 \qquad s = 0.194 \qquad F = 38.3$$

where MR_i = molar refractivity (usually considered a measure of size) of a substituent at position i, and I_2 is an indicator variable for the presence of an unsaturated substituent at position 2. It can be seen that the standard errors for three descriptors [MR_1, $(\text{MR}_1)^2$, and I_2] are almost equal to the values of their respective coefficients, and thus are statistically unacceptable. The QSAR also contravenes the Topliss–Costello rule [42] and has not been validated, either internally or externally.

A QSAR for the acute toxicity of new hypoglycemic agents [48] was internally cross-validated, but used LD_{50} instead of log LD_{50} as the dependent variable, and (more seriously) used LD_{50} values in $g \cdot kg^{-1}$, rather than in a molar unit such as $mmol \cdot kg^{-1}$.

A key requirement of QSAR is that the compounds used in the modeling and prediction processes should have the same mechanism of action, and for this reason most QSAR studies are made with congeneric series of compounds. However, if a diverse set of compounds can reasonably be assumed to have the same mechanism of action, QSAR modeling can justifiably be carried out. For example, Dearden et al. [43] developed a QSAR for the ratio of brain levels of 22 very diverse drugs in the wild-type mouse and the P-glycoprotein knockout mouse ($R_{+/-}$):

$$\log (R_{+/-}) = 0.104\ Ct_{SdssC} + 0.0435\ N_{circ} - 0.113\ {}^{3}\chi_{p}^{v} - 22.6\ \alpha/V + 0.317 \quad (19.6)$$

$$n = 22 \qquad r^2 = 0.854 \qquad q^2 = 0.788 \qquad s = 0.182 \qquad F = 24.9$$

where Ct_{SdssC} is the number of carbon atoms that form one double bond, N_{circ} is the number of all possible rings, ${}^{3}\chi_{p}^{v}$ is third-order valence path molecular connectivity, and α/V is polarizability per unit volume.

Even if a common mechanism of action cannot be assumed, Benigni and Giuliani [49] have argued that it may still be valid to subject a heterogeneous group of compounds to QSAR analysis, although they emphasize that a lower level of accuracy of fit and prediction will have to be accepted. There are, in fact, numerous examples of QSARs concerning toxicity of heterogeneous data sets, which means that the diverse compound libraries generated by combinatorial chemistry and high-throughput screening could well be amenable to QSAR analysis [28].

Three examples concerning toxicity of heterogeneous data sets are given below. The first [50] relates to mutagenicity to *Salmonella typhimurium* of aromatic and heteroaromatic nitro-compounds:

$$\log \mathrm{TA98} = 0.65 \log \mathrm{P} - 2.90 \log(\beta \mathrm{P} + 1) - 1.38\ E_{\mathrm{LUMO}} + 1.88\ I_1 - 2.89\ I_a - 4.15 \quad (19.7)$$

$$n = 188 \qquad r^2 = 0.810 \qquad s = 0.886 \qquad \log \beta = -5.48 \qquad F = 48.6$$

where TA98 is the number of revertants/nmol, E_{LUMO} is the energy of the lowest unoccupied molecular orbital, and I_1 and I_a are indicator variables for the presence of three or more fused rings and acenthrylene structures, respectively. No validation of this QSAR was reported.

The FDA [51] has used the MDL QSAR software [19] to develop QSARs for the carcinogenic potential of pharmaceuticals and organic chemicals. These were validated using a test set of 108 compounds, with 72% correct prediction of carcinogens and 72% correct prediction of noncarcinogens.

Cardiac QT interval prolongation is a potentially fatal effect of a number of nonantiarrhythmic drugs, and several have had to be withdrawn from the market because of this. The hERG (*human ether-à-go-go*-related gene) potassium channel is expressed in the human heart; it is a major contributor to cardiac repolarization, and its inhibition generally leads to prolongation of the QT interval. hERG inhibition values for 60 diverse drugs and drug candidates yielded the following QSAR [52]:

$$\log IC_{50} = 0.411\,nO - 1.20\,Ed_{max} - 0.683\,({}^{3}\chi_{c} - {}^{4}\chi_{pc}) + 0.000148\,I_{Z} + 0.000635\,TE + 2.12 \quad (19.8)$$

$$n = 60 \qquad r^2 = 0.842 \qquad q^2 = 0.797 \qquad s = 0.614 \qquad F = 57.5$$

where nO is the number of oxygen atoms, Ed_{max} is the maximum hydrogen bond donor energy, $({}^{3}\chi_{c} - {}^{4}\chi_{pc})$ is the difference between third-order cluster and fourth-order path-cluster molecular connectivity, I_Z is the principal moment of inertia along the *Z*-axis, and TE is total molecular energy.

19.3.2 Other Correlation Techniques

Because of the drawbacks of MLR, a number of other approaches to correlation analysis have been employed [24]. One of these is principal components analysis (PCA), in which the descriptors are combined into a smaller number of terms, called principal components, that are orthogonal to (uncorrelated with) each other. Generally it is found that a small number of principal components accounts for a large percentage of the variation in the biological data. The principal components per se have no physicochemical significance, but they can be correlated with the original descriptors to determine which they best represent. The structure-toxicity relationship of naphthalene derivatives was investigated with PCA [53], and Ridings et al. [54] used the technique to investigate structure-toxicity relationships in a series of dopamine mimetics.

A refinement of PCA is partial least-squares (PLS) analysis, which allows the development of principal components and multiple regression in a single step. It has the advantages of being able to handle large numbers of descriptors and not being affected by high collinearities between descriptors. However, as with PCA, it does not yield a MLR-type regression equation. Bravi and Wikel [55] used PLS to model the binding of coumarins to cytochrome P450 2A5.

A widely used 3-D QSAR method that makes use of PLS is comparative molecular field analysis (CoMFA), in which a probe atom is used to calculate the steric and electronic fields at numerous points in a 3D lattice within which the molecules have been aligned. Poso et al. [56] used the technique to model the binding of coumarins to cytochrome P450 2A5, with similar results to those obtained by Bravi and Wikel [55]. Shi et al. [57] used it to model the estrogen receptor binding of a large diverse set of compounds, and Cavalli et al. [58] used it to develop a pharmacophore for hERG potassium channel-blocking drugs; both of these studies are of interest because the alignment requirement of CoMFA makes it difficult to deal with noncongeneric compounds.

CoMSIA (comparative molecular similarity index analysis) is a recent development from CoMFA and does not suffer from the alignment problem. It has been used to model hERG potassium channel inhibition by drugs [59] and the toxicity of phenylsulfonyl carboxylates [60], organophosphates [61], and polybrominated diphenyl ethers [62], with results comparable to those from CoMFA.

Molecular similarity has also been used directly to model toxicity. Bartlett et al. [63] found that the incidence of cutaneous rash from oral penicillins was a function of shape similarity to benzylpenicillin, and Basak et al. [64] used molecular similarity to model the mutagenicity of aromatic and heteroaromatic amines.

A similarity-related approach is k-nearest neighbor (KNN) analysis, based on the premise that similar compounds have similar properties. Compounds are distributed in multidimensional space according to their values of a number of selected properties; the toxicity of a compound of interest is then taken as the mean of the toxicities of a number (k) of nearest neighbors. Cronin et al. [65] used KNN to model the toxicity of 91 heterogeneous organic chemicals to the alga *Chlorella vulgaris*, but found it no better than MLR.

A widely used QSAR technique is that of artificial neural networks (ANNs) [66, 67]. An ANN comprises layers of discrete processing elements analogous to brain neurons. The input layer feeds in the data (biological activity and descriptor values), and one or more core (hidden) layers process the information and feed the response to an output layer. The hidden layers allow the network response to be nonlinear, thus increasing the modeling ability. The ANN is trained by first randomly initializing the connection weights between the neurons and then running the data through the network and comparing the output with the known biological responses. Repetition of this process allows the connection weights to be adjusted until a good response is achieved. The ANN can then be used for prediction. However, it is easy to overtrain the network, so that predictive ability declines.

There do not appear to be any published studies to date of ANNs being used for the prediction of drug toxicity, although they have been used for the prediction of toxicity of chemicals such as pesticides [68, 69].

So far, we have considered the QSAR modeling of continuous biological data, that is, where the toxicity value is a number such as an LD_{50}. However, some data are not continuous but are binary (e.g., toxic/ nontoxic); a common example is carcinogenicity, for which test results are almost invariably reported in this way. Clearly, one cannot perform, say, MLR on such classification data (although a method called fuzzy adaptive least squares [70] can be used). A number of methods are available for the modeling of classification data.

One of the best-known techniques for QSAR analysis of classification data is discriminant analysis [71, 72]. If a single descriptor is adequate to discriminate between toxic and nontoxic compounds, then the critical value of the descriptor is clear. If two descriptors are sufficient, a plot of one descriptor against the other should show a separation between toxic and nontoxic compounds. A good example of this is shown by the work of Barratt [73] to distinguish between compounds that are or are not skin corrosive; although Barratt used four descriptors, he reduced these to two principal components, and hence a two-dimensional plot sufficed to discriminate. If more than three descriptors are necessary for discrimination, then (unless one uses PCA) the toxic and nontoxic compounds are separated by a hyperplane in multidimensional space. Generally, of course, less than perfect discrimination is achieved, so that the results are expressed as the percentage of correct predictions for toxic compounds (sensitivity) and the percentage of correct predictions for nontoxic compounds (specificity). Rose and Jurs [74] used a total of 22 topological and molecular orbital-based descriptors to give 97% correct overall classification of the carcinogenicity of 150 nitrosamines. Helguera et al. [75] used a topological substructural approach to predict the carcinogenicity of 189 heterogeneous compounds and found 76.3% correct classification; leave-one-out cross-validation yielded the same percentage correct classification. Worth and Cronin [72] have discussed various types of discriminant analysis such as canonical and stepwise discriminant analysis.

Another classification technique is logistic regression [76], which is based on the assumption that a sigmoidal dependency exists between the probability of group membership and one or more predictor variables. It has been used [72] to model eye irritation data.

The above methods all assume that a clear spatial distinction can be made between toxic and nontoxic compounds. However, it is sometimes found that toxic compounds form a cluster embedded in a milieu of nontoxic compounds. In such cases, a different technique, embedded cluster modeling, can be used [77]. Cronin [78] has used the technique to model eye irritation data.

19.3.3 Expert Systems

The need for rapidly accessible estimation of toxicity has led to the development of software and other algorithms that will generate estimations of toxicity, usually for organic compounds [79]; such methodology is termed an expert system, which has been defined [34] as "any formalised system, not necessarily computer-based, which enables a user to obtain rational predictions about the toxicity of chemicals." Essentially, expert systems fall into two classes—those relying on statistical approaches and those based on explicit rules derived from human knowledge.

There are two commercially available expert systems that rely on a statistical approach: TOPKAT, which was developed by Health Designs Inc. but is now owned by Accelrys [18], and CASE/MultiCASE, developed at Case Western University [31].

Earlier versions of TOPKAT included the use of substructural fragments, but recent versions use only continuously variable descriptor, topological shape, and symmetry indices and electrotopological indices, which can take into account the steric and electronic environments of substructures. For toxicity end points with continuous measures (e.g., LD_{50}, LOAEL, lowest observable adverse effect level), linear regression equations are used to give predictions. For end points with dichotomous or binary measures (e.g., carcinogenicity, mutagenicity), linear discriminant regression functions are used to give predictions. The 16 end points covered include carcinogenicity, mutagenicity, developmental toxicity, irritation, skin sensitization, and acute toxicity. A valuable feature of TOPKAT is its ability to indicate whether or not a compound of interest is within the descriptor space (optimum prediction space) of the model and thus to give an indication of confidence in the prediction. There have been a number of publications dealing with the predictive ability of TOPKAT; for example, Enslein et al. [80] reported that its skin sensitization module yielded a cross-validated specificity of between 81% and 91%, and a cross-validated sensitivity of between 85% and 95%. It should be noted that some chemical classes are not well covered by certain TOPKAT modules [34].

The CASE approach is quite different. CASE decomposes a molecule into all possible fragments from two to ten heavy (nonhydrogen) atoms. With a statistical technique, these are then classified into biophores (allied to toxicity) and biophobes (not allied to toxicity). These are then combined into an equation:

$$\text{CASE units} = \text{constant} + a(\text{fragment 1}) + b(\text{fragment 2}) + \ldots (x)$$

Interaction between fragments is accounted for, because large fragments automatically encompass smaller fragments. The CASE software covers a range of end points similar to that of TOPKAT, but includes also CYP450 2D inhibition and cellular toxicity. There are numerous publications concerning the performance of CASE, for example, in carcinogenicity [81] and developmental toxicity [82] prediction. Clearly CASE does not require mechanistic knowledge to find structural alerts, but at the same time it does not attach any mechanistic significance to biophores. It should be noted that the US FDA uses a modified version of the CASE software in its regulatory procedures [83].

A Russian expert system, PASS (prediction of activity spectra for substances) [84], uses substructural descriptors called "multilevel neighborhoods of atoms" [85] to predict over 900 different pharmacological activities from molecular structure. These activities include a number of toxicity end points such as carcinogenicity, mutagenicity, teratogenicity, and embryotoxicity. The accuracy of prediction has been shown [86] to range from about 85% to over 90%. One-off predictions can be obtained free of charge on the PASS website [84].

OASIS (optimized approach based on structural indices set) has been developed by Mekenyan and co-workers [87]. Given the activities or toxicities of a set of compounds, it generates large numbers of structural indices for each and develops QSAR correlations. The approach has been used to model the acute toxicity of industrial chemicals [88]. It is claimed [89] that the method can be of use in elucidating mechanisms of action.

Turning to expert systems that use a rule base, a method that is finding increasing use for classification data is decision tree analysis [72]. This is based on the "if . . . then" approach and can involve a considerable number of sequential steps. The OncoLogic software [www.logichem.com] comprises four independent subsystems, each with an hierarchical decision tree assembly, for estimating the carcinogenicity of fibers, metals and metal-containing compounds, polymers, and organics [90]. It provides a mechanistically based justification for each evaluation. However, the user has to classify the chemical of interest into one of the predefined chemical classes, which can be difficult for multifunctional group compounds.

Purdy [91] used the technique to predict the carcinogenicity of organic chemicals in rodents, although his model was based on physicochemical and molecular orbital-based descriptors as well as on substructural features and it used only a relatively small number of compounds. His decision tree, which was manual rather than computer based, was trained on 306 compounds and tested on 301 different compounds; it achieved 96% correct classification for the training set and 90% correct classification for the test set.

The COMPACT (computer-optimized molecular parametric analysis of chemical toxicity) procedure, developed by Lewis and co-workers [92], uses a form of discriminant analysis based on two descriptors, namely, molecular planarity and electronic activation energy (the difference between the energies of the highest occupied and lowest unoccupied molecular orbitals), which predict the potential of a compound to act as a substrate for one of the cytochromes P450. Lewis et al. [93] found 64% correct predictions for 100 compounds tested by the NTP for mutagenicity.

A widely used knowledge-based expert system is DEREK (deductive estimation of risk from existing knowledge), originally devised by Derek Sanderson at Schering and now developed and marketed by Lhasa Limited [30]. It covers a number of toxicological end points, including carcinogenicity, mutagenicity, teratogenicity, irritation, skin sensitization, acute toxicity, and neurotoxicity, and also offers an estimate of skin permeability. Its main strengths lie in the prediction of carcinogenicity, mutagenicity, and skin sensitization [94]. For example, for a diverse data set of 266 compounds, DEREK correctly predicted 84% of mutagens [95]. Barratt et al. [96] have discussed the development of the DEREK rule base for the identification of photoallergens. Ongoing development of DEREK is aided by its users giving regular feedback to Lhasa; in addition, in-house data can be incorporated by users. One physicochemical property, namely log P, is also automatically calculated.

Although DEREK cannot of itself handle metabolism, a sister program, METEOR [97], allows the prediction of metabolites, which can then be assessed by DEREK.

CompuDrug Limited [32] have developed a versatile toxicity prediction program called HazardExpert [98]; it incorporates a version of its sister program MetabolExpert, which allows it to take account of metabolites, and it can also calculate log P and pK_a values of compounds, which allows estimates of bioavailability to be made. It operates by a combination of toxicological knowledge, QSAR models, and fuzzy logic; the last enables HazardExpert to simulate different exposure conditions. It offers a range of end points, including carcinogenicity, mutagenicity, teratogenicity, irritation, skin sensitization, immunotoxicity, and neurotoxicity, but not acute toxicity. Its chemical database and rule base are accessible to, and can be modified by, the user. In a test of its ability to predict carcinogenicity [99], it was found to be good at identifying noncarcinogens (81% correct predictions) but poor at identifying carcinogens (36% correct predictions). CompuDrug also offer ToxAlert, based on HazardExpert, which flags compounds in a screening library or other collections for hazards associated with specific pharmacophores.

What a prospective user of expert systems needs is independent evidence of the performance of available software in toxicity prediction. So far as I know, only two comparative tests have been carried out to date, both by the National Toxicology Program (NTP) of the US National Institutes of Health and both concerned with carcinogenicity prediction. Some years ago the NTP invited the developers of expert systems, and others concerned with prediction of carcinogenicity, to predict whether or not 40 substances (test 1) and 26 substances (test 2) that had not been subjected to carcinogenicity testing were carcinogenic. The NTP then carried out rodent carcinogenicity testing of the substances.

The prediction results were not, on the face of it, encouraging. Overall correct predictions (concordances) for test 1 were DEREK 59%, TOPKAT 58%, COMPACT 54%, and CASE 49%. For test 2 the figures were OncoLogic 67%, COMPACT 44%, DEREK 38%, Purdy 35%, and CASE 18%. However, it has been pointed out [100] that the substances that the NTP tested were not a random selection from the chemical universe, but included a majority of suspect substances; thus the goal was not to separate carcinogens from noncarcinogens (which is what the expert systems were designed to do) but rather to separate actual carcinogens from possible carcinogens. This is very difficult because of the plethora of molecular interactions that can modulate the carcinogenic potential of a primary structural feature such as an aromatic nitro group. It should also be noted that, because compounds with a given type of toxicity probably cluster in a relatively small region of descriptor space, it is generally easier to predict lack of toxicity than to predict toxicity.

The comments of Richard [101], writing in 1998, that "all of the current commercial methods for toxicity prediction are limited in very real ways by available data and knowledge, and we must be careful not to place unrealistic expectations on their predictive capabilities" are still apposite today, albeit to a somewhat lesser extent, because most of the expert systems discussed above are under continual development, and hence their predictive abilities continue to improve. For the present, however, it is recommended that a consensus approach be used if feasible; that is, the results of two or more expert systems should be combined. Consensus modeling has been found to give improved predictions for numerous end points. For example, Lewis et al. [102] found, for a small set of 14 human carcinogens, that although COMPACT alone gave 71% correct predictions, and HazardExpert alone gave 57% correct predictions, the two systems used in conjunction gave 100% correct predictions.

19.4 END POINTS MODELED

The conventional QSAR end points have come about through the availability of databases and data sets for modeling, rather than being driven by specific regulatory or commercial needs. There is no way around this somewhat pragmatic model development—if there are no data to model, no models can be developed. More recently the US FDA has been compiling and beginning to model data associated with adverse drug reactions. However, these models are not yet openly available for use.

End points particularly associated with toxicities relevant to pharmaceuticals include those described as "general human health" effects, for example, mutagenicity, carcinogenicity, and acute toxicity. There are a number of issues with these models, most notably that the training sets often have few pharmacologically active compounds in them, and also that these are complex end points and none of the mechanisms is properly considered. There is generally a lack of good *in silico* models in areas important for drug development, that is, those that require long-term and costly toxicological evaluation such as reproductive and chronic toxicity.

Over the past decade, there has been an increased emphasis on developing specific and localized models on toxicities more specifically related to drugs. An excellent example is hERG, particularly as it is related to QT interval prolongation. Recent progress in predicting hERG activity has recently been well reviewed by Norinder [103]. It is clear that the application of drug design techniques to toxicological QSAR is highly appropriate for modeling such an end point. However, it must be remembered that techniques such as CoMFA and CoMSIA are labor-intensive, not only in the development of the models but also in their usage. QT interval prolongation is an interesting end point for a number of reasons: It has already caused a number of drugs to be withdrawn from the market; it is clearly a receptor-binding phenomenon, and thus could be modeled by structural features [but see 52]. Aptula and Cronin [104] have provided structural rules and dimensions that are able to discriminate binders from nonbinders.

There are undoubtedly a large number of other end points, at the specific and mechanistic levels, that require both data and modeling in the future to make QSAR a truly useful science for the prediction of drug toxicity. It is to be hoped that such data will become available in the not-too-distant future, perhaps through data-sharing facilities such as VITIC [105].

19.5 ISSUES WITH TOXICITY PREDICTION

All predictions must be taken for what they are, namely, generalizations based on current knowledge and understanding. There is a temptation for a user to assume that a computer-generated answer must be correct. To determine whether this is in fact the case, a number of factors concerning the model must be addressed. The statistical evaluation of a model was addressed above. Another very important criterion is to ensure that a prediction is an interpolation within the model space, and not an extrapolation outside of it. To determine this, the concept of the "applicability domain" of a model has been introduced [106].

In the area of predictive toxicology the applicability domain is taken to express the scope and limitations of a model, that is, the range of chemical structures for which the model is considered to be applicable [106]. Although this issue has been fundamental to the use of QSAR (and indeed any predictive technique) since its conception, there remain few reliable methods to define and apply an applicability domain in predictive toxicology. The current status of methods to define the applicability domain for use in (Q)SAR has been assessed recently by Netzeva et al. [106].

There is currently debate on the best methods to define the applicability domain for a model in predictive toxicology. The ultimate solution is likely to be lacking for a number of years. However, there are some initiatives that are beginning to address the issue of applicability domain, which include the use of statistical measures and also mechanistic appreciation.

There are a growing number of tools to assess applicability domain, and a number of expert systems, for example, TOPKAT and MultiCASE, have their own measures of fit. These need to be developed and their application to larger drug libraries demonstrated.

19.6 GOOD PRACTICE AND RECOMMENDATIONS

The modern science of *in silico* toxicity prediction has made great strides since its inception in 1962 [13]. Nevertheless, there are still many problems to be overcome [107], and it is to be hoped that future work in this essential field will take into account the following recommendations:

- More toxicity data, of greater consistency, are required.
- A better mechanistic appreciation of drug toxicity is needed.
- The model user should consider use of a variety of techniques so as to build consensus answers, rather than simply relying on a single prediction.
- A consideration of whether or not a compound fits into the chemical and biological space of the model should be made by the model user.

ACKNOWLEDGMENTS

The author is grateful to Dr. Mark Cronin for constructive comments and advice on the manuscript.

REFERENCES

1. Kennedy T. Managing the drug discovery/development interface. *Drug Discov Today* 1997;2:436–44.
2. Ekins S, Boulanger B, Swaan PW, Hupcey MAZ. Towards a new age of virtual ADME/TOX and multidimensional drug discovery. *J Comput-Aided Mol Des* 2002;16:381–401.
3. Tute MS. History and objectives of quantitative drug design. In: Ramsden CA, editor, *Comprehensive medicinal chemistry*, vol. 4. Quantitative drug design. Oxford: Pergamon, 1990. p. 1–31.
4. Crum Brown A, Fraser TR. On the connection between chemical constitution and physiological action. I. On the physiological action of the salts of the ammonium bases, derived from trichina, brachia, thebaia, codeia, morphia, and nicotia. *Trans R Soc Edinburgh* 1868–9;25:151–203.
5. Richardson BJ. Physiological research on alcohols. *Med Times & Gazette* 1869;(ii):703–6.
6. Richet C. On the relationship between the toxicity and the physical properties of substances. *Compt Rend Soc Biol* 1893;(9)5:775–6.
7. Overton E. Osmotic properties of cells in the bearing on toxicology and pharmacology. *Z Physik Chem* 1897;22:189–209.
8. Meyer H. On the theory of alcohol narcosis. I. Which property of anesthetics gives them their narcotic activity? *Arch Exper Pathol Pharmakol* 1899; 42:109–18.
9. Hansch C, Leo A. *Exploring QSAR. 1. Fundamentals and applications in chemistry and biology*. Washington DC: American Chemical Society, 1995.
10. Ferguson J. The use of chemical potentials as indices of toxicity. *Proc R Soc Lond B* 1939;127:387–403.
11. Hansch C. Quantitative approaches to biochemical structure-activity relationships. *Acc Chem Res* 1969;2:232–9.

12. Hansch C, Clayton JM. Lipophilic character and biological activity of drugs. II. The parabolic case. *J Pharm Soc* 1973;62:1–21.
13. Hansch C, Maloney PP, Fujita T. Correlation of biological activity of phenoxy-acetic acids with Hammett subsistent constants and partition coefficients. *Nature* 1962; 194:178–80.
14. Livingstone D. *Data analysis for chemists: application to QSAR and chemical product design*. Oxford: Oxford University Press, 1995.
15. Walker JD, Jaworska J, Comber MHI, Schultz TW, Dearden JC. Guidelines for developing and using quantitative structure-activity relationships. *Environ Toxicol Chem* 2003;22:1653–65.
16. Pleiss MA, Unger SH. The design of test series and the significance of QSAR relationships. In: Ramsden CA, editor, *Comprehensive medicinal chemistry*. Vol. 4: Quantitative drug design. Oxford: Pergamon Press, 1990. p. 561–87.
17. Topliss JG, Edwards RP. Chance factors in studies of quantitative structure-activity relationships. *J Med Chem* 1979;22:1238–44.
18. www.accelrys.com
19. www.mdli.com
20. www.semichem.com
21. www.talete.mi.it/dragon.htm
22. software.timtec.net/hybot-plus.htm
23. www.eslc.vabiotech.com/molconn/
24. Livingstone DJ. Building QSAR models: a practical guide. In: Cronin MTD, Livingstone DJ, editors, *Predicting chemical toxicity and fate*. Boca Raton: CRC Press, 2004. p. 151–70.
25. Whitley DC, Ford MG, Livingstone DJ. Unsupervised forward selection: a method for eliminating redundant variables. *J Chem Inf Comput Sci* 2000;40:1160–8.
26. Wold S. Validation of QSARs. *Quant Struct-Act Relat* 1991;10:191–3.
27. Aptula AO, Jeliazkova NG, Schultz TW, Cronin MTD. The better predictive model: high q^2 for the training set or low root mean square error of prediction for the test set? *QSAR Comb Sci* 2005;24:385–96.
28. Perkins R, Fang H, Tong W, Welsh WJ. Quantitative structure-activity relationship methods: perspectives on drug discovery and toxicology. *Environ Toxicol Chem* 2003;22:1666–79.
29. Dearden JC. *In silico* prediction of drug toxicity. *J Comput-Aid Mol Des* 2003;17:119–27.
30. www.lhasalimited.org
31. www.multicase.com
32. www.compudrug.com
33. www.logichem.com
34. Dearden JC, Barratt MD, Benigni R, Bristol DW, Combes RD, Cronin MTD et al. The development and validation of expert systems for predicting toxicity. *ATLA* 1997;25:223–52.

35. Agrafiotis DK. A constant time algorithm for estimating the diversity of large chemical libraries. *J Chem Inf Comput Sci* 2001;41:159–67.
36. Tulsi B. Can SAR overcome its technological limits? *Drug Discov Dev* 2004;7:41–4.
37. Scherf U, Ross DT, Waltham M, Smith LH, Lee JK, Tanabe L et al. A gene expression database for the molecular biology of cancer. *Nat Genet* 2000; 24:236–44.
38. Bassett DE, Eisen MB, Boguski MS. Gene expression informatics—it's all in your mine. *Nat Genet* 1999;21(Suppl 1):51–5.
39. Kalocsai P, Shams S. Visualization and analysis of gene expression data. *J Assoc Lab Automation* 1999;4:58–61.
40. www.fda.gov/cder/Offices/OPS_IO/ICSAS.htm#ComToxProgram
41. Cronin MTD, Schultz TW. Pitfalls in QSAR. *J Mol Struct (Theochem)* 2003; 622:39–51.
42. Topliss JG, Costello RJ. Chance correlations in structure-activity studies using multiple regression analysis. *J Med Chem* 1972;15:1066–9.
43. Dearden JC, Al-Noobi A, Scott AC, Thomson SA. QSAR studies on P-glycoprotein-regulated multidrug resistance and on its reversal by phenothiazines. *SAR QSAR Environ Res* 2003;14:447–54.
44. Kier LB, Hall LH. *Molecular connectivity in structure-activity analysis.* New York: John Wiley & Sons, Inc., 1986.
45. Kier LB, Hall LH. *Molecular structure description: the electrotopological state.* San Diego: Academic Press, 1999.
46. Leo A, Panthananickal A, Hansch C, Theiss J, Shimkin M, Andrews AW. A comparison of mutagenic and carcinogenic activities of aniline mustards. *J Med Chem* 1981;24:859–64.
47. Schön U, Antel J, Brückner, Messinger J. Synthesis, pharmacological characterization, and quantitative structure-activity relationship analyses of 3,7,9,9-tetraalkylbispidines: derivatives with specific bradycardic activity. *J Med Chem* 1998;41:318–31.
48. Murcia-Soler M, Péréz-Giménez F, Naldo-Molina R, Salabert-Salvador MT, García-March FJ, Cercós-del-Pozo RA et al. QSAR analysis of hypoglycaemic agents using the topological indices. *J Chem Inf Comput Sci* 2001;41:1345–54.
49. Benigni R, Giuliani A. Quantitative structure-activity relationship (QSAR) studies of mutagens and carcinogens. *Med Res Rev* 1996;16:267–84.
50. Debnath AK, Lopez de Compadre RL, Debnath G, Shusterman AJ, Hansch C. Structure-activity relationship of mutagenic aromatic and heteroaromatic nitrocompounds—correlation with molecular orbital energies and hydrophobicity. *J Med Chem* 1991;34:786–97.
51. Contrera JF, Matthews EJ, Benz RD. Predicting the carcinogenic potential of pharmaceuticals in rodents using molecular structural similarity and E-state indices. *Regul Toxicol Pharmacol* 2003;38:243–59.
52. Dearden JC, Netzeva TI. QSAR modelling of hERG potassium channel inhibition with low-dimensional descriptors. *J Pharm Pharmacol* 2004;56 Suppl: S-82.

53. Schultz TW, Moulton MP. Structure-toxicity relationships of selected naphthalene derivatives. 2. Principal components analysis. *Bull Environ Contam Toxicol* 1985;34:1–9.
54. Ridings JE, Manallack DT, Saunders MR, Baldwin JA, Livingstone DJ. Multivariate quantitative structure-toxicity relationships in a series of dopamine mimetics. *Toxicol* 1992;76:209–17.
55. Bravi G, Wikel JH. Application of MS-WHIM descriptors: 1. Introduction of new molecular surface properties and 2. Prediction of binding affinity data. *Quant Struct-Act Relat* 2000;19:29–38.
56. Poso A, Juvonen R, Gynther J. Comparative molecular field analysis of compounds with CYP2A5 binding affinity. *Quant Struct-Act Relat* 1995;14: 507–11.
57. Shi LM, Fang H, Tong W, Wu J, Perkins R, Blair R et al. QSAR models using a large diverse set of estrogens. *J Chem Inf Comput Sci* 2001;41:186–95.
58. Cavalli A, Poluzzi E, De Ponti F, Recanatini M. Toward a pharmacophore for drugs inducing the long QT syndrome: insights from a CoMFA study of HERG K^+ channel blockers. *J Med Chem* 2002;45:3844–53.
59. Pearlstein RA, Vaz RJ, Kang J, Chen X-L, Preobrazhenskaya M, Shchekotikhin AE et al. Characterisation of HERG Potassium channel inhibition using COMSiA 3D QSAR and homology modeling approaches. *Bioorg Med Chem Lett* 2003;13:1829–35.
60. Liu XH, Yang ZF, Wang LS. Three-dimensional quantitative structure-activity relationship study for phenylsulfonyl carboxylates using CoMFA and CoMSIA. *Chemosphere* 2003;53:945–52.
61. Zhao JS, Wang B, Dai ZX, Wang XD, Kong LR, Wang LS. 3D-quantitative structure-activity relationship study of organophosphate compounds. *Chinese Sci Bull* 2004;49:240–5.
62. Wang YW, Liu HX, Zhao CY, Liu HX, Cai ZW, Jiang GB. Quantitative structure-activity relationship models for prediction of the toxicity of polybrominated diphenyl ether congeners. *Environ Sci Technol* 2005;39:4961–6.
63. Bartlett A, Dearden JC, Sibley PR. Quantitative structure-activity relationships in the prediction of penicillin immunotoxicity. *Quant Struct-Act Relat* 1995; 14:258–63.
64. Basak SC, Gute BD, Mills D, Hawkins DM. Quantitative molecular similarity methods in the property/toxicity estimation of chemicals: a comparison of arbitrary versus tailored similarity spaces. *J Mol Struct (Theochem)* 2003;622: 127–45.
65. Cronin MTD, Netzeva TI, Dearden JC, Edwards R, Worgan ADP. Assessment and modeling of the toxicity of organic chemicals to *Chlorella vulgaris*: development of a novel database. *Chem Res Toxicol* 2004;17:545–54.
66. Maddalena DJ. Applications of artificial neural networks to quantitative structure-activity relationships. *Expert Opin Ther Patents* 1996;6:239–51.
67. Livingstone DJ, Manallack DT. Neural networks in 3D QSAR. *QSAR Comb Sci* 2003;22:510–8.
68. Devillers J. A general QSAR model for predicting the acute toxicity of pesticides to *Lepomis macrochirus*. *SAR QSAR Environ Res* 2001;11:397–417.

69. Devillers J. Prediction of mammalian toxicity of organophosphorus pesticides from QSTR modeling. *SAR QSAR Environ Res* 2004;15:501–10.
70. Moriguchi I, Hirano H, Hirono S. Prediction of the rodent carcinogenicity of some organic compounds from their chemical structure using the FALS method. *Environ Health Perspect* 1996;104:1051–8.
71. Livingstone DJ. Pattern recognition methods in rational drug design. In: Largone JJ, editor, *Methods in enzymology*, vol 203. San Diego: Academic Press, 1991. p. 613–38.
72. Worth AP, Cronin MTD. The use of discriminant analysis, logistic regression and classification tree analysis in the development of classification models for human health effects. *J Mol Struct (Theochem)* 2003;622:97–111.
73. Barratt MD. The role of structure-activity relationships and expert systems in alternative strategies for the determination of skin sensitisation, skin corrosivity and eye irritation. *ATLA* 1995;23:111–22.
74. Rose SL, Jurs PC. Computer-assisted studies of structure-activity relationships of *N*-nitroso compounds. *J Med Chem* 1981;25:769–76.
75. Helguera AM, Pérez MAC, González MP, Ruiz RM, Díaz HG. A topological substructural approach applied to the computational prediction of rodent carcinogenicity. *Bioorg Med Chem* 2005;13:2477–88.
76. Hosmer DW, Lemeshow S. *Applied logistic regression*. New York: John Wiley & Sons, Inc., 1989.
77. Worth AP, Cronin MTD. Embedded cluster modelling: a novel QSAR method for generating elliptic models of biological activity. In: Balls M, van Zeller A-M, editors, *Progress in the reduction, refinement and replacement of animal experimentation*. Amsterdam: Elsevier, 2000. p. 479–91.
78. Cronin MTD. The use of cluster significance analysis to identify asymmetric QSAR data sets in toxicology. An example with eye irritation data. *SAR QSAR Environ Res* 1996;5:167–75.
79. Benigni R, Richard AM. Quantitative structure-based modeling applied to characterization and prediction of chemical toxicity. *Methods* 1998;14:264–76.
80. Enslein K, Gombar VK, Blake BW, Maibach HI, Hostynek JJ, Sigman CC et al. A quantitative structure-activity relationships model for the dermal sensitization guinea pig maximization assay. *Food Chem Toxicol* 1997;35:1091–8.
81. Cunningham AR, Klopman G, Rosenkrantz HS. Identification of structural features and associated mechanisms of action for carcinogens in rats. *Mut Res Fund Mol Mech Mut* 1998;405:9–28.
82. Gomez J, Macina OT, Mattison DR, Zhang YP, Klopman G, Rosenkrantz HS. Structural determinants of developmental toxicity in hamsters. *Teratol* 1999; 60:190–205.
83. Matthews EJ, Benz RD, Contrera JF. Use of toxicological information in drug design. *J Mol Graph Modell* 2000;18:605–15.
84. www.ibmc.msk.ru/PASS
85. Filimonov DA, Poroikov VV, Borodina Y, Gloriozova T. Chemical similarity assessment through multilevel neighborhoods of atoms: definition and comparison with the other descriptors. *J Chem Inf Comput Sci* 1999;39:666–70.

86. Poroikov VV, Filimonov DA, Borodina YuV, Lagunin AA, Kos A. Robustness of biological activity spectra predicting by computer program PASS for non-congeneric sets of chemical compounds. *J Chem Inf Comput Sci* 2000; 40:1349–55.
87. Mekenyan O, Karabunarliev S, Bonchev D. The microcomputer OASIS system for predicting the biological activity of chemical compounds. *Comput Chem* 1990;14:193–200.
88. Ivanov J, Karabunarliev S, Mekenyan O. 3DGEN: a system for exhaustive 3D molecular design proceeding from molecular topology. *J Chem Inf Comput Sci* 1994;34:234–43.
89. Mekenyan OG, Bonchev DG, Enchev VG. Modeling the interaction of small organic molecules with biomacromolecules (the Oasis approach). V. Toxicity of phenols to algae "Lemna minor". *Quant Struct-Act Relat* 1988;7:240–4.
90. Woo Y-T, Lai DY, Argus MF, Arcos JC. Development of structure-activity relationship rules for predicting carcinogenic potential of chemicals. *Toxicol Lett* 1995;79:219–28.
91. Purdy R. A mechanism-mediated model for carcinogenicity: model content and prediction of the outcome of rodent carcinogenicity bioassays currently being conducted on 25 organic chemicals. *Environ Health Perspect* 1996;104:1085–94.
92. Parke DV, Ioannides C, Lewis DFV. The safety evaluation of drugs and chemicals by the use of computer-optimised molecular parametric analysis of chemical toxicity (COMPACT). *ATLA* 1990;18:91–102.
93. Lewis DFV, Ioannides C, Parke DV. Validation of a novel molecular-orbital approach (COMPACT) for the prospective safety evaluation of chemicals, by comparison with rodent carcinogenicity and *Salmonella* mutagenicity data evaluated by the United States NCI NTP. *Mut Res* 1993;291:61–77.
94. Greene N. Computer systems for the prediction of toxicity: an update. *Adv Drug Deliv Rev* 2002;54:417–31.
95. Greene N, Judson PN, Langowski JJ, Marchant CA. Knowledge-based expert systems for toxicity and metabolism prediction: DEREK, StAR and METEOR. *SAR QSAR Environ Res* 1999;10:299–314.
96. Barratt MD, Castell JV, Miranda MA, Langowski JJ. Development of an expert system rulebase for the prospective identification of photoallergens. *Photochem Photobiol B Biol* 2000;58:54–61.
97. Testa B, Balmat AL, Long A, Judson P. Predicting drug metabolism—an evaluation of the expert system METEOR. *Chem Biodiversity* 2005;2:872–85.
98. Smithing MP, Darvas F. Hazardexpert: an expert system for predicting chemical toxicity. In: Finlay JW, Robinson SF, Armstrong DJ, editors, *Food safety assessment*. Washington DC: American Chemical Society, 1992. p. 191–200.
99. Brown SJ, Raja AA, Lewis DFV. A comparison between COMPACT and Hazardexpert evaluations for 80 chemicals tested by the NTP/NCI rodent bioassay. *ATLA* 1994;22:482–500.
100. Richard AM, Benigni R. AI and SAR approaches for predicting chemical carcinogenicity: survey and status report. *SAR QSAR Environ Res* 2002;13:1–19.

101. Richard AM. Structure-based methods for predicting mutagenicity and carcinogenicity: are we there yet? *Mut Res Fund Mol Mech Mut* 1998;400:493–507.

102. Lewis DFV, Bird MG, Jacobs MN. Human carcinogens: an evaluation study via the COMPACT and HazardExpert procedures. *Hum Exper Toxicol* 2002;21: 115–22.

103. Norinder U. *In silico* modelling of ADMET—a minireview of work from 2000 to 2004. *SAR QSAR Environ Res* 2005;16:1–11.

104. Aptula AO, Cronin MTD. Prediction of hERG K^+ blocking potency: application of structural knowledge. *SAR QSAR Environ Res* 2004;15:399–411.

105. Judson PN, Cooke PA, Doerrer NG, Greene N, Hanzlik RP, Hardy C et al. Towards the creation of an international toxicology information centre. *Toxicol* 2005;213:117–28.

106. Netzeva TI, Worth AP, Aldenberg T, Benigni R, Cronin MTD, Gramatica P et al. Current status of methods for defining the applicability domain of (quantitative) structure-activity relationships. The report and recommendations of ECVAM workshop 52. *ATLA* 2005;33:152–73.

107. Barratt MD, Rodford RA. The computational prediction of toxicity. *Curr Opin Chem Biol* 2001,5:383–8.

20

COMPUTATIONAL MODELING OF DRUG DISPOSITION

Cheng Chang and Peter W. Swaan

Contents

Computer Applications in Pharmaceutical Research and Development, Edited by Sean Ekins.
ISBN 0-471-73779-8

20.1 INTRODUCTION

Historically, drug discovery has focused almost exclusively on efficacy and selectivity against the biological target. As a result, nearly half of drug candidates fail at phase II and phase III clinical trials because of undesirable drug pharmacokinetics properties, including absorption, distribution, metabolism, excretion, and toxicity (ADMET). The pressure to control the escalating cost of new drug development has changed the paradigm since the mid-1990s. To reduce the attrition rate at more expensive later stages, in vitro evaluation of ADMET properties in the early phase of drug discovery has been widely adopted. Many high-throughput in vitro ADMET property screening assays have been developed and applied successfully [1]. For example, Caco-2 and MDCK cell monolayers are widely used to simulate membrane permeability as an in vitro estimation of in vivo absorption. These in vitro results have enabled the training of *in silico* models, which could be applied to predict the ADMET properties of compounds even before they are synthesized. Fueled by the ever-increasing computational power and significant advances of *in silico* modeling algorithms, numerous computational programs that aim at modeling drug ADMET properties have emerged. A comprehensive list of available commercial ADMET modeling software has been provided previously by van de Waterbeemd and Gifford [2].

Our discussion in this chapter focuses on *in silico* modeling of drug disposition including absorption, distribution, and excretion (Fig. 20.1). We begin with a summary of *in silico* techniques in modeling drug ADMET properties, followed by a discussion of current progress in modeling different aspects of drug disposition at the systemic level. Recent advancements in modeling a diverse array of active transporters as well as their impact on drug pharmacokinetic profiles are also reviewed. This chapter concludes with the challenges and future trends of *in silico* drug disposition property modeling.

20.2 MODELING TECHNIQUES

There are mainly two types of modeling approaches. The quantitative approaches represented by pharmacophore modeling and flexible docking studies investigate the structural requirements for the interaction between drugs and the targets that are involved in ADMET processes. These are especially useful when there is an accumulation of knowledge against a certain target. For example, a set of drugs known to be transported by a transporter would enable a pharmacophore study to elucidate the minimum required structural features for transport. The availability of a protein's three-dimensional structure, from either X-ray crystallization or homology modeling, would assist flexible docking of the active ligand to derive important interactions between the protein and the ligand. Three widely used automated

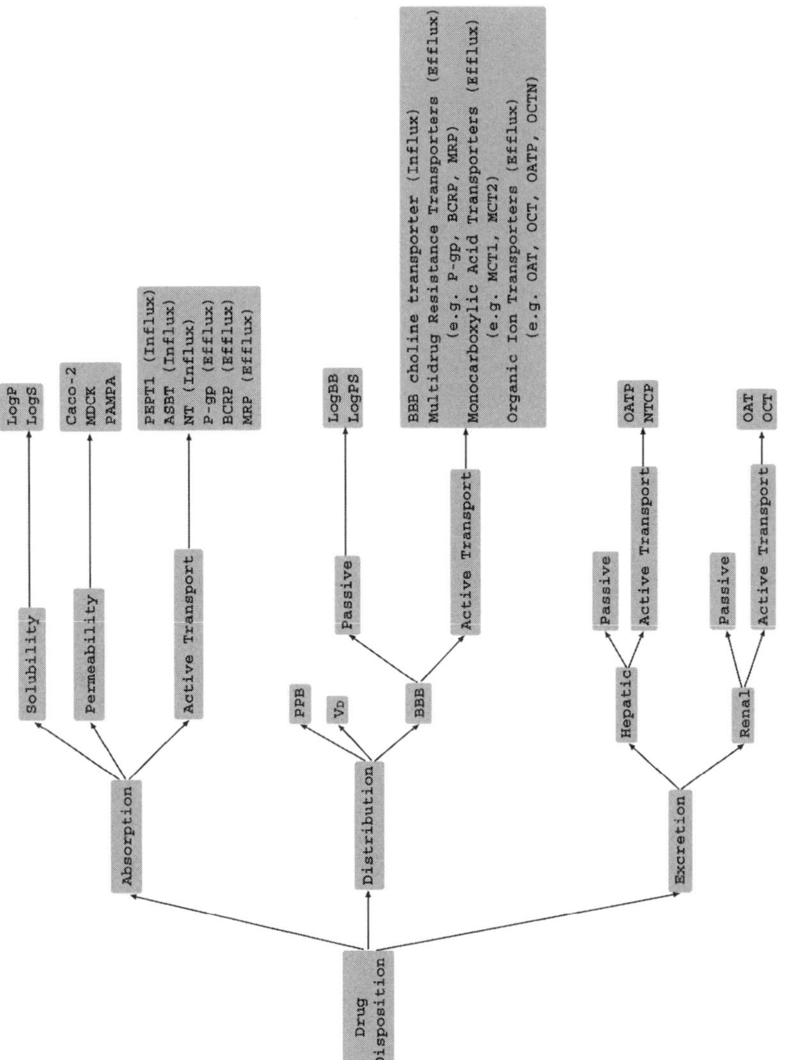

Figure 20.1 *In silico* modeling targets of drug disposition.

pharmacophore perception tools, DISCO (DIStance COmparisons) [3], GASP (Genetic Algorithm Similarity Program) [4], and Catalyst/HIPHOP [5], were critically evaluated and compared by Patel and colleagues [6]. All three programs attempt to determine common features based on the superposition of active compounds with different algorithms. The application of different flexible docking algorithms in drug discovery has recently been reviewed [7]. The essential interactions derived from either study can be used as a screen in evaluating drug ADMET properties.

The qualitative approaches represented by quantitative structure-activity relationship (QSAR) and quantitative structure-property relationship (QSPR) studies utilize multivariate analysis to correlate molecular descriptors with ADMET-related properties. A diverse range of molecular descriptors can be calculated based on the drug structure. Some of these descriptors are closely related to a physical property and are easy to comprehend (e.g., molecular weight), whereas the majority of the descriptors are of quantum mechanical concepts or interaction energies at dispersed space points that are beyond simple physicochemical parameters. When calculating correlations, it is important to select the molecular descriptors that represent the type of interactions contributing to the targeted biological property. In fact, a set of descriptors that specifically target ADME related properties has been proposed by Cruciani and colleagues [8]. The majority of published ADMET models are generated based on 2D descriptors. Even though the alignment-dependent 3D descriptors that are relevant to the targeted biological activity tend to generate the most predictive models, the difficulties inherent in structure alignment thwart attempts to apply this type of modeling in a high-throughput manner. This has prompted the development of alignment-independent 3D descriptors. However, most of these descriptors to date are still insufficiently discriminating.

A wide selection of statistical algorithms is available to researchers for correlating field descriptors with ADMET properties including simple multiple linear regression (MLR), multivariate partial least-squares (PLS), and the nonlinear regression-type algorithms such as artificial neural networks (ANN) and support vector machine (SVM). No one method can consistently perform better than the others. Just like descriptor selection, it is essential to select the right mathematical tool for most effective ADMET modeling. Sometimes it is necessary to apply multiple statistical methods and compare the results to identify the best approach, as illustrated in a recent solubility QSPR model [9].

20.3 DRUG ABSORPTION

Because of its convenience and good patient compliance, oral administration is the most preferred drug delivery form. As a result, much of the attention of *in silico* approaches is focused on modeling drug oral absorption, which mainly occurs in the human intestine. In general, drug bioavailability and absorption is the result of the interplay between drug solubility and intestinal permeability.

20.3.1 Solubility

A drug generally must dissolve before it can be absorbed from the intestinal lumen. Direct measurement of solubility is time-consuming and requires a large amount of (expensive) compound at the milligram scale. By measuring a drug's logP value (log of the partition coefficient of the compound between water and *n*-octanol) and its melting point, one could indirectly estimate solubility using the "general solubility equation" [10]. Even though the process is simplified, it still requires the synthesis of the compound. To predict the solubility of the compound even before synthesizing it, *in silico* modeling can be implemented. There are mainly two approaches to modeling solubility. One is based on the underlying physiological processes, and the other is an empirical approach.

The dissolution process involves the breaking up of the solute from its crystal lattice and the association of the solute with solvent molecules. Obviously, weaker interactions within the crystal lattice (lower melting point) and stronger interactions between solute and solvent molecules will result in better solubility and vice versa. For druglike molecules, solvent-solute interaction has been the major determinant of solubility and its prediction attracts most efforts. LogP is the simplest estimation of solvent-solute interaction and can be readily predicted with commercial programs such as CLogP (Daylight Chemical Information Systems, Aliso Viejo, CA), which utilizes a fragment-based approach. To recognize the contribution of solute crystal lattice energy in determining solubility, other approaches amended LogP values with additional terms for more accurate predictions [11, 12].

Empirical approaches, represented by QSPR, utilize multivariate analyses to identify correlations between molecular descriptors and solubility. Even though the calculation process ignores the underlying physiological processes, the molecular descriptor selection and model interpretation still requires understanding of the dissolution process. Selection of field descriptors that adequately describe the physiological process and the appropriate multivariate analysis is essential to successful modeling. The target property for most models is the logarithm of solubility (logS), and many models are trained and verified with the AQUASOL (http://www.pharmacy.arizona.edu/outreach/aquasol/) and PhysProp (http://www.syrres.com/esc/physprop.htm) databases. Lombardo and colleagues have provided a critical review of available solubility prediction algorithms [13].

20.3.2 Intestinal Permeation

Intestinal permeation describes the ability of drugs to cross the intestinal mucosa separating the gut lumen from the portal circulation. It is an essential process for drugs to pass the intestinal membrane before entering the systemic circulation to reach their target site of action. The process involves both passive diffusion and active transport. It is a complex process that is difficult to predict solely based on molecular mechanism. As a result, most current models aim to simulate in vitro membrane permeation of Caco-2, MDCK [14], or PAMPA [15], which have been a useful indicator of in vivo drug absorption [16, 17]. The current progress of intestinal permeation research has been reviewed by Malkia and colleagues [18].

20.3.3 Other Considerations

The ionization state will affect both solubility and permeability and, as a result, influence the absorption profile of a compound. Given the environmental pH, the charge of a molecule can be determined using the compound's ionization constant value (pK_a), which indicates the strength of an acid or a base. Several commercially and publicly available programs provide pK_a estimation based on the input structure, including SCSpKa (ChemSilico, Tewksbury, MA), Pallas/pKalc (CompuDrug, Sedona, AZ), ACD/pKa (ACD, Toronto, ON, Canada), and SPARC online calculator (http://ibmlc2.chem.uga.edu/sparc/index.cfm).

Both influx and efflux transporters are located in intestinal epithelial cells and can either increase or decrease oral absorption. Influx transporters such as human peptide transporter 1 (hPEPT1), apical sodium bile acid transporter (ASBT), and nucleoside transporters actively transport drugs that mimic their native substrates across the epithelial cell, whereas efflux transporters such as P-glycoprotein (P-gp), multidrug resistance-associated protein (MRP), and breast cancer resistance protein (BCRP) actively pump absorbed drugs back into the intestinal lumen.

To correctly predict overall oral absorption, drug metabolism in intestinal epithelial cells by cytochrome P450 enzymes should also be considered. The prediction of drug metabolism has already been covered in detail in Chapter 18.

Other than the different approaches mentioned above, commercial packages such as GastroPlus (Simulations Plus, Lancaster, CA) [19] and iDEA (LionBioscience, Inc. Cambridge, MA) [19] are available to predict oral absorption and other pharmacokinetic properties. They are both based on the advanced compartmental absorption and transit (CAT) model [20], which incorporates the effects of drug moving through the gastrointestinal tract and its absorption into each compartment at the same time (see also Chapter 22).

20.4 DRUG DISTRIBUTION

Distribution is an important aspect of a drug's pharmacokinetic profile. The structural and physiochemical properties of a drug determine the extent of its distribution, which is mainly reflected by three parameters: volume of distribution (V_D), plasma-protein binding (PPB), and blood-brain barrier (BBB) permeability. V_D is a measure of relative partitioning of drug between plasma and tissue, an important proportional constant that, when combined with drug clearance, could be used to predict drug half-life. The half-life of a drug is a major determinant of how often the drug should be administered. However, because of the scarcity of in vivo data and the complexity of the underlying processes, computational models that are capable of predicting V_D based solely on computed descriptors are still under development. However Lombardo and colleagues have proposed an approach to predicting V_D for neutral and basic compounds with two in vitro physicochemical parameters [21]. With additional data, this model was further expanded and the robustness of the approach was tested and validated [22]. This represents a step in the right direction in accurately predicting V_D.

Drugs bind to a variety of plasma proteins such as serum albumin. As unbound drug primarily contributes to pharmacological efficacy, the effect of PPB is an important consideration when evaluating the effective (unbound) drug plasma concentration. Several models have been proposed to predict PPB [23–27]. As suggested by Lombardo and colleagues [13], the model should not rely on the binding data of only one protein when predicting plasma protein binding because it is a composite parameter reflecting interactions with multiple proteins. Recently, Yamazaki and Kanaoka applied a nonlinear regression analysis over 300 drugs with experimental human PPB percent data. For neutral and basic drugs they found a sigmoidal correlation between logD (distribution coefficient) and PPB, and for acidic drugs the same sigmoidal correlation between logP and PPB. The model was validated with an external test set of 20 compounds. This work provides a useful approximation of PPB.

The BBB maintains the restricted extracellular environment in the central nerve system (CNS). The evaluation of drug penetration through the BBB is an integral part of the drug discovery and development process. For drugs that target the CNS, it is imperative they cross the BBB to reach their targets. Conversely, for drugs with peripheral targets, it is desirable to restrict their passage through the BBB to avoid CNS side effects. Again, because of the few experimental data derived from inconsistent protocols, most BBB permeation prediction models are of limited practical use despite intensive efforts [28–32]. Most approaches model log blood/brain (logBB), which is a measurement of the drug partitioning between blood and brain tissue. This measurement is an indirect implication of the BBB permeability, which does not discriminate between free and plasma protein-bound solute [33]. Pardridge suggests modeling of a more accurate parameter, log BBB permeability-surface area (logPS), which reflects the free drug level in brain [33]. This new concept was successfully adopted in two recent modeling studies [34, 35]. A recent review discusses key considerations for development and application of the BBB modeling [36]. In addition to forming complex tight junctions, the presence of efflux transporters and metabolic enzymes is another mechanism that the BBB employs to prevent xenobiotics from entering the CNS. Three types of drug efflux transporters have been identified from brain: multidrug resistance transporters, monocarboxylic acid transporters, and organic ion transporters. A large number of commonly prescribed drugs fall into the categories of substrates of these efflux transporters [37]. Failing to consider these active transport systems would greatly compromise accuracy of the BBB penetration prediction. Extensive substrate requirement studies have been performed for multidrug resistance transporters, especially P-gp, because of their influence on various aspects of drug discovery and development. The role of monocarboxylic acid transporters and organic ion transporters in the BBB is just being established through accumulating experimental evidence, and no computational models have been generated to date. We can expect to see such models with the accumulation of experimental data.

20.5 DRUG EXCRETION

The excretion or clearance of a drug is quantified by plasma clearance, which is defined as plasma volume that has been cleared completely free of drug per unit of time [38]. Together with V_D, it can assist in the calculation of drug half-life, thus determining dosage regime. Hepatic and renal clearances are the two main components of plasma clearance. No model has been reported that is capable of predicting plasma clearance solely from computed drug structures. Current modeling efforts are mainly focused on estimating in vivo clearance from in vitro data [39, 40]. Just like other pharmacokinetic aspects, the hepatic and renal clearance process is also complicated by the presence of active transporters. In a study performed by Sasaki and colleagues [40], the effect of active transport is incorporated by measuring in vitro data from MDCK cells that express organic anion transporting polypeptide (OATP) 4 and MRP2. However, to predict clearance for a given structure, knowledge of the structural requirements for these transporters is required.

20.6 ACTIVE TRANSPORT

Transporters should be an integral part of any ADMET modeling program because of their ubiquitous presence on barrier membranes and the substantial overlap between their substrates and many drugs. Unfortunately, because of our limited understanding of transporters, most prediction programs do not have a mechanism to incorporate the effect of active transport. However, interest in these transporters has resulted in a relatively large amount of in vitro data, which in turn have enabled the generation of pharmacophore and QSAR models for many of them. These models have assisted in the understanding of the complex effects of transporters on drug disposition, including absorption, distribution, and excretion. Their incorporation into current modeling programs would also result in more accurate prediction of drug disposition behavior. Readers are referred to a recent review for discussions of *in silico* strategies in modeling transporters [41].

20.6.1 P-gp

P-glycoprotein (P-gp) is an ATP-dependent efflux transporter that transports a broad range of substrates out of the cell. It affects drug disposition by reducing absorption and enhancing renal and hepatic excretion [42]. For example, P-gp is known to limit the intestinal absorption of the anticancer drug paclitaxel [43] and restricts the CNS penetration of human immunodeficiency virus (HIV) protease inhibitors [44]. It is also responsible for multidrug resistance in cancer chemotherapy. Because of its significance in drug disposition and effective cancer treatment, P-gp attracted numerous efforts and has become the most extensively studied transporter, with abundant experimental data [42].

Ekins and colleagues generated five computational pharmacophore models to predict the inhibition of P-gp from in vitro data on a diverse set of inhibitors with several cell systems, including inhibition of digoxin transport and verapamil binding in Caco-2 cells; vinblastine and calcein accumulation in P-gp-expressing LLC-PK1 (L-MDR1) cells; and vinblastine binding in vesicles derived from CEM/VLB100 cells [45, 46]. By comparing and merging all P-gp pharmacophore models, common areas of identical chemical features such as hydrophobes, hydrogen bond acceptors, and ring aromatic features as well as their geometric arrangement were identified to be the substrate requirements for P-gp. Similar transport requirements were reiterated in other works [47, 48]. More recently Cianchetta and colleagues combined alignment-independent 3D descriptors and physicochemical descriptors to model inhibition of calcein accumulation in Caco-2 cells [49]. Using a diverse set of 129 compounds, the authors derived a robust QSAR model that revealed two hydrophobic features, two hydrogen bond acceptors, and the molecular dimension to be essential determinants of P-gp-mediated transport. These identified transport requirements not only to help screen compounds with potential efflux related bioavailability problems, but also to assist the identification of novel P-gp inhibitors, which when coadministered with target drugs would optimize their pharmacokinetic profile by increasing bioavailability. In fact, a recent pharmacophore-based database screening has proposed 28 novel P-gp inhibitors from the Derwent World Drug Index [50]. Our own Catalyst pharmacophore searches of databases have also guided the identification of several currently prescribed drugs that are P-gp inhibitors (μM), which was previously unknown (Fig. 20.2, manuscript in preparation).

20.6.2 BCRP

Breast cancer resistance protein (BCRP) is another ATP-dependent efflux transporter that confers resistance to a variety of anticancer agents, including

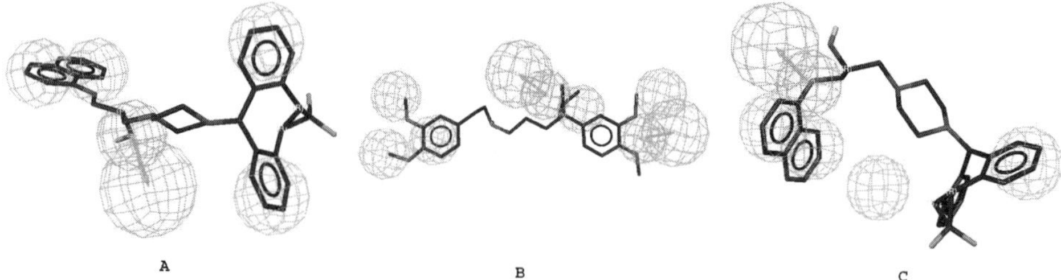

Figure 20.2 Pharmacophore models for P-gp inhibition. A. P-gp inhibition pharmacophore aligned with the potent inhibitor LY335979. B. P-gp substrate pharmacophore aligned with verapamil. C. P-gp inhibition pharmacophore 2 aligned with LY335979. Green indicates H-bond acceptor feature, and cyan indicates hydrophobic feature. See color plate.

anthracyclines and mitoxantrone [51]. In addition to a high level of expression in hematological malignancies and solid tumors, BCRP is also expressed in intestine, liver, and brain, thus implicating its intricate role in drug disposition behavior. Recently, Zhang and colleagues generated a BCRP 3D-QSAR model by analyzing structure and activity of 25 flavonoid analogs [52]. The model emphasizes very specific structural feature requirements for BCRP such as the presence of a 2,3-double bond in ring C and hydroxylation at position 5. Because the model is only based on a set of closely related structures instead of a diverse set, it should be applied with caution. Satisfying the transport model would render a compound susceptible to BCRP, but not fitting into the model does not necessarily exclude the candidate from BCRP transport. In fact, this caveat should be considered for all predictive *in silico* models, because no model can cover all possible chemical space.

20.6.3 Nucleoside Transporters

Nucleoside transporters transport both naturally occurring nucleosides and synthetic nucleoside analogs that are used as anticancer drugs (e.g., cladribine) and antiviral drugs (e.g., zalcitabine). There are different types of nucleoside transporters, including concentrative nucleoside transporters (CNT1, CNT2, CNT3) and equilibrative nucleoside transporters (ENT1, ENT2), each having different substrate specificities. The broad-affinity, low-selective ENTs are ubiquitously located, whereas the high-affinity, selective CNTs are mainly located in epithelia of intestine, kidney, liver, and brain [53], indicating their involvement in drug absorption, distribution, and excretion. The first 3D-QSAR model for nucleoside transporters was generated back in 1990 [54]. It is an oversimplified general model limited by the scarce experimental data at that time. A more comprehensive study generated distinctive models for CNT1, CNT2, and ENT1 with both pharmacophore and 3D-QSAR modeling techniques [55]. All models show the common features required for nucleoside transporter-mediated transport: two hydrophobic features and one hydrogen bond acceptor on the pentose ring. The individual models also reveal the subtle characteristic requirements for each specific transporter. The modeling results also support the previous observation that CNT2 is the most selective transporter whereas ENT1 has the broadest inhibitor specificity. More recently, we performed the same analyses and generated pharmacophore and 3D-QSAR models for CNT3 by assessing the transport activity of 33 nucleoside analogs [55a]. These studies represent a comprehensive evaluation of transport requirements of all three types of CNTs.

20.6.4 hPEPT1

The human peptide transporter (hPEPT1) is a low-affinity high-capacity oligopeptide transport system that transports a diverse range of substrates including β-lactam antibiotics [56] and angiotensin-converting enzyme (ACE) inhibitors [57]. It is mainly expressed in intestine and kidney, affecting drug absorption and excretion. A pharmacophore model based on three high-affinity substrates (Gly-Sar, bestatin, and enalapril) recognized two hydrophobic features, one hydrogen bond donor, one hydrogen bond acceptor, and one negative ionizable feature to be hPEPT1 transport requirements [58]. This pharmacophore model was subsequently applied to screen the CMC database with over 8000 druglike molecules. The antidiabetic repaglinide and HMG-CoA reductase inhibitor fluvastatin were suggested by the model and later verified to inhibit hPEPT1 with submillimolar potency [58]. This work demonstrated the potential of applying *in silico* models in high-throughput database screening.

20.6.5 ASBT

The human apical sodium-dependent bile acid transporter (ASBT) is a high-efficacy, high-capacity transporter expressed on the apical membrane of intestinal epithelial cells and cholangiocytes. It assists absorption of bile acids and their analogs, thus providing an additional intestinal target for improving drug absorption. Baringhaus and colleagues developed a pharmacophore model based on a training set of 17 chemically diverse inhibitors of ASBT [59]. The model revealed ASBT transport requirements as one hydrogen bond donor, one hydrogen bond acceptor, one negative charge, and three hydrophobic centers. These requirements are in good agreement with a previous 3D-QSAR model derived from the structure and activity of 30 ASBT inhibitors and substrates [60].

20.6.6 OCT

The organic cation transporters (OCTs) facilitate the uptake of many cationic drugs across different barrier membranes from kidney, liver, and intestine epithelia. A broad range of drugs or their metabolites fall into the chemical class of organic cation (carrying a net positive charge at physiological pH) including antiarrhythmics, β-adrenoreceptor blocking agents, antihistamines, antiviral agents, and skeletal muscle-relaxing agents [61]. Three OCTs have been cloned from different species, OCT1, OCT2, and OCT3. A human OCT1 pharmacophore model was developed by analyzing the extent of inhibition of TEA uptake in HeLa cells of 22 diverse molecules. The model suggests the transport requirements of human OCT1 as three hydrophobic features and one positive ionizable feature [62]. Molecular determinants of substrate binding to human OCT2 and rabbit OCT2 were recently reported [63]. Both 2D- and 3D-QSAR analyses were performed to identify and discriminate the binding requirements of the two orthologs. The models showed the same chemical features, highlighting their similarities. However, the orientation of a critical hydrogen bonding feature set the two orthologs apart. This work illustrates the sensitivity of *in silico* modeling in discriminating similar transporters.

20.6.7 OATP

Organic anion transporting polypeptides (OATPs) influence the plasma concentration of many drugs by actively transporting them across a diverse range of tissue membranes such as liver, intestine, lung, and brain [64]. Because of their broad substrate specificity, OATPs transport not only organic anionic drugs, as originally thought, but also organic cationic drugs. Currently 11 human OATPs have been identified, and the substrate binding requirements of the best-studied OATP1B1 were successfully modeled with the metapharmacophore approach recently [65]. Through assessing a training set of 18 diverse molecules, the metapharmacophore model identified three hydrophobic features flanked by two hydrogen bond acceptor features to be the essential requirement for OATP1B1 transport. Similar requirements were derived from another 3D-QSAR study based on rat Oatp1a5 [66].

20.6.8 BBB-Choline Transporter

The BBB-choline transporter is a native nutrient transporter that transports choline, a charged cation, across the BBB into the CNS [67]. Its active transport assists the BBB penetration of cholinelike compounds, and understanding its structural requirements should afford a more accurate prediction of BBB permeation. Even though the BBB-choline transporter has not been cloned, Geldenhuys and colleagues applied a combination of empirical and theoretical methodologies to study its binding requirements [68]. The 3D-QSAR models were built with empirical K_i data obtained from in situ rat brain perfusion experiments with a structurally diverse set of compounds. Three hydrophobic interactions and one hydrogen bonding interaction surrounding the positively charged ammonium moiety were identified to be important for BBB-choline transporter recognition. Even though the model statistical significance is not optimal ($q^2 < 0.5$), it does provide a useful estimation of BBB-choline transporter binding requirements. More accurate *in silico* models could be generated once higher-quality data from the cloned BBB-choline transporter are available.

20.7 CURRENT CHALLENGES AND FUTURE DIRECTIONS

Two years ago, several reviews [e.g., 2, 13] pointed out that data quality is the most limiting factor in ADMET modeling. We believe that data quality is still the weakest link, thereby effectively limiting the practical application of ADMET models. The major recent advancement in ADMET modeling is in elucidating the role and successful modeling of various transporters [45, 46, 48, 50, 52, 55, 58–60, 62, 63, 65, 66, 68, 69]. Incorporation of the influence of these transporters into current models is an ongoing task in ADMET modeling. Some commercial programs have already implemented the capability of modeling active transport, such as the recent versions of GastroPlus (Simulations Plus, Lancaster, CA), PK-Sim (Bayer Technology Services, Germany), and ADME/Tox WEB (Pharma Algorithms, Toronto, ON, Canada). A successful implementation of active transport as a filter is exemplified in the ADME/Tox WEB absorption prediction program [70]. Compounds are first screened against pharmacophore models of different active transporters. The compound that fits these models is removed from further predictions, which is based solely on physicochemical properties.

Importantly, the currently available transporter models only cover a small fraction of all transporters involved in drug disposition. Other than incorporating current stand-alone transporter models into systemic models to directly predict drug pharmacokinetic properties, continued efforts are still needed to investigate other transporters such as MRP, BCRP, NTCP, and OAT, to get a more complete understanding of the drug pharmacokinetic profile.

Not all pharmaceutical companies can afford the resources to generate their own in-house modeling programs, so the commercially available *in silico* modeling suites have become an attractive option. However, this leads to a potential problem: The chemical space that these commercial packages are developed from might not be directly related to the company's chemical scope. *In silico* models are most predictive when applied in the same chemical space as the training compounds. As a result, a decreased predictive power is to be expected when the model is applied to a different chemical space. The fact that the majority of these programs do not offer capabilities to customize parameters aggravates the above-mentioned problem. In answer to this, some modeling programs such as Algorithm Builder (Pharma Algorithms, Toronto, ON, Canada) are offering flexibility for customers to generate their in-house models with their own training set and the statistical algorithm of their choice. Additionally, we should expect more mechanism-based modeling algorithms that are easy to understand and implement owing to a more detailed understanding of underlying mechanisms for different aspects of drug disposition.

These trends will accelerate the shift of model building from computational scientists to experimental scientists.

As discussed above, all ADMET aspects are dependent on each other and should all be considered when making predictions. Integrated analysis of different aspects of drug pharmacokinetic profiles is yet another future trend. Ultimately, drug ADMET properties should be predicted based on an integration of a compilation of *in silico* models reflecting different aspects of the process.

REFERENCES

1. Ekins S, Nikolsky Y and Nikolskaya T. Techniques: Application of systems biology to absorption, distribution, metabolism, excretion, and toxicity. *Trends Pharmacol Sci* 2005;26:202–9.
2. van de Waterbeemd H and Gifford E. ADMET in silico modelling: towards prediction paradise? *Nat Rev Drug Discov* 2003;2:192–204.
3. Martin YC, Bures MG, Danaher EA, DeLazzer J, Lico I and Pavlik PA. A fast new approach to pharmacophore mapping and its application to dopaminergic and benzodiazepine agonists. *J Comput Aided Mol Des* 1993;7:83–102.
4. Jones G, Willett P and Glen RC. A genetic algorithm for flexible molecular overlay and pharmacophore elucidation. *J Comput Aided Mol Des* 1995;9: 532–49.
5. Clement OO and Mehl AT. HipHop: pharmacophore based on multiple common-feature alignments. In: Guner OF, editor, *Pharmacophore perception, development, and use in drug design.* San Diego: IUL, 2000. pp. 69–84.
6. Patel Y, Gillet VJ, Bravi G and Leach AR. A comparison of the pharmacophore identification programs: Catalyst, DISCO and GASP. *J Comput Aided Mol Des* 2002;16:653–81.
7. Schneidman-Duhovny D, Nussinov R and Wolfson HJ. Predicting molecular interactions *in silico*: II. Protein-protein and protein-drug docking. *Curr Med Chem* 2004;11:91–107.
8. Cruciani G, Pastor M and Guba W. VolSurf: a new tool for the pharmacokinetic optimization of lead compounds. *Eur J Pharm Sci* 2000;11 Suppl 2:S29–39.
9. Eros D, Keri G, Kovesdi I, Szantai-Kis C, Meszaros G and Orfi L. Comparison of predictive ability of water solubility QSPR models generated by MLR, PLS and ANN methods. *Mini Rev Med Chem* 2004;4:167–77.
10. Yang G, Ran Y and Yalkowsky SH. Prediction of the aqueous solubility: comparison of the general solubility equation and the method using an amended solvation energy relationship. *J Pharm Sci* 2002;91:517–33.
11. Butina D and Gola JM. Modeling aqueous solubility. *J Chem Inf Comput Sci* 2003;43:837–41.
12. Delaney JS. ESOL: estimating aqueous solubility directly from molecular structure. *J Chem Inf Comput Sci* 2004;44:1000–5.
13. Lombardo F, Gifford E and Shalaeva MY. *In silico* ADME prediction: data, models, facts and myths. *Mini Rev Med Chem* 2003;3:861–75.

14. Refsgaard HH, Jensen BF, Brockhoff PB, Padkjaer SB, Guldbrandt M and Christensen MS. In silico prediction of membrane permeability from calculated molecular parameters. *J Med Chem* 2005;48:805–11.
15. Fujikawa M, Ano R, Nakao K, Shimizu R and Akamatsu M. Relationships between structure and high-throughput screening permeability of diverse drugs with artificial membranes: application to prediction of Caco-2 cell permeability. *Bioorg Med Chem* 2005;13:4721–32.
16. Artursson P and Karlsson J. Correlation between oral drug absorption in humans and apparent drug permeability coefficients in human intestinal epithelial (Caco-2) cells. *Biochem Biophys Res Commun* 1991;175:880–5.
17. Irvine JD, Takahashi L, Lockhart K, Cheong J, Tolan JW, Selick HE, et al. MDCK (Madin-Darby canine kidney) cells: a tool for membrane permeability screening. *J Pharm Sci* 1999;88:28–33.
18. Malkia A, Murtomaki L, Urtti A and Kontturi K. Drug permeation in biomembranes: in vitro and in silico prediction and influence of physicochemical properties. *Eur J Pharm Sci* 2004;23:13–47.
19. Agoram B, Woltosz WS and Bolger MB. Predicting the impact of physiological and biochemical processes on oral drug bioavailability. *Adv Drug Deliv Rev* 2001;50 Suppl 1:S41–67.
20. Yu LX, Lipka E, Crison JR and Amidon GL. Transport approaches to the biopharmaceutical design of oral drug delivery systems: prediction of intestinal absorption. *Adv Drug Deliv Rev* 1996;19:359–76.
21. Lombardo F, Obach RS, Shalaeva MY and Gao F. Prediction of volume of distribution values in humans for neutral and basic drugs using physicochemical measurements and plasma protein binding data. *J Med Chem* 2002;45:2867–76.
22. Lombardo F, Obach RS, Shalaeva MY and Gao F. Prediction of human volume of distribution values for neutral and basic drugs. 2. Extended data set and leave-class-out statistics. *J Med Chem* 2004;47:1242–50.
23. Colmenarejo G, Alvarez-Pedraglio A and Lavandera JL. Cheminformatic models to predict binding affinities to human serum albumin. *J Med Chem* 2001;44:4370–8.
24. Kratochwil NA, Huber W, Muller F, Kansy M and Gerber PR. Predicting plasma protein binding of drugs: a new approach. *Biochem Pharmacol* 2002;64:1355–74.
25. Lobell M and Sivarajah V. In silico prediction of aqueous solubility, human plasma protein binding and volume of distribution of compounds from calculated pKa and AlogP98 values. *Mol Divers* 2003;7:69–87.
26. Mager DE and Jusko WJ. Quantitative structure-pharmacokinetic/pharmacodynamic relationships of corticosteroids in man. *J Pharm Sci* 2002;91:2441–51.
27. Yamazaki K and Kanaoka M. Computational prediction of the plasma protein-binding percent of diverse pharmaceutical compounds. *J Pharm Sci* 2004;93:1480–94.
28. Cabrera MA, Bermejo M, Perez M and Ramos R. TOPS-MODE approach for the prediction of blood-brain barrier permeation. *J Pharm Sci* 2004;93:1701–17.
29. Ecker GF and Noe CR. In silico prediction models for blood-brain barrier permeation. *Curr Med Chem* 2004;11:1617–28.

30. Li H, Yap CW, Ung CY, Xue Y, Cao ZW and Chen YZ., Effect of selection of molecular descriptors on the prediction of blood-brain barrier penetrating and nonpenetrating agents by statistical learning methods. *J Chem Inf Model* 2005;45:1376–1384.
31. Narayanan R and Gunturi SB. *In silico* ADME modelling: prediction models for blood-brain barrier permeation using a systematic variable selection method. *Bioorg Med Chem* 2005;13:3017–28.
32. Subramanian G and Kitchen DB. Computational models to predict blood-brain barrier permeation and CNS activity. *J Comput Aided Mol Des* 2003;17:643–64.
33. Pardridge WM, Log(BB). PS products and in silico models of drug brain penetration. *Drug Discov Today* 2004;9:392–3.
34. Abraham MH. The factors that influence permeation across the blood-brain barrier. *Eur J Med Chem* 2004;39:235–40.
35. Liu X, Tu M, Kelly RS, Chen C and Smith BJ. Development of a computational approach to predict blood-brain barrier permeability. *Drug Metab Dispos* 2004;32:132–9.
36. Goodwin JT and Clark DE., In silico predictions of blood-brain barrier penetration: considerations to "keep in mind". *J Pharmacol Exp Ther* 2005.
37. Taylor EM. The impact of efflux transporters in the brain on the development of drugs for CNS disorders. *Clin Pharmacokinet* 2002;41:81–92.
38. Toutain PL and Bousquet-Melou A. Plasma clearance. *J Vet Pharmacol Ther* 2004;27:415–25.
39. Ito K and Houston JB. Prediction of human drug clearance from in vitro and preclinical data using physiologically based and empirical approaches. *Pharm Res* 2005;22:103–12.
40. Sasaki M, Suzuki H, Aoki J, Ito K, Meier PJ and Sugiyama Y. Prediction of in vivo biliary clearance from the in vitro transcellular transport of organic anions across a double-transfected Madin-Darby canine kidney II monolayer expressing both rat organic anion transporting polypeptide 4 and multidrug resistance associated protein 2. *Mol Pharmacol* 2004;66:450–9.
41. Chang C, Ray A and Swaan P. *In silico* strategies for modeling membrane transporter function. *Drug Discov Today* 2005;10:663–71.
42. Lin JH and Yamazaki M. Role of P-glycoprotein in pharmacokinetics: clinical implications. *Clin Pharmacokinet* 2003;42:59–98.
43. Sparreboom A, van Asperen J, Mayer U, Schinkel AH, Smit JW, Meijer DK, et al. Limited oral bioavailability and active epithelial excretion of paclitaxel (Taxol) caused by P-glycoprotein in the intestine. *Proc Natl Acad Sci USA* 1997;94:2031–5.
44. Polli JW, Jarrett JL, Studenberg SD, Humphreys JE, Dennis SW, Brouwer KR, et al. Role of P-glycoprotein on the CNS disposition of amprenavir (141W94), an HIV protease inhibitor. *Pharm Res* 1999;16:1206–12.
45. Ekins S, Kim RB, Leake BF, Dantzig AH, Schuetz E, Lan LB, et al. Application of three dimensional quantitative structure-activity relationships of P-glycoprotein inhibitors and substrates. *Mol Pharmacol* 2002;61:974–981.

46. Ekins S, Kim RB, Leake BF, Dantzig AH, Schuetz EG, Lan LB, et al. Three-dimensional quantitative structure-activity relationships of inhibitors of P-glycoprotein. *Mol Pharmacol* 2002;61:964–73.

47. Pajeva IK and Wiese M. Pharmacophore model of drugs involved in P-glycoprotein multidrug resistance: explanation of structural variety (hypothesis). *J Med Chem* 2002;45:5671–5686.

48. Yates CR, Chang C, Kearbey JD, Yasuda K, Schuetz EG, Miller DD, et al. Structural determinants of P-glycoprotein-mediated transport of glucocorticoids. *Pharm Res* 2003;20:1794–803.

49. Cianchetta G, Singleton RW, Zhang M, Wildgoose M, Giesing D, Fravolini A, et al. A pharmacophore hypothesis for P-glycoprotein substrate recognition using GRIND-based 3D-QSAR. *J Med Chem* 2005;48:2927–35.

50. Langer T, Eder M, Hoffmann RD, Chiba P and Ecker GF. Lead identification for modulators of multidrug resistance based on in silico screening with a pharmacophoric feature model. *Arch Pharm (Weinheim)* 2004;337:317–27.

51. Mao Q and Unadkat JD. Role of the breast cancer resistance protein (ABCG2) in drug transport. *AAPS J* 2005;7:E118–33.

52. Zhang S, Yang X, Coburn RA and Morris ME. Structure activity relationships and quantitative structure activity relationships for the flavonoid-mediated inhibition of breast cancer resistance protein. *Biochem Pharmacol* 2005;70:627–39.

53. Aymerich I, Duflot S, Fernandez-Veledo S, Guillen-Gomez E, Huber-Ruano I, Casado FJ, et al. The concentrative nucleoside transporter family (SLC28): new roles beyond salvage? *Biochem Soc Trans* 2005;33:216–9.

54. Viswanadhan VN, Ghose AK and Weinstein JN. Mapping the binding site of the nucleoside transporter protein: a 3D-OSAR study. *Biochim Biophys Acta* 1990;1039:356–66.

55. Chang C, Swaan PW, Ngo LY, Lum PY, Patil SD and Unadkat JD. Molecular requirements of the human nucleoside transporters hCNT1, hCNT2, and hENT1. *Mol Pharmacol* 2004;65:558–70.

55a. Hu H, Endres CJ, Chang C, Umapathy NS, Lee EW, Fei YJ, et al. Electrophysiological Characterization and Modeling of the Structure Activity Relationship of the Human Concentrative Nucleoside Transporter 3 (hCNT3). *Mol Pharmacol* 2006; in press.

56. Snyder NJ, Tabas LB, Berry DM, Duckworth DC, Spry DO and Dantzig AH. Structure-activity relationship of carbacephalosporins and cephalosporins: antibacterial activity and interaction with the intestinal proton-dependent dipeptide transport carrier of Caco-2 cells. *Antimicrob Agents Chemother* 1997;41:1649–57.

57. Leibach FH and Ganapathy V. Peptide transporters in the intestine and the kidney. *Annu Rev Nutr* 1996;16:99–119.

58. Ekins S, Johnston JS, Bahadduri P, D'Souza VM, Ray A, Chang C, et al. In vitro and pharmacophore-based discovery of novel hPEPT1 inhibitors. *Pharm Res* 2005;22:512–7.

59. Baringhaus KH, Matter H, Stengelin S and Kramer W. Substrate specificity of the ileal and the hepatic Na^+/bile acid cotransporters of the rabbit. II. A reliable

3D QSAR pharmacophore model for the ileal Na^+/bile acid cotransporter. *J Lipid Res* 1999;40:2158–68.

60. Swaan PW, Szoka FC, Jr. and Oie S. Molecular modeling of the intestinal bile acid carrier: a comparative molecular field analysis study. *J Comput Aided Mol Des* 1997;11:581–8.
61. Wright SH and Dantzler WH. Molecular and cellular physiology of renal organic cation and anion transport. *Physiol Rev* 2004;84:987–1049.
62. Bednarczyk D, Ekins S, Wikel JH and Wright SH. Influence of molecular structure on substrate binding to the human organic cation transporter, hOCT1. *Mol Pharmacol* 2003;63:489–98.
63. Suhre WM, Ekins S, Chang C, Swaan PW and Wright SH. Molecular determinants of substrate/inhibitor binding to the human and rabbit renal organic cation transporters hOCT2 and rbOCT2. *Mol Pharmacol* 2005;67:1067–77.
64. Tamai I, Nezu J, Uchino H, Sai Y, Oku A, Shimane M, et al. Molecular identification and characterization of novel members of the human organic anion transporter (OATP) family. *Biochem Biophys Res Commun* 2000;273:251–60.
65. Chang C, Pang KS, Swaan PW, Ekins S. Comparative pharmacophore modeling of organic anion transporting polypeptides: a meta-analysis of rat Oatp1a1 and human OATP1B1. *J Pharmacol Exp Ther* 2005; 314:533–41.
66. Yarim M, Moro S, Huber R, Meier PJ, Kaseda C, Kashima T, et al. Application of QSAR analysis to organic anion transporting polypeptide 1a5 (Oatp1a5) substrates. *Bioorg Med Chem* 2005;13:463–71.
67. Allen DD and Smith QR. Characterization of the blood-brain barrier choline transporter using the in situ rat brain perfusion technique. *J Neurochem* 2001;76:1032–41.
68. Geldenhuys WJ, Lockman PR, McAfee JH, Fitzpatrick KT, Van der Schyf CJ and Allen DD. Molecular modeling studies on the active binding site of the blood-brain barrier choline transporter. *Bioorg Med Chem Lett* 2004;14:3085–92.
69. Zhang EY, Phelps MA, Cheng C, Ekins S and Swaan PW. Modeling of active transport systems. *Adv Drug Deliv Rev* 2002;54:329–54.
70. Zmuidinavicius D, Didziapetris R, Japertas P, Avdeef A and Petrauskas A. Classification structure-activity relations (C-SAR) in prediction of human intestinal absorption. *J Pharm Sci* 2003;92:621–33.

21

COMPUTER SIMULATIONS IN PHARMACOKINETICS AND PHARMACODYNAMICS: REDISCOVERING SYSTEMS PHYSIOLOGY IN THE 21ST CENTURY

PAOLO VICINI

Contents

21.1 INTRODUCTION

Perhaps no technology in human history has radically changed so many disciplines as the introduction of personal computing and the now-ubiquitous presence of the World Wide Web. What the joint application of these enabling technologies allows us to do is to instantaneously and efficiently exchange

Computer Applications in Pharmaceutical Research and Development, Edited by Sean Ekins.
ISBN 0-471-73779-8

robust, verifiable, and consistent information. An area that has benefited enormously from this is what is sometimes termed as "biocomputation," or the revolutionary transformation of biological and biomedical research from a painstaking endeavor often reserved for bench and field researchers to a discipline based on prompt availability of information and data mining (Fig. 21.1). However, clearly outlining what is exactly entailed by "biocomputation," or "biomedical simulations," is more often than not a challenge. Terms like "systems biology" and "bioinformatics" are increasingly used in multiple settings, but the multiple meanings behind them and especially the expectations associated with these technologies are not always clear. Some even draw a distinction between "biomedical informatics" and "bioinformatics," not unlike those who distinguish between "bioengineering" and "biomedical engineering." The very fact that biomedical computation has become so pervasive has made it difficult to draw clear boundaries between areas and to unambiguously define areas of expertise and/or influence for practitioners that are now extending computer modeling to virtually every aspect of the biomedical enterprise "from bench to bedside"[1], all the way from clinical record management to computer-aided drug design, through clinical trial simulation, therapeutic drug monitoring, pharmacogenomics, and molecular engineering.

The information revolution in biology has been facilitated, and in a very real sense motivated, by the emphasis placed on "discovery science"[2] projects such as the Human Genome Project and the various databasing efforts needed to somehow coordinate and manage the increasing amount of bioinformation being generated by thousands of laboratories worldwide. This has coincided with a scientific change of emphasis that is best tracked through the different interpretations and meanings associated with the phrase "systems biology" nowadays and a few decades ago. According to Guyton [3] and other holistic physiologists, a living homeostatic system was thought of as being comprised of a series of interacting parts, or subsystems, an understanding of which was deemed essential to comprehension of the complex dynamics of the whole. However, the starting point at that time was the intact system, as it was believed that only through information gathered on the macroscopic behavior of the whole could one understand the inner workings of the parts. Since Aristotle's proposal that "the whole is more than the sum of the parts," direct investigation of the living system was essential. The approach was "top to bottom." This point of view shifted with the advent of molecular biology, which brought within reach the possibility of looking directly at the parts themselves at an unprecedented level of biophysical detail. A clear, unambiguous, and validated understanding of the parts would in time, researchers argued, lead to an understanding of how they interact and how they conspire to shape the dynamic performance of the intact, living system. This in turn motivated a paradigm shift from clinical sciences to basic sciences, and in pharmaceutical sciences from clinical pharmacology to molecular pharmacology. This is the "bottom to top"

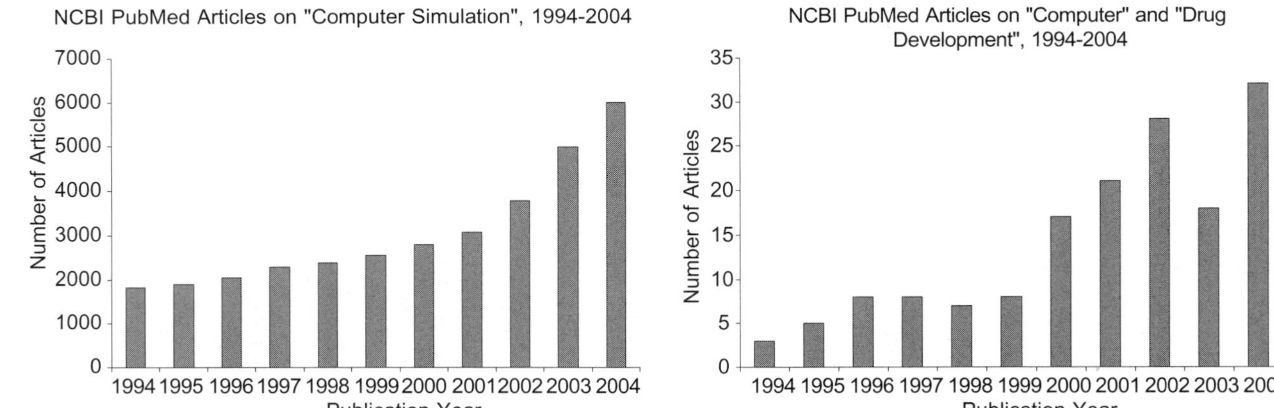

Figure 21.1 The emergence of computer simulation in the peer-reviewed biomedical literature as represented in NCBI's PubMed. The database is available at http://www.pubmed.org, and the searches were carried out on September 17, 2005.

approach to biomedical research. Clearly, with so much information at their fingertips, modern biologists should have more than enough ammunition to build comprehensive, testable models of biosystems: *Possunt quia posse videntur.* However, what could not be anticipated is that unexpected complexity lurked in the modalities of interactions of the ingredients that make up a living system, so that mathematical and computer representations of comparatively simple subsystems tend to be almost invariably much more complex than the whole, living system of which they are a part [4]. This has turned into a somewhat unsatisfactory situation for modern biological research, where the need to refocus is periodically felt, for example, through initiatives such as the NIH Roadmap [5] and changes to NIH peer review criteria [6].

The drug development process was also influenced by these changes in perspective, but in a slightly different way. Because drug development must remain focused on the clinical outcome, or, in other words, it has to generate drugs that are safe and effective, the shift to molecular pharmacology has, at least in the private sector, been accompanied by a continued presence of the tenets of clinical pharmacology, in a beneficial synergy that includes the best of both worlds [7]. This has not necessarily been the case in academia, where training programs in clinical pharmacology have become few and far between and the emphasis is on basic science, sometimes at the expense of traditional disciplines such as pharmacokinetics and pharmacodynamics [8].

What happens in drug development these days is a recasting of Guyton's all-encompassing, whole-system quantification approach, balanced by an increased awareness of the "parts list" that comes from molecular biology [9]. Thanks to the pragmatism that characterizes the drug development process, these two different emphases are both used to lead to the creation of better therapeutics. The FDA, for example, has been rather well positioned to take advantage of advances in biocomputation and has introduced recent developments in computational modeling in the development process through the issue of guidances and consensus documents [10]. The same is happening at other federal agencies. The EPA is becoming increasingly aware [11] of the potential advantage [12] of aggressively using computational representations of complex systems to predict likely system behavior, or at least narrow down the field of possibilities. DARPA has started a project, termed Virtual Soldier, to achieve the rather ambitious goal of creating physiological, mathematical, and software representations of individual soldiers [13].

In this chapter, we describe some of the advances in biocomputation that have impacted or potentially will impact pharmaceutical research and development. We list them by "biological size," going from the most to the least organized, or from the most complex to the least complex. We focus on clinical sciences in particular, because we feel that simplified, but useful representations of pharmacological interventions have the greatest potential for shortening the development process and weeding out potentially unsatisfactory candidates. The discussion is articulated along four levels, roughly following the idea of "biological size." which will carry us from whole organism to genetic networks through the analysis of biocomputation applications to isolated organs, cells, and molecules.

21.2 LEVEL 1: COMPUTER SIMULATION OF THE WHOLE ORGANISM

In a sense, being able to model the whole organism is the essential goal of biocomputing. In drug development, it provides the obligatory handle to lead to response from exposure (Fig. 21.2). Provided the intact organism can be mathematically represented, a whole series of possibilities can be brought into practice, such as the simulation of clinical trials and of the prospective behavior of entire populations. In drug development, whole body systems are usually represented in one of two ways. The first approach is through the formalization of a lumped-parameter PK-PD model [14], often coupled with a model of the disease process [15], whose parameters can be estimated from data. A relatively small number of differential equations, between one and ten, is used to predict the system's behavior over time [16]. Often, but not always, some variation of population PK-PD [17], predicated on nonlinear regression and nonlinear mixed-effects models [18], is used to estimate both the population parameter values and their statistical distribution. The same approach can be taken in reverse [19] by using models to generate synthetic data, ultimately performing a full clinical trial simulation from first principles [20]. The other approach to whole organism models is based on physiological modeling [21], brought into practice by physiologically based pharmacokinetic (PBPK) models [22]. These models are still based on ordinary differential equations, but they attempt to describe the organism and especially the interacting organs with more detail, often by increasing the number of differential equations (from 10 to perhaps 30) and building appropriate interactions between

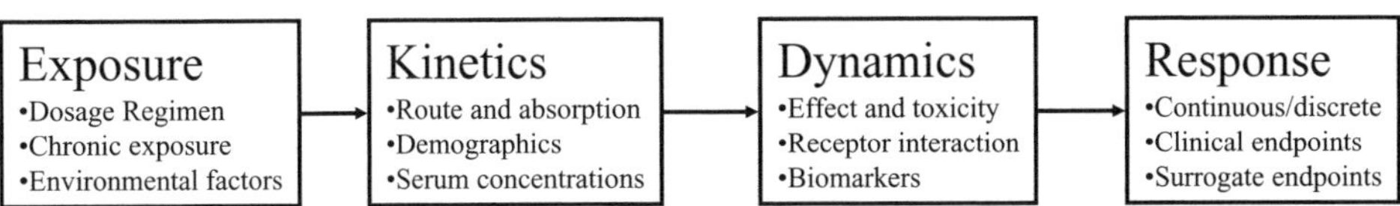

Figure 21.2 The exposure-response road map passes through pharmacokinetics and pharmacodynamics. This sequence of events is essentially the same as that which informs computer simulation of clinical trials, with the addition of complicating, but important, factors such as protocol adherence and dropouts.

the organs that resemble their physical arrangement in the organism being studied.

Although the representation of the intact organism provided by PK-PD and PBPK models is simplified, it does pose nontraditional challenges. For PK-PD, the purpose consists in finding the best (simplest?) model that can explain the observations [23]. Formally speaking, the concept of "best" is difficult to define unambiguously. More often than not, model selection is driven by some kind of parsimony criterion that balances model complexity with the actual information content provided by the measurements. A consensus workshop developed some time ago a set of "good practices" that can serve as guidance to model development, selection, and application [24]. PBPK models come at the problem from a different angle [25]. Because they embed previous knowledge about the organ kinetics, their arrangements, and their specific parameter values, the process of tailoring the model to the specific measurements at hand is not as crucial. On the other hand, PBPK models can suffer greatly in their predictive power if their parameterization is inaccurate, poorly specified, or not well tailored to the particular drug. Many researchers split PBPK model parameters and structures into "drug specific" and "not drug specific," thus implying that the model can indeed capture some underlying dynamics that are general for all drugs, and that further specification can be limited to the exclusive characteristics of a certain molecule. It is also very important to specify parameter and structure uncertainty when dealing with model-based predictions [26]. More detail on how these parameters can be specified is also provided below. The approach taken by PBPK modeling is not very dissimilar from the recently proposed Physiome Project [27], a "parts list" of the human organism whose development follows the broad strokes of the Human Genome Project. More often than not, the rate-limiting step for development of PBPK models is the availability of information on single-organ parameters, such as clearance rates and partition coefficients [28]. An exhaustive list of these such as the one that the Physiome Project may provide could certainly be of use to the biomedical investigator. As we have mentioned above, the EPA is also showing interest in computer-based prediction of individual pharmacokinetics and has recently released a document detailing the technology for public comment. Finally, it is worthwhile to note that there have been recent advances in the understanding of the mechanistic underpinnings of whole organism homeostasis [29] that have not yet been aggressively applied in drug development (where they would be most useful, one would expect, for between- and within-species scaling).

It is interesting to note that the foremost challenges for the detailed modeling of the intact organism (computing time, complexity of interactions, model selection) are very similar to those entailed by the analysis of proteomic or genomic data. In the clinical case, complexity shifts from the richness of the data set to the model formulation, whereas in the proteomic-genomic case the main source of difficulties is the sheer size of the data set; however, at least at present, interpretative tools are rather uncomplicated.

21.3 LEVEL 2: COMPUTER SIMULATION OF ISOLATED TISSUES AND ORGANS

The behavior of molecules in isolated organs has been the subject of extensive investigation. The heart [30] and the liver [31] were historically the organs most extensively investigated [32], although the kidney [33] and brain [34] have also been the subjects of mathematical modeling research. The liver in particular has been extensively researched both in the biomedical [35] and pharmaceutical [36] literature. Many of the computer simulations for the heart and liver were carried out with distributed blood-tissue exchange (BTEX) models [37], because the increased level of detail and temporal resolution certainly makes the good mixing and uniformity hypotheses at the basis of lumped parameter models less tenable [38]. The work of Goresky, Bassingthwaighte, and others has spearheaded this area of development for mathematical modeling, and in recent times drug development has rediscovered some of the analytical tools proposed by this research community [39]. It can be speculated that the integration of organ-specific modeling with the above whole-organism models would result in improvements for the PBPK approach through "better" (i.e., more physiologically sensible and plausible) models of individual organs. The main challenge in doing so is the required shift from lumped to distributed parameter models. The jump to partial differential equations is fraught with difficulties, especially because the average bench biologist often has a lot of trouble grasping the concepts behind ordinary differential equations as well. This motivates the question of which is the audience for these technologies, or who is expected to be a user for the various software and a reader for the papers. There is an enormous variety of software for pharmacokinetic and pharmacodynamic simulations, with a partial list available in Table 21.1 and more updated lists available elsewhere [40].

As an example of infrastructure endeavors, a new project funded by the National Institute for General Medical Sciences at the NIH, the Center for Modeling Integrated Metabolic Systems (MIMS) [41], has as its mission the development and integration of in vivo, organ-specific mathematical models that can successfully predict behaviors for a range of parameters, including rest and exercise and various pathophysiological conditions. The Microcirculation Physiome [42] and the Cardiome [43] are other multicenter projects focused on particular aspects of the Physiome undertaking. One prevalent concept that seems to emerge in these large-scale projects is that of interdisciplinary collaboration, and especially of the need to tap many areas of expertise for the solution of these problems. It seems widely accepted that the development of integrated computational representations of biological systems has to borrow from many fields, if nothing else because of the multidisciplinary complexity that some of these endeavors imply.

TABLE 21.1

Name	Manufacturer/Distributor	Web Site
acslXtreme	Xcellon and AEgis Technologies Group	http://www.aegisxcellon.com/
ADAPT II	Biomedical Simulations Resource (USC)	http://bmsr.usc.edu/
Berkeley Madonna	University of California-Berkeley	http://www.berkeleymadonna.com/
GastroPlus	Simulations Plus	http://www.simulations-plus.com
GNU Octave	University of Wisconsin	http://www.octave.org/
JSim	National Simulation Resource	http://nsr.bioeng.washington.edu/PLN/
Kinetica	Thermo Electron Corporation	http://www.thermo.com
MATLAB-Simulink	The MathWorks	http://www.mathworks.com/
MLAB	Civilized Software	Inc: http://www.civilized.com/
ModelMaker	ModelKinetix	http://www.modelkinetix.com/
NONMEM	University of California at San Francisco and Globomax ICON	http://www.globomaxservice.com
PhysioLab	Entelos	http://www.entelos.com/
PKBUGS	Imperial College at St Mary's Hospital London	http://www.mrc-bsu.cam.ac.uk/bugs/
PopKinetics	SAAM Institute	http://www.saam.com
R	The R Project Group	http://www.r-project.org/
SAAM II	SAAM Institute	http://www.saam.com
S-PLUS	Insightful	http://www.insightful.com/
Stella	isee Systems (formerly High Performance Systems)	http://www.hps-inc.com/
Trial Simulator	Pharsight Corporation	http://www.pharsight.com
USC*PACK	Laboratory of Applied Pharmacokinetics USC	http://www.lapk.org
WinNonlin	Pharsight Corporation	http://www.pharsight.com
WinNonMix	Pharsight Corporation	http://www.pharsight.com
XDA	Teranode	http://www.teranode.com

This table lists some currently available software tools, both academic and commercial, that can and have been used for pharmacokinetic and pharmacodynamic simulations, sometimes together with data integration and analysis results management. These tools run the gamut from very general modeling and data analysis tools to highly specialized population pharmacokinetic and pharmacodynamic programs. The reader should be aware that the list is not exhaustive, and the capabilities of most of these products, as well as their availability, are expected to change over time. No endorsement of these particular products is implied.

21.4 LEVEL 3: COMPUTER SIMULATIONS OF THE CELL

Cellular level computer simulations are complicated by the fact that there is no universal accord as to how several of the intracellular and membrane processes actually take place. Although the use of competing computer models would be an efficient way to select the best hypothesis among a slew of competing ones, this approach is rarely taken in cell biology, where experimental verification dominates the literature by and large [44]. At the same time, although understanding the cell, its receptors and channels, and the modalities of membrane transport may be a worthwhile endeavor from the scientific point of view, in drug development this has to be balanced against the constructive role of this information in accelerating the development process. Because many of these models await independent scientific validation, their use in drug development is perhaps not as widespread. These modeling paradigms are more aggressively used in the biomedical research arena. The Virtual Cell [45] is an online [46] repository of some of these models, which also makes available a computer simulation of the whole cell to its users' network [47]. Another online repository of biophysical models is at the CellML website [48].

The idea of "network" is very widespread in the models that focus on the cellular environment. Clearly, interactions between cells, or also within the intracellular milieu, can be viewed as complex networks of signals, and thus the computer implementation of oriented networks is a straightforward approach to modeling this kind of systems. Some very interesting work has been done in this regard in bacterial systems through a very creative approach based on the exhaustive enumeration of the biochemical reactions taking place within the cell [49]. The system is then studied at steady state, because the dynamic parameters determining the time-varying biochemistry are largely unknown and the stoichiometry of the reactions, in contrast, is reasonably well identified. However, far from being limiting, the study of the (structurally constrained) universe of possibilities [50] related to all steady states in such a system has allowed us to learn a great deal about the long-term behavior of simple organisms exposed to variable environmental conditions and has provided new avenues of investigation for the optimal design of bioreactors and, more in general, for how biological systems may choose to adapt in the face of changing environments [51] by redistributing energy to various sublocations of the overall reaction network. This has been described for simple organisms by models that integrate data at many levels, from gene to biochemistry to physiology [52].

A whole new level of complexity is provided by the investigation of signals within the cell. Signaling networks are increasingly complex with respect to the networks we have discussed that deal with material fluxes because the precise signaling modalities are largely unknown, and this is a significant source of difficulties. New tools are being developed for this purpose [53].

In the pharmacokinetics literature, there are still not that many examples of tight integration between cellular, in vitro information and whole system prediction. One example regarding a mechanistic model of the intracellular metabolism of methotrexate [54], which was then merged in an integrated model of in vitro and in vivo information [55], may serve as a possible case in point for the gains that can be reaped from the synergistic amalgamation (with predictive purposes) of cellular and whole-body models.

21.5 LEVEL 4: PROTEINS AND GENES

Computational protein design is an area of ever-increasing interest [56]. Its most intriguing feature is that it can lead to the design and laboratory creation of structures that are not present in nature [57]. From the standpoint of pharmacokinetics and pharmacodynamics computer simulations, the challenge is once again to achieve the blending of very heterogeneous information at many structural levels. There is no doubt that drug design can be accomplished through computer simulation of the expected behavior of new molecules designed to have specific physicochemical properties. The success story of antiretrovirals [58] testifies to that concept. At the same time, one of the most interesting contributions of computer simulation to pharmacotherapy was also in the field of HIV/AIDS treatment, through the development of models of HIV viral load [59] based on clinical data [60] that shed considerable light on the disease mechanism. One wonders how much stronger the impact would have been if such models could have been augmented with cellular and molecular quantitative information. As it often happens, the precise modalities of the interaction in question are not that clear. It seems, however, that tight collaboration between clinical and preclinical departments in industry, or between clinicians and bench biologists in academia, is essential to make significant progress in the development and applications of *in silico* biomedicine.

One example of such constructive cross talk can be found in the growing literature on quantitative structure-pharmacokinetic relationships (QSPKR). Reports on how to predict pharmacokinetics from molecular information, or how to link pharmacokinetic parameters with molecular features, have appeared in both the pharmacokinetic [61] and the toxicological [62] literature. Others are extending this to pharmacodynamics as well [63], and the approaches look promising.

Perhaps a common feature to these examples is that there does not seem to be an overarching, well-defined method for approaching the integration problem at the basis of preclinical to clinical simulations. It can also be said, however, that many different methodological developments are being aggressively tried. For example, information theory approaches are being tried to identify genes that lead to disease susceptibility [64], in a sense merging the smallest with the largest information items. Some recent contributions allow the mapping of genetic data onto a queryable network based on ordinary differential equations [65]. Which of these numerous methodological approaches will become the gold standard of tomorrow? This is hard to say as of now. Could it be that some of the new fields in the "new biology" are just not mature enough? By way of example, a PubMed search of "pharmacogenomics" reveals a research paper to review ratio of 2.40 (two and a half research papers for every review, 3128/1301); compare that with the 8.91 ratio obtained with "pharmacokinetics" (about nine research papers for every review, 246683/27691), or with the even higher ratio of a more established discipline such as "simulation" (22.12, or 71269/3222). This present "state of the literature" may be the hallmark of fields that are still trying to define themselves and their untapped potential.

21.6 CONCLUSION

We have attempted to provide a brief review of recent developments in biocomputation that are of (potential) relevance to drug development. The major challenge that seems to emerge is the need for quantitative, testable, and validated frameworks for the joint analysis of large data sets available in disparate formats and focused on different biological scales (Fig. 21.3). Clearly, the solution(s) to this problem will have to borrow from many disciplines, undoubtedly biology and pharmacology, but also (bio)-engineering, computer science, (applied) mathematics and physics, and (bio)statistics. It seems that biology is currently at a crossroads, where the "best" approaches to analyze and synthesize this rapidly growing corpus of information have not been developed yet. For drug development, the challenge is to formalize testable models of intact systems that would allow, for example, simulation and testing of all development steps of various therapeutic targets against the ever-changing landscape of human physiology. This will in turn require rapidly changing professional expertise that can quickly and efficiently adapt to the shifting objectives of modern biomedical investigation.

ACKNOWLEDGMENTS

This work was partially supported by Grant NIH P41-001975, "Resource Facility for Population Kinetics."

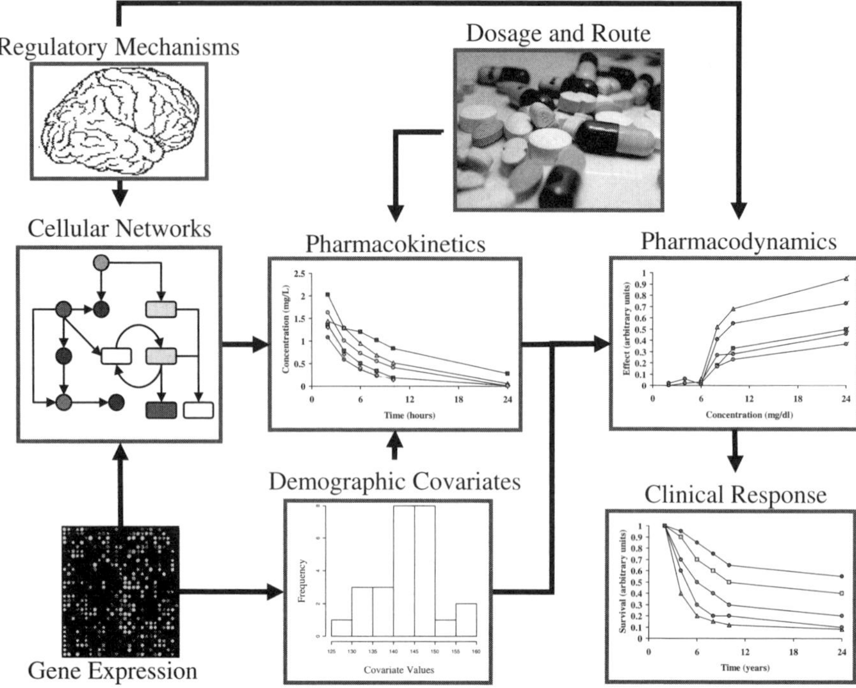

Figure 21.3 Modeling and simulation in the general context of the study of xenobiotics. The network of signals and regulatory pathways, sources of variability, and multistep regulation that are involved in this problem is shown together with its main components. It is important to realize how between-subject and between-event variation must be addressed in a model of the system that is not purely structural, but also statistical. The power of model-based data analysis is to elucidate the (main) subsystems and their putative role in overall regulation, at a variety of life stages, species, and functional (cell to organismal) levels. Images have been selected for illustrative purposes only. See color plate.

REFERENCES

1. Weinshilboum R, Wang L. Pharmacogenomics: bench to bedside. *Nat Rev Drug Discov* 2004;3:739–48.
2. Aebersold R, Hood LE, Watts JD. Equipping scientists for the new biology. *Nat Biotechnol* 2000;18:359.
3. Guyton AC. *Human physiology and mechanisms of disease*, 4th Ed. Philadelphia: W. B. Saunders, 1987.
4. Westerhoff HV, Palsson BO. The evolution of molecular biology into systems biology. *Nat Biotechnol* 2004;22:1249–52.
5. NIH Roadmap for Medical Research, http://nihroadmap.nih.gov/ (accessed October 1, 2005).

6. NOT-OD-05-002: NIH Announces Updated Criteria for Evaluating Research Grant Applications, http://grants.nih.gov/grants/guide/notice-files/NOT-OD-05-002.html (accessed October 1, 2005).
7. U.S. Department of Health and Human Services, Food and Drug Administration, Center for Drug Evaluation and Research (CDER) and Center for Biologics Evaluation and Research (CBER). *Guidance for Industry: Exposure-Response Relationships—Study Design, Data Analysis, and Regulatory Applications.* http://www.fda.gov/cder/guidance/5341fnl.pdf (accessed October 1, 2005).
8. Preusch PC. Integrative and organ systems pharmacology: a new initiative from the National Institute of General Medical Sciences. *Mol Interv* 2004;4:72–3.
9. Crampin EJ, Smith NP, Hunter PJ. Multi-scale modelling and the IUPS physiome project. *J Mol Histol* 2004;35:707–14.
10. U.S. Department of Health and Human Services, Food and Drug Administration, Center for Drug Evaluation and Research (CDER) and Center for Biologics Evaluation and Research (CBER). *Guidance for Industry: Population Pharmacokinetics.* http://www.fda.gov/cder/guidance/1852fnl.pdf (accessed October 1, 2005).
11. Notice: Approaches for the Application of Physiologically-Based Pharmacokinetic (PBPK) Models and Supporting Data in Risk Assessment E-Docket ID No. ORD-2005-0022. *Fed Reg* July 28, 2005;70 (144): 43692–43693.
12. Dourson ML, Andersen ME, Erdreich LS, MacGregor JA. Using human data to protect the public's health. *Regul Toxicol Pharmacol* 2001;33:234–56.
13. The Virtual Soldier Project, http://www.virtualsoldier.net/ (accessed October 4, 2005).
14. Sheiner LB, Steimer JL. Pharmacokinetic/pharmacodynamic modeling in drug development. *Annu Rev Pharmacol Toxicol* 2000;40:67–95.
15. Chan PL, Holford NH. Drug treatment effects on disease progression. *Annu Rev Pharmacol Toxicol* 2001;41:625–59.
16. Jang GR, Harris RZ, Lau DT. Pharmacokinetics and its role in small molecule drug discovery research. *Med Res Rev* 2001;21:382–96.
17. Sheiner LB, Ludden TM. Population pharmacokinetics/dynamics. *Annu Rev Pharmacol Toxicol* 1992;32:185–209.
18. Sheiner L, Wakefield J. Population modelling in drug development. *Stat Methods Med Res* 1999;8:183–93.
19. Gieschke R, Reigner BG, Steimer JL. Exploring clinical study design by computer simulation based on pharmacokinetic/pharmacodynamic modelling. *Int J Clin Pharmacol Ther* 1997;35:469–74.
20. Bonate PL. Clinical trial simulation in drug development. *Pharm Res* 2000;17:252–6.
21. Rowland M. Physiologic pharmacokinetic models: relevance, experience, and future trends. *Drug Metab Rev* 1984;15:55–74.
22. Nestorov I. Whole body pharmacokinetic models. *Clin Pharmacokinet* 2003;42:883–908.
23. Ludden TM, Beal SL, Sheiner LB. Comparison of the Akaike Information Criterion, the Schwarz criterion and the F test as guides to model selection. *J Pharmacokinet Biopharm* 1994;22:431–45.

24. Holford NHG, Hale M, Ko HC, Steimer J-L, Sheiner LB, Peck CC et al. *Simulation in Drug Development: Good Practices*. Draft Publication of the Center for Drug Development Science (CDDS) Draft version 1.0, July 23, 1999, http://cdds.georgetown.edu/research/sddgp723.html (accessed October 1, 2005)
25. Rowland M, Balant L, Peck C. Physiologically based pharmacokinetics in drug development and regulatory science: a workshop report (Georgetown University, Washington, DC, May 29–30, 2002). *AAPS PharmSci* 2004;6:E6.
26. Nestorov I. Modelling and simulation of variability and uncertainty in toxicokinetics and pharmacokinetics. *Toxicol Lett* 2001;120:411–20.
27. Hunter PJ, Borg TK. Integration from proteins to organs: the Physiome Project. *Nat Rev Mol Cell Biol* 2003;4:237–43.
28. Nestorov IA, Aarons LJ, Rowland M. Physiologically based pharmacokinetic modeling of a homologous series of barbiturates in the rat: a sensitivity analysis. *J Pharmacokinet Biopharm* 1997;25:413–47.
29. West GB, Woodruff WH, Brown JH. Allometric scaling of metabolic rate from molecules and mitochondria to cells and mammals. *Proc Natl Acad Sci USA* 2002;99 Suppl 1:2473–8.
30. Cousineau D, Rose CP, Lamoureux D, Goresky CA. Changes in cardiac transcapillary exchange with metabolic coronary vasodilation in the intact dog. *Circ Res* 1983;53:719–30.
31. Goresky CA. Kinetic interpretation of hepatic multiple-indicator dilution studies. *Am J Physiol Gastrointest Liver Physiol* 1983;245:G1–G12.
32. Goresky CA, Rose CP. Blood-tissue exchange in liver and heart: the influence of heterogeneity of capillary transit times. *Fed Proc* 1977;36:2629–34.
33. Kainer R. A functional model of the rat kidney. *J Math Biol* 1979;7:57–94.
34. Kassissia IG, Goresky CA, Rose CP, Schwab AJ, Simard A, Huet PM, Bach GG. Tracer oxygen distribution is barrier-limited in the cerebral microcirculation. *Circ Res* 1995;77:1201–11.
35. Goresky CA. A linear method for determining liver sinusoidal and extravascular volumes. *Am J Physiol* 1963;204:626–40.
36. Tirona RG, Schwab AJ, Geng W, Pang KS. Hepatic clearance models: comparison of the dispersion and Goresky models in outflow profiles from multiple indicator dilution rat liver studies. *Drug Metab Dispos* 1998;26:465–75.
37. Bassingthwaighte JB, Sparks HV. Indicator dilution estimation of capillary endothelial transport. *Annu Rev Physiol* 1986;48:321–34.
38. Bassingthwaighte JB, Wang CY, Chan IS. Blood-tissue exchange via transport and transformation by capillary endothelial cells. *Circ Res* 1989;65:997–1020.
39. Muzikant AL, Penland RC. Models for profiling the potential QT prolongation risk of drugs. *Curr Opin Drug Discov Devel* 2002;5:127–35.
40. Pharmacokinetic and Pharmacodynamic Resources, http://www.boomer.org/pkin/ (accessed October 1, 2005)
41. Center for Modeling Integrated Metabolic Systems (MIMS), http://www.csuohio.edu/mims/ (accessed October 1, 2005)
42. Popel AS, Pries AR, Slaaf DW. Microcirculation Physiome Project. *J Vasc Res* 1999;36:253–5.

43. Bassingthwaighte JB, Qian H, Li Z. The Cardiome Project. An integrated view of cardiac metabolism and regional mechanical function. *Adv Exp Med Biol* 1999;471:541–53.
44. Lazebnik Y. Can a biologist fix a radio? Or, what I learned while studying apoptosis. *Cancer Cell* 2002;2:179–82.
45. Loew LM, Schaff JC. The Virtual Cell: a software environment for computational cell biology. *Trends Biotechnol* 2001;19:401–6.
46. National Resource for Cell Analysis and Modeling (NRCAM), home of the Virtual Cell, http://www.nrcam.uchc.edu/ (accessed October 2, 2005)
47. Slepchenko BM, Schaff JC, Macara I, Loew LM. Quantitative cell biology with the Virtual Cell. *Trends Cell Biol* 2003;13:570–6.
48. CellML, http://www.cellml.org/ (accessed October 2, 2005).
49. Price ND, Papin JA, Schilling CH, Palsson BO. Genome-scale microbial *in silico* models: the constraints-based approach. *Trends Biotechnol* 2003;21:162–9.
50. Famili I, Forster J, Nielsen J, Palsson BO. *Saccharomyces cerevisiae* phenotypes can be predicted by using constraint-based analysis of a genome-scale reconstructed metabolic network. *Proc Natl Acad Sci USA* 2003;100:13134–9.
51. Ibarra RU, Edwards JS, Palsson BO. *Escherichia coli* K-12 undergoes adaptive evolution to achieve *in silico* predicted optimal growth. *Nature* 2002;420:186–9.
52. Schilling CH, Covert MW, Famili I, Church GM, Edwards JS, Palsson BO. Genome-scale metabolic model of *Helicobacter pylori* 26695. *J Bacteriol* 2002;184:4582–93.
53. Papin JA, Hunter T, Palsson BO, Subramaniam S. Reconstruction of cellular signalling networks and analysis of their properties. *Nat Rev Mol Cell Biol* 2005;6:99–111.
54. Panetta JC, Wall A, Pui CH, Relling MV, Evans WE. Methotrexate intracellular disposition in acute lymphoblastic leukemia: a mathematical model of gamma-glutamyl hydrolase activity. *Clin Cancer Res* 2002;8:2423–9.
55. Panetta JC, Yanishevski Y, Pui CH, Sandlund JT, Rubnitz J, Rivera GK et al. A mathematical model of in vivo methotrexate accumulation in acute lymphoblastic leukemia. *Cancer Chemother Pharmacol* 2002;50:419–28.
56. Park S, Yang X, Saven JG. Advances in computational protein design. *Curr Opin Struct Biol* 2004;14:487–94.
57. Kuhlman B, Dantas G, Ireton GC, Varani G, Stoddard BL, Baker D. Design of a novel globular protein fold with atomic-level accuracy. *Science* 2003;302:1364–8.
58. Erickson J, Neidhart DJ, VanDrie J, Kempf DJ, Wang XC, Norbeck DW et al. Design, activity, and 2.8 Å crystal structure of a C2 symmetric inhibitor complexed to HIV-1 protease. *Science* 1990;249:527–33.
59. Perelson AS, Neumann AU, Markowitz M, Leonard JM, Ho DD. HIV-1 dynamics in vivo: virion clearance rate, infected cell life-span, and viral generation time. *Science* 1996;271:1582–6.
60. Ho DD, Neumann AU, Perelson AS, Chen W, Leonard JM, Markowitz M. Rapid turnover of plasma virions and CD4 lymphocytes in HIV-1 infection. *Nature* 1995;373:123–6.

61. Van der Graaf PH, Nilsson J, Van Schaick EA, Danhof M. Multivariate quantitative structure-pharmacokinetic relationships (QSPKR) analysis of adenosine A1 receptor agonists in rat. *J Pharm Sci* 1999;88:306–12.
62. Fouchecourt MO, Beliveau M, Krishnan K. Quantitative structure-pharmacokinetic relationship modelling. *Sci Total Environ* 2001;274:125–35.
63. Mager DE, Jusko WJ. Quantitative structure-pharmacokinetic/pharmacodynamic relationships of corticosteroids in man. *J Pharm Sci* 2002;91:2441–51.
64. Sebastiani P, Ramoni MF, Nolan V, Baldwin CT, Steinberg MH. Genetic dissection and prognostic modeling of overt stroke in sickle cell anemia. *Nat Genet* 2005;37:435–40.
65. Meir E, Munro EM, Odell GM, Von Dassow G. Ingeneue: a versatile tool for reconstituting genetic networks, with examples from the segment polarity network. *J Exp Zool* 2002;294:216–51.

22

PREDICTIVE MODELS FOR BETTER DECISIONS: FROM UNDERSTANDING PHYSIOLOGY TO OPTIMIZING TRIAL DESIGN

JAMES R. BOSLEY, JR.

Contents

22.1 INTRODUCTION AND MOTIVATION

Successfully discovering and developing drugs that are safe and effective is a difficult task. The striking successes of the past are hard to match for reasons that are both commercial and technical. Many diseases are very well served by the current pharmacopoeia. Lower lifetime drug revenues result from shorter periods of exclusivity, competition from lower-cost

Computer Applications in Pharmaceutical Research and Development, Edited by Sean Ekins.
ISBN 0-471-73779-8

generics, and (in the US, the largest drug research and development center and market) reimported drugs [1]. These market trends all increase the pressure on pharmaceutical companies to be more efficient. The "low-hanging fruit" for therapeutic targets has now been picked. Where current treatments fall short, the disease process is usually complex (e.g., diabetes, obesity, and metabolic syndrome) and very often lacks good in vitro or animal model tests to facilitate discovery (e.g., Alzheimer disease). These difficulties lead to higher research costs [2, 3]. Clearly, if the drug and biotechnology industries are to maintain their historic high level of business success they must dramatically improve research productivity and efficiency. The US FDA has recognized the need for increased development efficiency and advocates changes in both industrial and regulatory practice: Its "critical path"[4] makes clear the expectation that modeling and simulation should be used to improve both the development process itself and industry-agency communication.

Creating a successful drug requires a series of favorable circumstances, each the result of many decisions. If enough of those decisions are correct (or at least not too incorrect) and decisions are well executed, government agencies allow a drug to be marketed. These decisions are difficult: Only three in ten marketed drugs have revenues that match or exceed average research costs [5]. Only one in two compounds entering clinical phase III trials is approved, so clearly one high-value decision that profoundly affects research cost and business success is the go/no-go gate before those trials. These gates also arise at many other points in the discovery and development process. "Killing losers early" avoids wasting time, personnel, and budget on compounds that will eventually fail. Just as important is efficiently generating and developing "winners" for the portfolio. Generating or acquiring at least one compound with the potential to be shown safe and effective is necessary and requires good resource allocation decisions. Whether we buy or make compounds, we can improve efficiency by properly targeting diseases, therapeutic areas, and specific targets that match organizational expertise, intellectual assets, market needs, and marketing access.

There are many other common decision topics ranging from in vitro basic science through clinical trials to the postmarketing phase of drug life including (for example) target selection, lead/follow-on compound prioritization, protocol design (dose, regimen, assays, clinical end points, and/or surrogate markers), portfolio optimization, labeling, label extension, marketing approach, resource allocation, portfolio optimization, drug and corporate valuation, and strategy. Organizational success therefore depends in part on choosing which targets, compounds, and markets to pursue and choosing which of these to avoid, ultimately deciding on the best allocation of resources and design of experiments to produce safe and effective therapies. How can these decisions best be made?

Optimal decisions depend, in part, on fully exploiting relevant data and knowledge. This ranges from physiological and pharmacological knowledge to business knowledge, and includes both public and proprietary information and data in the public domain.

The relevant information and data available can be sparse or overwhelming in data set size and complexity. Typically in a pharmaceutical company we have proportionally more in vitro data, less preclinical data, and very little clinical data. The quantity of each data type varies inversely to the cost of obtaining it, and often to its relevance and usefulness [6]. So we may have very sparse data directly relating to our goal of estimating whether a molecule, target, or trial is likely to be successful. In some cases, we may not have any data that are directly relevant to a decision during the drug discovery and development process. Worse, we may not even know it. At the other extreme, and perhaps the norm today, is the existence of enormous data sets. Managing the huge amount of data generated in our industry is a problem and an area of significant activity. Combinatorial chemistry, high-throughput screening, microarrays of various types, an ever-expanding palette of assays, and other new and existing techniques are used to generate these huge data sets. Physiology, whether cell or human, also shows dynamic effects requiring multiple sampling times. Each datum varies in degree of relevance to the problem at hand. In addition to proprietary data generated internally, pharmaceutical companies must acquire, read, understand, curate, and exploit data from scientific journals, public regulatory agencies, and competitors. Even mature science is expanding rapidly, as can be observed by comparing recent successive editions of biochemistry or molecular biology textbooks or the growth in size of available genomics and proteomics databases.

There is also a problem with the use of data on molecules, targets, or patients that share similarities with those of current interest. How can we best exploit data for previously investigated compounds that are analogs or homologs to our current molecule? How can we exploit physiological knowledge not related to any drug (e.g., blood perfusion in different tissues, body fat distribution by tissue, disease severity, and genetic differences) together with drug-specific characteristics (e.g., binding affinity, lipophilicity, pK_a of acid groups) and related data for similar compounds to better understand the likely behavior of a specific compound of current interest?

The information and data we have are often inconsistent, either with other data or with our mental model of how these data "should" behave. Inconsistencies may allow different conclusions and support opposite decision paths. This inconsistency can result from errors in experimental technique, from incorrectly assuming what the data mean, or from ignoring (or not knowing) the complete physiology. Data are generated, justified, and explained by fallible humans with specific fields of enthusiasm and expertise and with varying ability and motivation for advocacy. An approach allowing unbiased testing of different hypotheses to settle conflicts in data or theory would be ideal.

To make sense of large, complex, and conflicting data sets, humans have used mental models. Mental models for drug discovery and development have made manifest contributions. However, humans, even the brightest, can only simultaneously consider a small number ("seven, plus or minus two" [7]) of simultaneous quantities. But relevant physiology, with "chains" of effect (e.g., drug absorption, distribution, binding to cell receptor, increased second messenger, and so forth), parallel paths (e.g., multiple chemical mediators in inflammation), feedback loops (e.g., blood glucose increase, insulin release, glucose lowering by peripheral disposal, or the positive feedback of voltage-gated sodium channels), and multiple timescales (acute blood sugar increase caused by a meal, long-term increase caused by disease progression) requires simultaneously considering hundreds of interacting and time-varying quantities. The massive amounts of incomplete and inconsistent data of varying relevance and mind-numbing complexity focused through a limited human intellect argue strongly for the use of a better way to integrate our understanding of a particular physiology, disease, therapy, population, or market.

Even so, mental models are what we use to make decisions. Mental models that are relevant and correct facilitate better decisions. The systems of interest here (e.g., an experiment or a clinical trial) are complex. Creating a correct and relevant mental model for a complex system from diverse, conflicting, and incomplete data is nearly impossible without computational assistance. The author's experience has shown that not only does a quantitative computational model give "answers," but the process of creating and exercising such models facilitates formation of mental models that are correct, useful, and relevant. Additionally, creation and use of such models curates and stores knowledge and facilitates learning and communication between experts, offering competitive advantage.

Engineers have long relied on detailed mathematical models to design complex systems such as aircraft and spacecraft, optimize motor vehicle design, and operate and control nuclear and chemical reactors. The models quantitatively represent the quantities of interest in a way that is consistent with all available data. Where inconsistencies are found, the model(s) can be used to evaluate different explanatory hypotheses or to suggest experiments to resolve the conflict. Models containing no representation of physical mechanism can represent phenomena and data without bias and are excellent for statistically describing data sets and for interpolation. Models incorporating general knowledge and physical laws are called mechanistic. The constraints provided by physics (and physiology) essentially comprise additional general data and thus can better facilitate extrapolation beyond the range of specific data. Both phenomenological and mechanistic models can show gaps and inconsistencies in our data. An appropriate model allows us to test various hypotheses to explain inconsistent data and suggests experiments to eliminate gaps in our knowledge. Making sense of all we know about a complex system in a way that allows people to understand the relevant implications of choices and to make better decisions certainly involves mathematical modeling of one form or another.

This chapter includes a description of the goals of modeling and simulation, with some guidelines for successful projects. An overview of various model types is offered, followed by descriptions of two specific types of computer models that are being used more and more frequently in pharmaceutical discovery and development. The first of these is physiologically based models, both pharmacokinetic and pharmacodynamic (PBPK and PBPD). These are useful in integrating diverse data, in extrapolating data, and in learning of systems relationships that are not apparent from the usual reductionist scientific approach. Next we offer a case study of a successful industrial computer-aided trial design (CATD) project. The drug and therapeutic area of the study were deliberately disguised, but the major lessons of this study (failures, with attendant delays and costs, can be minimized) remain clear.

22.2 GOALS OF MATHEMATICAL AND COMPUTATIONAL MODELING AND SIMULATION

We can identify several goals of mathematical and computational models, all aimed at improving our decisions in the face of complexity, data overload, sparsity, and inconsistency. From the previous discussion, we see that models can be used to:

1. Integrate a wide variety of different data
2. Account for changes in a system over time
3. Account for interactions within systems (multiple parallel paths, feedback)
4. Account for variability and uncertainty
5. Exploit our knowledge of known physical/physiological relationships
6. Identify relevant gaps in our knowledge
7. Understand behavior within the range of original data
8. Predict system behavior outside the range of original data
9. Understand which drug effects, pathways, and targets are most important
10. Test different hypotheses about conflicting data (conflicting mental models)
11. Predict outcome for alternate designs (molecular, clinical trial) allowing optimization of portfolios, experiments, and trial protocols
12. Provide a fair umpire in disagreements between experts
13. Synthesize (in creating the math model) a correct and shared mental model
14. Communicate and store different expertise in a meaningful way

Not every model addresses every issue listed above—modeling projects focus on specific goals relevant to the decision at hand.

Modeling and simulation are often taken as synonymous. Here, we take modeling to mean the creation of a mathematical and statistical structure and the determination of parameters to be consistent with available data and knowledge. Modeling looks at existing data—the past. Simulation is prospective. Simulation uses a model to predict results for experiments we have not done. Where variability and uncertainty are included in the underlying model, simulation can be used to predict the likelihood of different outcomes from a given experimental design. This permits choosing the best existing alternative, or synthesizing an optimal design. Simulation predicts possible future occurrences. Bonate has characterized similar distinctions that are useful [8]. In this chapter "modeling" should be taken to mean either modeling or simulation, as the context indicates.

2.3 SUCCESS OF MODELING AND SIMULATION PROJECTS

Not every project requires a detailed mathematical or computational model of the disease, drug, trial, or market population. Creating models requires significant expertise, ability, time and a commitment of resources. Many technologists intuitively favor an approach to science involving modeling and simulation, but "modeling for modeling's sake" is expensive in several ways. The goals for a modeling project or initiative should be very clear. The following questions are suggested as essential in determining what modeling approach, if any, is appropriate:

1. What is the business goal of the modeling work?
2. What is (are) the technical goals? (Will the model be used to "confirm," or to "learn"?[9])
3. What decisions will be made with the modeling results?
4. What is the value (consequence) of a good decision or a poor one?
5. What are the timetables for the decision(s)?
6. Make or buy: Do we have all the expertise in-house, or will outside firms and consultants give a better return, faster results, or more confidence?
7. Who (individuals, functional groups) will create the model?
8. Who are stakeholders? Who will participate in the modeling project?
9. Who will generate results with the model, and who will interpret results?
10. Who will make the decision(s)?
11. How will the modeling and simulation results be communicated to decision makers?

12. What is the cost (budget, personnel, management and staff attention) of a model?
13. Is the model relevant to other decisions at other levels?
14. Will this model form the basis for future work? Will it build expertise, or does it lose relevance after the decision?
15. How will information be communicated among the project team?
16. How does modeling fit in with any corporate technology adoption initiatives? Should it?

The quality of front-end work in answering the questions above, when addressed by a broadly comprised project team, is directly related to project success. It is useful to keep in mind that the consequences of decisions (question 4) are often different for the firm, for departments, for research groups, and for individuals on the research team. Models can reduce ambiguity and arbitrary discretion. This is appreciated in successful projects.

Given the growth in acceptance (and the regulatory trend toward insisting on) mathematical modeling of drugs and disease, most major companies either have developed internal competence or have significant initiatives to build internal competence in modeling and simulation. This adoption process has its own set of factors critical for success and is beyond the scope of this discussion.

22.4 TYPES OF MODELS USED IN DRUG DISCOVERY AND DEVELOPMENT

Models can be characterized in many ways, in what might be called dimensions. Some dimensions are a matter of degree. These include ranges such as simple to complex, phenomenological to mechanistic, descriptive to predictive, and quantitative to qualitative. Other dimension types are discrete and either/or: steady-state or dynamic, deterministic or stochastic. Using these descriptive dimensions facilitates understanding the differences between models and their fitness for specific uses.

Analysis of most (perhaps 65%) pharmacokinetic data from clinical trials starts and stops with noncompartmental analysis (NCA). NCA usually includes calculating the area under the curve (AUC) of concentration versus time, or under the first-moment curve (AUMC, from a graph of concentration multiplied by time versus time). Calculation of AUC and AUMC facilitates simple calculations for some standard pharmacokinetic parameters and collapses measurements made at several sampling times into a single number representing exposure. The approach makes few assumptions, has few parameters, and allows fairly rigorous statistical description of exposure and how it is affected by dose. An exposure response model may be created. With respect to descriptive dimensions these dose-exposure and exposure-response models are fairly simple (as opposed to complex), have few parameters (rather than many), are phenomenological (not physiological), do not represent time variations in concentration (they are not dynamic), and are quantitative in representing central tendency and in facilitating determination of confidence intervals. This approach is often used to describe data and to confirm high-level hypotheses.

Model equations can be augmented with expressions accounting for covariates such as subject age, sex, weight, disease state, therapy history, and life-style (smoker or nonsmoker, IV drug user or not, therapy compliance, and others). If sufficient data exist, the parameters of these augmented models (or a distribution of the parameters consistent with the data) may be determined. Multiple simulations for prospective experiments or trials, with different parameter values generated from the distributions, can then be used to predict a range of outcomes and the related likelihood of each outcome. Such dose-exposure, exposure-response, or dose-response models can be classified as steady state, stochastic, of low to moderate complexity, predictive, and quantitative. A case study is described in Section 22.6.

Adding explicit representation of time-varying absorption, distribution, metabolism, and elimination increases model complexity in a different dimension—the model is now "dynamic." A multicompartment model assumes (usually) that simple rate laws govern elimination or transfer of drug between compartments. Compartments typically represent the time-varying amount of drug in the gut, in the blood, and possibly (in "link" pharmacodynamic models [10]) in the biophase (that is, the site of action). The resulting differential equation model requires more assumptions than NCA or dose response. More free parameters exist, and hence more data are required to support strong statistical conclusions and tight parameter confidence intervals. We benefit from a more detailed insight into some mechanisms, time dependencies, and a better understanding of variability assignable to specific parameters (e.g., interpatient variability in drug clearance), inputs, and outputs of the model, as well as the ability to allocate uncertainty accordingly. Such a model is more complex than the NCA model above, it is more physiological, it is dynamic, and it is more mechanistic. Given enough data, the model retains excellent descriptive properties and the ability to confirm but also might be used to predict and extrapolate—to learn.

Standard commercial software packages allow for NCA and low-order compartmental pharmacokinetic modeling. In some cases these have been augmented to include capability for more advanced modeling (e.g., what is called mixed-effect modeling in Kinetica™, from ThermoElectron Corporation, www.thermoelectron.com) or have companion products that allow such modeling (WinNonMix™, which complements WinNonLin™, both from Pharsight Corporation, www.pharsight.com) and simulation (Trial Simulator™, also from Pharsight). NONMEM™ (Globomax, www.globomax.com) is a venerable and powerful modeling package, although it is dated and requires significant expertise. Modules within statistically oriented packages such as SAS (SAS Institute, www.sas.com) and S-plus (Insightful Corporation, www.insightful.com) and R (The R Foundation, www.r-project.org) offer experts the ability to do powerful modeling. General-purpose modeling packages such as MATLAB/Simulink (www.mathworks.com), Extend (www.imaginethatinc.com), and Vissim (www.vissol.com) can be used. Ekins et al. discuss these software packages and others in the context of predicting absorption, distribution, metabolism, excretion, and toxicology (ADME) [11].

Useful discussions reviewing PK model structure [12] and PK correlations [13] and describing applications or PK models [14,15] are recommended. Comprehensive reviews of pharmacokinetic modeling are given by Lin and Lu [16] and Sheiner and Steimer [17].

What are called physiologically based pharmacokinetic (PBPK) and pharmacodynamic (PBPD) models are more mechanistically complex and often include more compartments, more parameters, and more detailed expressions of rates and fluxes and contain more mechanistic representation. This type of model is reviewed in more detail in Section 22.5. Here, we merely classify such models and note several characteristics. PBPK models have more parameters, are more mechanistic, can exploit a wider range of data, often represent the whole body, and can be used both to describe and interpolate as well as to predict and extrapolate. Complexity of such models ranges from moderate to high. They typically contain 10 or more compartments, and can range to hundreds. The increase in the number of flux relationships between compartments and the related parameters is often more than proportional to compartment count.

The description of these models has been in terms of dimensions. These dimensions are summarized in Table 22.1. In addition to the questions suggested in Section 22.3, it is often useful to consider these dimensions to clarify thinking about a modeling project. Although some of the rows of this table are related and correlated, each can and should be considered separately.

22.5 PHYSIOLOGICALLY BASED MODELS

Physiologically based models often use nonclinical data, or clinical data about a different drug, to predict a drug's uptake, disposition, and effect. This is extrapolation. Another common use is to understand and predict disposition by organ or tissue. Excellent reviews are available for physiologically based pharmacokinetic and pharmacodynamic models. These include descriptions by Nestorov [18], Nestorov et al. [19], and Blakey et al. [20] of whole-body pharmacokinetic models. Andersen [21] describes the use of PBPK and PBPD models in toxicology and risk assessment, and Clewell et al. [22] give an example, which was analyzed by Bois [23]. Poulin and Theil provide a discussion of the creation of a PBPK model, using three drugs with different chemical characteristics [24]. Examples of PBPK models for capecitabine [25], cyclosporin A [26], midazolam [27], and pravastatin [28] offer useful insights. Because PB models typically have many parameters that depend on the drug properties, predictions of these properties from chemical structure are essen-

TABLE 22.1 Models Can be Described Using Dimensions, As Stated in the Text. Here, Some of these Dimensions are Described by Stating their Extremes

Descriptive Dimension Extremes		Comments
Phenomenological	Mechanistic	
Few compartments	Many compartments	
Steady state, or time averaged	Dynamic	
Deterministic	Stochastic	Variability and uncertainty representation is useful for prediction
Qualitative	Quantitative	
Subsystem (gene, pathway, cell, tissue, organ)	Whole body	Need whole body if feedback and multiple pathways affect disease state
Focused (purpose built)	Broadly applicable	
Few parameters	Many parameters	The more parameters, the more data required
Few assumptions required	Assume some physiological laws constrain the model	
Uses data from a specific experiment	Uses data from a wide range of experiments	
Tractable to rigorous statistics	Limited statistical rigor	
Limited physiological insight	Physiologically rigorous	
Useful for confirmation (e.g., $P < 0.05$)	Useful for learning and exploring	
Descriptive	Predictive	
Can interpolate	Can both interpolate and extrapolate	

tial. Several approaches [29–31] for *in silico* prediction of the ADME properties useful for PB models have been described. Ekins [32] has described *in silico* prediction of drug binding properties, useful in understanding drug interactions. Leahy [33] describes how predicted PK parameters might be captured and utilized in PB models. Obach et al. [34] offer a detailed approach to predicting PK parameters from in vitro and preclinical measurements. Houston and Carlile [35] describe how useful hepatic clearance parameters can be elucidated from liver tissue, cell, and cell-component tests. In 1985, Charnick et al. [36] offered a perspective of PBPK models in drug development and discovery. It is interesting to contrast the work of Charnick et al. to the comprehensive view offered by Theil et al. [37] in 2003. A PBPK workshop convened by Malcolm Rowland and Carl Peck under the auspices of Georgetown University attracted many leading practitioners and a useful summary has been published [38]. A collection of papers on physiologically based modeling is available [39] and contains contributions by eminent researchers.

PBPK is not new. Some thoughtful early examples of models that may be classified as physiologically based pharmacokinetics (PBPK) were generated early in the last century [40, 41]. In the 1960s two chemical engineers at the University of Delaware, Ken Bischoff and Bob Dedrick [42–45], exploited newly available computer power to advance this science. Early examples represented drug distribution to different tissues and organs with blood perfusion data [46] and simple flux laws based on diffusion and affinity. Figure 22.1A shows the schema for such a "multiorgan model.". The version shown has been augmented to include a modern approach to drug absorption after a drawing in Theil et al. [37]. Each tissue type is represented by a vascular and an extravascular volume separated by a membrane regulating transport (Fig. 22.1B). Each extravascular volume is modeled as a compartment, as are arterial and venous blood pools. Blood flow at rate Q (taken from a tabulation of experimentally determined values) and concentration C_{Arterial} (determined by a dynamic mass balance accounting for absorption and clearance) enters the tissue. Drug flux varies according to a driving force and some rate law, for example, the Renkin flow-diffusion equation [47]:

$$\text{CL}_\text{I} = Q\,(1 - e^{-P \cdot S/Q})$$

Here CL_I is the intercompartmental clearance of drug from the vascular flow, Q is the blood flow rate, and P and S are the drug-specific permeability and drug-independent transvascular surface area, respectively. The total flux is $\text{CL}_\text{I} \times C_{\text{Arterial}}$. The driving force is determined by considering relative affinity of the drug between blood and the extravascular tissue (e.g., a lipophilic drug will have a higher equilibrium concentration in adipose tissue, and hence there are a higher driving force and flux from blood to adipose in this case) and the concentration of drug in the plasma and extravascular compartment. Protein binding in the blood and tissue can be included as necessary.

In sum, the time-varying concentration or amount of a drug (and potentially of its metabolites) in a compartment is calculated by considering absorption, flux into and out of the compartment, and clearance in the compartment. The fluxes and clearances are calculated based on correlations describing physical principles of transport (diffusion, carrier-mediated transport, passive or active transport) and enzymatic reactions (Michaelis–Menton or Hill kinetics). The driving force for fluxes can vary with relative affinity between blood, blood proteins, and tissue. If good correlations for this driving force and for transport are available, PBPK models allow prediction of distribution of drug into various organs of the body.

In PBPK models tissue blood perfusion and tissue composition can be characterized independently of the drug; thus such a model can be created once and reused for many different drugs. Furthermore, because physical laws (mass conservation, diffusion, or facilitated transport mechanisms) are incor-

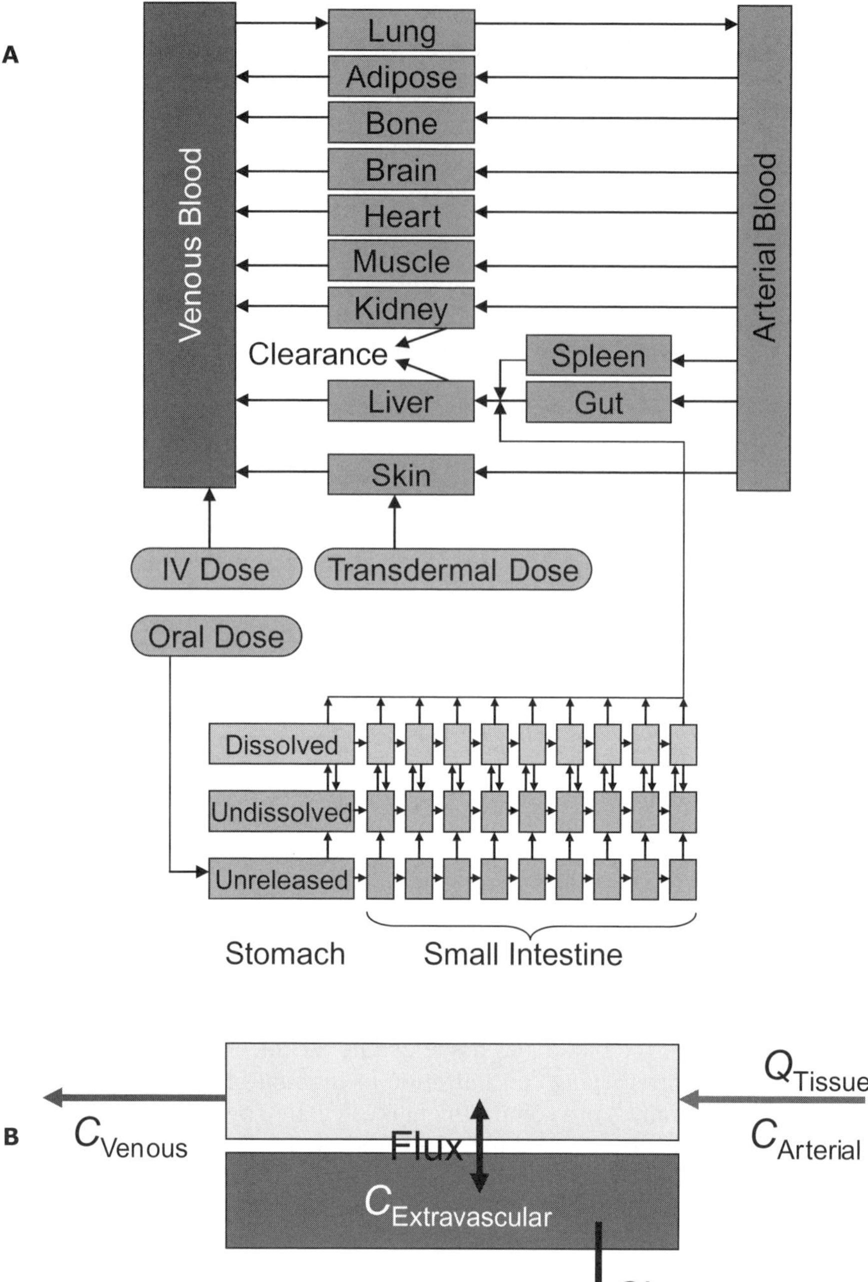

Figure 22.1 A. Schema for a physiologically based pharmacokinetic model incorporating absorption in the stomach and intestines and distribution to various tissues. B. Each organ or tissue type includes representation of perfusion (Q) and drug concentrations entering and leaving the tissue. Fluxes are computed by the product of an appropriate rate law, and permeable surface area accounts for the affinity (e.g., lipophilic drugs absorbing more readily into adipose tissue). Clearance is computed for each tissue based on physiology and is often assumed to be zero for tissues other than the gut, the liver, and the kidneys.

porated, usually as simple expressions requiring few parameters, the data specific to a drug that is required to model PK may actually be quite modest, comprising such items as molecular weight, solubility, lipophilicity (usually as a partition coefficient), pH characterizations (pK_a), and intestinal cell (Caco-2) permeability. Because components of physiological interest are represented by idealized physical systems that are the same (with different parameter values) for different subjects and species, data from these different sources can be used to improve the model's predictive power for the animal or human of interest. That is, we can exploit results from animals, or from in vitro experiments with intestinal tissue, to improve clinical predictions. The goal is to use relatively simple, fast, and inexpensive experiments or *in silico* molecular structure-activity relationships to predict the range of results that are likely for expensive tests such as clinical trials.

A good body of early and current PBPK literature describes anticancer drugs. These drugs are cytotoxic, and this toxicity is often not specific to diseased tissue. Cancer cells are more susceptible to these drugs, but the therapeutic index can be low. For this reason, the distribution of these drugs between tissues containing target and nontarget cells in the patient is of high interest. PBPK models can be used to predict this. Table 22.2 [after 48] contains some early examples of anticancer and other compounds for which PK results were analyzed with PBPK techniques during the 1970s. The environmental toxin PCB is included in the table to emphasize that PBPK is an important tool for industrial toxicologists and many advances have been contributed by this discipline [49, 50].

One observation the author heard many times from experts attending the 2002 PBPK workshop [38] was that much of the current PB work was centered on pharmacodynamics. In general, this work strives to develop good correlations between concentrations in one compartment of standard low-order compartmental models and a clinical end point. Schaddelee et al. provide an example [51]. The approach keeps the model order low, facilitating clearer determination of model parameters and making statistical treatment tractable. The correlations may not have a physical basis, or if a basis exists (e.g., using the Hill equation to represent saturation of effect observed at high drug concentrations), the physical significance (what metabolic pathway is saturated?) is not made clear. This may not be important in many applications.

TABLE 22.2 Early Examples of PBPK Models

Anticancer Drugs	Other Drugs
Actinomycin D (1977)	Cephalosporins (1978)
Adriamycin (1978)	Digoxin (1977)
ARA-C (1978)	Salicylate (1978)
Cyclocytidine (1977)	Thiopental (1968, 1975)
Cisplatin (1978)	Pentobarbital (1968)
Mercaptopurine (1977)	Environmental Toxins
Methotrexate (1971, 1978)	PCB (1977)

If it is necessary to understand and represent the mechanism of the detailed physiology, then a different approach is taken. Historically, physiological models have focused on a specific cell type, tissue type, organ, or physiological subsystem. Isolating specific subsystems to understand basic phenomena is time-honored in science, and this reductionist approach has yielded great advances. An interesting early example, Hodgkin and Huxley's [52] experimental and modeling work describing action potential generation and transmission in nerve cells in vitro, has contributed enormously to understanding of ion channel function. It is interesting to note that these authors (who won a Nobel Prize for their work) did not feel that they understood the physiology until their model could duplicate their observations. There is an overwhelming abundance of isolated models of cells or physiological subsystems in the literature, and a book reviewing a wide variety of models is recommended [53]. But health and disease are states that result from complex interactions between different cells, tissue types, and physiological systems. Feedback and parallel signaling paths in a range of systems cannot be considered in isolation and cannot be representative of whole organism behavior. This has led to a "systems" or "top-down" approach to modeling complex diseases. In this approach, the model begins by phenomenologically representing clinical observations ("what the doctor observes"). Model detail and structure are added as needed to represent both system behavior and disease components of most interest. Specific sections of the model acquire high physiological fidelity. Other sections of the model, included to ensure a complete description of relevant signaling paths and feedback loops, can be very much "black box". All elements affecting the disease physiology or health are represented quantitatively. The approach does not abandon the results from the "bottom-up" reductionist approach, but rather exploits them by integrating them with the constraints of physical laws or known relationships. Examples include the law of mass conservation, enzyme metabolism rates described by the Hill equation, and simple Fickian or facilitated diffusion used to describe the absorption, distribution, metabolism, and excretion of drugs, nutrients, and endogenous compounds. Knowledge of drug-receptor binding curves, second messengers, and the resulting effect on metabolic pathway fluxes can be incorporated. The behavior of components and subsystems is tested with all available data. Parameters in the integrated model can be set to match a widely diverse and rich subset of clinical test results. These typically include both normal and pathophysiological states and different individuals with different genotypes and environmental and lifestyle influences. Often, parameters from in vitro results must be adjusted to match whole-organism results. The resulting model and set of parameters can be tested against a different set of diverse clinical results. Such models are extremely complex, highly parameterized, and very faithful to physiological laws and both subsystem and whole-organism data. Creating such models involves significant resources and expertise.

The best-known examples of this approach have been the diabetes/obesity, asthma, and rheumatoid arthritis models created by the firm Entelos. These models, called PhysioLabs™, each include hundreds of compartments and thousands of parameters [54]. Such models are expensive to create, but they yield unique benefits. For example, these models contain a quantitative representation of all known possible targets. By simulation of the effect of up- or downregulating pathways associated with each target (essentially assuming that we have a perfect drug for that target), the effects of feedback and of parallel pathways can be seen. In many cases, the target of interest can be shown to have no clinical effect even when a simulated "perfect" drug has achieved exactly the desired modulation of the pathway related to the target. This can identify new targets with high potential and rule out those targets that are likely to fail for physiological reasons. This allowed Johnson & Johnson to stop work on a target predicted to fail, according to Richard Ho, Head of Medical Informatics. "Other pharmaceutical companies have been working on this target for the last five years at least," says Ho. "I presume they are still." [55]. Uehling has compiled a list of "supermodels," which is available on-line [56].

Because model structure as well as drug-independent parameters are reusable for many different drugs and therapies, commercial modeling software packages are available. Some examples include ADMET Plus™ and Gastroplus™ (Simulations Plus, www.simulationsplus.com), which respectively allow prediction of absorption properties from compound characteristics and simulate absorption given those properties and data from various in vitro and preclinical tests. PK-Sim™ [57] (Bayer Technology Services, http://www.research.bayer.com/medien/pages/2999/pharmacokinetics.pdf) offers the ability to do whole-body PBPK simulation. A comparison of GastroPlus with IDEA™ (Trega Biosciences) [58] is available. SimCYP Limited (www.simcyp.com) is a consortium applying knowledge of liver enzyme activity and variability within populations to PBPK models, allowing dose and trial design optimization and identification.

Classic parameter estimation techniques involve using experimental data to estimate all parameters at once. This allows an estimate of central tendency and a confidence interval for each parameter, but it also allows determination of a matrix of covariances between parameters. To determine parameters and confidence intervals at some level, the requirements for data increase more than proportionally with the number of parameters in the model. Above some number of parameters, simultaneous estimation becomes impractical, and the experiments required to generate the data become impossible or unethical. For models at this level of complexity parameters and covariances can be estimated for each subsection of the model. This assumes that the covariance between parameters in different subsections is zero. This is unsatisfactory to some practitioners, and this (and the complexity of such models and the difficulty and cost of building them) has been a criticism of highly parameterized PBPK and PBPD models. An alternate view assumes that decisions will be made that should be informed by as much information about the system as possible, that the assumption of zero covariance between parameters in different subsections is based on physiological knowledge and is likely a good one, and that this assumption is at least explicit and its effect can be tested. This is a variation of the Frequentist-Bayesian conflict, and is unlikely to be settled here to the satisfaction of either side. The author's prejudice is likely clear, so one observation is offered. Decisions often need to be made regarding very complex system and widely ranging data, and the alternatives to reaching this decision are either many experts arguing, arbited only by etiquette and a program manager, or those same experts arguing, but refereed by an unbiased science- and data-based model they helped create. For very complex systems with much available data, the alternative to modeling is guessing.

D'Sousa and Boxenbaum [59] commented on PBPK models: "At their best, they allow us to understand the accumulation of thought in pharmacokinetics and pharmacodynamics, and help with the integration of data and improvement of experimental design." The author emphatically agrees—there is no other technology or approach that accepts such a wide range of data while giving quantitative predictions that facilitate improved experiments and trials. The ability to facilitate and stimulate communication between diverse experts, and the ability to adjudicate between conflicting hypotheses in an unbiased manner, are additional benefits.

22.6 COMPUTER-AIDED TRIAL DESIGN (CATD)

Clinical trials are the most expensive and time-consuming single expense in getting a drug to market. The protocol for a trial is developed before it starts, and data are often unavailable until the trial is complete and the data are "locked." It is not known whether the trial has failed until it is over, and millions of dollar equivalents and months or perhaps years of development are sunk. It is clear that improving the odds of successfully showing safety and efficacy of a drug has real and provable value. Consider a $50 million phase III clinical trial lasting 12 months for a drug with significant market potential. Simple calculations show more than $1 million of increased expected value for every percent that the likelihood of success is increased. Of course, not every drug entering a trial is safe and effective, and a successful trial should reveal those drugs with flaws. Clearly any definition of success must include trial results that are correct and unambiguous. Trials that are efficient—unambiguous at minimum cost—are also desired. Ethically we require that trials be as safe and humane as possible. Part of this is minimizing nonessential risks to trial subjects, and part is ensuring that the risks regarding adverse events and effects in the population to be treated are minimized.

Trial objectives may also incorporate commercial imperatives. The marketing department may suggest that "the treatment regimen must be once per day to be successful in the market." This requirement affects optimal dose and regimen for the trial and may even determine feasibility for the drug. Conversely, trial results can inform commercial decisions such as label strategy, marketing approach, and go/no-go decisions for the tested compounds as well as others.

Modeling data and simulating trials can be used to increase the likelihood of trial success and safety and can ensure that trial design delivers adequate information for decisions in other areas such as marketing or resource allocation.

Holford et al. have reviewed the use of simulations in clinical trials [60]. A recent collection of papers [61] discusses this topic from a PK/PD modeling perspective. Burman et al. [62] offer an industrial overview. The thesis of Abbas [63] contains a (Spanish language) review of the use of models in trial design and an extensive albeit idiosyncratic bibliography. A concise but useful commented bibliography is offered on-line [64]. Detailed examples of designing clinical trials and of optimizing trial design and conduct exist. Wientjes et al. [65] improved a trial design by modeling both exposure of bladder cancer cells to mitomycin C and efficacy of treatment. Their simulations suggested that nondose protocol elements, such as complete bladder emptying, low liquid intake, and alkalization of urine, improved positive outcome by as much as 20%. Mandema and Stanski [66] applied population pharmacokinetics to clinical trial data and derived a model for postoperative pain relief. An optimal Ketorolac dose was derived from this. Gebski et al. [67] used models on data from a partially completed trial to suggest an earlier-than-normal closure for a breast cancer study.

A case study is used here to illustrate the benefits of CATD and to emphasize some of the points we have outlined. The example is of simulation applied to a clinical trial. All aspects of the trial have been deliberately disguised. It is hoped that the benefits and results given here are useful and motivating.

A clinical phase III trial was about to begin. The estimated cost was about $50 million, with a duration of between one and two years. The market was a lucrative one and a market-leading competitor existed, so the trial strategy was positioning. Demonstrating noninferiority was the goal. Several clinical phase II studies demonstrated some efficacy, but these trials had different end points, did not include a comparator, and had been conducted over different (more or less broad) dose ranges. Doses that showed some efficacy were selected for the forthcoming trial, and power calculations were used to determine the number of subjects in each arm. A new lead physician (with competitor experience) was concerned that the trial protocol as designed would fail. She had no way of quantifying the likelihood of failure or of reducing it. She engaged experts in trial simulation to analyze the design and to advise her project team.

Specific analysis objectives were to estimate the best dose(s) to show noninferiority, to evaluate the design and synthesize alternatives, and to evaluate the likelihood of success for each alternative design.

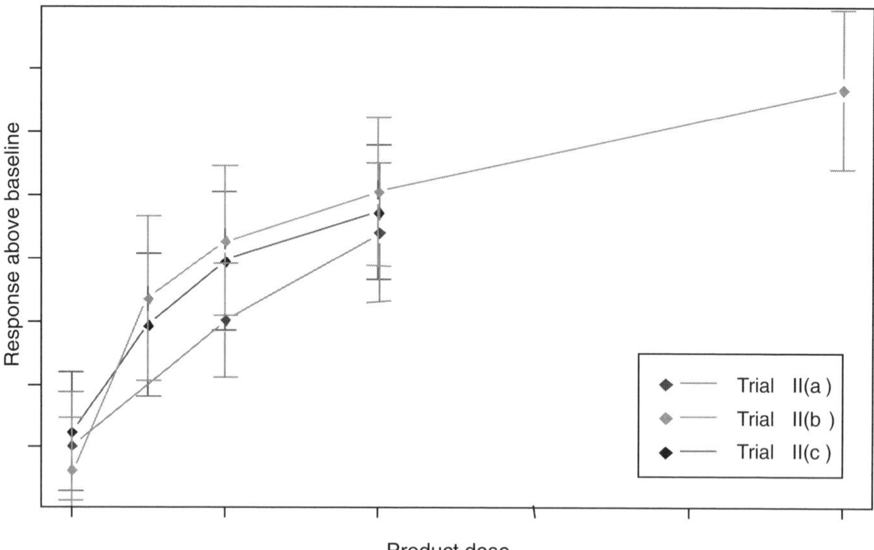

Figure 22.2 Three different clinical phase II trials, each with slightly different end points, are compared on an equal footing. This comparison is made possible by using these diverse data to derive a single model with a uniform end point. It is clear that the maximum effect was approached in only one trial. Modeling and analysis of the data would likely have suggested phase II trials that included more data at higher doses.

The modeling approach began by creating a dose-response model for each of the phase II trial results and by integrating these, using assumptions about the different clinical end points used. Figure 22.2 shows representative dose-response curves. This graph makes clear that at higher doses data were sparse, with the result that the maximum drug effect was not certain. Simulation analysis in earlier trials might have indicated this early enough for the researchers to get more high-dose data in the phase II trials. In this program, hand-offs between groups led to an uncoordinated approach and lost knowledge. Again, a model incorporating important data can act as a communication tool and can prevent knowledge "leaks" as team members leave the project.

The next step was to augment and expand the model to be able to predict the dose response for the comparator. Comparator data, from SBA (summary basis for approval data submitted to the FDA), yielded one model that predicted both candidate and comparator performance. The model accounted for age, disease baseline, and trial differences. Differences based on sex, weight, and other covariates were estimated to be negligible. The addition of the comparator data improved the predictive ability of the model for both drugs (Fig. 22.3).

The initial trial design tested two doses of drug, nominally low/medium and high, against a very high dose of comparator. Failure was defined as an

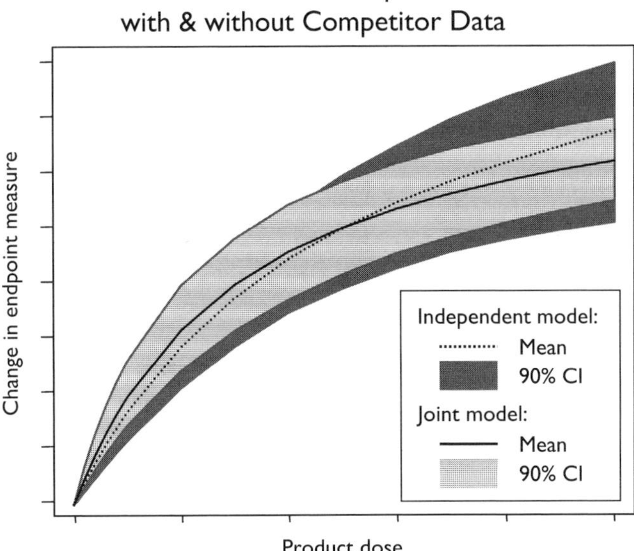

Figure 22.3 The drug dose-response model was augmented by using data for the comparator drug. Because the mechanism of the drugs was the same, this comprised additional data for the model. This enhanced the predictive power of the model, in a better estimate for central tendency (solid line compared with dotted line) but also in smaller confidence intervals. This is especially pronounced at the higher doses—precisely where data on the drug were sparse. See color plate.

measure difference of specific amount or greater between drug and comparator. Figure 22.4 shows simulation results for the high drug dose compared to the very high comparator dose. Probability of success was about 33%. For the low/medium drug dose this probability (not shown) was approximately zero. Likelihood of overall success of the trial as defined by the company was estimated to be approximately 3%—almost certainly a failure.

This suggested selecting a different dosing strategy for the trial design. The new design was simulated and showed that the success and failure likelihoods were reversed—the new trial was estimated to have about a 98% chance of success. At this point, the model was used in an interesting way. The company wanted to lower the 2% chance of failure even further. To do this, the team looked to the model itself. It is often useful to analyze models by varying parameters across their range of uncertainty and observing the effect on the end point of interest. These effects can be arranged in descending order and represented as a "tornado diagram": horizontal bars with lengths proportional to the range of effect associated with the parameter. Such a diagram shows parameters with variability most likely to affect predicted outcome. The model contained a parameter that was identified as key: relative potency,

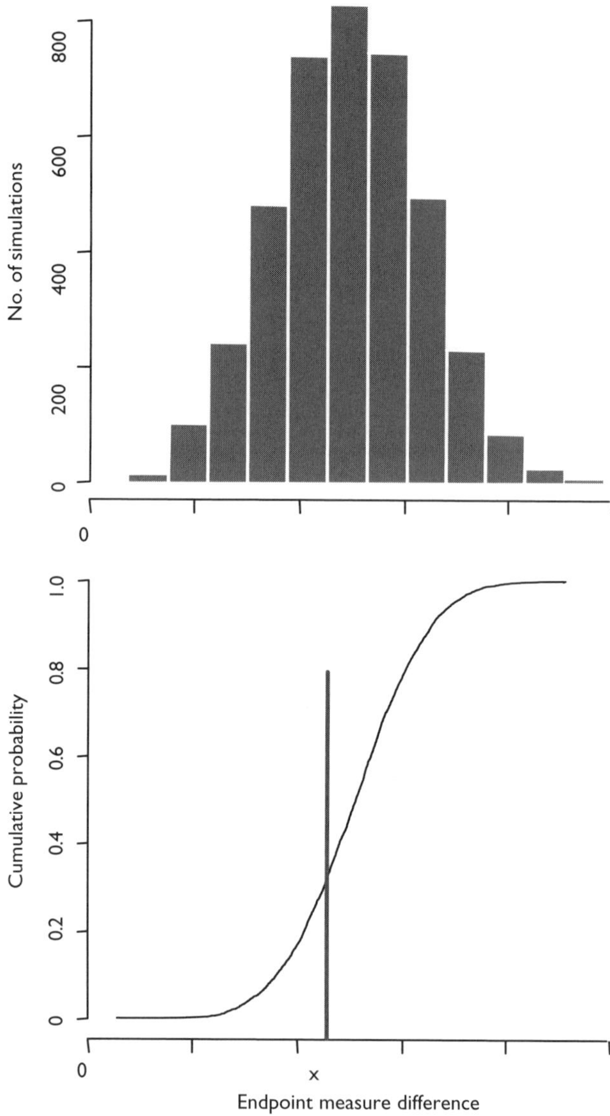

Figure 22.4 Monte Carlo techniques were used to simulate different hypothetical individuals for different instances of the trial design, using variability and uncertainty distributions from the model analysis. The result is a collection of predicted outcomes, shown as a binned histogram (top figure). Success was defined as a difference in end point measurement of "X" or smaller between drug and comparator. Likelihood of success (shown in the bottom figure as a cumulative probability) for this example (low/medium drug dose and high comparator dose) is seen to be low, about 33%.

which is the ratio of the dose of the drug creating 50% of maximum effect (ED_{50}) with the ED_{50} of its competitor. This suggested a crossover study that minimized the effect of interpatient variability. Simulations confirmed that the crossover design increased success likelihood. In fact, simulations confirmed that the number of patients could be drastically reduced for this design (approximately from 550 to 125) without significant loss of power. A side benefit was that crossover design allowed recruitment of nonnaive patients. Requiring fewer patients from a broader pool of candidates shortened the recruitment period by months. Finally, analysis of the simulations and consideration of the model suggested stratification between patient types. Simulations confirmed that all of these design changes improved the likelihood of success.

The trial was run, and FDA approval, on the basis of the results, was obtained. The drug is currently commercially successful. Were it not for the new team member who commissioned this work, this trial would have failed—at a cost of $50 million and the loss of two years of revenue. Moreover, other efficiencies (fewer patients, faster recruiting, better understanding of patient and market stratification) would not have been realized. The cost (in time and resources) for modeling projects should be balanced by the benefits of increased likelihood of success (for a drug that will be successful) and of possibly avoiding a trial for a compound that cannot succeed.

22.7 CONCLUSION

In this chapter motivation for creating mathematical models and for using them in simulations has been offered. An example of successful use of trial simulation was given. The need to make decisions in the face of incomplete, inconsistent, variably relevant, sparse, or overwhelmingly large sets of data was emphasized. The use of models was suggested as a proven way to make sense of and exploit these data to make good decisions. Specifically, physiologically based models allow the appropriate use of a wide variety of disparate data and knowledge. Incorporating physical laws essentially adds additional data, allowing physiological models to predict outcomes outside the range of the original data used to create them and offering a scientifically sound, data-based alternative to guessing. Because much of the model structure (especially for PBPK models) and its parameters are drug independent, the models can be used and reused. In fact, model structure between species is similar (except for size and geometry parameters), allowing better prediction of human results from animal tests. In vitro tests such as Caco -2 cell permeability are more directly applied to such models. Because many other drug-dependent parameters are based on physical measurements (molecular weight, solubility, lipophilicity, pK_a) the goal of a predictive human PK model based on in vitro measurements is moving closer to reality. PBPD models have many of the same advantages but give better insight into drug and disease effects on individual metabolic and signaling pathways. Models accurately representing the phenomena revealed by data can be used predictively to improve in vitro, preclinical, and clinical experiments.

ACKNOWLEDGMENT

Many ideas in this work developed in conversations with Dr. Sam Holtzman and Dr. Ron Beaver.

REFERENCES

1. Pharmaceutical Research and Manufacturers of America. Annual Report, 2003–04 (Washington, DC: PhRMA, October 2003).
2. DiMasi, JA, Hansen RW, and Grabowski, HG. The price of innovation: new estimates of drug development costs." *J Health Econ* 2003:22:151–85.
3. Office of Technology Assessment. "Pharmaceutical R&D: costs, risks, and rewards," OTA-H-522 (February 1993).
4. US Food and Drug Administration. Challenge and Opportunity on the Path to New Medical Products, March, 2004, http://www.fda.gov/oc/initiatives/criticalpath/whitepaper.html
5. Grabowski H, Vernon J, and DiMasi J. Returns on research and development for 1990s new drug introductions. *Pharmacoecon* Dec 2002; suppl. 3, 20:11–29.
6. Polidori D. "Modeling Diabetes for Pharmaceutical R and D Applications", Talk presented at: Center for Integrative Multiscale Modeling and Simulation Focused Workshop on Uncertainty Management in Engineering Design, California Institute of Technology, Jerrold E. Marsden, Director, May 2002.
7. Miller, G. A. The magical number seven, plus or minus two: some limits on our capacity for processing information. *Psych Rev* 1956;63:81–97.
8. Bonate P. Clinical trial simulation in drug development. *Pharm Res* 17:252–6.
9. Sheiner LB. Learning versus confirming in clinical drug development. *Clin Pharmacol Ther* 1997 Mar;61(3):275–91. Review.
10. Gabrielsson J and Weine, D. *Pharmacokinetic and pharmacodynamic data analysis: concept and applications,* 3rd Edition. Stockholm: Swedish Pharmaceutical Society, 2000.
11. Ekins S, Nikolsky Y, Nikolskaya T. Techniques: application of systems biology to absorption, distribution, metabolism, excretion and toxicity. *Trends Pharmacol Sci* 2005 Apr;26(4):202–9.
12. Wagner J. *Pharmacokinetics: past developments, present issues, future challenges, in pharmacokinetics: regulatory-industrial-academic perspectives*, Welling PG and Tse FLS, editors. New York: Marcel Dekker, 1988.
13. Hochhaus G, Barrett JS, Derendorf H. Evolution of pharmacokinetics and pharmacokinetic/dynamic correlations during the 20th century. *J Clin Pharmacol.* 2000 Sep;40(9):908–17.

14. Jang GR, Harris RZ, Lau DT. Pharmacokinetics and its role in small molecule drug discovery research. *Med Res Rev* 2001 Sep;21(5):382–96. Review.
15. Sheiner LB. PK/PD Approach to Dose Selection. Presented at the Esteve Foundation Symposium IX: Optimal Dose Identification, Lloret de Mar, Spain, October 2000.
16. Lin JH and Lu AYH. Role of pharmacokinetics and metabolism in drug discovery and development. *Pharm Rev* 1997;49(4):403–49.
17. Sheiner LB and Steimer J-L. Pharmacokinetic/pharmacodynamic modeling in drug development. *Annu Rev Pharmacol Toxicol* 2000; 40:67–95.
18. Nestorov I. Whole body pharmacokinetic models. *Clin Pharmacokinet* 2003; 42(10):883–908. Review.
19. Nestorov IA, Aarons LJ, Arundel PA, Rowland M. Lumping of whole-body physiologically based pharmacokinetic models. *J Pharmacokinet Biopharm* 1998 Feb;26(1):21–46.
20. Blakey GE, Nestorov IA, Arundel PA, Aarons LJ, Rowland M. Quantitative structure-pharmacokinetics relationships: I. Development of a whole-body physiologically based model to characterize changes in pharmacokinetics across a homologous series of barbiturates in the rat. *J Pharmacokinet Biopharm* 1997 Jun;25(3):277–312. Erratum in *J Pharmacokinet Biopharm* 1998 Feb;26(1): 131.
21. Andersen ME. Toxicokinetic modeling and its applications in chemical risk assessment. *Toxicol Lett* 2003 Feb; 18;138(1–2):9–27. Review.
22. Clewell HJ 3rd, Gentry PR, Covington TR, Gearhart JM. Development of a physiologically based pharmacokinetic model of trichloroethylene and its metabolites for use in risk assessment. *Environ Health Perspect* 2000 May;108 Suppl 2:283–305.
23. Bois FY. Statistical analysis of Clewell et al. PBPK model of trichloroethylene kinetics. *Environ Health Perspect* 2000 May;108 Suppl 2:307–16.
24. Poulin P, Theil FP. Prediction of pharmacokinetics prior to in vivo studies. II. Generic physiologically based pharmacokinetic models of drug disposition. *J Pharm Sci* 2002 May;91(5):1358–70.
25. Tsukamoto Y, Kato Y, Ura M, Horii I, Ishitsuka H, Kusuhara H, Sugiyama Y. A physiologically based pharmacokinetic analysis of capecitabine, a triple prodrug of 5-FU, in humans: the mechanism for tumor-selective accumulation of 5-FU. *Pharm Res* 2001 Aug;18(8):1190–202.
26. Kawai R, Mathew D, Tanaka C, Rowland M Physiologically based pharmacokinetics of cyclosporine A: extension to tissue distribution kinetics in rats and scale-up to human. *J Pharmacol Exp Ther* 1998 Nov;287(2):457–68.
27. Bjorkman S, Wada DR, Berling BM, Benoni G. Prediction of the disposition of midazolam in surgical patients by a physiologically based pharmacokinetic model. *J Pharm Sci* 2001 Sep;90(9):1226–41.
28. Hatanaka T. Clinical pharmacokinetics of pravastatin: mechanisms of pharmacokinetic events. *Clin Pharmacokinet* 2000 Dec;39(6):397–412. Review.
29. van de Waterbeemd H, Gifford E. ADMET in silico modelling: towards prediction paradise? *Nat Rev Drug Discov* 2003 Mar;2(3):192–204. Review.

30. Dickins M, van de Waterbeemd H, Simulation models for drug disposition and drug interaction. *Drug Discov Today: Biosilico* 2004; 2(1):38–45
31. Ekins S, Wrighton SA. Application of in silico approaches to predicting drug-drug interactions. *J Pharmacol Toxicol Methods* 2001 Jan–Feb;45(1):65–9. Review.
32. Ekins S. Predicting undesirable drug interactions with promiscuous proteins in silico. *Drug Discov Today* 2004 Mar 15;9(6):276–85. Review.
33. Leahy D. Drug discovery information integration: virtual humans for pharmacokinetics. *Drug Discov Today* 2004;2(2):78–84.
34. Obach RS, Baxter JG, Liston TE, Silber BM, Jones BC, MacIntyre F, Rance DJ, Wastall P. The prediction of human pharmacokinetic parameters from preclinical and in vitro metabolism data. *J Pharmacol Exp Ther* 1997 Oct;283(1): 46–58
35. Houston JB, Carlile DJ. Prediction of hepatic clearance from microsomes, hepatocytes, and liver slices. *Drug Metab Rev* 1997 Nov;29(4):891–922.
36. Charnick SB, Kawai R, Nedelman JR, Lemaire M, Niederberger W, Sato H. Perspectives in pharmacokinetics. Physiologically based pharmacokinetic modeling as a tool for drug development. *J Pharmacokinet Biopharm* 1995 Apr;23(2):217–29. Review.
37. Theil FP, Guentert TW, Haddad S, Poulin P. Utility of physiologically based pharmacokinetic models to drug development and rational drug discovery candidate selection. *Toxicol Lett* 2003 Feb 18;138(1–2):29–49. Review.
38. Rowland M, Balant L, Peck C. Physiologically based pharmacokinetics in drug development and regulatory science: a workshop report (Georgetown University, Washington, DC, May 29–30, 2002). *AAPS PharmSci* 2004 Feb; 9;6(1):E6.
39. Reddy M, Yang RSH, Clewell HJ, Andersen ME (eds). *Physiologically based pharmacokinetic modeling.* Zurich: Wiley VCH, 2005.
40. Haggard HW, Greenberg LA, Turner JA. The physiological principles governing the action of acetone together with determination of toxicity. *J Ind Hyg Toxicol* 1944;26:133–51.
41. Teorell T. Kinetics of distribution of substances administered to the body. *Arch Intern Pharmacodyn* 1937;57:205–40.
42. Bischoff KB, Dedrick RL. Thiopental pharmacokinetics. *J Pharm Sci* 1968 Aug;57(8):1346–51.
43. Bischoff KB, Dedrick RL, Zaharko DS, Longstreth JA. Methotrexate pharmacokinetics. *J Pharm Sci* 1971 Aug;60(8):1128–33.
44. Zaharko DS, Dedrick RL, Bischoff KB, Longstreth JA, Oliverio VT. Methotrexate tissue distribution: prediction by a mathematical model. *J Natl Cancer Inst* 1971 Apr;46(4):775–84.
45. Dedrick R, Bischoff KB, Zaharko DS. Interspecies correlation of plasma concentration history of methotrexate (NSC-740). *Cancer Chemother Rep* 1970 Apr;54(2):95–101.
46. Guyton AC, *Textbook of medical physiology*, 2nd ed. Philadelphia: W. B. Saunders, 1964.
47. Atkinson AJ, Daniels CE, Dedrick RL, Grudzinskas CV, Markey SP. *Principles of clinical pharmacology.* San Diego: Academic Press, 2001

48. Chen HS, Gross JF. Physiologically based pharmacokinetic models for anticancer drugs. *Cancer Chemother Pharmacol* 1979;2(2):85–94. Review.
49. Lutz RJ, Dedrick RL, Matthews HB, Eling TE, Anderson MW. A preliminary pharmacokinetic model for several chlorinated biphenyls in the rat. *Drug Metab Dispos* 1977;5:386–396
50. Fujita M, Takabatake E. Mercury levels in human maternal and neonatal blood, hair and milk. *Bull Environ Contam Toxicol* 18:205–209 (1977).
51. Schaddelee MP, Collins SD, DeJongh J, de Boer AG, Ijzerman AP, Danhof M. Pharmacokinetic/pharmacodynamic modelling of the anti-hyperalgesic and anti-nociceptive effect of adenosine A1 receptor partial agonists in neuropathic pain. *Eur J Pharmacol* 2005 May 9;514(2–3):131–40.
52. Hodgkin AL, Huxley AF. A quantitative description of membrane current and its application to conduction and excitation in nerve cells. *J Physiol* 1952;117: 500–44.
53. Bower JM, Bolouri H. *Computational modeling of genetic and biochemical networks*. Cambridge, MA: MIT Press, 2001.
54. Stokes CL. Biological systems modeling: powerful medicine for biomedical eR&D. *Am Inst Chem Eng J* 2000;46:430.
55. Uehing MD. Model patient. *Bio-IT World*, November 1, 2005, http://www.bio-itworld.com/archive/121503/trials.html
56. Uehing MD. Supermodels: a gallery. *Bio-IT World*, November 1, 2005, http://www.bio-itworld.com/archive/121503/trials_sidebar_3918.html
57. Willmann S, Lippert J, Sevestre M, Solodenko J, Fois F, Schmitt W. PK-Sim®: a physiologically based pharmacokinetic "whole-body" model. *Biosilico* 2003;1(4): 121–4
58. Parrott N, Lave T. Prediction of intestinal absorption: comparative assessment of GASTROPLUS™ and IDEA™. *Eur J Pharm Sci* 2002;17:51–61
59. D'Sousa RW, Boxenbaum H. Physiological pharmacokinetic models: some aspects of theory, practice, and potential. *Toxicol Ind Health* 1988;4:151–91.
60. Holford NH, Kimko HC, Monteleone JP, Peck CC. Simulation of clinical trials. *Annu Rev Pharmacol Toxicol* 2000;40:209–34.
61. Duffal SB, Kimko HC (eds). *Simulation for designing clinical trials: a pharmacokinetic-pharmacodynamic modeling perspective (Drugs and the pharmaceutical sciences*, Vol 127). New York: Marcel Dekker, 2003
62. Burman C-F, Hamrén B, Olsson P. Modelling and simulation to improve decision-making in clinical development. *Pharm Stat* 2005;4(1):47–58.
63. Abbas I. *Integración de los Modelos de Simulación en el Diseño de los Ensayos Clíninos*, Doctoral Thesis, December, 2003, Polytechnic University of Barcelona.
64. Bibliography for Computer-Assisted Trial Design, at www.pharsight.com/solutions/soln_catd_bibliography.php
65. Wientjes MG, Badalament RA, Au JL. Use of pharmacologic data and computer simulations to design an efficacy trial of intravesical mitomycin C therapy for superficial bladder cancer. *Cancer Chemother Pharmacol* 1993;32(4): 255–62.

66. Mandema JW, Stanski DR. Population pharmacodynamic model for ketorolac analgesia. *Clin Pharmacol Ther* 1996 Dec;60(6):619–35.
67. Gebski V, McNeil D, Coates A, Forbes J. Monitoring distributional assumptions and early stopping for a prospective clinical trial using Monte Carlo simulation. *Stat Med* 1987 Sep;6(6):667–78.

PART VI

COMPUTERS IN DEVELOPMENT DECISION MAKING, ECONOMICS, AND MARKET ANALYSIS

23

MAKING PHARMACEUTICAL DEVELOPMENT MORE EFFICIENT

Michael Rosenberg and Richard Farris

Contents

23.1 INTRODUCTION

The need to improve the efficiency of the discovery and development process is reflected most visibly by the high cost of developing new drugs and the pace at which those costs have outstripped inflation. Between 1987 and 2001, the cost of developing a single new drug increased from $138 million to $802

Computer Applications in Pharmaceutical Research and Development, Edited by Sean Ekins.
ISBN 0-471-73779-8

million. Had this increase paced inflation, the number would have been $318 million (in 2002 dollars) [1]. These figures include direct research costs as well as those of discovery, attrition, and cost of capital. The largest single component, direct cost of clinical assessment, has increased sharply, because of increases in the number and size of clinical trials [2], regulatory demands, chronic and complex indications, difficulty in recruiting and retaining patients, and programs that are increasingly global. Even more dismaying is the fact that despite considerably greater investments in research efforts, the number of newer products is shrinking [3].

There is thus little question of the urgent need to improve the efficiency of clinical development, defined by the time and cost of getting a new drug to market. Recognizing that only about one of every five candidates that enter clinical testing will eventually make it to the marketplace, the means of improved efficiency must lie in improved decision making, primarily in the form of the ability to kill unpromising candidates early and speed the progress of those that are promising. Cutting development time by half is estimated to reduce the development costs by 30%, and improving clinical success rates to one in three would reduce costs by 27% [4]. The key to improved decision making can only lie in improved data handling—earlier decisions enabled by more data, of better quality, earlier in the process than is currently possible.

Decision making is the linchpin of efficiency. Even a small change—killing an unpromising candidate even a few days earlier—will substantially impact development costs. This capability will increasingly be a key differentiator for any company developing pharmaceutical products, from the largest multinational to the smallest biotech firm. It may well be the single capability that best predicts market dominance in the next decade. Large companies have dominated drug discovery in the past because of the enormous resources required, but technology dramatically changed this by enabling even very small companies to effectively compete through effective use of inexpensive technology. For development, the same message is clear: Smaller companies will become formidable competitors through effective leveraging of technology. The lesson in every business is to change or die.

Industry's challenge is how to use the demonstrated capability of existing communications and computer technology to improve data handling and decision making. Despite widespread recognition of these developments, the industry has made little leeway in implementing meaningful changes. This chapter discusses the context, approach, and tools by which the efficiency of development of pharmaceuticals can be markedly improved.

23.2 TECHNOLOGY, PAST AND PRESENT

Pharmaceutical development traditionally involves a linear, sequential series of structured events. This is true on both a macro (program) level as well as a micro (study) level. In both cases, there is an extraordinary amount of highly structured data—a single clinical trial alone may involve several million data points, and a development program may include as many as 30 or more studies. One of the challenging aspects of pharmaceutical development is the fact that this enormous quantity of data must be handled accurately, with accountability from the first place a result was recorded to the final database, along with each change along the way.

The legacy of this process is that what began as a paper-and-pencil process remains essentially unchanged today, despite considerable advancement in communications and data handling over the past several decades. Few would argue that computers and the Internet have materially altered the way businesses communicate and access information, but few would argue that these advances have similarly altered the way pharmaceutical research is conducted. As demands for more studies of larger size have mounted, the disappointing effect has been a drop in efficiency reflected in the hard figures cited above.

The basic processes that have been utilized in collecting and analyzing data over the past few decades remain essentially unchanged. A major bottleneck remains simply getting data into the system: The majority of data are still recorded with a pen on a piece of paper, and then those figures are manually entered into a computer. Discrepancies are resolved mostly by faxing sites and manually entering corrections. On a more strategic level, each step is completed before the next step is started: Each query must be resolved before a database can be locked, analysis cannot start until a database is locked, and decisions cannot be made before analysis is completed.

Also notable is the limited impact of the handful of new technologies that have been adopted. Web-based electronic data collection (commonly called EDC systems, although this term actually refers to any electronic system that handles data, regardless of how data are collected), which allows some edit checks to be done in the field, is an example. Even this tool has been hobbled by tradition: This technology still requires that data are recorded first on a piece of paper, then transferred to a worksheet, and then manually entered by keyboard at the site level. Although some edit checks (primarily those that check range validity) are done, checks on the most frequent source of discrepancies, inconsistency with other parts of the questionnaire and past data, are batched and run periodically rather than as the user enters data. The requirement for manual data entry also extracts a price—site personnel are clinicians (such as nurses), which means they are not necessarily skilled at data entry. The result is that data entry is slow and expensive. In addition, because the task is onerous to many, the work simply gets delayed. The importance of such pragmatic issues is reflected by the fact that only a fraction of clinical practices participate in clinical trials more than once. All of these considerations belie the larger problem—the technology is simply not being designed and used well. This is reflected by the observation that even with the adoption of web-based data collection, the median time between critical clinical trial milestones has been increasing since 1977 [5]. So long as these systems continue to focus on getting data into a database—the data management function—rather than decision making, they will never contribute materially to improving the overall efficiency of drug development.

Although technology has the potential to revolutionize drug development, its application has been stunted by an industry that seeks to apply it without changing the underlying processes. Yes, technology has improved some elements of data collection and handling, most notably validation. This task is eminently suited to computerization because it is demanding, tedious, and stultifyingly repetitive. However, technology's potential lies in allowing new processes that better leverage information flow.

Two major areas are ripe for improvement: more efficient processes enabled by technology and the ability to make better decisions earlier, a capability enabled by the availability of more data, or better quality, earlier than previously possible. The former can be understood from the standpoint of incrementalism: The benefit of technology is to allow processes to be improved, so the full advantage of technology will not be enjoyed until they change. Indeed, this "bolt electronic data collection on the front end" approach taken by industry so far has indeed failed to improve overall timelines despite a considerable financial cost, in the same way that after Watt's invention of the steam engine it took a number of years to realize that the mills need no longer be located at the stream—usually next to the waterwheels that powered the mills before the steam engine. From a technical perspective, implementation of technology without revisiting the underlying processes often results in reduced efficiency over manual processes, user frustration, and ultimately, failure of the technology. Failure also taints future technology development because the unrealized promise of the past makes users reluctant to try new things in the future—especially in an industry that is decidedly resistant to change.

The most important but currently absent component is the focus on decision making. This is an area rife with examples from other industries in which processes were changed to focus on the important aspects of business. In pharmaceutical development, there is none that is more important than decision making, on both a tactical as well as a strategic level. Strategic decisions (those focusing on big-picture issues such as advancing to a higher dose, weighing safety information against efficacy data, progressing from one phase of development to the next) are built on a foundation of tactical decisions (data and tight management of studies) decisions.

23.3 TACTICAL DECISION MAKING

The practical aspects of computers lie in their ability to collect, simplify, and provide access to massive amounts of data easily The traditional approach of patiently waiting for field data, where entry often takes weeks to months, does not take advantage of currently available technology. Even with web-based data collection, data availability remains a bottleneck to effectively managing studies.

Tactical decisions focus on two key elements, data and performance. The data component is the traditional focus of study efficiency, as evidenced by the first application of technology (even as ineffective as it has been) to this step. Although it is clear that clean data are an essential element of any development program, technology has for the most part not been applied to the effective management of its collection. Thus, although the current focus of technology is getting data into a database, it is actually the performance measures that determine the speed and accuracy with which data are collected. For example, slow response times at the site (reflected by measures such as interval between data collection and entry and between query receipt and response) best predict future data quality. Systems that focus on a range of performance indices allow fundamental management decisions about the magnitude and reasons for sub-optimal performance and allow measures to improve.

The focus of technology has been largely in data entry. Since the adoption of web-based data entry systems (commonly called EDC, though the term is much more broad) over the past five years, the promise of faster development times has been found to be elusive. As with previous technologies (such as faxback systems) that made the same promise, product timelines have not improved. Overall, development timelines continue to increase, and some companies have forayed into this technology with disastrous results, most often the consequence of inadequate planning and failure to appreciate the changes that must surround technology itself. The high cost of such systems has also made them prohibitive for smaller research groups, and a lesson from industry's experience is that it takes a good deal of training and change of processes to make these systems work well. For example, training must be provided to sites and internal staff, technical and user support must be available, and conflicts with current processes must be quickly identified and resolved, to name just a few requirements. Few companies are able to effectively do these things, and as a result, few are able to appreciate a beneficial return on investment.

23.4 STRATEGIC DECISION MAKING

If the day-to-day management of studies can be considered tactical, the strategic use of information is the real—and largely unrealized—promise of computers and technology. Assuming that the tactical side provides for a reliable stream of information, strategic decisions can then be made as data accumulate rather than waiting until a project's completion. After the last patient visit, data need to be cleaned, then analyzed, then acted upon, usually to design and finalize the next step of research. This process generally takes weeks to months.

This application has numerous examples. One is early rising-dose escalation studies that are generally conducted during phase I of a product's development. These involve sequentially increasing administered dose to find the maximum tolerated dose for subsequent testing in patients. The industry currently conducts such studies by completing each dose level, analyzing the data collected, and deciding about the next higher dose, a process that averages about six weeks.

However, technology allows this same six-week interval to be trimmed down to a matter of days by careful planning and use of technology. A patient group is dosed in the morning, data are collected in the afternoon and evening, and they are summarized and analyzed that evening and posted to a website. The individuals involved with making the decision about whether to proceed to the next higher dose level are able to examine and discuss the data regardless of where they are in the world and what time it is there. Once a decision is made, the next dosing can be administered the following day.

During a study, this same process can be repeated for other study areas. For example, a typical phase II study might involve several dosing arms. These studies are designed at the outset to determine a single, sometimes two, doses that will be used in the large, costly phase III studies that serve as the basis of application to regulatory authorities to market a drug. Rather than awaiting the end of the study, data are made available as they are collected. Halfway through the study, a pharmaceutical company would have half of the data and half of the knowledge they would have if they waited to the end of the study. Because issues such as study duration and magnitude of effect of a drug under test are at best roughly estimated, it may be that when you are only three-quarters of the way through a planned study sufficient information exists that you can make a decision. It may be that one dosing arm is clearly not working, and a decision to stop enrollment in that arm can be made; it may be that a decision is effectively and efficiently made to stop the study entirely. Another scenario is that the end of the study provides insufficient information. Early detection of this impending problem will allow for quick decisions on extension of the study before its anticipated end, thus eliminating the need to repeat the study or to regroup at the study conclusion, wasting time and resources

Finally, one major and unappreciated advantage is the ability to reduce the between-study timelines, one of industry's traditional Achilles' heels. The sequential, linear model that remains the industry norm involves completion of a study, cleanup, and analysis. After this, the next study is designed and implemented. The entire process generally takes several months, often longer if the project is complex. If technical capabilities allow greater ability to manage tactical aspects (tight study management) but broad strategic processes (speed of making key decisions, especially on safety, moving between studies and phases) are not modified, then potential remains unrealized. Most companies find that use of these systems most often reflects difficulty not so much in adopting technology (which is easy to install and use) but in the process of process reengineering that really matters. Most innovators find that that the full benefits of technology are most often limited by the ability to accommodate the technology in a manner that fully leverages its potential.

In contrast, current computational technology allows a steady stream of information that builds as the study evolves. When the study is half completed, indications of many aspects of drug safety and performance become obvious. At that point, the next study can be roughed out. This plan can be refined as the study progresses and greater knowledge is gained. If the study is not blinded, the need for this process is self-evident; if it is blinded, then there is still much to be gained. A wealth of safety information is generated, key because safety often drives development as well as being a general indication of drug efficacy. For example, if there is a single treatment arm, efficacy can be indicated by subtracting the expected performance of the comparison arm (placebo or standard use therapy) from the pooled effect estimate. The same principle can be used to guide the extensive preparation that precedes preparation of regulatory submissions after Phase III studies.

23.5 SYSTEMS INTEGRATION

Decision making and management requires (1) a means of quickly collecting both data and performance indicators on a wide variety of measures, (2) being able to quickly and automatically summarize those data, in different forms for different functional responsibilities, and (3) providing a means of reacting to that information. Decision making is thus the culmination of the technology's value—transforming a vast stream of raw data into meaningful information and further refining to knowledge. Oversight and intervention at each stage are important, as is understanding the mechanisms of how data are summarized and simplified and the ability to drill down as required.

A system designed with these principles has been in use for more than a decade [6, 7]. The system, which has been continually refined and expanded during the 15 years since it was first used, involves a series of component modules designed to work together and that can be rapidly and flexibly customized.

The system currently includes (Fig. 23.1):

- Multiple options for data input, the most important of which are machine read and thus obviate the bottleneck that often occurs in data entry. The two main options are Optical Mark Read (bubble) forms, and SmartPen™, a special pen with an optical sensor that records each keystroke (Fig. 23.2). Both utilize paper case report forms, for which sites have indicated a strong preference over the requirement to enter data on a keyboard.

- An automated system that immediately validates and flags areas where human intervention is required, coupled with a second layer of more extensive validation executed by data management specialists
- Patient randomization and tracking of study subjects through an electronic master log
- A online query management system that allows sites to receive queries within minutes of data submission and resolution to be handled and documented immediately (Fig. 23.3)
- Links to document management system for regulatory reports and submissions
- A full range of reports reflecting both data and performance indices, available over the web, that can be easily modified and supplemented

The system differs from others in having all the components designed at the outset to work as part of a single integrated unit that selectively evaluates a stream of information that reflects site performance, data quality, and product performance. One of the benefits is that the reporting is oriented around the information needed by different performance roles: Monitors normally get a different set of reports than project managers, and medical monitors see different status indicators than executive-level reviewers. These roles are, however, only a starting point: With different permissions, any team member can view whatever information is needed. A second major benefit is that the reports can be altered quickly in response to changing requirements during a study. The system's evolution has been guided by users, based on the premise

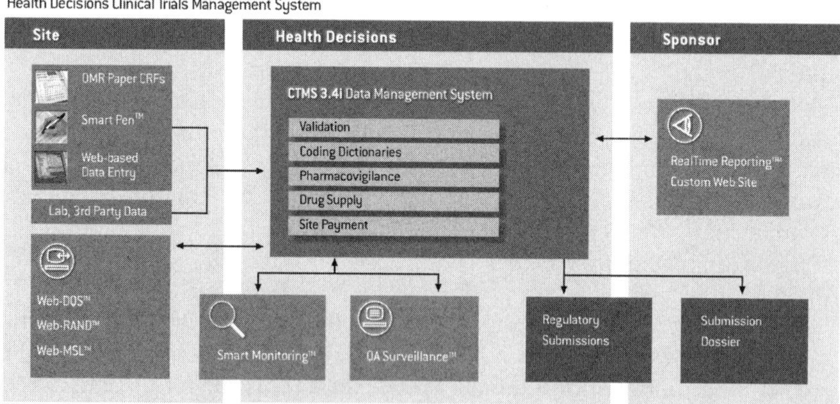

Figure 23.1 Components of the integrated system from the perspective of the clinical site, the data management group, and project management. The function of each of these components is built around complementary capabilities of others in the system to allow timely communications, tasking, and management. (Copyright 2001–6, Health Decisions, Inc.) See color plate.

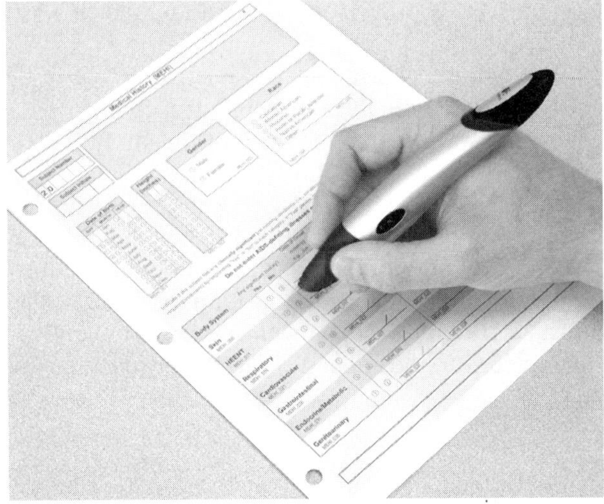

Figure 23.2 The SmartPen™ system is a pen with an optical sensor that records each keystroke on a special form. The pen is docked at a computer or data can be wirelessly transmitted, and data from anywhere in the world are immediately sent for validation. Queries are generated within minutes, closing the feedback loop and markedly reducing query rates as compared to conventional systems.

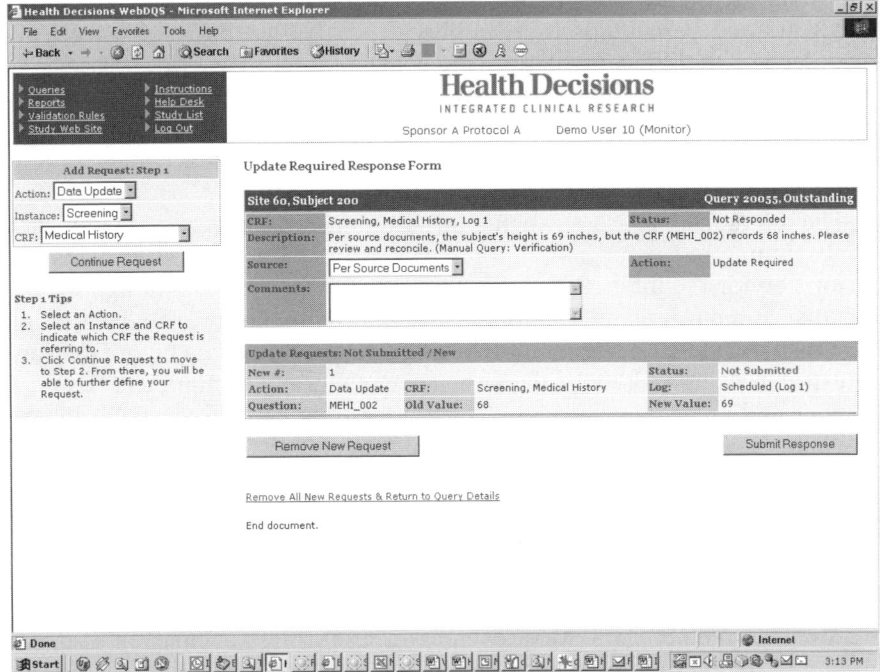

Figure 23.3 The Data Query System™ is a web-based management tool that sites use to receive and manage queries. See color plate.

that technology must be appropriately applied and its success measured by user return on investment.[8]

This ability to provide a continuous perspective of key indicators, essentially as they are generated, enables multiple decision processes to proceed in parallel rather than waiting until the end of the study. The approach also has a number of other benefits that may not be immediately apparent but can significantly affect both cost and timelines for development.

The success of this approach is illustrated by the multiple industry benchmarks it has established, but none more clearly than its use on a large multinational evaluation involving 1500 patients for a drug for Alzheimer disease. Measured against starting project goals, the system was central to the ability to complete the project 1.6 years ahead of the 5-year schedule and $32 million under budget [9].

23.6 THE BOTTOM LINE: EXAMPLES

23.6.1 Improving Efficiency of Monitoring

Stringent regulatory requirements dictate that the integrity of each piece of information be verified, from the first time it is recorded and at each step along the way until the final database. Perhaps the most demanding of these requirements is the industry practice of field monitoring, which requires highly trained individuals to visit sites to verify that data are accurately recorded and that FDA regulations are being followed. This process accounts for approximately one-third the cost of a study, which can run into the tens of millions of dollars for each study. In addition, the traditional approach is that data collected at the site remain there until the monitor comes by, normally every few weeks, to examine the data and bring them back.

The monitoring process is being improved in two major ways: First, sites are beginning to submit unmonitored data between monitor visits. This is a major step for the industry but one that is eminently sensible in light of the fact that computers do a far more reliable and comprehensive job of checking data than individuals. The relic of having monitors check data before they are returned harkens back to the days when computers and communications were complicated and expensive and did not effectively exist in the field. Just as computer programmers learn that the quickest way to debug a program is to allow debugging applications to handle the preliminary evaluations, the industry is learning—slowly, some argue—that computers are also much better at sorting through and highlighting areas of concern in data.

The second improvement comes from the potential that computers have, in conjunction with newer processes, to dramatically reduce the cost and time required to monitor data. Most of monitoring involves comparing a source document, defined as the first place a piece of data was recorded, with what was written. Because data are often recorded by first entry in a patient record, then abstracting to a case report form, and then manual entry, substantial potential for error exists. This is why the traditional practice of carefully checking at each step is reasonable. However, the advent of newer technology such as an optical pen (SmartPen™) means that data can, for the first time, be recorded on a form that will be the source document. Indeed, it is electronically recorded as it is written. This aspect alone could substantially impact both the cost and time required for a development program.

23.6.2 Improved Quality and Timeliness of Data

A major complaint of clinical sites is the difficulty and time required for data entry (when they have to enter the data through a keyboard) and the effort required to resolve queries, which are often returned weeks or even months after a patient visit. Machine-read data, whether collected by optical mark read or SmartPen™, ensure that data are both entered and validated, with queries returned, in a matter of minutes after they are recorded. Coupled with a quick feedback loop, this system ensures that query rates are typically about one-tenth those for web-based EDC systems and even lower for paper-and-hand entry systems. This system also highlights recurring problems and areas of potential improvement that may impair study timeliness and quality.

23.6.3 Site Performance Tracking

Close tracking of data entry means that performance measures can be tracked and managed. Such measures typically include query rates (which can be tracked by site, investigator, quesiton, and any comparators), time to respond to queries, rate of query rejection, and the like, and they provide an opportunity to identify and correct performance issues, whether associated with an individual site or study or a program. This capability alone provides a powerful tool by which sites throughout the world can be closely monitored.

23.6.4 The Changing Role of Clinical Research Associates

The availability of a range of performance measures and the ability to do many more routine tasks by computer (notably those related to source verification) mean that the Clinical research associate (CRA)'s role changes from box-checker to manager. The CRA, and a newer layer of submanagers who specialize in monitoring performance data, can then focus on identifying and addressing performance issues. The traditional requirement to go to a site to fully understand what is occurring is substantially reduced, and monitoring can be more effectively conducted while spending less time traveling.

23.6.5 Patient Recruitment

The rate of recruitment is one of the most frequent factors limiting the speed of clinical evaluations. Particularly in some areas, such as oncology, finding an adequate supply of patients even in a large geographical area such as the US frequently is the main constraint on study speed. Traditionally, a strategy is put in place and followed for the life of a project.

Newer systems, however, offer the possibility of evaluating performance on a daily basis and the opportunity for midcourse corrections. Tracking screen failures, enrollment (reflected by integrated web-based randomization and online master subject logs), and dropout rates failure all measures that directly affect study duration and underlying assumptions about statistical power, directly reflect study experience. The ability to link performance metrics at each step allows successful strategies to be differentiated from those that are less successful and to have the more successful quickly shared and the less successful reduced or eliminated. As an example, use of this strategy has consistently allowed the establishment of industry benchmarks in enrolling studies in diverse geographical and therapeutic areas, including enrollment in studies of breast cancer, vaginal microbiocides, and Alzheimer disease.

23.6.6 Reduced Time to Database Lock

This event is one of the most visible in a study, representing the culmination of efforts spanning months or years and often representing the future of a product or even a company. Locking the database requires that every query and all outstanding discrepancies regarding data be resolved.

The key to rapid database lock is minimizing the number of outstanding queries. With electronic systems, the number of queries generated can be minimized through the use of systems that provide rapid feedback to sites and systems to rapidly identify and resolve those that do occur. Our experience with such systems shows that rapid feedback is the major element in query reduction. Using the integrated system shown in Figure 23.1, those queries that are generated are resolved as they are generated (sites normally have 2 weeks to complete resolution, with that time progressively reduced toward the end of a study). With careful planning, the integrated system enables database lock on the same day as the last patient visit (LPLV), a task that is regularly accomplished with minimal extra effort. On average, this system produces database lock within five to seven days after LPLV.

Although web-based data collection systems have been credited with reducing database lock times as compared with those of five years ago, today there is a high degree of variability between companies on time to database lock. One of the promises of web-based data collection is rapid database lock; this promise, however, has gone unrealized because of the high number of queries that typically remain even with web-based data collection systems. Database lock times typically range between several weeks and several months, with the average probably around eight weeks. This variability probably reflects whether and how electronic systems are used internally, emphasizing the need for processes that build on the capabilities of electronic systems.

23.6.7 Management of Geographically Diverse Studies

The confluence of communications and data processing technology provides their greatest synergy in the management of complex, diverse studies, especially those that may be additionally complicated by globalization. Properly designed, the electronic systems described here can operate with minimal intervention, providing a steady stream of data and performance indices, especially those systems that allow data to be machine read and at least partial validation to be automated.

23.7 CONCLUSIONS

There can be little doubt that utilization of technology is necessary to even keeping pace in the expanding-complexity world of pharmaceutical development. This is true not only because of the increasing number and size of studies with development programs but also because a global perspective and the ability to effectively conduct complex studies throughout the world, often concurrently, are becoming the norm. The challenge then becomes one of implementing a system that facilitates collection of high-quality data and continuous monitoring of performance data, along with management tools to continuously improve performance. That tactical ability to tightly manage complex studies enables a strategic ability of earlier, better, and more nimble decisions.

The technology and processes to improve decision making exist today and have been demonstrated in large clinical studies to be capable of significantly reducing both expense and timelines [9]. As with any technology, it is the processes that are enabled by the technology, rather than the technology itself, that will most centrally determine a company's ability to effectively improve efficiency. Just as the automobile industry underwent a profound change when Japanese competitors entered the market, the pharmaceutical industry is likely to change in coming years to favor those competitors who can embrace new technology and processes that make them more nimble and efficient than those who cannot.

REFERENCES

1. DiMasi JA, Hansen RW, Grabowski HG. The price of innovation: new estimates of drug development costs. *Pharmacoeconomics* 2003;22:151–85.
2. Centre for Medicines Research. *Describing Dossiers: Characterising Clinical Dossiers for Global Registration*. R&D Briefing 25, CMR International, Surrey, UK, 2000.
3. Centre for Medicines Research. *R&D Pharmaceutical Investment and Output Survey*. CMR International, Surrey, UK, 2003.

4. DiMasi JA. The value of improving the productivity of the drug development process: faster times and better decisions. In: The cost and value of new medicines in an era of change. *Pharmacoeconomics* 2002;20(Suppl 3):1–10.
5. Centre for Medicines Research, *2004 Global Clinical Performances Metrics Programme Report*, Industry Report, July 2004.
6. Rosenberg MJ, Haldi JR. Accelerating drug development with electronic data collection and processing. *Sci Computing Automation* 1995;11:13–17.
7. Rosenberg MJ. The promise and practice of technology: implementing electronic development systems. *Curr Drug Discov* 2001;25–8.
8. Rosenberg M, Farris F. Electronic systems and decision making. *Curr Drug Discov* 2003;3:1–4.
9. Schoenberger C. An Alzheimer's drug goes on trial, *Forbes Magazine*, March 20, 2000, pp. 94–6.

24

USE OF INTERACTIVE SOFTWARE IN MEDICAL DECISION MAKING

RENÉE J. GOLDBERG ARNOLD

Contents

Computer Applications in Pharmaceutical Research and Development, Edited by Sean Ekins.
ISBN 0-471-73779-8

24.1 INTRODUCTION

Interactive software, encompassing automated programs using individual computers, the Internet, and interactive voice response (IVR/telephone), has a valuable place in health outcomes research, disease management, and decision making in clinical and marketing settings. Rather than being static (i.e., a one-time calculation), automated models offer the major advantage of enhanced external validity (generalizability), the ability to project outcomes beyond a limited time horizon, and the ability to examine multiple groups and perform subanalyses.

The use of evidence-based medicine, that is, using the best data or evidence available to inform scientific decisions, has garnered interest recently because it can help propel development of interactive programs to help inform multiple potential end users. These end users include (1) patients, who can use such programs for self-management of chronic illnesses; (2) health care providers, in terms of their decisions on individual patients or groups of patients to provide an improved patient experience and enhanced patient-provider responsiveness; and (3) clinical and marketing members of the pharmaceutical company team, to use actual, rather than anecdotal, trends and outcomes to help determine future directions that are likely to be fruitful in the clinical development arena and to satisfy regulatory requirements for postmarketing data.

24.2 METHODOLOGIES OF SOFTWARE AND MODEL DEVELOPMENT

A variety of institutional and commercial off-the-shelf (COTS) products are available to facilitate development of health economic or other models to aid in decision making. Some, such as Decision Maker® and U-Maker® (personal communication, Frank Sonnenberg, M.D.), are available primarily through educational institutions and for research uses only. Examples of COTS tools include programs such as Microsoft® Excel and DATA™ (TreeAge Software, Inc.). Some advantages and disadvantages of each of these methods are enumerated in Table 24.1. These tools are used to develop decision trees (decision-analytic models), create mathematical spreadsheets, develop simulation models, and perform cost enumeration, among others, for cost-effectiveness analyses, creation of dynamic treatment protocols, development of patient education models, as pharmaceutical sales tools, patient and health care provider shared decision making, and go/no-go decisions by pharmaceutical manufacturers. Some of these applications are summarized below.

24.2.1 Cost-Effectiveness Analyses

Cost-effectiveness analyses first came of interest in the 1970s and have assumed greater importance through the development of more sophisticated analytic

TABLE 24.1 Interactive Software Tool Features

Feature	Program	
	DATA™	Microsoft Excel
Ease of use (learning curve)	+	++
Sensitivity analyses	++	+
Time sensitivity	++	O/+
Creation of diagrams	++	+
Dissemination of interactive build (via Internet or CD-ROM)	+(requires TreeAge Pro)	+
Purchasing	By license only	Purchase
Compatibility with Excel	Some versions incorporate Excel	N/A

techniques [1, 2]. Because of the increasing prominence of these analyses in worldwide drug registration, formulary decision making, therapeutic guideline determination [3], and individual patient decisions, it is incumbent upon end users to understand the basic tenets of health economic (HE) analyses, a major use of interactive software. The science of HE is more far-reaching than the question of which therapeutic options should be available within a particular setting. In fact, these analyses are currently being conducted in some institutions to help determine which health professionals should initially be treating patients (e.g., generalist versus specialist [4–8]) and even which setting should be recommended [6, 9]. Many influential groups, including the American Heart Association, support the tenet that cost-effectiveness, in addition to clinical effectiveness, must be determined to allow for appropriate treatment while maximizing allocation of scarce medical resources [10].

An effective HE or cost-effectiveness analysis is designed to answer certain questions, such as: Is the treatment effective? What will it cost? and How do the gains compare with the costs? By combining answers to all of these questions, the technique helps decision makers weigh the factors, compare alternative treatments, and decide which treatments are most appropriate for specific situations. Typically, one chooses the option with the least cost per unit of measure gained; the results are represented by the ratio of cost to effectiveness (C:E). With this type of analysis, called a cost-effectiveness analysis (CEA), various disease end points that are affected by therapy (risk markers, disease severity, death) can be assessed by corresponding indexes of therapeutic outcome (mmHg blood pressure reduction, hospitalizations averted, life years saved, respectively). It is beyond the scope of this chapter to elaborate further on principles of cost-effectiveness analyses. A number of references are available for this purpose [11–13].

Decision-analytic models are structured methods of incorporating probabilities and costs of likely events for expected therapeutic pathways and provide a framework for evaluating these data. These models use a tree structure and principles of expected outcome to calculate both cost and effectiveness. Numerous evaluations have utilized this method for determining the most cost-effective strategy [14–17]. These analyses can be accomplished with either software designed specifically for decision-analytic modeling (e.g., DATA™, Decision Maker™) or spreadsheet software such as Excel.

24.2.2 DECISION MODELING SOFTWARE

Continuous risk and uncertain timing of events may need to be considered in clinical decision-making. Special types of decision-analytic models, such as Markov models [18], account for issues of time sensitivity. For example, Lewis and colleagues [17] employed a Markov model to discern the relative cost-effectiveness of Sandimmune® (an older formulation of cyclosporine) versus Neoral® (a newer formulation of cyclosporine) in the first three months after renal transplantation (Table 24.2). Patients went on to experience one of five "health states" (see Fig. 24.1), namely, (1) NOREJCT: patient experienced no previous rejection; (2) FUNCGR1: patient experienced one episode of rejection; (3) FUNCGR2: patient experienced two or more episodes of rejection; (4) DIALYSIS: patient returned to permanent dialysis because of graft failure; and (5) DEAD: patient died. With results from one of the multiple sources that informed the model, detailed in Section 24.3.2 on "informing models," Neoral was shown to be both more effective and less costly than Sandimmune for both effectiveness criteria—functioning graft and rejection-free clinical course; thus Neoral was the dominant strategy (Fig. 24.2, Table 24.2), a result that the pharmaceutical manufacturer would embrace. The practical application of these data for the health care providers would be that

TABLE 24.2 Results of Renal Transplant Model Using Multiple Data Sets (Adapted from Lewis et al. [17])

Strategy	Cost	Probability of Functioning Graft	Probability of Being Rejection Free	Cost per Functioning Graft	Cost per Rejection-Free Clinical Course
Neoral (Europe)	$77,669.22	0.922	0.460	$84,239.93	$168,846.12
HCFA (No AA)	$87,618.09	0.943	0.430	$92,914.20	$203,763.00
Neoral (USA)	$76,127.01	1.000	0.572	$76,127.01	$133,089.17
HCFA (All)	$88,271.04	0.938	0.430	$94,105.59	$205,281.48

AA = African–Americans, HCFA = Health Care Financing Administration (now CMS)

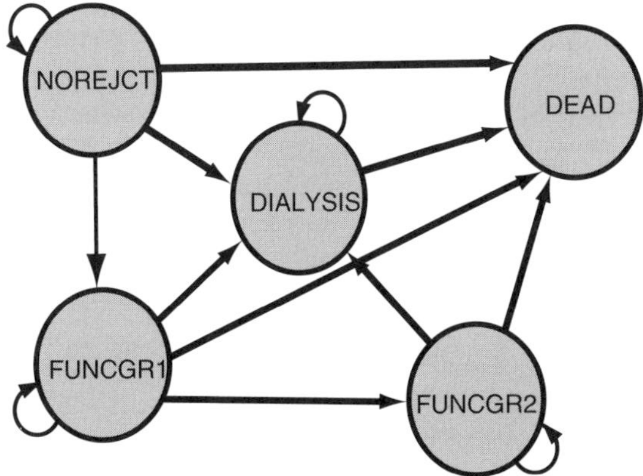

Figure 24.1 A health state model depicting all five transitional health states for patients undergoing renal transplant.

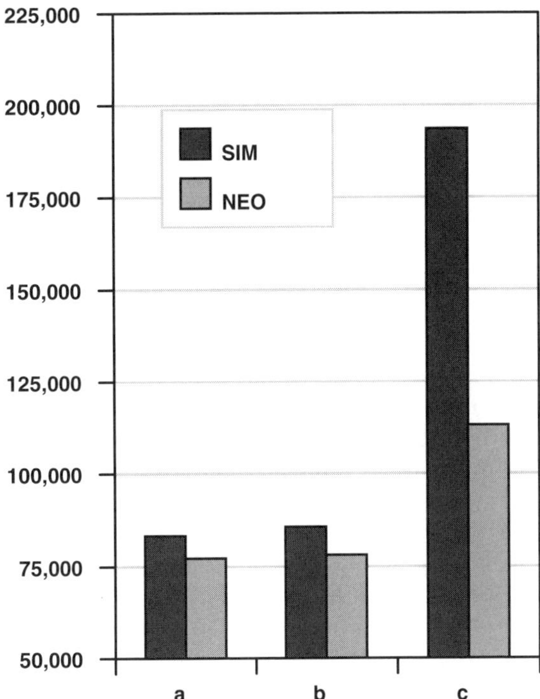

Figure 24.2 The Markov decision-analytic model shows cost and cost-effectiveness evaluations for patients undergoing renal transplant [17]. a = cost; b = cost per functioning graft; c = cost per rejection-free clinical course.

with a $10 million budget it would be possible to transplant 115 patients on Sandimmune or 124 patients on Neoral; 49/115 (43%) patients on Sandimmune vs. 84/124 (68%) patients on Neoral would have a rejection-free clinical course.

The increasing prevalence of managed care (MC) plans has fueled the demand for cost-effective diagnostic modalities. In particular, ultrasound (US) may become a "diagnostic gatekeeper" because of its relatively low cost and widespread availability. That is, it may be used to reduce the proportion of patients undergoing more costly procedures. The development of agents to enhance the quality of US imaging may result in fewer false-positive, indeterminate, or equivocal studies, obviating the need for further diagnostic testing. The result may be more cost-effective patient management. To test this hypothesis, a Markov model that employed a Bayesian approach was developed to compare US enhanced by SonoRx®, an oral contrast agent, with US alone in evaluating patients with abdominal pain suspected of having pancreatic disease (Fig. 24.3) [14]. This statistical method (Bayesian analysis) is used to account for uncertainty in a diagnosis/prognosis and to allow the incorporation of differential specificity and sensitivity of diagnostic tests into the decision about which diagnostic method to employ [19]. In the analysis, SonoRx®-enhanced US was less expensive ($714 vs. $808 for SonoRx®-enhanced and unenhanced US, respectively, using Medicare costs; $1612 vs. $1878 for SonoRx®-enhanced and unenhanced US, respectively, using non-Medicare costs) and as effective (0.785 vs. 0.782 for SonoRx®-enhanced and unenhanced US, respectively) as US alone. SonoRx®-enhanced US was the most cost-effective strategy ($909 vs. $1034 for SonoRx®-enhanced and unenhanced US, respectively, using Medicare costs; $2052 vs. $2401 for SonoRx®-enhanced and unenhanced US, respectively, using non-Medicare costs).

24.2.3 Mathematical Spreadsheets

These models calculate the cost and cost-effectiveness of therapeutic strategies by multiplying the probability of an event by its cost. An example of a decision-analytic model that illustrates the need to consider temporal effects of the drug(s) and disease is the economic analysis carried out by Arnold and colleagues [20] to evaluate the financial implications associated with use of the direct thrombin inhibitor argatroban for early treatment (<48 hours after thrombocytopenia onset), compared with delayed treatment (≥48 hours after thrombocytopenia onset), of immune-mediated heparin-induced thrombocytopenia (HIT) with or without thrombosis. The decision-analytic model (see Fig. 24.4), developed with Excel™, shows the strategies that were examined. The total per-patient cost included hospital days, diagnostic tests, heparin, argatroban, major hemorrhagic events, and patient outcomes (i.e., amputation, new thrombosis, stroke, or death), multiplied by the probability of each event. The incremental cost-effectiveness ratio (ICER) was calculated by dividing the incremental cost between patients with and without argatroban

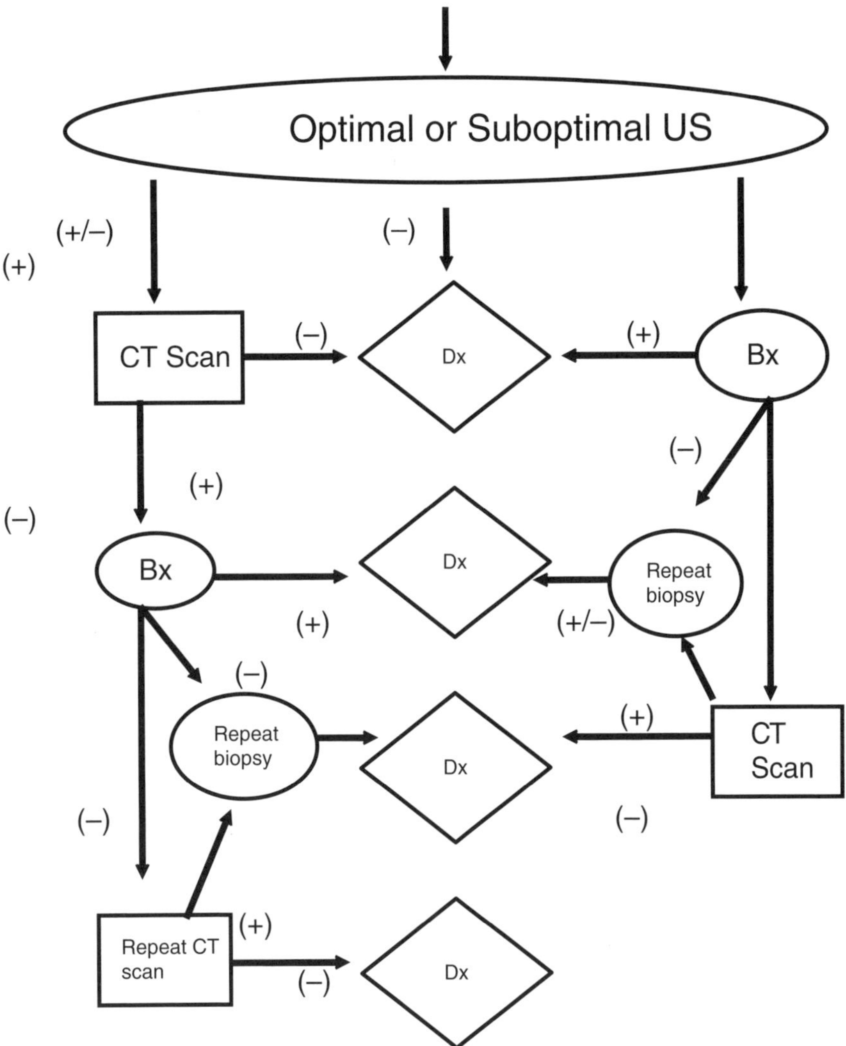

Figure 24.3 Strategic pathway of Bayesian Markov model showing decision points for diagnosis of pancreatic cancer [14]. Bx = biopsy; Dx = diagnosis.

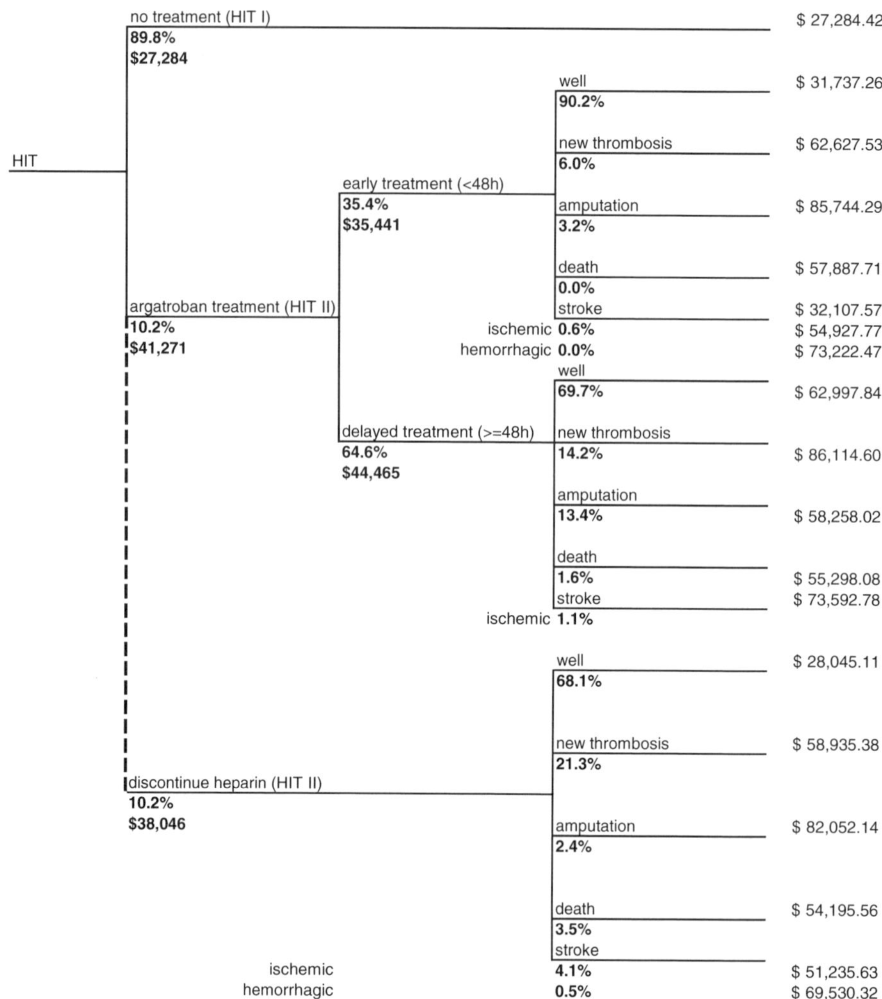

Figure 24.4 The decision-analytic model shows the three strategies that were examined by Arnold and researchers [22] to evaluate the financial implications of the direct thrombin inhibitor argatroban for early treatment (<48 hours after thrombocytopenia onset), compared with delayed treatment, of heparin-induced thrombocytopenia (HIT) with or without thrombosis.

treatment by the incremental effectiveness, or the cost per new thrombosis event avoided. The evaluation indicated that the mean cost per HIT patient without thrombosis decreased by 6.85% for patients who were treated earlier with argatroban therapy, representing a $2605 saving per patient compared with those not treated with argatroban. For those receiving delayed argatroban therapy, the mean cost increased by $9024 per patient compared with those receiving early treatment with argatroban.

Another economic model was developed to allow members of a pharmaceutical company team to evaluate potential total costs of managing patients with mild-to-moderate hypertension who were treated with a variety of medications. The cost analysis evaluated the average total cost per evaluation period to initially and subsequently control blood pressure for each of the agents and an investigational agent. In this analysis, cost was calculated as the sum of the cost of treating hypertension during the evaluation period, costs of treating adverse drug events, and drug acquisition costs. Two analyses were completed with this model: (1) a consultant-based analysis, which consisted of a literature review and an advisory panel (three primary care practitioners and three cardiologists) survey, and (2) a pharmacy benefits management (PBM) database-dependent evaluation. In the second analysis, actual drug utilization data were obtained via linkage of medical claims and drug utilization data. The least expensive agent was the investigational agent in the consultant-based analysis, whereas it was a marketed drug in the PBM-based analysis. The likely primary reason for the different ranking between the analyses was the small number of patients in the PBM database with costly and resource-intensive adverse drug events reported by the consultants and the literature for the marketed drug. In addition, only clinical trial data were available for the investigational drug, which is not likely to correspond to a "real-world" setting.

24.2.4 Internet-Based Programs

An Internet-based program for evaluation of clinical, humanistic, and economic outcomes of patients with type 2 diabetes, the Avandia Worldwide Awareness Registry (AWARe®), was developed to capture laboratory and clinical outcomes data from diabetes practice settings worldwide [21]. The data collection methods involved the electronic linkage of clinical information and quality of life (QoL) forms at the time and place of care delivery. As providers entered patients' clinical information into the patients' electronic health records (EHRs), the data elements of interest were automatically transmitted to a secure Internet site where the data were stored and continuously updated. Data collected in AWARe® included demographic information, prescription use, HbA1c, fasting plasma glucose, total cholesterol, triglycerides, LDL, HDL, blood pressure, liver function tests, the SF-36, and results of the Diabetes and Treatment Satisfaction Questionnaire (DTSQ). Every six months, participants used hand-held devices to complete the electronic versions of the SF-36 and the DTSQ. The results from these surveys were instantaneously transmitted via wireless technology to Evidence-Based Health (EB-Health™). AWARe® permits immediate retrieval of all data from an Internet-based registry. Information on patients' clinical progress may be continuously transmitted to EB-Health™, allowing researchers, clinicians, and administrators to perform "real-time" analyses of the clinical effectiveness of antidiabetic therapy, as well as to determine its impact on patients' QoL and satisfaction with treatment.

Finally, a system linking the Internet with other readily available interactive voice response (IVR) technologies (cellular phones, pagers, and e-mail) —EB-Health™—was developed to empower patients with chronic illnesses to self-manage and to facilitate communication between health care providers and patients [22, 23]. The system was designed to improve health outcomes in the population at large and to reduce health care costs stemming from chronic illnesses [24, 25]. This disease management support system is being deployed in adult and pediatric populations and has demonstrated statistically significant pre/post improvements in personal best peak flowmeter readings ($P < 0.01$, paired t-test), the number of emergency department (ED) visits ($P < 0.01$, paired t-test) and the number of patients with an ED visit ($P < 0.01$, McNemar test), the number of office visits ($P < 0.01$, paired t-test) and the number of patients with office visits ($P < 0.01$, McNemar test) and the number of participants requiring steroid (prednisone) therapy to control their asthma ($P < 0.05$ overall, McNemar test). In addition to being used by patients and health care practitioners, it is a valuable resource to pharmaceutical companies by providing a longitudinal database to quantify patient outcomes on different therapeutic options, patient drug compliance, and long-term adverse events.

24.3 INPUTS AND OUTPUTS

24.3.1 Graphical User Interfaces

Interactive programs based on rigorous economic models can be designed with user-friendly interfaces. These programs are customized to perform setting-specific analyses. For example, a user-friendly model was developed for use by clinicians at different hospital locations and for presentations to the Center for Medicare and Medicaid Services (CMS) to aid in price negotiations. In another case, a model is being developed to allow specialty pharmaceutical representatives to, once again, enable customization of analytical outcomes with customer-specific data (see Fig. 24.5).

24.3.2 Informing Models

A variety of data sources are available to inform interactive programs, including prospective data sets, retrospective databases, expert opinion, and unpublished/published literature. Time horizon, that is, the length of time into the future considered in the analysis over which costs and outcomes are projected, is very important here [26]. For example, if a clinical trial or the published literature only report short-term results for a chronic condition, the outcomes may come into question. This is where decision-analytic models may come

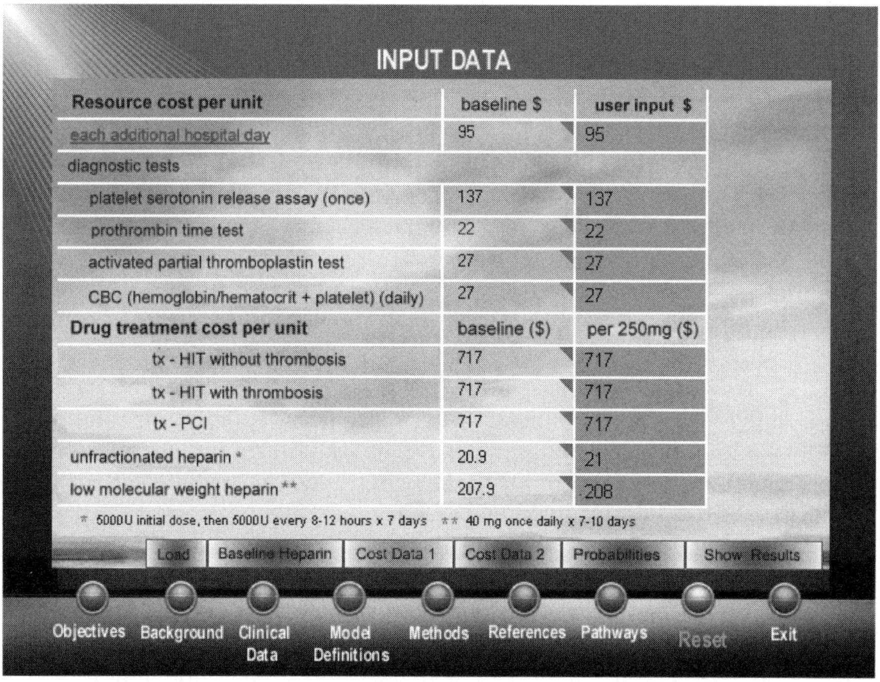

INPUT DATA

Resource cost per unit	baseline $	user input $
each additional hospital day	95	95
diagnostic tests		
platelet serotonin release assay (once)	137	137
prothrombin time test	22	22
activated partial thromboplastin test	27	27
CBC (hemoglobin/hematocrit + platelet) (daily)	27	27
Drug treatment cost per unit	baseline ($)	per 250mg ($)
tx - HIT without thrombosis	717	717
tx - HIT with thrombosis	717	717
tx - PCI	717	717
unfractionated heparin *	20.9	21
low molecular weight heparin **	207.9	208

* 5000U initial dose, then 5000U every 8-12 hours x 7 days ** 40 mg once daily x 7-10 days

Load | Baseline Heparin | Cost Data 1 | Cost Data 2 | Probabilities | Show Results

Objectives | Background | Clinical Data | Model Definitions | Methods | References | Pathways | Reset | Exit

Figure 24.5 Input screen from interactive model. See color plate.

into play, allowing one to project study results onto clinically realistic time frames. In addition, these models can help in projecting thresholds (see Section 24.3.6 on robustness) [27].

24.3.3 Prospective Sources

Prospective sources include encounter data, which may or may not be contained in EHRs; patient data input; and randomized, prospective clinical trials. Advantages of prospective sources to inform interactive software include the ability to control and monitor the circumstances of data collection; reduction (as a result of randomization) of sources of bias; potential minimization of missing data; potential to modify design of data collection; ability to verify data accuracy; and ability to validate and further test assumptions and modify existing programs.

24.3.4 Retrospective Sources

A number of interactive program developers advocate retrospective analyses and modeling as alternatives to prospective data sources. These sources include patient charts [28, 29], individual or meta-analyses of clinical trials in the literature [30–34], medical and pharmacy claims data [35, 36], Medicare data bases [37], and other large, publicly available data sets, such as the National Center for Health Statistics' National Health Care Survey (NHCS) and National Health Interview Survey (NHIS) and the Agency for Healthcare Research and Quality's Medical Expenditure Panel Survey (MEPS) and Healthcare Cost & Utilization Project (HCUP), among others. Claims or administrative databases have, in particular, recently gained favor as they are frequently computerized and reflect actual charges and payments for specific plans and populations. The advantages of these databases are displayed in Table 24.3 [38]. The disadvantages of these databases are reflected in Table 24.4 [39, 40]. Indeed, in two comparisons of clinical and insurance claims databases for patients with ischemic heart disease, claims data failed to identify more than one-half of patients with prognostically important conditions, including mitral insufficiency, congestive heart failure, peripheral vascular disease, old myocardial infarction (MI), hyperlipidemia, angina, and unstable angina [41, 42]. Similar inconsistencies were noted in a coronary artery bypass surgery study in which miscoding of diagnoses could be linked with the lack of specificity for an ICD-9-CM grouping and lack of reporting of coexisting conditions on discharge abstracts and claims [41, 42], using the HCUP database [43]. Given the current state of these types of analyses, collection of original data for a representative percentage of the patient population should be undertaken to validate the clinical information contained therein.

TABLE 24.3 Advantages of Retrospective Data Sets for Informing Interactive Software

Relatively inexpensive
Quickly done
Reflective of different populations
Encompass a realistic time frame
Organizationally specific
Can be used for benchmarking purposes
Include large sample sizes
Can capture real-world prescribing patterns

TABLE 24.4 Disadvantages of Retrospective Data Sets for Informing Interactive Software

Missing data
Inability to retrospectively interpret data
Diagnosis and procedure codes may reflect reimbursement strategies instead of clinically accurate diagnoses
Limited information on important covariates
Sparse outcomes data
Lack of representativeness
Lack of structure for research purposes

24.3.5 Expert Opinion

Expert opinion is a source, frequently elicited by survey, that is used to obtain information where no or few data are available. For example, in our experience with a multicountry evaluation of health care resource utilization in atrial fibrillation, very few country-specific published data were available on this subject. Thus the decision-analytic model was supplemented with data from a physician expert panel survey to determine initial management approach (rate control vs. cardioversion); first-, second-, and third-line agents; doses and durations of therapy; type and frequency of studies that would be performed to initiate and monitor therapy; type and frequency of adverse events, by body system and the resources used to manage them; place of treatment; and adverse consequences of lack of atrial fibrillation control and cost of these consequences, for example, stroke, congestive heart failure. This method may also be used in testing the robustness of the analysis [30].

24.3.6 Robustness (What-If Analyses)

In all analyses, there is uncertainty about the accuracy of the results that may be dealt with via sensitivity analyses [1, 2]. In these analyses, one essentially asks the question "What if?" These allow one to vary key values over clinically feasible ranges to determine whether the decision remains the same, that is, if the strategy initially found to be cost-effective remains the dominant strategy. By performing sensitivity analyses, one can increase the level of confidence in the conclusions. Sensitivity analyses also allow one to determine threshold values for these key parameters at which the decision would change. For example, in the previous example of a Bayesian evaluation embedded in a decision-analytic model of pancreatic cancer, a sensitivity analysis (Fig. 24.6) was conducted to evaluate the relationship

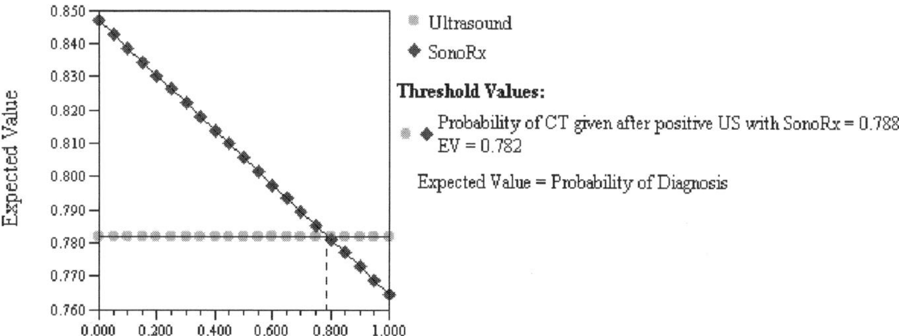

Figure 24.6 Sensitivity analysis on probability of CT after optimal positive US with SonoRx®.

between the probability of a CT scan and effectiveness [14]. The probability of performing a CT scan after an optimal positive US with SonoRx® was varied between 0% and 100%. This analysis showed that the threshold probability of a CT scan after an optimal positive US with SonoRx® was 79% (at this point, the effectiveness value for both the SonoRx®-enhanced US and unenhanced US strategies was 0.782). Thus the SonoRx®-enhanced US strategy was more effective than US alone when the probability of a CT scan after an optimal positive US with SonoRx® ranged from 0% to <79%.

24.4 FUTURE

Interactive programs are used in a variety of settings, including as decision aids and for assisting in reimbursement strategies for national formularies. In fact, the US, Belgium, Australia, Israel, the UK, France, the Netherlands, Finland, and Canada have implemented guidelines for economic technology assessment [44, 45]. Except for Australia, these and other countries do not yet require HE studies and interactive models for drug registration. However, they are used in determining formulary inclusion and pricing, with many countries strongly suggesting that these analyses be undertaken. For example, in Canada interactive models are used to "inform programmatic decision-making in regard to the appropriateness of health care interventions" [45]. Moreover, Canada and the US require portability of results, and the UK requires a National Health Service perspective. Finally, Belgium, Canada, the UK, and the US require that HE analyses be conducted to allow for capture of long-term cost and effect outcomes. The use of interactive software can help to improve generalizability, allow for inclusion of subgroup data sets, and facilitate sensitivity analyses. These programs are useful for policy makers who are concerned with health care resource allocation on an individual, institutional, statewide, federal, or country-specific level. End users for interactive programs may include insurance companies, pharmaceutical manufacturers (who are interested in demonstrating the comparative cost-effectiveness of their agents in relation to gold standards and/or the most commonly used therapeutic options and also for pricing and reimbursement strategies), government agencies (for establishing levels of reimbursement), managed care (MC) executives (to aid in establishing therapeutic guidelines), employers (who use these analyses as an aid in benchmarking the MC organizations they are evaluating for their employees' health plans), and pharmacy benefits managers (PBMs) (who also wish to demonstrate that they have evaluated MC plans to offer the most cost-effective plan to employers). Similarly, individual clinicians are becoming increasingly interested in documenting that they have systematically identified the most cost-effective therapeutic option for their patients.

24.4.1 Internet and Other Media

The advent of the Internet has enabled availability and dissemination of interactive software, with the only limitation being Internet access. Besides educating practitioners, interactive multimedia software products are available for patient use and education. Several researchers have used computers (Health Buddy, [46] Health-e-Pal©, [23]) perhaps in conjunction with a telephone-based (Health-e-Pal©, [23]) self-management program, to especially enable children to assess and monitor their asthma symptoms while simultaneously alerting health care providers to potential disease decompensation that might result in unscheduled clinic or emergency visits. Gustafson et al. [47, 48] have developed a Web-based health information and support system—Comprehensive Health Enhancement Support System (CHESS)—that includes modular programs on breast cancer, AIDS/HIV infection, sexual assault, alcoholism, and academic crisis. Functionality includes disease information, a treatment decision aid, an opportunity to contact health care providers via e-mail, testimonials from patients, and a patient forum to exchange information and to solicit social support. Despite its sophistication, the CHESS system lacks the capacity to present information in a targeted and tailored manner based on specific patient characteristics.

24.4.2 Personalized Programs

Just as genomics offers the seductive potential of customizing medications to specific patient characteristics, interactive software will increasingly accomplish this feat. Targeted interventions could take advantage of existing health-based infrastructures while providing a personalized level of education and care that could help increase patients' self-management abilities.

24.4.3 Transparency

It is essential that, with the use of evidence-based medicine to inform decisions in health care, the processes used in program development be as transparent as possible. Information about the limited evidence and inherent uncertainty should be disclosed and available for scrutiny, even within the software itself. In fact, in an attempt to maximize transparency, some have advocated open source development and publication of interactive software models [49, 50]. Certainly, details of methodologies, sources, and other techniques employed for development of the underlying models must be acknowledged. However, the proprietary nature of many of these programs must be taken into consideration and measures put into place to ensure confidentiality. Requested publication of all NIH-sponsored research online (in PubMed) [51] within a reasonable time frame after journal acceptance will help to ensure that these data are available in the public domain in short order.

24.5 CONCLUSIONS

Use of interactive, iterative programs in decision making by multiple stakeholders in the health care system has many advantages. The utility of interactive programs in assisting in these decisions depends to a great extent on the assumptions made and the quality of the data used for the analyses (e.g., the degree to which the data are evidence based) [52]. Just as continuous quality improvement (CQI) has helped to transform the "business" of health care, assessment of health impact [53] with limited data sets, prospective validation of the outcomes, and adjustment of the underlying structure based on the newest evidence will help health care providers and pharmaceutical company executives to identify the most cost-effective therapeutic pathways for individual and population health improvement. Continual software reevaluation and refinement, via usability testing, [54] as well as updating of methodologies of software development, will result in the availability of the most useful technology.

Analysis of therapies is a timely topic, especially in light of the fact that a number of governmental regulatory agencies are attempting to set reimbursement guidelines based on these data. At this time, numerous studies have been completed for a variety of therapeutic options. However, there are no standardized guidelines for these studies; inclusion of resource use (e.g., direct, indirect), effectiveness criteria (e.g., CHD event avoided, quality-adjusted life years), centralized cost sources, perspective, and incorporation of sensitivity analyses into the evaluation are quite variable. This underlies clinicians' concerns about premature efforts by regulatory agencies to dictate therapeutic options based on an incomplete understanding of the true costs to payers and society as well as the benefits to the patient. Moreover, in addition to the societal and governmental perspectives regarding these analyses, there is inadequate information for the individual clinician attempting to treat an individual patient in terms of cost, general estimates of life expectancy, and overall likelihood of success of one particular treatment regimen versus another. Furthermore, as newer and potentially more expensive therapies become readily available, decisions based on state-of-the-art analyses will be required to determine their place in therapy.

Although interactive software analyses will have an increasingly important role in individual and population health care decisions, there are some limitations to the underlying models [9]. As mentioned throughout this chapter, although the decision-analytic technique is an objective and well-established methodology, many other questions persist regarding basic issues such as uncertainty about costs and benefits, attribution of resources (e.g., if an adverse event requires a therapeutic switch, should future costs be attributed to the initial agent or to the switch agent?), perspective, appropriateness of retrospective (e.g., claims) databases, appropriate time horizon and projection to clinically relevant time frames, QOL utility measurements (e.g., health states worse than death), and discount rate (e.g., same for benefits as for costs, which value should be used), among others.

Despite these limitations, sensitivity analyses and ongoing updated evaluations will allow the creation of interactive software programs to aid health care stakeholders and patients in making the most informed decisions about treatments amid a milieu of cost containment.

REFERENCES

1. Eisenberg JM, Freund D, Glick H, et al. Clinical economics education in the International Clinical Epidemiology Network. INCLEN Economics Faculty. *J Clin Epidemiol* 1989;42:689–95.
2. Weinstein MC, Stason WB. Foundations of cost-effectiveness analysis for health and medical practices. *N Engl J Med* 1977;296:716–21.
3. Pare D, Freed M. Clinical practice guidelines for quality patient outcomes. *Nurs Clin North Am* 1995;30:183–96.
4. Winslow R. Study compares role of doctors in cardiac cases. *Wall Street J* 1995.
5. Goldstein S, Pearson T, Colwill J, et al. Task Force 4: The relationship between cardiovascular specialists and generalists. *J Am Coll Cardiol* 1994;24:304–12.
6. Greenfield S, Nelson E, Zubkoff M, et al. Variations in resource utilization among medical specialties and systems of care. Results from the medical outcomes study. *JAMA* 1992;267:1624–30.
7. Jaussi A. Continuing importance of the clinical approach. Observations on a regional collaboration between general practitioners, internists and cardiologists. *Schweiz Med Wochenschr* 1994;124:2049–52.
8. Mills P, Michnich M. Managed care and cardiac pacing and electrophysiology. *Pacing Clin Electrophysiol* 1993;16:1746–50.
9. Tarlov A, Ware J, Jr., Greenfield S, et al. The Medical Outcomes Study. An application of methods for monitoring the results of medical care. *JAMA* 1989;262:925–30.
10. Dustan H, Francis C, Allen H, et al. Principles of access to health care. Access to Health Care Task Force, American Heart Association. *Circulation* 1993;87:657–8.
11. Detsky AS, Naglie IG. A clinician's guide to cost-effectiveness analysis. *Ann Intern Med* 1990;113:147–54.
12. Goldberg Arnold R, Kaniecki D. Health economic considerations in cardiovascular drug utilization. In Frishman W, Sonnenblick E, editors, *Cardiovascular pharmacotherapeutics*. New York: McGraw-Hill, Inc., 2003. pp. 43–55.
13. Weinstein M, Fineberg H, Elstein A, et al. Clinical decisions and limited resources. In Weinstein M, editor, *Clinical decision analysis*. Philadelphia: Saunders, 1980. pp. 228–265.
14. Bree RL, Arnold RJ, Pettit KG, et al. Use of a decision-analytic model to support the use of a new oral US contrast agent in patients with abdominal pain. *Acad Radiol* 2001;8:234–42.

15. Arnold R, Kim R, Zhou Y, Tang B. Budgetary impact of heparin-induced thrombocytopenia with thrombosis and treatment with the direct thrombin inhibitor Argatroban (P401E). ASHP 39th Midyear Clinical Meeting. Orlando, FL, 2004.
16. Quenzer RW, Pettit KG, Arnold RJ, Kaniecki DJ. Pharmacoeconomic analysis of selected antibiotics in lower respiratory tract infection. *Am J Manag Care* 1997;3:1027–36.
17. Lewis R, Canafax D, Pettit K, et al. Use of Markov model for evaluating the cost-effectiveness of immunosuppressive therapies in renal transplant recipients. *Transpl Proc* 1996;28:2214–17.
18. Beck J, Pauker S. The Markov process in medical prognosis. *Med Decis Making* 1983;3:419–58.
19. AIME'01 Workshop: Bayesian Models in Medicine. The European Conference on Artificial Intelligence in Medicine (AIME'01). Cascais, Portugal, 2001.
20. Arnold R, Kim R, Tang B. The cost-effectiveness of argatroban treatment in heparin-induced thrombocytopenia: the effect of early versus delayed treatment. Cardiol Rev 2005;14:7–13.
21. Bakst A, Meletiche D, Arnold R, et al. The Avandia Worldwide Awareness Registry (AWARe®): an Internet-based program for evaluation of clinical, humanistic and economic outcomes of patients with type 2 diabetes. International Society for Pharmacoeconomics and Outcomes Research Sixth Annual International Meeting. Philadelphia, Pennsylvania, 2001.
22. Arnold R, Kaniecki D, Rosen J. Web-enabled asthma application for personalized medical communication within a multi-group practice setting. ISPOR 9th Annual International Meeting. Washington, DC, 2004.
23. Arnold R, Kaniecki D, Rosen J. Web-enabled asthma application for personalized medical communication within a multi-group practice setting. *Value in Health* 2004;7:310.
24. Arnold R. Implementing automated chronic disease management support systems in asthma: the promise and the pitfalls. Critical Issues in eHealth Research Conference. Bethesda, MD, 2005.
25. Arnold R, Stein-Albert M, Serebrisky D, et al. Use of an automated chronic care management system in underserved pediatric asthmatic patients. American Academy of Pediatrics (AAP) Council on Clinical Information Technology, AAP National Conference and Exhibition. Washington, DC, 2005.
26. Detsky A, Naglie I. A clinician's guide to cost-effectiveness analysis. *Ann Intern Med* 1990;113:147–54.
27. Beck J, Salem D, Estes N, Pauker S. A computer-based Markov decision analysis of the management of symptomatic bifascicular block: the threshold probability for pacing. *J Am Coll Cardiol* 1987;9:920–35.
28. Arnold RJ, Kaniecki DJ, Frishman WH. Cost-effectiveness of antihypertensive agents in patients with reduced left ventricular function. *Pharmacotherapy* 1994;14:178–84.
29. Jubran A, Gross N, Ramsdell J, et al. Comparative cost-effectiveness analysis of theophylline and ipratropium bromide in chronic obstructive pulmonary disease. A three-center study. *Chest* 1993;103:678–84.

30. Podrid PJ, Kowey PR, Frishman WH, et al. Comparative cost-effectiveness analysis of quinidine, procainamide and mexiletine. *Am J Cardiol* 1991;68:1662–7.
31. Oster G, Epstein AM. Cost-effectiveness of antihyperlipemic therapy in the prevention of coronary heart disease. The case of cholestyramine. *JAMA* 1987;258:2381–7.
32. Krumholz HM, Pasternak RC, Weinstein MC, et al. Cost effectiveness of thrombolytic therapy with streptokinase in elderly patients with suspected acute myocardial infarction. *N Engl J Med* 1992;327:7–13.
33. Barrett B, Parfrey P, Foley R, et al. An economic analysis of strategies for the use of contrast media for diagnostic cardiac catheterization. *Med Decis Making* 1994;14:325–35.
34. Goldberg Arnold R, Kaniecki D, Tak Piech C, et al. An economic evaluation of HMG-CoA reductase inhibitors for cholesterol reduction in the primary prevention of coronary heart disease. 11th International Conference on Pharmacoepidemiology. Montreal, Quebec, Canada, 1995.
35. Goldman L, Weinstein MC, Goldman PA, Williams LW. Cost-effectiveness of HMG-CoA reductase inhibition for primary and secondary prevention of coronary heart disease. *JAMA* 1991;265:1145–51.
36. Larsen GC, Manolis AS, Sonnenberg FA, et al. Cost-effectiveness of the implantable cardioverter-defibrillator: effect of improved battery life and comparison with amiodarone therapy. *J Am Coll Cardiol* 1992;19:1323–34.
37. Altman DG, Flora JA, Fortmann SP, Farquhar JW. The cost-effectiveness of three smoking cessation programs. *Am J Public Health* 1987;77:162–5.
38. Arnold R, Kotsanos J. Proceedings of the Advisory Panel Meeting and Conference on Pharmacoeconomic Issues: Panel 3: Methodological issues in conducting pharmacoeconomic evaluations-retrospective and claims database studies. *Value Health* 1999;2:82–7.
39. Using administrative data for clinical (disease) management. *Tutorial on Disease Management Methodologies.* 17th Annual Meeting of Society for Medical Decision Making. Scottsdale, AZ, 1995.
40. Lewis NJ, Patwell JT, Briesacher BA. The role of insurance claims databases in drug therapy outcomes research. *Pharmacoeconomics* 1993;4:323–30.
41. Jollis JG, Ancukiewicz M, DeLong ER, et al. Discordance of databases designed for claims payment versus clinical information systems. Implications for outcomes research. *Ann Intern Med* 1993;119:844–50.
42. Romano PS, Roos LL, Luft HS, et al. A comparison of administrative versus clinical data: coronary artery bypass surgery as an example. Ischemic Heart Disease Patient Outcomes Research Team. *J Clin Epidemiol* 1994;47:249–60.
43. Berthelsen CL. Evaluation of coding data quality of the HCUP National Inpatient Sample. *Top Health Inf Manage* 2000;21:10–23.
44. Hjelmgren J, Berggren F, Andersson F. Health economic guidelines—similarities, differences and some implications. *Value Health* 2001;4:225–50.
45. Tarn TY, Dix Smith M. Pharmacoeconomic guidelines around the world. *ISPOR Connections*, Vol. 10, 2004.
46. Guendelman S, Meade K, Benson M, et al. Improving asthma outcomes and self-management behaviors of inner-city children: a randomized trial of the Health

Buddy interactive device and an asthma diary. *Arch Pediatr Adolesc Med* 2002; 156:114–20.

47. Gustafson DH, Bosworth K, Hawkins RP, et al. CHESS: a computer-based system for providing information, referrals, decision support and social support to people facing medical and other health-related crises. *Proc Annu Symp Comput Appl Med Care* 1992:161–5.
48. Gustafson DH, Hawkins RP, Boberg EW, et al. CHESS: 10 years of research and development in consumer health informatics for broad populations, including the underserved. *Int J Med Inform* 2002;65:169–77.
49. Open source. http://en.wikipedia.org/wiki/Open_sourcesoftware
50. Weinstein M, O'Brien B, Hornberger J, et al. Principles of good practice of decision analytic modeling in health care evaluation: Report of the ISPOR Task Force on Good Research Practices-Modeling Studies. *Value Health* 2003;6:9–17.
51. http://grantsl.nih.gov/grants/guide/notice-files/NOT-OD-05-022.html
52. Fletcher AE, Bulpitt CJ. Pharmacoeconomic evaluation of risk factors for cardiovascular disease: an epidemiological perspective. *Pharmacoeconomics* 1992;1:33–44.
53. Parry J, Stevens A. Prospective health impact assessment: pitfalls, problems, and possible ways forward. *BMJ* 2001;323:1177–82.
54. U.S. Department of Health and Human Services. Usability: methods for designing usable web sites. http://www.usability.gov/methods/usability_testing.html

PART VII

COMPUTERS IN CLINICAL DEVELOPMENT

25

CLINICAL DATA COLLECTION AND MANAGEMENT

MAZEN ABDELLATIF

DISCLAIMER

The opinions expressed in this chapter are solely those of the author and do not necessarily reflect those of the Department of Veterans Affairs (DVA), the VA Cooperative Studies Program (VACSP), or the Hines VA Cooperative Studies Program Coordinating Center (CSPCC).

Contents

Computer Applications in Pharmaceutical Research and Development, Edited by Sean Ekins.
ISBN 0-471-73779-8

25.1 INTRODUCTION

Clinical trial data management involves a set of processes that must be executed successfully to turn out reliable clinical, control, and administrative data to a central location such as a coordinating center, a data center, or a resource center. In the literature, these processes are lumped together under the name clinical data management or clinical trial data management. The title of this chapter, Clinical Data Collection and Management, was chosen to emphasize two of the major aspects in conducting clinical trials: data collection and data management. These complement each other to achieve the ultimate goal of turning out reliable master databases to a central location. These aspects are accomplished and coordinated through a set of communication tools, a central ingredient of any clinical trial, used to develop a data collection and management system. Figure 25.1 illustrates the integration of the communication aspect before data collection begins, during data collection, during data management, and after data collection.

The development of comprehensive and reliable data collection and management systems is fundamental for conducting successful clinical trials. The design and implementation of such systems affects all aspects of conducting clinical trials including data collection, editing, managing, monitoring, reporting, analyzing, archiving, and sharing. It is thus extremely important that close attention be given to the development of these systems in terms of their design and the hardware and software selections made.

The astonishing advancement in computer hardware and software technology has had tremendous impact on clinical trial data collection and management. Although the design and conduct of sound clinical trials have been well understood and appreciated from scientific and ethical points of view, most of the processes used to collect and manage data before this technological advancement were not fully automated and somewhat primitive. Before the explosion of information technology (IT), clinical trials relied on either manual methods or somewhat limited computer hardware and software. The

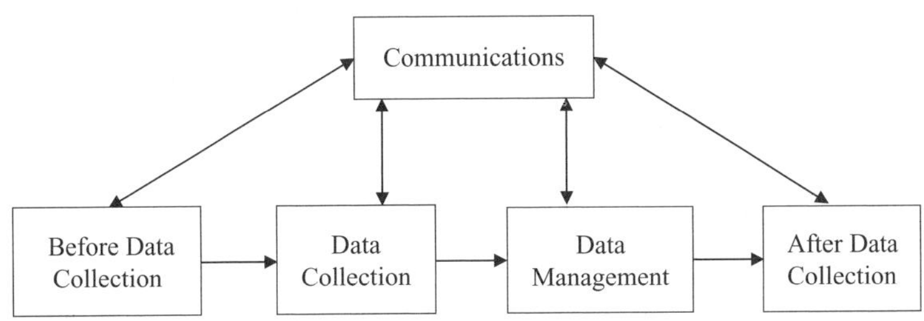

Figure 25.1 The integration of the communication aspect with other aspects.

obvious shortcomings of this reliance are demonstrated by the tendency these methods to be error prone and time consuming.

New developments in computer hardware and software technology have made clinical trial data collection and management timely, effective, and reliable, the cornerstones for conducting a successful clinical trial. With the ongoing and rapid advancement in computer hardware and software technology, and the wide range of newly available commercial databases, proprietary software vendors, design tools, and security applications, clinical trial data collection and management have become widely attainable, much easier, less time consuming, more reliable, more secure, and more scaleable than ever.

Although these attributes assure a greater confidence in the results of clinical trials, new challenges have arisen with this technological advancement, which must be addressed. Some of these are cost, learning curve, shifting responsibilities, and dealing with unforeseeable events.

This chapter presents the application of computer hardware and software technologies in clinical trial data collection and management. The chapter is organized into eleven major sections: (1) introduction, (2) data collection versus management, (3) communication in clinical trial data collection and management, (4) pure paper-based data collection and management systems, (5) electronic-based data collection and management systems, (6) hybrid data collection and management systems, (7) acquiring e-clinical software from vendors, (8) processes before data collection, (9) processes during data collection, (10) processes after data collection, and (11) final comments.

25.2 DATA COLLECTION VERSUS DATA MANAGEMENT

The term "clinical trial data management" does not fully describe how computers are used in conducting clinical trials. The two major, and distinct, computer applications in conducting clinical trials are data collection and data management. Each of these applications has a distinct role in clinical trials. For that reason, the term "clinical trial data collection and management" will be used. This does not imply that these two aspects are independent of each other. Although each one can be accomplished as a separate system, they should be integrated, thus the term "data collection and management system." Another aspect that is also integrated in each of these two aspects is data security. Data security tools and procedures are necessary during data collection and data management.

25.2.1 Data Collection

Data collection in clinical trials consists of the processes of collecting reliable clinical, control, and administrative data from the trial's participating sites with agreed-upon methods and procedures to record the collected data and send them to a central location.

25.2.2 Data Management

There are several definitions of data management. One is "all the disciplines related to managing data as a valuable resource, including acquisition, database administration, storage, backup, security, and quality assurance" [1]. Another definition is "work that involves the planning, development, implementation, and administration of systems for the acquisition, storage, and retrieval of data" [2]. These definitions, however, include data acquisition as a part of data management. The official definition given by the Data Management Association (DAMA) is "the development and execution of architectures, policies, practices and procedures that properly manage the full data lifecycle needs of an enterprise" [3]. A layperson's definition of data management is the process of accumulating collected data into a master database in a central location while ensuring their security, validity, and completeness by generating quality assurance reports to monitor the progress of the trial.

Some data collection and management systems have been developed to enable data collection and management of several trials being conducted simultaneously using a shared system. This presents security issues, including providing participating sites with secure access to data associated with their trial while restricting them from accessing data of other sites or trials and providing participating sites, the coordinating center, and other participating entities with the appropriate access to reports and queries. These security challenges are met by using secured socket layer technology (SSL).

25.2.3 Integration

Clinical trial data collection and management is, therefore, the integration of data collection and data management. The data management system depends on the data collection method. Data collection methods are of three major types: The first method is pure paper-based systems. With this approach data are collected on paper forms and sent to a central location. There they are entered into electronic files by the traditional double-key high-speed data entry method. The resulting electronic files are read into a centralized database through a data management system using specific computer hardware and software. The second method is electronic-based systems in which data are entered electronically into a computer system. The system can be centralized or distributed at participating sites. Electronic-based systems can utilize various technologies for data entry. Laptops and desktops use modem connections to transfer remotely collected data to the centralized location, whereas some handheld and pen-based devices use wireless communications to transfer the data. In Portable Data Files (PDF)-based systems, collected data are entered on electronic PDF forms, which are sent on a read-only CD to the centralized location or transferred to a centralized File Transfer Protocol (FTP) web site. The newest trend in data collection is direct data entry into a centralized system on the Internet with web-based data collection systems. This approach is essentially paperless. All data handling is computerized at both the participating sites and the centralized location. The third method is hybrid systems that integrate various methods and techniques for collecting and managing data. A good example of this approach employs specially designed forms that can be faxed from the participating sites to a centralized location, where a host computer equipped with Optical Markup Recognition (OMR) and/or Optical Character Recognition (OCR) software receives images of the faxed forms. This software reads and interprets the recorded data, flags data errors, and adds clean records to the master database. These specially designed forms can also be shipped to the centralized location to be scanned centrally by a high-speed scanner that is connected to a computer equipped with OMR or OCR software. Table 25.1 shows the computer hardware and software requirements at the participating sites and

TABLE 25.1 Types of Data Collection Systems

Type	Participating Sites	Coordinating Center
Pure paper-based	No computer hardware/software Complete paper forms. Send hard copies of completed forms to CC.	Computer hardware/software Enter forms into electronic files with double-key high-seed data entry. Process electronic raw data files through a computer system.
Pure electronic-based	Computer hardware/software Enter data directly into a computer system.	Computer hardware/software Process electronic batch files through a computer system.
Hybrid paper-based	*Method 1*: Complete paper forms: No computer hardware/software. Complete paper forms. Send hard copies of completed forms to a central location.	Computer hardware/software. 1. Enter forms directly into a centralized computer system. 2. Enter forms into electronic raw data files with double-key high-seed data entry and process them through a computer system.
	Method 2: Complete e-forms: Computer hardware/software Enter data into a computer system. Send electronic records.	Computer hardware/software Receive electronic files. Process electronic files.

the centralized location for these three groups, in addition to the data entry methods and the data transfer/receipt methods for each group.

Integrated systems using multiple technologies in the areas of communications, data collection, and management have been developed that allow patients to perform and report critical tests at home (Jones et al. [4]).

25.3 COMMUNICATION

Communication is the process of sending information from one location to another or from one person to another by means that enable the sender to send the information to the intended recipient and the intended recipient to receive, retrieve, and interpret the information. Locations and individuals can be geographically dispersed or within the confines of an organization, where information can flow between individuals with various types of communication including direct contact.

Communication is the backbone of clinical trial data collection and management. Planning, conducting, and ultimately reporting the results of a clinical trial require that trial personnel be connected throughout the duration of the trial to ensure successful completion. Efficient communication facilitates the conduct of clinical trials, especially multicenter clinical trials. Clinical trial staff have available many communication tools that have revolutionized the way they are able to share comments, exchange ideas, send and receive data, and solve unexpected problems. Trial staff are typically grouped into entities that include a coordinating center, sponsors, study leadership, resource centers, and participating sites. Examples of the types of communications between these entities have been described [5] and include direct contact meetings, regular mail carrier, telecommunication (voice communication such as telephones, pagers), teleconferencing (online meetings, a combination of sound and picture), and data communication (digital file sharing and transfer) using fax, e-mail, web site posting and FTP.

25.3.1 Direct Contact Meetings

The direct contact meeting method of communications is the first step in the development phase of a clinical trial data collection and management system. Once a trial is approved, the principal investigator (PI) meets with the appropriate coordinating center staff, which includes the biostatistician, computer programmer, and project manager, to review and finalize the drafted data collection forms and their data points before they are sent to the form designer for production. The programmer at the coordinating center meets with the biostatistician to get answers to questions regarding the trial's protocol and to set up a development plan, assign tasks, and resolve problems.

Computers are also used in this setting of communications during the trial's kickoff meeting to train the site coordinators (SCs) on the use of the system. The protocol, the manual of operations (MOP), drug-dispensing procedures, and any other important issues are presented, using various presentation packages such as MS PowerPoint through a projection device.

25.3.2 Mail Carrier

In clinical trials that solely or partially rely on paper forms and pure paper-based data collection systems, participating sites use a mail carrier to send batches of hard copies of completed forms to the coordinating center. With this approach to data, forms and computer programs are necessary to keep track of received batches of completed forms.

The mail carrier is also used as a means of communications to transfer special electronic files saved on diskettes, CDs, or tapes among resource centers, participating sites, or the coordinating center. Such electronic files may contain collected clinical data or system update batches. For example, in the VA Cooperative Studies Program (CSP) #399 trial (Singh et al. [6]), transtelephonic monitoring (TTM) data were extracted from the Transtelephonic Center database at the Washington, DC VA hospital, saved on diskettes, and sent monthly to the Hines VA Cooperative Studies Program Coordinating Center (CSPCC). In the VA CSP #7 trial, Anderson et al. [7] reported a system in which tape cartridges were used to send the entire database monthly from the coordinating center at the Seattle VA to the Hines VA CSPCC, the data center for the trial. In both cases, FedEx was used as the mail carrier. The files may be system updates, as in the distributed data collection and management system of the Glucosamine/Chondroitin Arthritis Intervention Trial (GAIT) (Abdellatif et al. [8]), or files containing verbatim adverse events to a centralized location, such as a pharmacy coordinating center (PCC) for coding to a standardized coding dictionary [9]. This approach to communications, however, does not provide instant access to the information.

25.3.3 Telephone

The telephone is still one of the primary means of communication for clinical trial personnel. The telephone is used for both voice and digital communications. Voice communication is the normal person-to-person telephone call. Data communication with the telephone is the transmission of digital data from one location to another. Various software packages have been developed for this purpose. Using a voice modem connected to a telephone, a user on a local computer can connect to another remote computer that has a modem connected to a telephone and download or upload data files. Local and remote users can also communicate with text messages. The local computer operator can even control the remote computer for trouble-shooting or system update.

The telephone is also utilized in the development of interactive voice response (IVR) systems that support touch-tone or speech recognition responses. IVR systems have been developed for subject randomization, drug assignment, and survey data collection.

25.3.4 Fax

With fax technology, documents can easily be transmitted to trial participants either from hard copies with a fax machine or as an electronic file directly from a computer. Fax technology enables distribution of reports from the coordinating centers to the participating sites [10] and allows for definition of groups of recipients according to the type of reports they need. For example, fax groups can be set up for SCs, the executive committee, the chairperson's office, the data and safety monitoring board (DSMB), and so on. Fax technology is also used to fax data collection forms as an image to a computer equipped with OMR or OCR software that can receive the image, interpret recorded data, flag bad entries, and add the data to a centralized database [11].

Fax technology has the advantages of transmitting text as images as well as electronic files if the receiving end is equipped with appropriate software and hardware. Its drawbacks include the impracticality of faxing large volumes of printed or electronic pages.

25.3.5 E-Mail

E-mail has many applications in clinical trial data collection and management. It is used as stand-alone software or integrated within a data collection and management system. With e-mail, text messages and attachment files can be sent to the trial's personnel instantaneously. When integrated in a data collection and management system, it can be programmed to send messages automatically [12].

E-mail as a communication tool has a number of drawbacks. First, it is vulnerable to being intercepted. This is a major security problem, especially when sensitive files are attached. Second, intended recipients may not access their e-mail on a timely basis, thus delaying any action that might need to be taken. Third, there is the possibility of sending files inadvertently to the wrong recipient.

25.3.6 Web Sites

The widespread acceptance and use of the Internet as a means for communication in clinical trials has revolutionized the way clinical trials information is disseminated among the various individuals and collaborating organizations running and monitoring these trials. A trial's web site provides trial personnel an easy, secure, and timely mechanism for getting critical trial information. Web sites have been developed as a means of providing trial personnel real-time access to information that includes operational issues, clinical procedures, data collection forms, data management, system manuals, training documents, phone directories, contact lists, calendars, reference documents, policies, protocol, MOPs, meeting agendas, and meeting minutes [10].

25.3.7 File Transfer Protocol

File transfer protocol (FTP) technology is a data communication tool that allows sending, accessing, and sharing files quickly and easily through a secure environment. The user logs onto the FTP site with a valid account name and a valid password. This method allows participants to share data files instantly.

25.3.8 Videoconferencing

In a videoconference, two or more people in different locations can see and hear each other at the same time, sometimes even sharing computer applications for collaboration. A video call is similar to a telephone call. After connecting, participants are able to view each other in color video and may be able to transfer files or collaborate via options such as document sharing or whiteboarding [13].

As an interactive communication medium, two-way video stands out in a number of ways. Most importantly, the visual communication provides a feeling of direct contact that enhances understanding and helps participants feel connected to each other. This can be critical in building relationships in a way that e-mail, telephone, or online chat systems cannot, supporting collaboration among traditionally isolated institutions. A videoconference can improve retention of study personnel and appeal to a variety of learning styles by including diverse media such as video or audio clips, graphics, animations, and computer applications.

A videoconference system must have audio-visual equipment (monitor, camera, microphone, and speaker) as well as a means of transmitting information between sites. Videoconferencing connections may be limited to a closed network such as a local area network (LAN) or may use public networks such as regular phone lines. Integrated services digital networks (ISDNs) are also widely used because of their economical solution for high-quality videoconferencing. ISDNs work over regular telephone lines, transmit at 128 Kbps per line, and provide dedicated bandwidth for smooth audio and video (15–30 frames per second).

In contrast, an Internet-based connection (as with CU-SeeMe) has to share bandwidth with other Internet data, which may cause audio clipping or delays as well as jerky video [14].

Videoconferencing can be a key component that facilitates the communications processes between the clinical trial entities, and it can be integrated as a part of a network system [15].

25.4 PURE PAPER-BASED SYSTEMS

Until recently, pure paper-based data collection systems have predominated in clinical trials. However, they are still being used by many contract research organizations (CROs) either because of financial constraints that prevent them from investing in newer technology or because they deal with small clinical trials that do not justify that investment. Other CROs consider the paper-based data collection method to be the safest and most reliable approach to data collection.

25.4.1 Suitability and Hardware/Software Requirements

Pure paper-based data collection systems are most suitable for small and short-term studies. Their advantages are that no computer hardware or software is needed at the participating sites because data are recorded manually on paper forms that are transferred to the centralized location in batches. A major drawback is that participating sites do not have real-time access to their data because no database is created locally. However, both hardware and software are needed at the centralized location for the data management system. The type of hardware and software used is determined by the configuration of the centralized computer. The most commonly used platforms include Open VMS, Unix, or PC, and one of the most widely used software packages is SAS® [16].

25.4.2 Design and Implementation

Pure paper-based data collection systems use paper forms that can be designed with any graphical or word processing software such as Adobe PageMaker, Microsoft Word, or MS PowerPoint. Like any other type of data collection system, forms should be finalized before the data collection phase begins. However, another advantage of this system is a certain degree of flexibility in that even after data collection begins minor changes to the forms, although not recommended, can be accommodated. Forms consisting of records of 80 columns long are standard, but they can be longer. A header is repeated for every record that contains identifying information, such as site code, patient ID, visit or encounter number, date, form number, and record number. These identifiers must contain sufficient information to uniquely identify each line or record of data entered into the database. Each collectable data element exists in a specific record of a specific form and can be further identified by the column or space number(s) within the record.

Validation of the data management system is typically done in two rounds. First, correctly completed data forms are entered to ensure that the system is not flagging any good data. In the second round, completed data forms with intentional data errors are entered. All errors must be identified by the system.

Personnel who will be doing the actual data collection must be trained in understanding the protocol and in the completion and submission of the data forms before actual data collection.

In paper-based systems it is important to establish a routine schedule for submission of data forms to the central location. A shipping log is included with each submission to record the actual forms being submitted. Figure 25.2 shows an example of a shipping log form.

25.4.3 Managing Data

Pure paper-based data collection systems are inefficient in that they require large data editing overhead. Personnel at the central location must perform visual inspections of forms, compare them against the shipping log, convey submission errors and omissions to the participating sites, visually edit the major identifiers, visually inspect for completion and legibility, log the received forms, and send the received forms that pass visual inspections to data entry

Adobe Acrobat - [FORM(91)-SHIPPING-LOG.PDF]

File Edit Document Tools View Window Help

Sudden Hearing Loss Multicenter Treatment Trial (SSNHL)

Shipping Log (FORM 91) — Site: 1 — Patient ID#: 4 — Patient Initials: 7 — Visit: 10

Form: 12 9 1 — Record: 14 0 1 — Date of Visit: 16 MM / DD / 2 0 YY

FORM #	Form Name	Form in Package YES	NO
00	Self Report	25 1	2
01	Eligibility Checklist	26 1	2
02	Baseline Physician (ptI-Clinical exclusions) (ptII-Baseline H + P)	27 1	2
03	Audiology Data	28 1	2
04	Audiology Eligibility	29 1	2
05	Baseline Participant Questionnaire	30 1	2
06	Baseline Lab Measures	31 1	2
07	Retrocochlear R/O	32 1	2
08	Pain Scale	33 1	2

1 of 1 8.5 x 11 in

Figure 25.2 An example of shipping log form for a fictitious trial.

staff. The data entry staff enters the data into electronic text files with double-key data entry software. Then these files are released to the trial data management programmer.

The trial programmer develops customized programs to read the text files, perform data checking for accuracy and consistency, rectify data errors, and add edited data to the master database. These programs constitute the data management system. A data management system may consist of four major applications: (1) Check for missing and duplicate records. All problems found are rectified before proceeding to the next application, (2) Create and maintain a summary file. The summary file contains key variables for each subject in the trial. The summary file record is created by the entry of a key form, such as a screening form, and is updated for each patient as subsequent forms are processed. The summary file variables are used to perform cross-form and cross-visit consistency checks, validate the forms' major identifiers, and determine whether submitted forms are expected. A summary file may contain information such as the subject's ID, screening date, eligibility, randomization or enrollment date, treatment assignment, date of last visit, vital status, and expected ancillary forms (laboratory, physical exam, etc.). As forms are processed, summary file flags are turned on/off, and "and/or" variables are updated. The summary file is used to create overdue reports and monitor accrual. (3) Check for specific data range validity and consistency: Once a form has passed the summary file application, it undergoes routine range and within-form consistency checks. Errors found during this edit are sent to a master error file, the field in question is marked to indicate that the data are in question, and clean records are included in the trial's text master file. The error file is cumulative and provides an audit trail for all changes to the data. The error file record created during the validity/consistency checks contains the subject ID, the date of the form, the form number, record, card columns of the variable in question, the original value submitted, and the reason the variable failed the edit checks. (4) Rectify the errors in the error file: The error file is used to create queries, which are sent to the participating sites for verification or rectification. The corrected queried data are processed through the error File application. The revised values are reedited, and, if they pass the edit, the master is updated, their error flags are turned off, and the new values are retained. If a submitted correction fails the reedit, a new error record is created and the process is repeated. The master file is the repository for all data that have successfully passed through the data management system.

25.5 ELECTRONIC-BASED SYSTEMS

Electronic-based data collection and management systems have revolutionized data collection and management. The advantages of such systems over the traditional pure paper-based data collection and management systems include their ability to (1) provide cleaner data faster, thus significantly reducing query rates and eliminating double data entry, (2) provide up-to-date interim progress reports in a timely fashion, and (3) dramatically reduce the time from last patient visit to final database lock out. These advantages provide for quick access of up-to-date data for feedback to the appropriate stakeholders, which allows them to make timely critical decisions and enables them to easily monitor protocol compliance, enrollment rates, and performance metrics of participating sites. Analysis has underlined the value of electronic data capture (EDC) as a cost- and time-saving approach in modern clinical research [17, 18].

Electronic-based data collection and management systems rely heavily on computer hardware and software at both the participating sites and the coordinating centers. The hallmark of the electronic-based data collection and management systems is the elimination of paper data collection forms. Instead of recording data on paper forms, data collectors enter data directly into a computer system where an electronic data record is generated for each form. The method of data transfer to the central location depends on the type of the electronic-based data collection and management system.

Situations in which proposed trials must await approval and funding before development of the electronic-based data collection and management system can begin present a real challenge to developers in terms of being able to complete the system before the initiation of data collection. Development of a basic system that is easily adaptable will aid in decreasing the time needed for development.

Electronic-based data collection and management systems use various computer hardware and software technologies. Although some organizations design and develop their own systems, others purchase well-established e-clinical trials software from a wide range of vendors.

In some clinical trials, sponsors may choose to compensate participating sites for completed clinical visits, medical tests, and other procedures. Electronic-based data collection and management systems provide a way for integrating electronic accounts payable systems. The data collection and management systems of the GAIT trial include such a system. Figure 25.3 shows an example of the trial's accounts payable report generated for each participating site after each download.

25.5.1 Centralized Systems

Centralized systems reside at a central location and are accessed through a local area network (LAN), a wide area network (WAN), or a virtual private network (VPN).

The user logs into the system with valid user id and password credentials from any computer connected to the network. The instantaneous access of the user to the centralized database enables direct entry of the data into a centralized database, whether with LAN, WAN, or VPN. Remote data entry

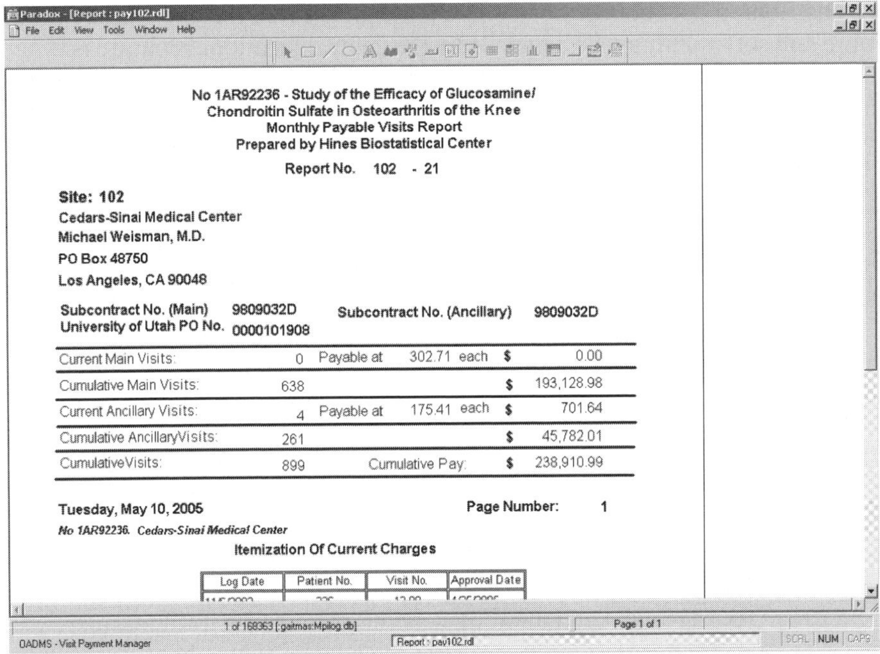

Paradox - [Report : pay102.rdl]

File Edit View Tools Window Help

No 1AR92236 - Study of the Efficacy of Glucosamine/
Chondroitin Sulfate in Osteoarthritis of the Knee
Monthly Payable Visits Report
Prepared by Hines Biostatistical Center

Report No. 102 - 21

Site: 102
Cedars-Sinai Medical Center
Michael Weisman, M.D.
PO Box 48750
Los Angeles, CA 90048

Subcontract No. (Main) 9809032D Subcontract No. (Ancillary) 9809032D
University of Utah PO No. 0000101908

Current Main Visits:	0	Payable at	302.71 each	$	0.00
Cumulative Main Visits:	638			$	193,128.98
Current Ancillary Visits:	4	Payable at	175.41 each	$	701.64
Cumulative AncillaryVisits:	261			$	45,782.01
CumulativeVisits:	899		Cumulative Pay:	$	238,910.99

Tuesday, May 10, 2005 Page Number: 1

No 1AR92236. Cedars-Sinai Medical Center

Itemization Of Current Charges

Log Date	Patient No.	Visit No.	Approval Date

1 of 168363 [:gaitmas:Mplog.db] Page 1 of 1

OADMS - Visit Payment Manager Report : pay102.rdl NUM

Figure 25.3 An example of the GAIT's accounts payable report.

does not necessarily require the purchase of any computer hardware and software for the participating sites because the system is centralized and participating sites can use existing computers to access it.

25.5.2 Distributed Systems

In distributed systems, each participating site must be equipped with a desktop or a laptop computer loaded with the distributed data collection system software to collect and enter data locally. In addition, each site is provided with necessary storage devices such as tapes, zip diskettes, and CDs and peripheral devices such as printers. Collected data are transferred periodically to the central location as files saved on storage devices, via phone modems, by FTP, or through wireless communications, where they are managed by a centralized data management system.

There are a variety of off-the-shelf relational database software that support Graphical User Interface (GUI) and scripting languages, which can be used to develop distributed data collection systems. Some of these include Microsoft Access using Visual Basic, Visual Basic Scripts, or Visual Basic for Application, and Paradox using its Paradox Application Language (PAL) as the scripting language.

Distributed data collection is very challenging. First, the appropriate hardware and software must be acquired by the central location. Separate licenses for required software are needed for each participating site. Each computer must be configured and tested. The system must be loaded on each computer before the initial training of personnel doing the data collection. Finally, the computer must be shipped to the participating sites.

The selection of the hardware and software is a function of the trial design and budget. The first step in the selection is to determine the minimum requirements needed to support the system and to outline a list of specifications. Supplier's web sites (such as www.Gateway.com and www.Dell.com) are useful in making the appropriate selections for the trial's requirements and budget. An itemized list of the costs of all the components required aids in constructing a budget estimate for all the hardware and software for the entire trial. One or two spare units should be included in this estimate for emergency situations such as the breakdown of a unit at a participating site.

Desktop computers have the advantage of stability and security over laptops, whereas laptops have the advantage of mobility. However, laptops are fragile and are prone to theft and damage. Safeguards must be put in place to prevent this from happening.

System testing and validation start while the system programmers are developing it. Peer programmers perform the next level of validation after the system has been completed. The last step is the testing of the system by the data collectors during training. Errors or suggestions resulting from any of these steps are resolved before the equipment is shipped to the participating sites to start data collection.

Training of the data collectors is an important step in ensuring reliable data collection. Trainees will have different levels of computer competency but all must be comfortably competent with the system before data collection can start. Entry of practice data for each form is recommended during training. Strict guidelines for the use of the trial computer hardware and software must be established at the outset to ensure system integrity. Table 25.2 illustrates a list of these guidelines.

Electronic data transfer is achieved by scheduled data download from the participating sites' local computers to the centralized location computer. Various software packages are available to transfer data from the participating sites to the central location. One example of this software is PCAnywhere32 from Semantic, which allows for downloading and uploading data from and to the participating sites in addition to remote control sessions. It supports three levels of encryption for transferred data. If modems are used for data transmission, it is recommended for security reasons that the local and host computers be stand alone and not connected to the organization's internal network or local intranet or the Internet.

System software maintenance presents some challenges. System updates may be needed to fix a glitch, incorporate protocol amendments, respond to changes in business rules, add, change, or disable reports, forms, or variables,

TABLE 25.2 Rules and Regulations for Distributed Systems

Area	Rules/Regulations
Environment	The PC should be placed in a secure room. The room should be leakproof. The room should be locked when trial personnel are away.
Usage	The PC access should be limited to the authorized personnel only. The PC should be used for the conduct of the trial only. The PC should not be left on while unattended. The PC should be covered with the protective cover when idle. We recommend the use of a password-protected screen saver.
Installing new software	Installing new software on the PC is prohibited.
Removing existing software	Removing existing software from the PC is prohibited.
Changing default settings	Changing any default settings of the trial PC is prohibited unless authorized by the Data/Biostatistical Center.
Eating/drinking near the PC	Eating and drinking near the PC are prohibited.
Password security	Sharing your password with others is prohibited. Posting passwords on sticky notes is prohibited.

correct misspelled or incorrect variable labels, correct variables' displayed unit of measurement, modify reference ranges, and add or modify existing consistency checks. Depending on the complexity and the extent of the update, system maintenance is achieved by uploading update batches to the participating site's computers or making the changes to the system directly with telecommunication software. If the update is urgent, it is accomplished by mailing update batches on floppy disks along with an installation program and instructions to the participating sites. Procedures are set to ensure that the update diskettes are received and implemented immediately. Each user is instructed to acknowledge the receipt and the installation of the system update. It is also very important to make sure that the local users are educated and trained on any system update.

System hardware maintenance also presents some challenges. Trial personnel at the Central location first attempt resolution of hardware malfunctions. If they are unable to resolve the problem, personnel at the central location try to resolve the problem, and if that does not solve the problem a repair order is requested from the vendor as long as there is an active warranty. If the problem persists, the participating site is instructed to ship the device to the central location. If the device is the computer, the site coordinator (SC) is instructed to back up the database before shipping the computer. Personnel at the central location try to repair the device, restore the system and the database, and then ship it back to the site. If the computer or its peripheral cannot be fixed and it is out of warranty, one of the spare systems is used or a new one is purchased.

The local user performs data entry by directly entering data into the system's database stored on the local computer with customized electronic forms. The system performs edit checks, which include range, across-form, and across-visit checks at the time of entry. This feature greatly reduces data error rates.

Site closeout can be challenging when distributed data collection systems are used. The closure of participating sites involves several processes that must be completed before the sites' funding is ended and their SC leaves. These processes include (1) final download of new and changed data, (2) processing the last collected data and resolution of all new and outstanding errors, (3) a comprehensive download of the entire database, (4) removal of the entire data collection system, including the database, (5) reclaiming all system update diskettes, and back-up CD/tapes, and (6) reclaiming hardware/software licenses as required.

25.5.3 Wireless Systems

The use of wireless computer systems has gain popularity in data collection for clinical trials. They have been used as a substitute for normal paper-based patient diaries (Koop et al. [19]) to increase data quality and shorten the time needed to close the database. They have also been used for mobile interviewing [20] and for bedside data collection [21]. In patient-directed data entry, subjects are given handheld computers to answer the trial's questions (Clarke et al. [22]).

In comparison to laptops and desktops, hand-held computers have much smaller screens. They have limited memory space and computational capability. For these reasons they cannot be used to enter large amounts of text data or perform sophisticated edit checks. The bulk of edit checks are done centrally by a centralized DMS. They are prone to loss or damage, but they have an advantage over laptops and desktops in their ease of mobility.

25.5.4 PDF-Based Systems

This method of data collection uses Portable Document Format (PDF) Forms. This approach is flexible and inexpensive. A number of commercial software packages such as Adobe Acrobat, LaText, and Microsoft Word and free software such as Python and R are used to create the PDF forms. Paper copies of the PDF forms may be used as an intermediate data collection. Electronic versions are completed at each site with Adobe Reader software. Completed forms are submitted on a CD or faxed as Extended Markup Language (XML) data files to the coordinating center, where data points are extracted and added to the database by a DMS.

Python has been used to extract data elements from submitted PDF files and create automated analysis data sets using R, where created tables and graphs were combined into reports generated automatically in LaText [23] Adobe Acrobat's built-in JavaScript capabilities have also been used to create an online user interface that dynamically generates the appropriate forms for a specified clinic visit [24]. In addition, annotated PDF study forms can be placed on a trial's web site [25] for immediate access. PDF technology is used at the DMS back end of the data collection and management system to disseminate laboratory information from the coordinating center to the participating sites. This has been accomplished with various telecommunication tools such as auto-fax server or through a web site over the Internet [26].

25.5.5 Web-Based Systems

With the increased acceptance of the Internet and the huge innovations in web development tools, web-based data collection and management systems have become the choice of many CROs because of their capability for collecting clinical trial data in real time and disseminating critical clinical trial information to the participating sites and various oversight committees [27].

Many languages are used to develop web-based data collection and management systems, including the design of dynamic data collection e-forms. These languages include tag-based and script-based languages. The most common of the tag-based languages is Macromedia ColdFusion Markup Language (CFML) using Macromedia ColdFusion Studio or Dreamweaver UltraDev. The most common script-based languages include Active Server Pages (ASP) from MS, which runs on Microsoft Internet Information Server (IIS), and Java Server Pages (JSP) from Sun Microsystems. Perl language has also been used to generate dynamic e-forms on the fly.

Web-based data collection and management systems provide a mechanism for remote data entry, where entered data are added to a centralized database once the submit button is pressed. They can be designed to automate the various aspects of clinical trials such as eligibility evaluation, data collection, and tracking specimens. They also serve as a resource site for participating sites to access trial-specific information, facilitate communication, track data queries and their resolutions, and allow administrative management of trials [28, 29]. For these reasons, they play an important role in facilitating the conduct of international clinical trials.

Such systems can reside on the organization's intranet or over the Internet. Various types of hardware and software are needed to host a website. The hardware includes switches, gateways, and routers. Software includes, among others, application servers, database servers, web servers, authentication servers, and firewalls. On the other hand, the only hardware and software needed at each participating site is a computer with access to the Internet and a web browser such as Internet Explorer and Netscape Navigator.

25.5.6 Direct Systems

There has been a push for direct data collection (DDC) as an alternative to remote data capture (RDC). In this approach most of the required clinical data are acquired directly from existing patient record systems such as MRI machines, ECG, EEG, TTM, laboratories, and other measurement equipment. This approach eliminates the need for paper transcription and reentry to another system. It promises error-free and resource-efficient data capture, which allows early locking of the database and therefore potentially earlier product launch [30].

25.6 HYBRID SYSTEMS

Hybrid systems are those systems that employ various strategies to collect data. In such systems, data may be collected on paper forms as patient self-administered questionnaires, while additional data may be downloaded from centralized databases.

25.6.1 Paper Data Collection with Centralized Interactive Data Entry

In this design, data are collected on paper forms and shipped to the coordinating center where data coordinators enters them directly into a centralized data management system. SCs complete the paper forms and ship them to the coordinating center. The data coordinator visually checks received forms as in pure paper-based DMS. However, forms are not entered by double-key high-speed data entry. Instead, they are entered directly into a customized data management system through computerized screens. A second data coordinator reviews the fully marked entered forms and compares the entries against the paper forms, flagging any discrepancies. The first data coordinator checks and rectifies these discrepancies. Range and consistence errors flagged upon entry are reported to the SCs for rectification as monthly error reports. Corrections are then applied to the database and added to the audit trail. Flagged entries that are valid are marked as "uncorrectables" so that they will not be flagged again.

This method was used in VA Cooperative Study # 418A [31]. Although this approach yielded a reliable database, it was time consuming because entering data into the computerized screens by one person and for all the data forms received from all participating sites takes time. The computerized screens cannot be designed for high-speed data entry, although they were designed to reduce data entry by implementing automatic skipping. In addition, a second person had to verify the entered data against their forms.

25.6.2 Paper Data Collection with Centralized Batch Data Entry

In this approach data are collected on paper forms. Completed forms are mailed to the coordinating center, where they go through visual inspections. Forms that pass the visual inspections are sent to the data entry department, where they are entered with high-speed double-key data entry. Created text data batches are processed through a customized centralized data management system. Range and consistency errors flagged upon entry are reported to the SCs for rectification as monthly error reports. Corrections are then applied to the database and added to the audit trail. Flagged entries that are valid are marked as "uncorrectables" so that they will not be flagged again.

This method is also being used at the Hines VA CSPCC for a number of trials. It appears to be superior to the paper data collection with centralized interactive data entry. It is not time consuming because data are entered with high-speed double-key data entry, which expedites processing of received forms and thus the accumulation of the master database. Another major advantage is that only one person is needed to run the system.

25.6.3 Paper Data Collection with Direct Data Transfer to Centralized DMS

Another approach is the use of facsimile (fax) transmission to a dedicated computer equipped with software such Teleform® software that can be customized to fit the needs of the clinical trial. Scannable forms are designed with specialized software and distributed to the participating sites to complete. SCs are equipped with fax machines to fax the completed forms to the central location. Advantages of this technology include the speed at which forms can be sent to a coordinating center and the fact that fax communications are very much standardized. Its drawbacks include the discipline required in form development and transmission.

Another approach is the use of scanners to scan completed forms, using specialized software to create an image of the paper forms and read their data fields into a database. Completed forms may be scanned at the local sites, and the resulted electronic data are sent to a central location or are scanned centrally.

25.6.4 Integration of Distributed Systems with Remote Servers over the Internet

In web-based application models that use web browsers to display information sent by the application server, the largest part of the data management applications reside on the server. This model has many advantages over the distributed model, but it has important limitations: (1) All participating sites must have an Internet connection; (2) it requires the ability to constantly be connected to the Internet; (3) the Internet connection makes it less portable; (4) it generates a large amount of network traffic; (5) it creates difficult issues of data validation and data integrity; and (6) there can be browser incompatibilities. Existing distributed systems can be modified into web-enabled systems. In this approach, the distributed application installed on the client PC at each of the participating sites communicates with a remote server over the Internet. This approach is inherently faster because only data and integrity check records need to be transmitted via the web, and the bulk of processing is performed locally, not on the server [32].

25.7 ACQUIRING PROPRIETARY E-CLINICAL SOFTWARE

25.7.1 The New Trend

Contract research organizations (CROs) may choose to acquire one of the many already established and well-developed proprietary data collection and management systems known as e-clinical software from various vendors in the field as an alternative to developing their own systems in-house. These systems tend to be comprised of integrated components using various technologies that allow flexibility in the methods of data entry, data submission, and data management. They can support paper-based and interactive data collection. Data submission can be done through fax technology or through the Internet. Data management aspects such as error reporting and correction depend on the type of the system and the way it is configured. Some vendors indicate that their products comply with FDA regulations for computerized systems, including 21 CFR Part 11 [33]. A CRO might ask the vendor to customize its system to address issues that were not addressed in the vendor's original design. So a great deal of effort must be expended by the CROs to really know what systems are available and to pick the best fit for the type of trials they conduct. The CROs must work with the selected vendors to provide live demos of their products and finally decide what CRO personnel should attend the demo to ask questions and get clarifications.

Most e-Clinical software consists of integrated suites of applications that support the clinical research process, including various ways of data entry that include in-house data entry, remote data capture, batch data load, and scan forms. These suites enable customers to quickly and easily design studies, capture clinical data, and automate workflow. Some e-clinical software systems are also Internet based.

25.7.2 e-Clinical Software Examples

Searching Google.com for "e-clinical" provides many vendors. Some of these are Oracle Clinical v4i® from Oracle Corporation [34], DataLabsXC® from DataLabs, Inc. [35], TrialMaster® from OmniComm Systems [36], and ClinPlus® Data Management (CPDM) by DZS Software Solutions, Inc. [37].

25.7.3 Questions to Ask the Vendors

Many questions should be asked before deciding on a particular e-clinical software package. Table 25.3 lists some of the general questions. A live demo of the software gives the audience the best opportunity to ask specific questions about issues that are important to them.

Some e-clinical software interfaces rely solely on "point and click" approaches to select a patient to work with. However, it is possible that the user can inadvertently point to and click on the wrong patient and thus enter the data of an intended patient. If the user wants to enter new or modify existing data, the new data or the updates of the intended patient are entered for the wrongly selected patient. This might not be realized until later, or not at all. Therefore, the specific question that needs to be asked is what safeguards, if any, does the software support to ensure that the user is entering data for the intended patient. When recording adverse events (AEs), it might be useful to also capture their resolution status and carry over "unresolved" AEs to subsequent visits. The specific question here is whether or not the software supports this. Entries flagged as out of reference range could be valid entries. Therefore, it is good to know whether the software provides a mechanism for the user to attach notes to such entries to indicate their validity to suppress their generated queries. Also, it is good to know whether the software supports a built-in report to list these entries for further inspection. Verifying eligibility at the time of randomization is of a highest importance. Therefore, it is essential to ask whether the software performs any eligibility checking before allowing the user to randomize a screened patient, and if so how it works. Some software packages rely solely on the inclusion and exclusion criteria reported on a screening form that consists of yes/no questions. However, it might also be necessary to verify the answers to any question with a corresponding entry on another baseline form.

Another important specific question to ask is how the software schedules patient visits. Does it schedule all visits when a patient is enrolled in the study, or is this done at specific phases (event)? For example, first, screening visits are scheduled, and then follow-up visits are scheduled after the patient is randomized. Related to this is how the software handles event-driven visits. For example, if a specific event occurs, additional visits at predefined intervals from the date of the event are expected. So the question here is whether the software can be configured to schedule these additional visits automatically as protocol visits or the user needs to schedule them as interim visits.

25.8 PROCESSES BEFORE DATA COLLECTION

All processes for data collection and management are defined, addressed, and accomplished before data collection begins. These processes include determining the type of the data collection and management systems, developing the systems, defining procedures for subject recruitment, registration, screening, randomization, and treatment dispensing.

TABLE 25.3 General Questions to Ask Vendors

Area	Question
Cost	How much does it cost?
	Do you provide technology transfer?
Regulation	Is it 21 CRF Part 11 compliant?
Configuration	What is special hardware needed?
	What is special software needed?
Delivery	How long does it take to install?
	How long does it take to be trained?
	How long does it take to set up a new trial?
Database	What is the underlying database?
	Can it integrate data from other databases?
	Can it convert the database to a different database type?
Data entry	What modes of data entry does it support?
	Can we purchase only the mode that we desire?
	How completed records are locked?
	Does it support automatic skipping?
Edit checks	How are entered data checked against reference ranges?
	How are entered data edited for accuracy?
	How are error reports printed?
	How are corrections resolved and applied to the database?
Coding capability	What are the coding capabilities?
	Does it support MedDRA dictionary?
	Does it support other coding dictionaries?
Audit trail	Does it support a full audit trail system?
Management	How is patient status tracked?
	How is visit status tracked?
	How is forms status tracked?
Maintenance	What kind of support do you provide?
	At what cost?
Documentations	Is there a user's manual?
	Is there a technical manual?
	Are these manuals online?
	How comprehensive are they?
Performance	What is the limit to the number of simultaneous users?
	Does it go down or slow down as more users are using it?
	Does it go down or slow down as database grows?
Flexibility	How are protocol exceptions handled?
	Does it allow for the registration of interim visits?
	What are the business rules for handling required and as-needed forms?
	How easy is it to incorporate protocol or form changes?
Metrics	What metrics does it support to assess its performance?
Reports	What kind of reports does it generate?
	Can new reports be generated as needed?
Security	What security features does it support?
	How reliable are its security features?
Standardization	Does it come with a standard global question library?

25.8.1 Choosing a Data Collection and Management System

Depending on the size of the CRO and the nature of the trial, the system may be acquired in one of the following ways: (1) developed in-house by the organization's staff with off-the-shelf commercial software, (2) outsourced to outside contractors, (3) with open source/free software (OSS/FS), and (4) purchased from e-clinical proprietary vendors.

The approach selected depends on various factors. The trial-related factors are usually derived from the trial's protocol. A summary of the trial's characteristic is identified and used to make a decision on the method to be used for data collection. These characteristics may include (1) kickoff date, (2) sample size, (3) length of subject intake, (4) length of follow-up, (5) trial duration, (6) number of participating sites, (7) number of data collection forms, (8) type of data collection, forms, (9) length of data collection forms, (10) complexity of data collection forms, and (11) type of collected data. Depending on these protocol characteristics, a decision can be made regarding the type of the data collection and management system. While paper-based systems are more suitable for small and short-term studies, electronic-based systems are more suitable for intricate trials that have complex rules and quick decision-making requirements. On the other hand, Internet-based systems are more suitable for studies that collect categorical data. In any case, several questions should be asked and answered before choosing a data collection and management system.

Other factors include available resources in terms of money and manpower to develop the system in-house, outsource, or purchase from e-clinical proprietary vendors, reliability, flexibility, and security. Some coordinating centers have chosen OSS/FS over proprietary vendors based on the criteria of cost, reliability, flexibility, and security [38]. The rationale is that although both have service comparability, proprietary software licensing costs, both for initial purchases and annual licensing, are significant.

The VA Cooperative Studies Program Persian Gulf trial was mandated by Congress and had to start right away. Therefore the pure paper-based data collection approach was chosen. The VA Cooperative Studies Program Parkinson's Trial started with pure paper-based data collection, and, as resources became available, data collection was migrated to DataLabs. The VA Cooperative Studies Program Diabetes Mellitus trial [39] was a very large trial. The limited manpower and financial recourses prohibited using an electronic-based system, so the pure paper-based system was used.

25.8.2 Hardware and Software Selection

Various issues must be considered before deciding on the type of the data collection and management system. The wide range of computer programming languages, database management, proprietary software, and hardware provide for the ability to select the most appropriate system design for a trial.

The type of system chosen determines the types of hardware and software needed. It also determines the processes for acquiring the necessary hardware and software. The hardware selection may include desktops, laptops, printers, scanners, fax machines, and storage devices, and the software selection includes the system development software, the database management software, the data communication software, the data conversion software, specialized proprietary software, servers, and firewalls.

25.8.3 Form and System Design

The success of any clinical research trial depends greatly on the quality of its collected data. Collecting high-quality data begins with developing well-designed data collection forms. Well-designed forms simplify the data collection and management processes. They also simplify the building of analysis data sets. All of these are essential to the success of any clinical trial. They greatly reduce the time and effort of data collection and management and drastically simplify the data analysis phase. Forms should be designed to accurately and consistently capture the data points defined by the protocol and provide ease of review, data entry, and analysis.

Protocols submitted for approval and funding usually start with sketchy form drafts. Therefore, several processes must be undertaken to finalize these sketchy drafts and have them in a layout compatible with the chosen data collection and management system approach. Some of these processes include (1) formalizing major identifiers, (2) grouping related section, (3) splitting unrelated sections, (4) avoiding duplication of data fields, unless necessary, (5) minimizing the number of across-form and across-visit edit checks, (6) assigning form numbers according to the forms' completion order, (7) redesigning as needed, (8) normalizing fields (i.e., mutually exclusive, categorical, yes/no, etc.), and (9) defining range and consistency checks.

Computer applications allow for defining and managing several important nonclinical data types that are managed by the system itself. Such data are referred to as metadata or control data. These are information such as domain-specific descriptions, application conditions, parameters, and methods in a repository. Control data fields can be part of the data collection forms or in system-defined tables. Some of these control fields include electronic signatures, form status, transmission date, transmission number, field completed, and memo fields (large text format). The database contains tables for reference ranges, visit schedule, form schedule, labels, and drug codes.

25.8.4 Protocol and System Rules

Protocol rules, also known as business rules, are the rules that reflect the trial design. For examples, a protocol rule states that up to 99 interim visits can be scheduled between two protocol visits, visits may occur before or after their expected dates given a predefined leeway, and if the trial has multiple screening visits, subjects are advanced to a subsequent screening visit only if they passed the previous one.

System rules deal with how the system is set up and used. When developing a data collection and management system, one can add and implement as many rules as necessary. The following are some of the rules that were implemented in the GAIT distributed data collection and management system: (1) A valid system password is required; (2) only one window (screen) can be active at a time; (3) minimizing or restoring screens is not allowed; (4) the entire system may be minimized; (5) screens can only be closed with a customized close button or command; (6) the visit/form manager (the grid) can be accessed only for one subject at a time; (7) a subject's verification is required to access his/her records; (8) all fields in a form must be filled completely before it is considered complete; (9) screening form fields must be filled individually at the initial screening visit; (10) screening form fields may be filled collectively with customized buttons at subsequent screening visits, if subjects meet all inclusion/exclusion criteria; (11) SCs must sign completely filled forms before they can be closed; (12) SCs cannot sign forms that have one or more blank fields; (13) PIs must approve completed forms before they can be transferred to the coordinating center; (14) PIs can approve only forms signed by SCs for transmission; (15) SCs cannot delete transmitted forms; (16) a deletion reason must be specified before a nontransmitted form can be deleted; (17) log records of required forms cannot be deleted; (18) log records of as-needed forms can be deleted; (19) if an as-needed form exists, its log record cannot be deleted; (20) a visit is considered missed if it has not taken place before the next protocol visit; (21) subject's verification is required to grant a request to insert the withdrawal form; (22) screening visits are scheduled one at a time; (23) all follow-up visits are scheduled when the randomization number is recorded; (24) the randomization date is used to calculate the expected dates of follow-up visits; (25) only new and changed forms are transmitted; (26) the coordinating center initiates the download session as a remote PC; (27) SCs make data changes locally at the site; and (28) participating sites are to back up the entire system daily.

25.8.5 System Development

A great deal of planning is required for system development. The development phases depend on the start of the trial and the type of the system. Very often the development of a fully functioning system may not be possible before the start of the trial. Therefore, system modules are identified and assigned priorities according to their functions with reference to the trial. For example, in pure paper-based systems, the highest priority is given to the development of the module that reads the raw data batches created by the double-key data entry staff. Next in line is the module that checks the major identifiers. Then the module that performs the range and consistency checks is developed, and so on. Integrated systems such as distributed and Internet-based systems usually consist of discrete database modules for data management functions such as registration, randomization, and data entry. Modules can be categorized based on their users. Most often, system users consist of the participating sites and the coordinating center. So, to meet the startup of the trial, the modules for the participating sites are developed first. Then the modules for the coordinating center are developed. In some cases other entities such as the pharmacy center, the chairperson's office, and a resource center may need to use the system and therefore other groups of modules are needed, as was the case in the GAIT distributed data collection and management system [40].

25.8.6 System Validation

Before a data collection and management system is implemented, it has to be validated. For a newly developed application, the validation processes consist of various layers of testing. The first layer is testing the components of the system as it is being developed. This validation ensures that the programming segments of the system are error free and work as expected. The next layer of validation takes place after the system is completed and before it is put into production. This validation involves entering dummy data with indented range and consistency errors into the system and making sure every component of the system works properly and that it catches the errors. If the system is electronic, another layer of validation takes place during trial kickoff when end users are trained on the system. During each layer, examples of what might be discovered include (1) a system module is not working properly; (2) a skip pattern is not working properly; (3) the system omits some edit range or consistency checks; (4) wrong reference ranges are applied to range check some variables; (5) consistency checks are not working properly; (6) some variables are labeled incorrectly; and (7) some variables have incorrect units of measurement.

Although it is possible to identify and test every scenario of consistency checks, a business decision has to be made as to the depth of the checks. However, it is essential that all serious scenarios that could affect data analysis be tested. This is true for any type of data collection system. However, for a system to be one hundred percent reliable, every scenario must be tested and dealt with appropriately. A scenario that cannot be predicted at the time of development may be incorporated into the system or handled as an exception and dealt with accordingly when it occurs.

25.8.7 Staff Training

No matter what type of system is used, staff training is a must. In distributed data entry settings, SCs are typically trained on the developed system during the kickoff meeting of the trial. The training involves going through the protocol, regulatory requirements, data collection forms, medication dispensing

TABLE 25.4 NIH GAIT System Training Outline

Training Outline
Turning the PC on and off
Launching the system
Closing the system
A quick tour of the major control screens
Registering a new subject
Completing the first screening form
Excluding the subject at the first screening visit
Registering a second subject
Completing the first screening form at the first screening visit and passing the subject
Scheduling the second screening (randomization) visit
Completing the second screening form at the randomization visit and passing the subject
Checking subject's eligibility
Randomizing the subject and recording the randomization number
Examining the constructed follow-up schedule for the randomized subject
Withdrawing the subject
Clearing the subject's future visits after withdrawal
Preparing for monthly data transmission
Backing up the system
Opening and completing all CRFs

procedures, and hands-on training on the usage of the system. Table 25.4 shows the training outlines for the GAIT distributed data collection and management system, and Table 25.5 lists the various training points for the users to evaluate their level of understanding based on three level criteria: (1) high, (2) medium, and (3) low.

25.9 PROCESSES DURING DATA COLLECTION

25.9.1 System Evaluation

A good way of finding out the effectiveness and user-friendliness of the system is to have the end users evaluate it after a short period of data collection. Such evaluation ensures that the system is working as intended, and that the end users understand it and are comfortable with it. It also provides feedback from the end users to correct any glitches and enhance the system. Typical evaluation may include the following major criteria: hardware, general design features, case report forms, report generation, user-friendliness, performance, system training, technical support, and user's manual. In addition, the end users may be asked to rate the system as a whole, compare it to other data collection systems that have been used or known, describe whether they fill

TABLE 25.5 NIH GAIT User System Understanding Criteria

Training Note
Rules and regulations
Turning the computer on and off
Launching and closing the system
How the mouse works
Registering a new subject
Printing a list of all registered subjects
Working with a specific registered subject
Scheduling subsequent screening visits
Scheduling the randomization visit
Recording the randomization number for eligible subjects
When and how to request an "as-needed" form
Scheduling an interim visit
The various visit types
The difference between forms' records and forms' log records
When and how to delete forms' records and forms' handles
When/how to remove future visits from the system for a withdrawn subject
How to restore the future visits of a mistakenly withdrawn subject
Generating and using the list of waiting fields report
Generating and using the upcoming visits list report
Reading the subjects' status summary cross tabulation report
The forms', visits', and subject's status codes
When and how to prepare the PC for remote control session or data transmission
Backing up the system
Signing completed forms
Monitoring the numbers of forms ready for the PI's review and signature
Completing fields with the "Waiting" or "Unobtainable" code
When and how the "Inapplicable" field codes are assigned
Completing the memo field
Attaching, resolving, archiving, and printing sticky notes
Displaying data history for a given field
Printing forms or reports
When to click the quick "Fill" buttons found on some of the forms
The purpose and the usage of the "Forms Overdue Report"
The various log fields of the "Form Manager Table Frame"
Moving from one field to another
Using the keyboard versus the mouse right button to enter categorical data
When to request and how to complete the Missed Visit form
When to request and how to complete the Missed Forms form
How to complete all other forms

out paper forms in an electronic-based data collection system before entering the data into the system, and how often, and state how much the type of the system impacted their workload. With built-in controlled fields, additional evaluation of the system can be done centrally to check for its performance by examining various data-related criteria. These may include the frequency with which a completed form is modified, the number of days it takes to lock it, the number of days it takes before it is added to the centralized database, the centralized error detection rate, the rate of unobtainable data, and the rate of deleted forms [8].

25.9.2 Subject Management

The first aspect in subject management is recruitment. Various strategies are used to enhance recruitment, including physician referrals, newsletters, and advertising in local media. Computers play a major role in identifying prospective subjects for enrollment in certain clinical trials. Keeping Health Insurance Portability and Accountability Act (HIPAA) privacy regulations in mind, computer applications are written to access existing centralized databases to locate subjects who meet the trial's inclusion criteria and thus have potential for entering the trial. For example, computer applications were developed to identify subjects with recent onset of the studied disease. Some VA Cooperative Studies Program trials used scripts written in the M programming language, formally known as MUMPS, to access the local patient databases, known as VISTA, and identify potential patients for a specific clinical trial. This practice may not be allowed any longer because of the HIPAA standards. The Internet is also being widely utilized to publicize clinical trials and solicit subjects.

Recruited subjects that have potential for qualification are registered for a formal screening visit. Subject registration is accomplished by completing a paper registration form or interactively in a computerized system [41]. Each subject is assigned a unique screening number. Several standards are used to assign screening numbers. In multicenter clinical trials, a unique site number is assigned for each site, typically three digits long, and a subject ID for each screened subject is also generated.

In randomized clinical trials, a sound randomization scheme must be adopted to generate and assign randomization numbers for treatment assignments to qualified subjects. Various computerized randomization methods and procedures have been developed to generate randomizations that could accommodate any clinical trial's design. Subject randomization has also evolved from using person-to-person telephone calls between the participating sites and the coordinating center to having subjects assigned with computerized voice systems, dedicated randomization web sites, or from the data collection and management systems. Some computerized systems can dynamically generate and assign randomization numbers after a call to the voice system or a valid access to the web site is made and valid data are entered.

In the traditional approach of person-to-person telephone call, the SC indicates the subject to be randomized and is asked protocol-specific questions collectively known as the randomization form. An eligible subject whose informed consent has been received and verified for accuracy and completeness is assigned the next randomization number from the pregenerated randomization lists. Control information such as subject ID, SC initials, and date of randomization is recorded on the list for each assigned randomization number. Code-break information is also recorded for blinded trials. In this approach, the randomization numbers are pregenerated with various computer programs. SAS provides various ways of constructing randomization numbers. SAS macros [42] have been written to generate randomization lists. Figure 25.4 depicts a sample list generated for a two-arm trial by a SAS macro using permuted blocks randomization (Abdellatif [43]).

Coordinating centers that prefer this approach use it because first, they feel they can ensure the validity of the subject-consenting process before randomizing, and second, they feel they can exert full control over the randomization processes to ensure their validity. This is achieved by requiring participating sites to fax signed informed consent forms to the coordinating center to enable review for completeness and validity before randomization.

Automated randomization systems have been developed using voice response [44] and telephone touch-tone technology [45, 46]. Others have used a preloaded password-protected system with hidden encrypted randomization files into the trial's laptop or desktop computers that are used as distributed data collection devices [47] or have developed centralized computer programs that dynamically randomize subjects [48].

RANDOMIZATION LIST FOR PAGE: 1
Polesteriding versus Walking for PAD Rehabilitation

HOSPITAL 578: 578 Hines, IL

PATIENT NUM.	RAND.#	TREATMENT	DATE OF RAND. MM/DD/YY	YOUR INIT.	CODE BREAK INFORMATION DATE MM/DD/YY	COMMENT
____	5789405	Walking	__/__/__	____	__/__/__	________
____	5789971	Polestriding	__/__/__	____	__/__/__	________
____	5789900	Walking	__/__/__	____	__/__/__	________
____	5789168	Polestriding	__/__/__	____	__/__/__	________
____	5789210	Polestriding	__/__/__	____	__/__/__	________
____	5789413	Walking	__/__/__	____	__/__/__	________
____	5789637	Walking	__/__/__	____	__/__/__	________
____	5789410	Polestriding	__/__/__	____	__/__/__	________
____	5789614	Walking	__/__/__	____	__/__/__	________

Figure 25.4 Sample randomization list.

Dedicated web sites have been developed for randomizing subjects over the Internet. Internet-based systems have also been widely used for subject enrollment and randomization. Some of these systems employ dynamic randomization number allocation [49, 50], whereas others use pregenerated randomization numbers. Various issues must be addressed when using the Internet for randomization, such as the availability of Internet access and the need for a backup system to ensure the continuation of operation when the web site is inaccessible [51].

Another approach used to automate the randomization process is by embedding pregenerated randomization lists in the data collection and management system. The main disadvantage of this approach is the security of the randomization lists. This can be remedied by having the system dynamically generate randomization numbers.

The use of electronic-based data collection and management systems allows the easy tracking of patient progress in the trial. Patient, visit, and form status are tracked. Patient status can be "in screening," "excluded," "randomized," "withdrew," or "completed study." Similarly, status codes can be assigned to protocol scheduled visits to indicate whether the visit occurs or not. Form status depends on the type of the data collection system. For example a form in a distributed data collection system can be "incomplete," "filled," "completed," "altered," or "transmitted."

The explosion of graphical software and the ability of database management systems to store graphical data provide a mechanism for designing and implementing clip art to convey certain meaning to the user. For example "traffic lights" have been used to convey the status of data collection forms.

25.9.3 Data Quality Assurance

From the moment data collection begins to the closing of the trial, monitoring the progress of the trial is essential for maintaining its integrity and successful completion. Various computer software and programs have been developed for that purpose, to enable the trial staff to be aware of every single development and indicate how to respond to it throughout the trial. Some of the things that should be monitored include (1) adherence to the protocol, (2) adherence to the system rules, which include terms for the use of computer equipments and backup procedures, (3) recruitment and randomization eligibility, (4) data transmission, (5) received forms in terms of completion, overdue, unobtainable fields, waiting fields, National Clinical Coordinator (NCC) notes resolution, data errors, and data changes, (6) drug dispensing and compliance, and (7) safety data and adherence to established regulatory standards. Monitoring clinical trials is usually accomplished by generating various customized routines that generate monitoring reports. For example, a SAS macro [52] was developed to generate routine reports of data completeness rates for predefined dimensions and subdimensions of data points in VA CSP #5 (formally CSHS #5) [53]. The macro was customized to output results into text files linked to Harvard Graphics® templates. The output for each dimension consists of a text file for the dimension and a text file for each of its subdimensions.

25.9.4 Treatment Dispensing

Clinical trials that involve drug dispensing or device assignment require a robust mechanism for distributing the drugs or devices to the participating sites and ensuring that the correct drug regimens or devices are assigned to the correct subjects based on their randomization numbers. Computers play a very vital role in making sure that this is done in a timely manner and accurately to enable the pharmacy coordinating center to track the distribution status at each participating site. This also enables accounting what has been dispensed and what has been returned.

Computer-controlled systems [54] are commonly used in clinical trials to control dispensing and manage site inventories of trial supplies. Such systems are implemented with telephone voice-based or Internet web-based systems.

In the telephone voice-based systems SCs call the PCC and follow the system voice prompt to enter the required information. Typical required information must include subject ID and randomization number. Based on that information, the system assignes the correct drug supply kit or device to the subject. With Internet web-based systems, the processes are similar, but the user interaction is with a computer.

25.9.5 Handling Unexpected Events

Unexpected events may occur that need to be taken care of during the clinical trial. Some of these events may require actions to be taken with regard to the data collection and management system. For example, there is always the possibility for a subject to move from one participating site to another. If the subject is willing to continue to be followed at the new site, his/her records must be transferred from the old to the new participating site. The subject is assigned a new subject number that reflects the new site number and the next sequential subject number at the new site. The randomization number for the subject remains the same. The processes needed to accomplish this depend on the type of the data collection and management system. In distributed data collection and management systems, this may be accomplished by the following three processes: (1) extract/export subject's records from old site; (2) import subject's extracted records to the new site; and (3) recreate subject's records with the new site number and subject number identifiers at the coordinating center. In centralized systems, this situation can be resolved by simply changing the subject's records in the centralized database to reflect the new site.

25.9.6 Data Transformation

Various computer software and programs have been developed and used to simplify the transformation, manipulation, and analysis of trial data, to speed up and increase the accuracy of reporting the trial's findings. If data are collected in a format other than that required by the analysis software, the data must be transformed. There are several data conversion software packages that can be used to transform the collected data from the original format to the analysis format. Examples of these include DBMSCopy and Stat/Transfer.

25.10 PROCESSES AFTER DATA COLLECTION

25.10.1 Data Lockout

Relatively little has been written about the practicalities of the closeout of large, multicenter clinical trials, but this aspect of trial conduct and design is important and requires careful planning to be accomplished in a timely and orderly fashion [55].

25.10.2 Data Retention

Data collected at each participating site must be stored in a read-only format at that site for future reference. The Institutional Review Board (IRB) at each participating site requires that the site retain its local database after trial closeout. Data retention can be achieved in various ways. However the method should ensure that (1) participating sites are not be able to modify retained data; (2) data are presented in a way that allows sites to easily locate any data form for any subject at any trial visit; and (3) the site PI is solely responsible for the retained data.

Abdellatif et al. reported a method for data retention [56] in which collected electronic data forms of each participating site are saved on a read-only CD as PDF files after the site's database has been locked. SAS Output Delivery System (ODS), PROC Template, and PROC Forms were used to construct a read-only CD of the data forms in a PDF format for each site and then sent to the site's PI.

25.10.3 Data Archiving

After the data collection phase of a clinical trial is completed and its collected data are analyzed, collected data are archived centrally, usually at the coordinating center, for future reference. The data archive method depends on the data collection system. In paper-based data collection system, the physical paper forms may need to be archived for a specified period of time. Scanning technology allows for storing paper forms as images. In electronic-based data collection, the electronic forms are stored. In either case, the computerized database is archived.

25.10.4 Data Sharing

Computers facilitate data sharing among researchers. The Internet provides an effective method for designing and implementing data repositories of completed clinical trials. The repository software may be designed to classify users as follows. (1) Administrative users have full access to the repository. (2) Casual researchers are able to read descriptions of the site and associated organizations and legal notices. These first-time visitors will be invited to establish accounts by supplying their names and e-mail addresses. Once this has happened, these users become a part of the "casual" user group and are able to examine descriptions of the repository contents. (3) Serious researchers, for whom more complete information about themselves and their institution are required, may submit a research proposal containing the identification of a principal investigator, IRB, associated researchers, research problem and hypothesis, objectives, requested data, and a justification for the data requested.

25.11 FINAL COMMENTS

In summary, advancement of IT has had a great impact on the conduct of clinical trials. A discussion was held during the Society for Clinical Data Management's (SCDM) Spring Forum in Atlanta, GA, March 13–15, 2005, that examined the role of technology and standards in the future clinical data management. The participants articulated that "CDM will be dramatically transformed by new uses of technology, and by the emergence of industry wide standards." Others anticipated a more "gradual impact." The complete list of the discussion results have been reported elsewhere [57].

ACKNOWLEDGMENTS

I would like to acknowledge Dr. Domenic J. Reda, Hines VA CSPCC, and Nancy Ellis, Hines VA CSPCC, for their insightful review of this chapter.

REFERENCES

1. http://www.tech-encyclopedia.com/data-management.htm
2. www.dcri.duke.edu/patient/glossary.jsp

3. http://www.dama.org/public/pages/index.cfm?pageid=71
4. Jones MS, Pontzer JF, DelCurto B, Badgett CA, Sather MR. Integrating interactive voice response system and web based systems to support home international normalization ratio testing. *Clin Trials* 2005;2:S73.
5. Bumendtein BA, James KE, Lind BK, Herman EM. Functions and organization of coordinating centers for multicenter studies. *Controlled Clin Trials* 1995; 16:4S–29S.
6. Singh S, Singh B, Reda D, et al. [Abdellatif M]. Comparison of sotalol vs. amiodarone in maintaining stability of sinus rhythm in subjects with atrial Fibrillation (Sotalol-Amiodarone Atrial Fibrillation Effectiveness Trial [SAFE-T]). *Am J Cardiol* 2003;92:468–72.
7. Anderson S, Abdellatif M, Schreiner S, McDonell M, Reda D, Fihn S. Information system for a multi-hospital trial using optical scanning and hospital database downloads. *Controlled Clin Trials* 1995;16:3S:76S.
8. Abdellatif M, Reda D. A Paradox-based data collection and management system for a multi-center randomized clinical trials. *Comput Methods Prog Biomed* 2004;73:145–64.
9. Swanson K, Abdellatif M, Fye C, Reda D, Williams D, Harris C, Clegg D. Adverse event reporting and monitoring system for the Glucosamine/Chondroitin Arthritis Intervention Trial (GAIT). *Clin Trials* 2005;2:S49.
10. Chen J, Meloro L, Eng H, Wisniewski S. Using SAS to create and e-mail individualized reports in a multi-center randomized clinical trial. *Clin Trials* 2005;2: S64.
11. Terrin ML, Forman S, Fick S, Clarke E, Gross R, Gerstenblith G, et al. Facsimile copy (fax) transmission data entry direct from clinical sites in the CHF team study. *Controlled Clin Trials* 1999;20:2S–91S.
12. Thompson GS, Quan K, DuChene A. Case report form image management system for large multicenter clinical trials. *Controlled Clin Trials* 2001:P34.
13. http://info.csd.org/newlinks/whatisvidconf.htm
14. http://www.cmsdnet.net/ito/videoconferencing/whatisvideoconferencing.htm
15. Nixon DW, Zang EA, McShane P, Ferretti A, Ferguson L, Gardnet R. The South Carolina prostate cancer prevention and telehealth program. *Controlled Clin Trials* 2003:P31.
16. SAS/BASE is a registered trademark or trademark of SAS Institute Inc. in the USA and other countries. ® Indicates USA registration.
17. Spink C. Electronic Data Capture (EDC) as a means for e-clinical trial success. IBM Global Services, Pharmaceutical Clinical Development 2002. http://www8.ibm.com/services/pdf/IBM_Consulting_Pharmaceutical_clinical_development.pdf
18. Green JA. The EDC value proposition to the pharmaceutical industry. A detailed comparison of EDC versus paper model costs for four different clinical research projects (Phase I–IIIb). Datatrak International, Inc., 2001.
19. Koop A, Mösges R. The use of handheld computers in clinical trials. *Controlled Clin Trials* 2002;23:469–80.
20. Wilson R, Fulmer T. Initial experiences with wireless, pen-based computing. *Public Health Nurs* 1998;15(3):225–32.

21. Karshmer JF, Karshmer AI. Hand-held computing in the patient care setting. A pilot project. *The Annual Symposium on Computer Applications in Medical Care* 1995:7–11.
22. Clarke WL, Cox DJ, Gonder-Frederick LA, Julian D, Schlundt D, Polonsky W. The relationship between no routine use of insulin, food, and exercise and the occurrence of hypoglycemia in adults with IDDM and varying degrees of hypoglycemic awareness and metabolic control. *Diabetes Educator* 1997;23:55–8.
23. Cox TA. Clinical data collection using free software. *Controlled Clin Trials* 2004: P56.
24. Gatt R. Web-based dynamic forms packet generator using Acrobat and Java Script. *Controlled Clin Trials* 2004:P48.
25. Beiser JA, Hornbeck E, Morrison D, Gordon MO, Goldberg J. De-identification of shared datasets. *Controlled Clin Trials* 2004:P36.
26. Grover NB. Reporting laboratory results to clinical centers through the study website. *Controlled Clin Trials* 2004:P39.
27. Speas C, Rushing S, Backfield M. Web based data entry in a hormone replacement therapy clinical trial for a data coordinating center. *Controlled Clin Trials* 2000;20:2S–91S.
28. Winget M, Kincaid H, Lin P, Li L, Kelly S, Thornquist M. A web-based system for managing and coordinating multiple multisite studies. *Clin Trials* 2005; 2:42–9.
29. Schmidt JR, Vignati AJ, Pagash RM, Simmons VA, Evans RL. Web-based distributed data management in the Childhood Asthma Research (CARE) network. *Clin Trials* 2005;2:50–60.
30. Hyde AW, Amersham N. The changing face of electronic data capture: from remote data entry to direct data capture. *Drug Inform J* 1998;32:1089–1092:0092-8615/98.
31. Bratt G, Martinez C, Wilson R, Takahashi G, Kricos P, [Abdellatif M]. Long-term findings from the NIDCD/VA hearing aid clinical trial. Research platform presentation at the American Speech-Language-Hearing Association (ASHA), 2004. http://search.asha.org/db/convention.html?col=conv&tb=Paper&trackingid=1437&charset=iso-8859-1
32. Kolova T, Younes N. "Fat-Client" web-enabled remote data management systems: an alternative to "Thin-Client" web data entry. *Controlled Clin Trials* 2004: P49.
33. FDA. Electronic Records; Electronic Signatures; Final Rule. Code of Federal Regulations, Title 21, Food and Drugs. Part 11. *Fed Reg* 1997;62:13429–66.
34. http://www.oracle.com/industries/life_sciences/clinicalds.pdf
35. http://www.datalabs.com/
36. http://www.omnicomm.com/trialmaster/easy.html
37. http://www.clinplus.com/products/data_management.htm
38. Christopher EF, Daniel S. Open source versus proprietary software in clinical trial coordinating center operations. *Clin Trials* 2005;2:S77.
39. Duckworth WC, McCarren M, Abraira C. Glucose control and cardiovascular complications: the VA diabetes trial. *Diabetes Care* 2001;24(5):942–5.

40. Abdellatif A, Motyka D, Williams D, Reda D, Kucmeroski D, Fye C, Clegg D. A data collection and management system for clinical trials in osteoarthritis. *Clin Trials* 2005;2:S71.
41. Pogash RM, Haak T, Grella V, Zimmerman R, Doty L. Using the web for securely managing the asthma Clinical Research Network (ACRN) and the Childhood Asthma Research And Education (CARE) network. *Controlled Clin Trials* 2004;l.1.4:387–98(12).
42. SAS/MACRO is a registered trademark or trademark of SAS Institute Inc. in the USA and other countries. ® Indicates USA registration.
43. Abdellatif M. A SAS macro for generating randomization lists in clinical trials using permuted blocks randomization. *SUGI 29 Proceeding* 2004:147–29.
44. Assman SF, Bodnya A, Smith SS, Tighe F. An interactive voice response system for randomizing subjects. *Controlled Clin Trials* 1996;17:2:S68–S69.
45. Spence ER, Horney A. Automated telephone randomization system. *Controlled Clin Trials* 1999;20:2S:88S.
46. Anthony S, Reece S, Rushing S, Margiti S, Albright C. Challenges in implementing a telephone touch-tone randomization system in the primary care setting. *Controlled Clin Trials* 1997;18:3:S156–7.
47. Swanson A. Computerized bedside randomization in a randomized clinical trial. *Controlled Clin Trials* 2003;24:3S:166S.
48. Palmar M, Broekhoven M, Garrah A, Tu D. CTASSIST: a computer program for subjects randomization and tracking of drug distribution. *Clin Trials* 2000; 21:2S:110S.
49. Kiuchi T, Ohashi Y, Konishi M, Bandai Y, Kosuge T, Kakizoe T. A world wide web-based user interface for a data management system for use in multi-institutional clinical trials—development and experimental operation of an automated subjects registration and random allocation system. *Controlled Clin Trials* 1996;17:6:476–93.
50. Campbell K, Radcliffe C, Thomas RG, Grundman M, Thal L. Online subject randomization and drug ordering system using the web linked to central data base. *Controlled Clin Trials* 1999;20:2S:91S.
51. Gillespie HA, Moke P, Beck R, Lester LA. Lessons learned in using web-based randomization in the community-based amblyopia treatment study. *Controlled Clin Trials* 2001;22:2S–80S.
52. Abdellatif M, Thottapurathu L, Reda D, Moritz T. Using PROC Means to report data completeness rates of predefined dimensions and subdimensions of variables. *SUGI Conference Proceedings* 1996;1031-1-36.
53. Marshal G, Grover FL, Henderson WG, Hammermeister KE. Assessment of predictive models for binary outcomes: an empirical approach using operative death from cardiac surgery. *Stat Med* 1994;13:1501–11.
54. Peterson M, Byrom B, Dowlman N, Mcentegart D. Optimizing clinical trial supply requirements: simulation of computer-controlled supply chain management. *Clin Trials* 2004;1.4:99–412.
55. Dinnett EM, Mungall MMB, Kent JA, Ronald ES, Gaw A. Closing out a large clinical trial: lessons from the Prospective Study of Pravastatin in the Elderly at Risk (PROSPER). *Clin Trials* 2004;1.6:545–52.

56. Abdellatif M, Thakkar B, Motyka D. Constructing data retention CDs for the VA CSP #399 participating sites after trial completion. Hines VA Research Day 2003:P39.
57. Clinical Data Management: Envisioning the future. SCDM Spring Forum 2005.

26

REGULATION OF COMPUTER SYSTEMS

SANDY WEINBERG

Contents

26.1 INTRODUCTION

The Federal Drug Administration (FDA) describes the biopharmaceutical industries as "self-regulated," retaining for itself the responsibility of assuring and checking on that self-regulatory process. Not surprisingly, then,

Computer Applications in Pharmaceutical Research and Development, Edited by Sean Ekins.
ISBN 0-471-73779-8

FDA resources are expended in areas based not on their absolute importance but on the lack of industry capability to control a particular concern. When manufacturing processes were primitive, unclean, and uncontrolled, the FDA issued the "Good Manufacturing Practices" and eventually the "Good Laboratory Practices," "Good Clinical Practices," and "Good Tissue Practices." Together these Practices provide standards for the industry operations.

In modern times, as most companies invested in compliance with these good practices, the FDA focused a step back, at the computers that controlled procedures in manufacturing, laboratory analysis, clinical testing, and tissue tracking. In 1989 the FDA issued a call for system validation (actually, the FDA issued a general call for system validation and then tacitly endorsed *System Validation Standards* [1], a call for the validation of computer systems used in all regulated areas). Over the next fifteen years field investigators increasingly asked to see evidence of the testing and validation of computer systems. By 1998 computer validation issues represented the largest category of FDA-issued "483s" (Notice of Adverse Findings).

In the late 1990s the biopharmaceutical industry began agitating for FDA acceptance of "electronic signatures," intended to make possible approval and retention of documents in electronic form. The impetus was in the clinical testing area: Hospitals had long been utilizing electronically signed patient records. To incorporate these records in FDA submissions, requirements calling for a written signature had to be updated.

A joint industry-agency committee was formed to propose guidelines for the use of electronic signatures. In the preliminary committee discussion it quickly became apparent that any new guideline should appropriately incorporate system validation requirements, because now the electronic signature would be unacceptable unless the system generating and storing that signature was reliable and properly controlled.

The first draft of the new requirement had draconian security requirements, softened (as is common) after a comment period: Demands for biometric identifiers were replaced with password control options. But the revised "final" regulation was still broad in scope and necessitated extensive documentation and testing for all systems used in the industry (with even stronger controls if the user opted for electronic signatures).

The United States Federal Regulation identified as 21 CFR Part 11 focuses on electronic records. While emphasizing the approval and long-term review of those records with guidance regarding electronic record archiving and electronic signature approval, the regulation incorporated standards for system validation and all previous guidance related to computer systems.

When Mark McClellan assumed the directorship of the FDA 2001, he was charged with developing strategies for minimizing drug development costs while maintaining high levels of quality and safety. One of the first targets of his cost containment campaign was 21 CFR Part 11: Cost of compliance was high, but was the benefit proportional?

Consider this example. There are two manufacturing facilities in central North Carolina facing each other on opposite sides of the street. One facility manufactures implantable pacemakers; the other cuts stripped pine into tongue depressors. Both utilize the same software package to track shipments and potentially to recall problem deliveries. A pacemaker recall must be perfect and timely, or a patient death is the likely result. A tongue depressor recall (hard to imagine) has little or no impact on health and safety.

Yet under the original requirements of 21 CFR Part 11 both companies would have had to conduct extensive test on the software; to write and implement eight to ten standard operating procedures; to document the requirements, development, and change history of the code; and to record and archive all records. In this case, as in so many, such an investment in time and dollars would have been justified for the pacemakers but wasted in the case of the tongue depressors.

When his analysis uncovered this and other similar situations, McClellan took two unusual steps. First, he suspended Part 11, calling for reconsideration. And second, four months later, he re-released 21 CFR Part 11 with some major changes in interpretation.

Because of the broad sweep of Part 11, the FDA offered two recommendations for prioritizing compliance efforts. First, the agency identified three areas that it will choose to de-emphasize; (1) well-established prior systems, (2) systems without direct impact on product safety (inventory, financial, etc.), and (3) systems that parallel but do not replace manual records. Second, and perhaps of greater impact, the agency urged the use of a risk assessment to identify situations in which potential dangers are most probable and most severe. Organizations are urged, with a multitiered validation and compliance protocol, to document the systems and subsystems in high, medium, and low classifications of risk. Each level implies differing standards of testing and control and appropriately differing levels of regulatory scrutiny. In the absence of such an assessment all systems are considered to be high risk, but with appropriate evaluation it is possible to fine-focus Part 11 on the areas of greatest concern.

Currently, Part 11 serves as a guideline for industry control of all computer systems (actually, of course, the regulation applies to all systems under FDA purview, effectively excepting financial systems, human resource systems, and other business systems) and as a requirement for high-risk systems directly affecting human health and safety. Responsibility for classifying and defending a system as falling outside the high-risk requirement circle falls on the regulated organization.

26.2 REVIEW OF 21 CFR PART 11

One of the great values of computer systems lies in their flexibility: Through targeted programming, the same computer using the same language code can be used for a variety of different functions. That very flexibility, however, makes regulation unusually complex: System requirements in effect customize a system in ways much more complicated than the functionality of a mixer or single factor analyzer.

Because of the complexity of computer hardware and software and because of the intricacy of a risk assessment, the FDA has to all intents and purposes adopted an indirect regulatory posture. Regulated companies are informally urged to conduct independent audits of Part 11 compliance, utilizing in-house or consultant expertise. The agency can then review the details of the audit report and the credentials for experience, expertise, and independence of the auditor. Follow-up investigation of specific points can then be laser-focused on specific areas of concern.

The audit also emphasizes the self-regulated nature of the industry and the ideal relationship between the agency and the industry. In theory and effective practice, a biomedical company utilizes its quality assurance (QA) unit (in this case, supplemented by credible Part 11 auditors) to maintain control of safety, effectiveness, and quality. The FDA can then review the quality system (QS) and spot-check the other systems such as laboratory or production for most efficient regulatory oversight. In effect, the QA regulates the company and the FDA regulates the QA.

The effectiveness of a QA-related independent Part 11 audit is dependent on the checklist or audit plan utilized. Here, provided as a model, is a two-part audit checklist. The depth of the evidence and support required is dependent on the results of the risk assessment: All high-, medium-, or low-risk systems should be subject to the same general questions.

The checklist also serves as a summary of and operationalization of the complex Part 11 requirement. When an auditor—either an independent expert or an FDA investigator—can check as compliant all identified issues, the system is de facto operating under the letter and spirit of 21 CFR Part 11. Any issue that emerges as questionable, unclear, noncompliant, or absent requires investigation, explanation, and remediation.

Presented is a model checklist divided into two parts: a general checklist of 21 CFR Part 11 requirements and a 21 CFR Part 11 software evaluation checklist for closed systems that do not use biometrics.

26.3 GENERAL CHECKLIST—21 CFR PART 11

26.3.1 Subpart B—Electronic Records

11.10 Controls for Closed Systems

11.10(a) Procedures and controls shall include validation of systems to ensure accuracy, reliability, consistent intended performance, and the ability to discern invalid or altered records.

11.10(b) Procedures and controls shall include the ability to generate accurate and complete copies of records in both human readable and electronic form suitable for inspection, review, and copying by the agency.

11.10(c) Procedures and controls shall include protection of records to enable their accurate and ready retrieval throughout the records retention period.

11.10(d) Procedures and controls shall include limiting system access to authorized individuals.

11.10(e) Procedures and controls shall include use of secure, computer-generated time-stamped audit trails to independently record the date and time of operator entries and actions that create, modify, or delete electronic records. Record changes shall not obscure previously recorded information. Such audit trail information shall be retained for a period at least as long as that required for the subject electronic records.

11.10(f) Procedures and controls shall include use of operational system checks to assure integrity of data.

11.10(g) Procedures and controls shall include use of authority checks to ensure that only authorized individuals can use the system, electronically sign a record, access the operation or computer system input or output device, alter a record, or delete a record.

11.10(h) Procedures and controls shall include use of device (e.g., terminal) checks to determine, as appropriate, the validity of the source of data input or of data transport.

11.50 Signature Manifestations

11.50 Signed electronic records shall contain information associated with the signing that clearly indicates the following:

- The printed name of the signer;
- The date and time when the signature was executed; and
- The version of the document signed (or indication that the document was locked once signed).

11.70 Signature/Record Linking

11.70 Electronic signatures and handwritten signatures executed to electronic records shall be linked to their respective electronic records to ensure that the signatures cannot be excised, copied, or otherwise transferred to falsify an electronic record by ordinary means.

26.3.2 Subpart C—Electronic Signatures

11.100 General Requirements

11.10 Controls for Closed Systems

11.100(a) Each electronic signature shall be unique to one individual and shall not be reused by, or reassigned to, anyone else.

11.200 Electronic Signature Components and Controls

11.200(a)(1) Electronic signatures shall employ at least two distinct components such as an identification code and password.

When an individual executes a series of signings during a single, continuous period of controlled system access, the first signing shall be executed using all electronic signature components; subsequent signings shall be executed using at least one electronic signature component that is only executable by, and designed to be used only by, the individual.

When an individual executes one or more signings not performed during a single, continuous period of controlled system access, each signing shall be executed using all of the electronic signature components.

11.200(a)(2) Electronic signatures shall be used only by their genuine owners.

11.200(a)(3) Electronic signatures shall be administered and executed to ensure that attempted use of an individual's electronic signature by anyone other than its genuine owner requires collaboration of two or more individuals.

11.300 Controls for Identification Codes/Passwords

11.300(a) Identification codes/passwords controls shall include maintaining the uniqueness of each combined identification code and password, such that no two individuals have the same combination of identification code and password.

11.300(b) Identification codes/passwords controls shall include ensuring that identification code and password issuances are periodically checked, recalled, or revised (e.g., to cover such events as password aging).

11.300(d) Identification codes/passwords controls shall include use of transaction safeguards to prevent unauthorized use of passwords and/or identification codes, and to detect and report in an immediate and urgent manner any attempts at their unauthorized use to the system security unit, and, as appropriate, to organizational management.

11.300(e) Identification codes/passwords controls shall include initial and periodic testing of devices that bear or generate identification code or password information to ensure that they function properly and have not been altered in an unauthorized manner.

26.4 21 CFR PART 11 SOFTWARE EVALUATION CHECKLIST FOR CLOSED SYSTEMS THAT DO NOT USE BIOMETRICS

Only those sections of 21 CFR Part 11 that describe technical controls required for 21 CFR Part 11 compliance of closed systems are included in this checklist (Table 26.1). Sections that describe only procedural controls [11.10(i), (j), (k); 11.100(b), (c); 11.300(c)] that cannot be implemented by a software product or additional controls for open system (11.30) are not included. Procedural controls can only be exercised during the implementation of a 21 CFR Part 11-compliant system of which the software is a component.

26.5 SUMMARY

The United States Food and Drug Administration issued 21 CFR Part 11, the requirement for the use of electronic signatures and archives (the equivalent guidelines issued by the EMEA is known as "GAMP4," the fourth revision of the European Good Automated Manufacturing Practices), after a lengthy period of FDA concern about the reliability, quality, and control of computer systems; the emergence and evolution of requirements for system validation; and increasing industry reliance on computers in laboratory, manufacturing, and clinical environments. Further emerging concerns about the relative cost and benefit of Part 11 led to its recall and revision, incorporating a risk assessment to focus the regulation on areas of greatest risk to health and safety.

To ensure 21 CFR Part 11 compliance an organization should:

a) Adopt a multitier protocol or operating procedure, detailing the evidence to be provided in support of high-, medium-, and low-risk systems or subsystems.
b) Adopt an audit checklist; identify the key issues of Part 11 compliance.
c) Conduct a Risk Assessment; utilizing dimensions of probability (likelihood of future occurrence and/or incident of past occurrence) and severity (risk to human health and safety) to classify all reasonable system dangers or missed performances.

TABLE 26.1 21 CFR Part 11 Software Evaluation Checklist for Closed Systems That Do Not Use Biometrics

Section	Regulatory Requirements	Functionality To Be Demonstrated
11.10(b)	Procedures and controls shall include the ability to generate accurate and complete copies of records in both human readable and electronic form suitable for inspection, review, and copying by the agency.	Demonstrate the functionality to generate accurate and complete copies of records in both human-readable and electronic form suitable for inspection, review, and copying by the agency. Include: • Methods • Sequences • Raw data • Results, both data and graphs • Reports • Other (?) In "review," can the agency regenerate results from raw data? How? Can the agency query the data (not simply to visually inspect)? Demonstrate retention of metadata. What is the relationship of the "single file" to the database?
11.10(c)	Procedures and controls shall include protection of records to enable their accurate and ready retrieval throughout the records retention period.	Demonstrate the functionality to accurately and readily retrieve archival records throughout the record retention period (e.g., backup and restore or archive/retrieve or other). Include: • Methods • Sequences • Raw data • Results, both data and graphs • Reports • Calibrations • Standards • Event logs • Other (?) Can the agency regenerate results from raw data? How? Do all metadata remain? Links between files? Audit trails? Are records protected during record retention period? Accessible by database commands, SQL, etc.?

TABLE 26.1 *Continued*

Section	Regulatory Requirements	Functionality To Be Demonstrated
		Are original HW and SW required for access/query?
11.10(d)	Procedures and controls shall include limiting system access to authorized individuals.	Demonstrate that functionality exists to limit user access to authorized individuals: • From the operating system (Windows NT/2000/XP, etc.) • From within the software • For application start-up • For direct access to files for edit, rename, delete Demonstrate setup of users and privileges. Demonstrate that administrative changes to users and privileges are subject to audit trail. Demonstrate that the logged-in user ID is displayed on all screens. Demonstrate that stored passwords are encrypted, and that encryp tion uses at least suggested standards. Demonstrate that the Admin password can be changed.
11.10(e)	Procedures and controls shall include use of secure, computer-generated time-stamped audit trails to independently record the date and time of operator entries and actions that create, modify, or delete electronic records. Record changes shall not obscure previously recorded information. Such audit trail information shall be retained for a period at least as long as that required for the subject electronic records and shall be available for agency review and copying.	Demonstrate that data cannot be overwritten. Demonstrate that audit trails are secure. Demonstrate that audit trails are created and maintained for: Date and time of operator entries and actions that create, modify, or delete electronic records (methods, sequences, raw data, results, reports, calibrations, standards, event logs) • Admin changes to privileges • Admin changes to passwords Demonstrate that audit trail is linked to data files during retention period. Demonstrate that audit trail is available for agency review and copying.

TABLE 26.1 *Continued*

Section	Regulatory Requirements	Functionality To Be Demonstrated
		Demonstrate that audit trail is available for query.
11.10(f)	Procedures and controls shall include the use of operational system checks to enforce permitted sequencing of steps and events, as appropriate.	Demonstrate that the system uses operational system checks to enforce permitted sequencing of steps and events, as appropriate. • Does the system enforce running blanks or standards before a sample? • Does the system employ "required" fields? • Does the system require all method and sequence data to be defined before a run? (For example, can the sample name, concentration, volume, etc. be changed after data are acquired?)
11.10(g)	Procedures and controls shall include use of authority checks to ensure that only authorized individuals can use the system, electronically sign a record, access the operation or computer system input or output device, alter a record, or perform the operation at hand.	Demonstrate functionality for authority checks for: • System use (access) • Electronic signature • Access to computer system input or output device (Can input or output devices be altered without authority checks in a manner that will predictably affect results?) • Record alteration • Individual operation • Does the system require the use of a stored system user ID and PW to access shared storage devices and perform system operations?
11.10(h)	Procedures and controls shall include use of device (e.g., terminal) checks to determine, as appropriate, the validity of the source of data input or operational instruction.	Demonstrate that the system uses device checks to identify (and record) the source of input data. Demonstrate that the system does not allow data acquisition from unidentifiable or incorrect sources. Demonstrate that the system uses checks for the validity of operational instructions. (For example, must instructions come

TABLE 26.1 *Continued*

Section	Regulatory Requirements	Functionality To Be Demonstrated
		from the application, or can they be overridden by a keypad?)
11.50	Signed electronic records shall contain information associated with the signing that clearly indicates the following: • The printed name of the signer; • The date and time when the signature was executed; and • The meaning (suchas review, approval, responsibility, or authorship) associated with the signature. These items are subject to the same controls as for electronic records and shall be included as part of any human readable form of the electronic record (such as electronic display or printout).	Demonstrate that the signed electronic records contain information associated with the signing that clearly indicate: • The printed name of the signer (not just the user ID) • The date and time when the signature was executed (traceable to the time zone) • The meaning of the signature Demonstrate that the electronic signature information has access controls, data integrity, audit trails, and record retention. Demonstrate that the name, date/time, and meaning are included as part of any human readable form of the electronic record, including display and printed report.
11.70	Electronic signatures and handwritten signatures executed to electronic records shall be linked to their respective electronic records to ensure that the signatures cannot be excised, copied, or otherwise transferred to falsify an electronic record by ordinary means.	Demonstrate that electronic signatures are linked to their respective electronic records in a manner that prevents excision, copying, modifying, or otherwise transferring to falsify an electronic record by ordinary means (e.g., by opening in WordPad to edit, or by simple file operations). Demonstrate that handwritten signatures executed to electronic records ("hybrid systems") are linked to their respective electronic records. Demonstrate that the printed, hand-signed copy has sufficient information to link the report to a unique electronic record (date, time printed, name of person printing report, file name, date/

TABLE 26.1 *Continued*

Section	Regulatory Requirements	Functionality To Be Demonstrated
		time file creation, unique file identification, location, etc.).
11.100(a)	Each electronic signature shall be unique to one individual and shall not be reused by, or reassigned to, anyone else.	Demonstrate that user ID (an essential element of user ID/PW combination comprising the electronic signature) is not reusable by deletion/recreation, overwrite, or other means. Demonstrate that the system does not allow redundant user IDs.
11.200(a)(1)	Electronic signatures shall employ at least two distinct components such as an identification code and password. When an individual executes a series of signings during a single, continuous period of controlled system access, the first signing shall be executed using all electronic signature components; subsequent signings shall be executed using at least one electronic signature component that is only executable by, and designed to be used only by, the individual. When an individual executes one or more signings not performed during a single, continuous period of controlled system access, each signing shall be executed using all of the electronic signature components.	Demonstrate that electronic signatures employ at least two distinct components (user ID and password). Demonstrate that the user ID of the person logged on to the system is displayed across all screens that allow user inputs. Demonstrate that the first signing of a continuous session uses all electronic signature components. Demonstrate that user ID is displayed at the time of application of the password to execute an electronic signature (i.e., at least one electronic signature component that is only executable by, and designed to be used only by, the individual). Demonstrate that each signing not performed in a continuous session uses all electronic signature components. Demonstrate that the system performs logout after a configurable interval to end an unattended session.
11.200(a)(2)	Electronic signatures shall be used only by their genuine owners.	Demonstrate that passwords (one of the two components of electronic signatures) can only be known to the genuine owners, and cannot be viewed by anyone, including administrators of the account (at operating system and application level).

TABLE 26.1 *Continued*

Section	Regulatory Requirements	Functionality To Be Demonstrated
		Demonstrate that administrator password management privileges extend only to the ability to reset a password. Demonstrate that the user must change the reset password at initial subsequent login.
11.200(a)(3)	Electronic signatures shall be administered and executed to ensure that attempted use of an individual's electronic signature by anyone other than its genuine owner requires collaboration of two or more individuals.	See 11.200(a)(2). Refer also to demo that use of invalid password does not allow access to system or permit electronic signature.
11.200(b)	Electronic signatures based on biometrics shall be designed to ensure that they cannot be used by anyone other than their genuine owners.	N/A—System does not employ biometrics.
11.300(a)	Identification codes/ passwords controls shall include maintaining the uniqueness of each combined identification code and password, such that no two individuals have the same combination of identification code and password.	Demonstrate (refer to earlier demo) that user IDs are unique (cannot be deleted or redundant). If a user ID has been inactivated, can it be reactivated? Would these actions be audit trailed? If reactivation is not possible, how would a new user ID for a returning employee be linked to the past ID so all records created or signed by an individual could be queried? (Does the system provide a technical solution, or would this be handled by a procedure?)
11.300(b)	Identification codes/ passwords controls shall include ensuring that identification code and password issuances are periodically checked, recalled, or revised (e.g., to cover such events as password aging).	Demonstrate controls include such configurable parameters as: • The password expiration period • Whether reuse of a previous password is allowed • The password minimum length • Whether numeric or special

TABLE 26.1 *Continued*

Section	Regulatory Requirements	Functionality To Be Demonstrated
		characters must be included in the password • The number of failed login attempts allowed before system lockout occurs Does the system allow configuration to exclude common (dictionary) terms from use as passwords?
11.300(d)	Identification codes/ passwords controls shall include use of transaction safeguards to prevent unauthorized use of passwords and/or identification codes, and to detect and report in an immediate and urgent manner any attempts at their unauthorized use to the system security unit, and, as appropriate, to organizational management.	Demonstrate that the system includes controls to detect multiple attempts at unauthorized use (e.g., repeated login attempts/failed password entry on login and electronic signature). Demonstrate that such attempts at unauthorized use can be reported in an immediate and urgent manner to the system security unit and, as appropriate, to organizational management.
11.300(e)	Identification codes/ passwords controls shall include initial and periodic testing of devices that bear or generate identification code or password information to ensure that they function properly and have not been altered in an unauthorized manner.	Does the system employ devices that bear or generate ID codes? Does the system employ such codes/passwords for instruments? For the system, servers, other?

d) Utilizing a highly credible team or individual (with significant Part 11 experience; system, regulatory, and Part 11 expertise and a separate reporting chain from the IT and user departments) conduct an audit against the preestablished audit checklist and collect evidence in appropriate depth and detail as established by the risk assessment.

The results of this four-step procedure, presumably utilizing the included checklist or equivalent to operationalize Part 11 for a specific computer system environment, will lead to regulatory compliance and to safe and effective utilization of the system in a laboratory, manufacturing, or clinical facility.

REFERENCE

1. Weinberg S, Romoff RM, Stein GC. *Handbook of System Validation*. Weinberg, Spelton and Sax Inc. 1993; Weinberg S. *Validation Compliance Annual*, in Weinberg S, Editor, *International Validation Forum*. Marcel Dekker; New York, 1995.

27

A NEW PARADIGM FOR ANALYZING ADVERSE DRUG EVENTS

Ana Szarfman, Jonathan G. Levine, and Joseph M. Tonning

DISCLAIMER

The opinions expressed in this chapter are solely those of the authors and do not necessarily reflect those of the United States Food and Drug Administration.

Contents

Computer Applications in Pharmaceutical Research and Development, Edited by Sean Ekins.
ISBN 0-471-73779-8

27.1 INTRODUCTION

Only a generation ago, 107 people in 15 states died within a few weeks after a new drug was placed on the market. Many of the victims were children. One victim was the best friend of the doctor who had prescribed the drug for him. The S.E. Massengill Company, which marketed the drug, had been looking for a solvent to dissolve sulfanilamide, a new antibiotic. A company chemist chose diethylene glycol, a chemical normally used as antifreeze. Diethylene glycol was effective in dissolving sulfanilamide but caused renal failure in the unsuspecting patients. The company owner shirked responsibility, stating, "We have been supplying a legitimate professional demand and not once could have foreseen the unlooked-for results." And how could they have foreseen the results? One doesn't find what one doesn't look for. The drug was completely legal. At that time, in 1937, the U.S. Food and Drug Administration (FDA) did not require drug products to be tested for safety [1].

The passage of the Food, Drug, and Cosmetic Act in 1938 greatly helped to improve drug safety. However, challenges in systematically gaining access and understanding of drug safety data in real time persisted and continue to persist to the present day. Computer technology was decades away in 1938. The FDA did not develop a computerized repository of postmarketing voluntary adverse event reports until 1968. FDA scientists analyzed adverse events with paper, pen, typewriter, and perhaps a mechanical calculator. Even in the 1980s, FDA scientists had little more at their disposal to review adverse event data than a typewriter or dedicated word processor. In the 1990s, personal computers and software programs made it possible to eliminate many of the paper processes involved in adverse event analysis. However, there were still no uniform data standards and interoperable systems in place, hindering efforts to truly analyze adverse events in a systematic, computerized way. To rectify this situation, the FDA and the pharmaceutical industry began constructing a computerized repository of premarketing and postmarketing clinical trial data that would enable more efficient data analysis and decision making.

27.2 CURRENT PARADIGMS OF ANALYSIS

The typical product of a traditional analytical method is a static, paper report. Such reports usually consist of a vast number of discrete, personal, ad hoc processes that cannot typically be used to perform subsequent comprehensive *reproducible* analyses as soon as additional analyses are needed. Having an analytical method that can be subsequently audited and *reproduced* is absolutely critical because essential drug safety decisions are made from these analyses. Unfortunately, many drug safety organizations still verify the accuracy of the data they analyze by manual, ad hoc methods when comparing the data stored in a database with the primary medical records. Auditing is done by a second-party review, again by manual ad hoc methods.

Current computerized analyses of adverse events still typically consist of a vast number of discrete, often personal, ad hoc processes that mimic paper and pencil methods. Some commercial-off-the-shelf (COTS) software tools (e.g., Adobe Acrobat®, Microsoft Word®, Excel®) do have the capability to search for specific terms in electronic documents/case reports and do have navigational tools with hyperlinks and fullfull-text indexing that enable researchers to create their own hyperlinks. Some other COTS software tools (e.g., SAS®, Excel®, Access®, JMP®) allow importation of electronic case report tabulations (ECRT) for more detailed analysis.

However, many of these tools, while enabling markedly faster and more detailed analysis than paper-based methods, still mimic static, one-by-one "paperlike" reports with no real-time auditing capability. Moreover, these COTS do not have integrated data analysis and automated data screening capabilities and are not optimized for systematic analyses. Furthermore, the ad hoc analyses that these COTS produce lack interactive, automatic auditing *reproducible* functions. Thus these tools are often used to produce the same dense, unwieldy paper tables of counts and percentages that were created manually before personal computers became ubiquitous.

Humans should use computers to do functional work for them in the most efficient manner possible. However, we must not delude ourselves into thinking that the mere use of a computer to analyze adverse events will magically analyze these events in a systematic, efficient way. Computers do not *automatically* produce coherent, auditable results that can be subsequently reproduced with ease. Computers must be *actively* programmed through an iterative process involving tight communication between analysts and software developers until these processes are totally functional.

27.3 WHY WE NEED A PARADIGM CHANGE

A new paradigm for computer-assisted analysis of adverse drug events is sorely needed. Critics of the current paradigm emphasize the need for more transparency in the data review process, claiming that there is the potential for suppressing negative results or for hiding safety issues in both interventional and observational studies. It is often necessary to reanalyze the data in light of new information about a particular adverse event or class of events for a drug or class of drugs months—or even years—after the initial analysis. In many such situations, it is critical to have ready access to all preclinical,

clinical trial, and postmarketing data. The findings from these updated analyses are potentially so influential that they can impact drug therapy recommendations for decades. However, ready access to all of the actual data and results is still lacking in many situations.

To properly assess drug safety, we must be able to systematically tap the information captured in the massive amounts of medical data collected in both premarketing and postmarketing settings. In addition, as stated above, we must also be able to *reproduce* findings in different repositories of medical data in an auditable way. However, two major issues in studying drug safety confront us.

The first issue lies in the whole realm of the human disease process itself. Many adverse drug events mimic diseases and vice versa. Is an "adverse event" really an adverse event, or is it merely a natural occurrence of a disease process that is entirely independent of drug exposure? The science of drug safety is often complicated by the lack of objective markers of drug toxicity that can systematically separate a disease process from an adverse drug event process [2]. Clinical trials, often viewed as the gold standard to assess efficacy, are simply too limited in scope to answer safety questions in a systematic way.

The second issue involves the whole process of data collection, transformation, and presentation. At the study level, important information needed to assess the safety of a new drug is often presented in idiosyncratic ways. For example, concomitant medications are often not translated into standard drug names, and there are often subtle errors in coding of events (which we discuss further). This lack of standards hinders the creation of an integrated safety database. Later, the data that may come from numerous preclinical, clinical, and postmarketing studies are often not collected with a common data standard and are not systematically integrated into a single cumulative database before analysis. Various personnel working in different organizations or in different sections of the same organization may perform analytical tasks with nonstandardized and nonintegrated data. Even when the premarketing adverse event data of a new drug *are* incorporated into an integrated summary of clinical trial safety data, the *totality* of the safety data from *all* pre- and post-marketing marketing research are usually *not* integrated into a coherent, analyzable database that can be used for a comprehensive, real-time analysis.

It is therefore easy to see why this current drug safety paradigm, with its lack of standards in data collection and analysis, hinders the analysis of adverse events. Without data standards in place, it is difficult to build practical, reusable tools for systematic safety analysis. With no standard tools, truly standardized analyses cannot occur. Reviewers may forget their initial analytical processes if they are not using standardized data and tools. Comprehensive reproducibility and auditability, therefore, become nearly impossible. In practice, the same data sets and analytical processes cannot be easily reused, even by the same reviewers who produced the original data sets and analyses. Not using standardized tools slows the real-time systematic analysis and reanalysis of the data because of the large number of restructuring steps needed to perform these analyses and reanalysis These obstacles restrict the ability of analysts and senior decision makers to gain a full understanding of the entire data and the results in a timely manner. The end result is that analysts cannot routinely access the *computerized* prepreclinical, clinical, and clinical data that supported the marketing approval of a drug, a new indication, or a new dosage schedule.

27.4 A NEW PARADIGM: INFORMATICS

We need to transition from quasi-computerized methods, in which the different elements of the analytical process are treated as discrete, "paper report" tasks, to a comprehensive *informatics approach*, in which the entire data collection and analysis is considered as a single reusable, extensible, auditable, and reproducible system. Informatics can be defined as the science of "storing, manipulating, analyzing, and visualizing information using computer systems."[3]

To analyze adverse drug events from an informatics framework, six major infrastructure elements must be in place:

- *Data standards and interoperable systems*. When interoperability is in place, standard, automated software tools for systematically analyzing the data can be constructed.
- *High-quality data.* Miscoding, duplicate records, missing data items, and other data problems must be kept to a minimum.
- *Restructuring capabilities.* There must be the capability of restructuring the data for various types of analyses in a transparent way.
- *Systematic analysis.* The data must be systematically analyzed to gain insight regarding the associations between various treatments and medical conditions. This knowledge can assist in causality assessments.
- *Reproducible capabilities.* The data and analyses must be electronically accessible in real-time, easily reanalyzable, and easily reproduced, even years after the adverse event data were collected.
- *Maintenance.* The database and software that comprise the data systems must be maintained.

27.4.1 Data Standards and Interoperable Systems

The foundation of any efficient computer-assisted data analysis system is the creation and use of data standards. Data standards consist of standard data file names for each predefined file, standard data elements in each data file, standardized names for each data element, and standard definitions for each data element.

Data standards are exceedingly important because they allow for the use of "interoperable systems." The concept of interoperable systems can be illustrated by the situation that prevailed in the American railroad industry during the nineteenth century. At that time, there were many small, local railroad companies throughout the country. Each company, however, utilized different standards of rail gauges, that is, the distance between the two parallel rails on a track. The Baltimore and Ohio Railroad used a 4 foot, 8-1/2 inch gauge; railroads in the South used a 5 foot, 0 inch gauge; the Erie and Lackawanna Railroad used a 6 foot, 0 inch gauge, and so forth. The onset of the Civil War exposed the absurdity of the lack of rail gauge standards when such inconsistencies made it nearly impossible to accomplish very fundamental tasks, such as materiel transport. [4]. At the 2005 FDA Science Forum, Secretary of Health and Human Services Michael O. Leavitt recounted the story of rail gauge inconsistencies to emphasize the need for interoperability to advance health information technology [5]. It becomes obvious, therefore, why standardized, unique codes for all data values across all stages of drug development and during the entire postmarketing period are so essential. Comprehensive data standards allow for the creation and systematic implementation of reusable software for analyzing medical records and adverse event data. These reusable tools enable the creation of standard analysis tools that can be shared among safety analysts for enhanced communication and learning and refined as existing analytical techniques are evaluated and extended.

All data fields (patient identification, date, sex, drug names, narratives, etc.) require rules regarding the data, because some characters, such as tabs and return characters, can interfere with attempts to store, read, and/or reorganize the data. For example, if the data are being migrated from Oracle® into other data analysis software and data fields in Oracle® contain tabs and return characters, the data from these fields may be split into several columns and rows upon migration into the other software. This fact is extremely important because information that is misplaced in a data file may not be readily apparent to the user without the use of systematic approaches for analysis. This missing information may have profound and unpredictable influences at all levels of drug safety analysis, including studies using preapproval and postapproval pharmacoepidemiological data.

Ideally, the data from the whole drug development program, including accumulating postmarketing data, would be integrated into a single database. This integration would simplify the process of answering important, but previously *unforeseeable* questions (remember the sulfanilamide example). For instance, is a new dose increase as safe as the previously approved dosages? Is it enough to compare the two highest dosages with each other? A better answer could be obtained if the entire integrated clinical trial data across all dosages are studied. However, as mentioned above, drug safety data from multiple sources are not usually integrated into a single database. Compounding this problem is that many people tasked with managing data are focused on preparing a small portion of the data for a specific purpose and are not trying to create a single database that integrates all of the data. Integration of the entire safety data for a drug would enable better and faster communication among decision makers in various organizations (industry, regulatory agencies, etc.)

27.4.2 High-Quality Data

It is essential to have high-quality data in place for interoperable systems to function efficiently. Standard data structures can only be used to full advantage if they are combined with standard terminology for values populating a data element. Yet there are many potential pitfalls in data collection and configuration for analysis. Some of the more common pitfalls are discussed here, but this list is by no means comprehensive.

Errors and Inconsistencies in Patient Identification. Whatever system is used to identify patients in a database, it is essential that a single, unique identifier be used for each patient. This identifier must be consistent throughout the database. Errors and inconsistencies in patient identification can significantly interfere with adverse event analysis. Examples include situations in which hyphens, commas, additional zeros, or other characters are not used consistently for identifying patients. In some cases, the *same* patient in a study may have *different* patient identification numbers listed in various tables [5] (Table 27.1). In such situations, correctly merging patient data from multiple sources/tables becomes essentially impossible, because some of the data for the same patient either will be treated as missing or will appear as data for the wrong patient. In one New Drug Application (NDA) submitted to the FDA, a sponsor built a "unique patient identifier" for some tables by concatenating the study identification number plus the study site identification number plus the patient within-site identification number, whereas in other tables the numbers were concatenated in a different sequence. In another NDA, a sponsor separated the concatenated identifiers by hyphens in some tables but not in others. In yet another NDA, a sponsor concatenated numeric with character identifiers (the latter with leading zeroes) in some tables, but

TABLE 27.1 An Example of Different Types of Unique Patient Identifiers for the Same Patients in a Clinical Trial

Unique Patient Identifier in Data Tables	Unique Patient Identifier in the Narrative Table
8023007	Patient 08-023-007 is a 48-year-old Caucasian male, etc.
8031011	Patient 08-031-011 is a 61-year-old Hispanic female, etc.

not in others. In our experience, such problems are easier to detect when systematic approaches for analysis are in place.

Errors and Inconsistencies in Categorical Variables. For categorical variables such as sex, race, diagnosis, etc. it is essential that the values used to designate the different categories be precisely defined and consistently used. Precise variable value definitions and their consistent use greatly simplify the analysis at hand and also future analyses. For example, a human being can readily tell that "M," "m," "Male," "male," "hombre," "homme," etc. all refer to the same sex. A computer, on the other hand, cannot readily make this distinction (unless specifically programmed to do so) and will therefore treat these items as different values for sex. In one FDA submission, a sponsor coded "male" by using the code "1" in some studies and the code "2" in other studies, resulting in the finding of "pregnancies in men." In another submission, a similar problem resulted in males developing "female breast carcinomas."

Errors and Inconsistencies in Formatting Dates. It is also necessary to use standardized formats to record dates. For example, Oracle® stores a date as the number of seconds since January 1, 4712 BC, and then uses various functions to display the dates in more human-friendly formats. There are many different and personal ways for recording dates; one of the authors (AS) has noted at least 25 different ways in a single clinical trial submitted for FDA review! Should February 1, 2007 be recorded as 1 February 2007, 1 Feb 2007, 1 Feb 07, or 02/01/07? This problem still exists when data for numerical dates are extracted into software programs such as Excel® that do not force the user to select a unique format for dates.

Errors and Inconsistencies in Adverse Event Coding. Adverse events are also subject to errors and inconsistencies by coders and data entry personnel. Many of these inconsistencies become very important when adverse events are analyzed by automated software.

Adverse events need to be coded consistently with respect to letter case. Problems can occur when there is discordant coding using all capital letters, all lower-case letters, or combinations thereof, as computer software will interpret these capitalization variations as different events. Letter case sensitivity can be important when two or more words are used to describe an adverse event. For example, some databases utilizing the Medical Dictionary for Regulatory Activities (MedDRA) coding dictionary employ a coding system in which only the first letter of the first word of an adverse event is capitalized (e.g., "Atrioventricular block complete"). Failing to adhere to uniform letter case conventions across the data can result in severe errors in data analysis.

Proper interpretation and coding of events are also extremely important so that drug safety data can be appropriately analyzed. However, investigators and coders vary widely with respect to their health care training to properly interpret and code these events. Individual investigators may choose different terms to code the same adverse event. Subjectivity in coding may be due to personal preferences of coders in the selection of terms versus the granularity of coding dictionaries that offer the coder a considerable array of terms to classify the reported adverse event. For example, kidney stones may be coded with a number of terms such as "kidney stones," "nephrolithiasis," "renal calculi," and "renal calculus not otherwise specified." There can also be variations in spelling of the exact same event code, such as the British spelling of "gynaecomastia" versus the American "gynecomastia."

Coding dictionaries also change over time (sometimes even before a study is completed) because of revisions in coding terminology. In one NDA submitted to the FDA, the data were coded with different versions of the same coding dictionary without properly integrating the terms into a single coding version. Such a scenario may lead to partitioning events into too many terms and therefore mischaracterization of adverse events. Again, this misclassification, although not readily apparent, may have a profound impact on the results of the analysis performed.

It is especially difficult to code events when they occur as a constellation of signs, symptoms, and laboratory findings, because a coder may inadvertently minimize or exaggerate the severity of an adverse event, depending on the selection of terms to code that event. The use of only one or two seemingly benign terms such as "muscle cramps" and "pain in limb" to describe rhabdomyolysis would not provide a comprehensive picture of the event. On the other hand, categorizing an isolated case of elevated transaminases (with no other associated laboratory findings) as acute liver failure would be inappropriate. Potential signals of adverse events may be obscured or distorted depending on how the events are grouped. Splitting events into multiple terms or grouping unrelated terms may erroneously underestimate the magnitude of a signal.

Errors and Inconsistencies in Drug Names. Drug naming conventions are also exceedingly important. Although it may be expected that multiple names of the same medications would occur in postmarketing safety databases, this problem is also often seen in *premarketing* data. In one NDA submitted to the FDA, the data contained 900 different names for 150 unique concomitant drugs. Another NDA recorded 34,000 drug names for 2,000 concomitant drugs mentioned in the study because contractors in different countries had submitted different names for the same medications.

Errors and Inconsistencies in Numerical Data. It is also important to understand that *character* and *numeric* data are not interchangeable. Errors can occur when there is not a clear understanding between coding with characters versus coding with numbers. A variable may be inadvertently entered with character data in one study and numerical data in another study. For example, studies measuring the effects of a 30mg dose of a drug may utilize a "30mg" code in some studies and a "30" code in other studies. The "30 mg" code is treated as character data, but the "30" code is treated as numerical data. Efforts to successfully combine and analyze these studies may be hindered. The "30mg" and "30" will be treated as two different doses if the numerical variable is treated as a character. If the combined variable is treated as a number, the data for the character variable will be treated as missing in some types of further analyses (e.g., regression analyses).

Missing Information. Both premarketing and postmarketing collections of data are perpetually plagued by missing information. In premarketing and postmarketing clinical trials, patients can be lost to follow-up because of:

- Undocumented beginning and/or end of a medication or an adverse event (see Figure 27.1)
- Undocumented death
- Undocumented serious adverse events
- Undocumented nonserious adverse events
- Failure to assess adverse events that occur more than 30 days after the last dose of a drug
- Failure to assess adverse events occurring outside a scheduled time window
- Loss of interest of a patient or unwillingness to continue in a study
- Geographical moves by patients
- Loss of insurance coverage (in a postmarketing case control study)
- Missing records due to technical errors during data migration (see below)

Even when patients remain in a study, information regarding adverse events may not be complete. The event itself may not be coded, even when the narrative includes relevant laboratory or other data (e.g., renal failure may not be coded, even though the narrative mentions abnormal blood urea nitrogen and creatinine levels and the need for dialysis). Moreover, adverse event data (such as laboratory tests, radiological reports, biopsy reports, and hospital records) collected outside a scheduled time window, outside of the study center, or after the study is completed *might not* be included in the final database for the study. This issue is important because unexpected adverse events do not occur at known prespecified time windows. "Tight windows" of adverse event data collection can also be a problem with drugs that have a very long half-life or the potential for causing a delayed, but serious condition.

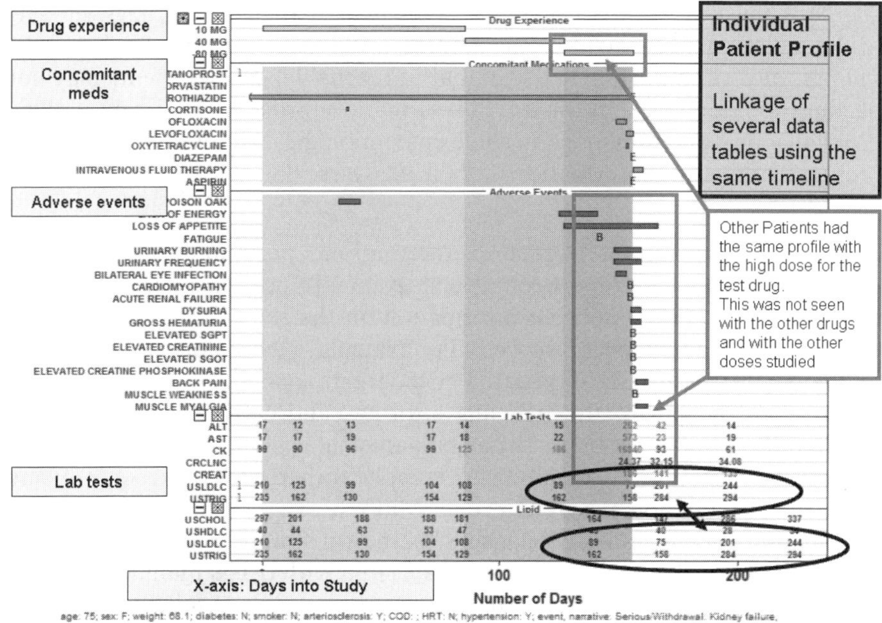

Figure 27.1 An example of New Drug Application (NDA) data graphically displayed for an individual patient in a dose escalation clinical trial. This graph displays and links drug exposure information, clinical adverse events, concomitant medications, clinical laboratory values, demographic information, and narratives. The graph is divided into 4 major sections: The x-axis for all 4 sections depicts time, and the y-axis the labels for each section. The top section displays drug exposure data for the test drug used in various doses (color coded). The second section displays exposure to concomitant medications over time. The third section displays adverse events over time. The bottom sections display when laboratory tests were conducted and the results. Note in the highlighted red squares that clinical and laboratory adverse events were associated with the high dose of the test drug. Other patients had the same profile with the high dose for the test drug. This was not seen with the other drugs and with the other doses studied. Note that the beginning of an adverse event is displayed (B) but not the end for many adverse events. Note that the end of a concomitant medication is displayed (E) but not the beginning for some medications. Observe highlighted in black the areas showing discrepancies in the timing of the same laboratory results in different tables, making it difficult to assess whether these values occurred before or after an adverse event or a concomitant drug. See color plate.

The problem of missing data is even more pervasive in postmarketing drug safety databases. Most of these systems rely on voluntary reporting for which there are no well-defined protocols. Additionally, there are significant challenges in interpreting such data because of the wide variability of reporting sources (physicians, pharmaceutical companies, patients, attorneys, etc., as well as submissions from different countries). With electronic medical records, the presence of important relevant, but unreachable, data elements may not become apparent without the use of systematic approaches for analysis. This problem may be compounded in some epidemiological studies that ignore the presence of missing information in their analyses.

Duplicate Information. Both premarketing and postmarketing databases may contain duplicate reports of adverse events. In postmarketing databases of voluntary reports, duplicate information on the same adverse event case may be submitted by several sources. For example, submission of information on the same event may be duplicated by the treating physician, the dispensing pharmacist, the nurse, the patient's attorney, and/or the patient himself. Submission of information by drug companies may compound the problem, even though they are attempting to comply with regulatory requirements mandating submission of adverse events. Multiple drug companies may submit information on the same case, using their own unique patient identifiers, especially when the adverse event is associated with drugs manufactured by several different companies. There may also be a series of follow-up reports for the same case as additional information becomes available. However, updated patient identifiers for the same patient may not be linked to the original patient identifier. Duplicated information on the same event may also come from several teams working for the same drug company. Despite these problems, removal of duplicate reports is absolutely essential (though challenging) because superfluous information may result in false positive signals of adverse events and wasted analysis time.

In postmarketing electronic longitudinal medical records, redundant and potentially contradictory information may come from several sources, (e.g., reports from medical residents, their supervisors, the attending physicians). In these cases time stamping of each event may help to delineate the important sequences in understanding the adverse events.

Other Inconsistencies. Inconsistencies in drug safety data due to difficulties in standardization also include a subject's primary diagnosis, differential diagnoses, relevant medical history, relevant physical exam findings, pertinent information from hospital records, and follow-up information (all of which may be subjective). There may also be a lack of consistency in the narrative summaries for individual patients and the data supporting the narratives. Indeed, it is difficult to clearly describe in the narratives the sequence of adverse events, medication, and laboratory results by using case report forms or line listings as source information. In complex patient records, case report forms and line listings may generate uneven temporal sequences of adverse events, concomitant medications, dosages, etc. that cannot readily be comprehended. Such data need to be visualized by tools capable of displaying the complex, interrelated information on a common time line (Figure 27.1).

Additional examples of variability in data collection (which, in turn, affects data interpretation) include questionnaires and physical exam forms. Questionnaires often utilize open-ended questions that allow great variability in the type and extent of adverse event information gathered. Physical exam forms—even when designed in a checklist format—may elicit variable collection of adverse event data; what is a serious event to one clinician may not be serious to another.

27.4.3 Restructuring Capabilities

Reconfiguration of Data. Drug safety data from different sources are often pooled or combined in databases. Reasons for combining data vary. In the case of premarketing studies, data from different sites are routinely combined because one site may not be able to recruit enough patients for a study. Data from different studies are often combined to increase sample size and therefore statistical power for detecting an uncommon adverse event.

In postmarketing safety surveillance databases, data from different countries or from different sources (physicians, patients, drug companies) may be combined in the same database in an attempt to obtain as much information about approved drugs as possible. Pooling or combining data can allow explorations of drug toxicity among various subgroups. Having a large database allows studying possible drug-drug, drug-disease, and drug-demographic associations.

When reconfiguring the data, several issues must be borne in mind. Combining data from different data sources can obscure potentially meaningful signals of adverse drug events [6]. For example, combining data for the term "colitis" with "ischemic colitis" may obscure the presence of ischemic colitis. Also, the criteria for reporting and coding an adverse event may differ among various data sources (e.g., countries with disparate regulatory requirements and different coding dictionaries). Reference ranges for normal values may vary, depending on the reporting source. When reference ranges vary, changes from baseline grouped by treatment assignment may provide useful information. Patient populations may also vary in different study arms or in different countries where studies are conducted. Different populations may tolerate drugs differently or have varying levels of drug sensitivity. Study design may vary among sites, especially in terms of how outliers are handled and follow-up information is obtained. The selection of analytes and biomarkers of toxicity to measure may vary depending on the reporting source and when the data were collected (criteria for toxicity and case definition may be site specific and can change over time). Duration of drug exposure (as well as drug dose) may vary among studies. Because so many factors can influence the results, the process of transforming and combining data from different sources should be documented in a way that is easy for subsequent investigators to understand.

Reconfiguration of Databases. Not only must data from different sources be preprocessed ("cleaned"), reconfigured, and validated before analysis, but entire databases must also sometimes be reconfigured and validated. This is especially the case if the database has evolved and has been maintained over a long period of time.

A good example of an evolving database is the FDA's Adverse Event Reporting System (AERS) database containing reports of spontaneously submitted adverse events. AERS has undergone several configurations since its inception in 1968. This database was known as the Spontaneous Reporting System (SRS) from 1968 to 1997. Adverse events were coded into SRS with the COSTART (Coding Symbols for Thesaurus of Adverse Reaction Terms) dictionary. Only 1200 event codes were present in the COSTART dictionary. COSTART was replaced by the much more granular MedDRA (Medical Dictionary for Regulatory Activities) system of coding in 1997. MedDRA contains over 15,000 preferred term event codes, of which 10,000 are currently in use in the database. When SRS was modified to build AERS, adverse events coded with COSTART terms were mapped to MedDRA terms. Moreover, drug names in AERS have been and are still collected in free text form. There is substantial variation among reporting sources regarding the manner in which drug names are ultimately listed in adverse event reports. Drugs may be listed by their generic or trade names, with numerous and creative variations in spelling, abbreviations, spacing, and punctuation (see Section 27.4.2 on high-quality data). Thus what is now termed the AERS database is really a data set containing data that have undergone several organizational changes during more than three decades of data collection. This mapping, recoding, organizational reconfiguration, and validation of the database has been necessary to provide a uniform format for data analysis, yet this entire process has, understandably, been labor intensive and challenging.

With electronic medical records, multiple clinical records for the same patient may be treated as belonging to different patients during anonymization and migration of electronic medical records, tainting analytical conclusions. This problem may be difficult to untangle once the anonymized data migration takes place.

Sound analytical assessments require that analysts understand the manner in which the data were collected, reconfigured, migrated, and combined. These processes should be documented in a transparent way so that future investigators can readily understand the anonymization and migration in real time.

27.4.4 Data Analysis

Current practices require that all the data collected be "cleaned," reconfigured, and standardized in order to perform analytical and integrative tasks. These processes are complex, time consuming, and error prone—especially when there are many different personal standards in place. This process of "data cleaning" [7], reconfiguration, standardization, and integration must be done because the data are typically collected by several different contract research organizations, each with their own independent personal data collection standards. Because of personal standards in data cleaning and reconfiguration, many investigators end up analyzing only a small portion of the safety data, resulting in missed rare but serious adverse events or risk factors. If systematic data cleaning and reconfiguration are not done initially, then even seasoned investigators will still waste time constructing a new integrated database prior to analysis.

Size of the Database. Database size is important in assessing drug safety in both premarketing and postmarketing settings. During clinical trials in the premarketing period, the number of subjects in a drug safety database often depends on the intended use of a product. For products intended for long-term treatment of non-lifelife-threatening conditions, subjects studied may number in the thousands. For products intended for *short-term* treatment of *rare or life-threatening* conditions for which there are few effective treatment options available, a "smaller" number of subjects are studied, but there can be great subjectivity in defining the word "small" in such cases. This subjectivity is in part a reflection of the wide spectrum of disease severity for which such products might be indicated. For products intended for *chronic* treatment of *life-threatening* conditions, the number of subjects would need to be greater, but again, there is great potential for subjectivity.

Larger databases can help with risk-benefit decisions, but how can we achieve consensus on the exact size of the number of subjects needed for the database? A clinical trial database that contains limited information on a small number of subjects will likely lack the statistical power needed to detect differences in adverse events between control and treatment groups. A researcher may specify criteria for the minimum differences of adverse event rates between the two groups in an attempt to identify important safety signals, but ultimately these criteria are arbitrary. Even when a study enrolls a large number of subjects and records a large volume of data in a database, it is difficult to adequately identify all potential risks associated with a product. Some risks will only become apparent once a product is approved, that is, when hundreds of thousands or even millions in the general population are exposed. Adverse events in the postmarketing period are often collected in a voluntary manner through the use of spontaneous reporting systems such as FDA's previously described AERS database or drug registries (e.g., clozapine). Yet extracting safety information from these databases—even if they are large—can still be challenging because background rates for various events can be difficult to obtain systematically. What is the background rate for headache, rash, decreased appetite, appendicitis, and fatigue—events that frequently occur in the population independent of drug therapy? Moreover, how does one assess the background rate of an event in a prespecified, but non-drugdrug-exposed population compared to the rate of the same adverse event in a similar, but drug-exposed population? For example, how does one assess the risk of confusion in elderly diabetic patients due to the effects of a drug prescribed for diabetes from baseline rates of confusion in elderly diabetic patients who are not receiving the same diabetes drug and concomitant drugs?

High-Dimensional Aspect of Data. The high-dimensional aspect of data collected in a study can make the analysis of these data challenging. Even a simple clinical trial may have recorded dozens of measurements for each patient. More sophisticated studies may have hundreds of measurements per patient. Complex tests measuring the physiology of a specific system, such as pulmonary function tests or echocardiograpy, may be impossible to standardize over many different treatment groups or over a period of time because of technological changes and interpretation of findings. Pathological specimens (e.g., biopsies) may also be difficult to classify in a systematic and objective way. Other high-dimensional data include pharmacokinetic and pharmacodynamic information in phase III clinical trials, both of which are crucial in anticipating potential safety problems, especially in patients with impaired hepatic and renal function or in patients taking many concomitant medications. The challenge then lies in how to analyze such high-dimensional data. Unfortunately, we often do not have systematic methods for reducing the dimensionality of the data to find the subset of variables for which the treatments differ and the key statistics that describe the differences without losing important interdependent information.

Variations Among Subjects. In the premarketing phase of assessing drug safety, it is important to have a study population that is not only representative of the target population but also sufficiently diverse in terms of demographics. This diversity will bolster the generalizability of the safety analysis. Diversity in the study population can be enhanced by including both males and females and also patients in different age, racial, body weight, and risk factor groups. Yet this same variability that is so necessary in increasing generalizability also presents challenges in analyzing data. For example, there may be a great deal of variability in renal and hepatic function among elderly patients. Plasma levels of a drug can also vary greatly if patients are given the same dose regardless of body weight, body surface area, or renal and hepatic function. There may also be great differences in sensitivity to the effect of a particular drug among individual patients. These issues may also taint the analysis of postmarketing safety data, including electronic medical records. Computerized safety analysis systems (discussed below) can aid in studying the effect of these variations by automatically generating stratified analyses to adjust for the impact of these patient attributes on adverse events.

Temporal Relationships of Adverse Events. The temporal relationship between duration of product exposure and development of an adverse event is important in assessing causality. But how can data on temporal relationships be systematically summarized in a database containing thousands or even hundreds of thousands of subjects? Temporal relationships cannot be clearly elicited if only frequencies of adverse events between treatment and control groups are compared. There can be many disparities in the subjects' time of exposure or time at risk. Toxic manifestations of drugs may not occur until several months or even years after the initial exposure to the drug. How do we systematically assess delayed toxicity of a previously prescribed drug from the effect of a newly prescribed drug? Such a scenario occurred with reported cases of pancreatitis associated with valproic acid therapy, in which some cases appeared several years after therapy [2].

Sometimes an adverse event that occurs with a different frequency in the treatment group than in the control group is also qualitatively different in the two groups. For example, suppose a rare but serious vascular event occurs more frequently and earlier in the treatment group than the control group and is more likely to lead to discontinuation in the treatment group than in the control group. We need to describe that the event occurs more frequently and earlier in the treatment group and that it is more likely to cause discontinuation of treatment. This information is difficult to convey with tabular data, but often becomes clear when the data are presented in graphical form [8 (Figure 27.2), 9].

Effect of Concomitant Medication. Assessing drug-drug interactions is absolutely critical in evaluating the safety profile of a drug. Interactions can occur when one drug affects the absorption, distribution, metabolism, or excretion of another drug or drugs, producing additive or antagonistic effects on the other drugs. Various foods and dietary or herbal supplements (e.g., St. John's Wort) can also interact with drugs. Yet how do we systematically assess adverse events from one drug as opposed to adverse events from concomitant drugs or supplements?

Effect of Preexisting Disease. The adverse event profile of a drug can be confounded because of the effects of underlying disease for which the drug may or may not be prescribed. Comorbidity can affect a drug's potential for inducing an adverse event. However, it is often difficult to separate the influence of preexisting disease when assessing the potential toxicity of a drug. How do we systematically separate the effects of a drug from a disease, the progression of that disease, or multiple diseases syndromes—each with its own varying rate of progression?

Preexisting disease, such as renal or hepatic disease, can especially influence the metabolism and excretion of certain drugs. In clinical trials, and in electronic longitudinal medical records, it is important to have sufficient variability in disease states and concomitant diseases among subjects in both the

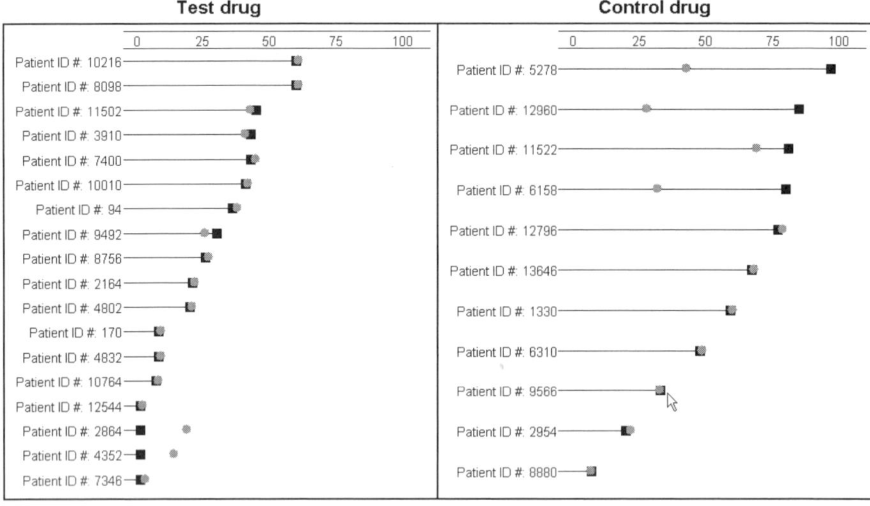

Figure 27.2 A display that summarizes the duration of treatment (black squares) and the timing of serious vascular events (circles) for the subset of patients who withdrew from treatment because of an adverse event. Each line represents a single patient's experience over time in days for the test (left panel) and the control drug (right panel). Patients are sorted by decreased duration of treatment. In this 1:1 randomized clinical trial there were 18 withdrawals due to a severe vascular adverse event with the test drug. This is in contrast with the control drug, with 11 withdrawals. Withdrawals with the test drug occurred sooner than with the control drug.

study and control groups. Investigators need to consider whether the adverse events that occur are due to abnormalities in the distribution, metabolism, and excretion of drugs as a result of underlying disease. These analyses could be systematically facilitated by having standardized ways of measuring blood (and in some cases, tissue) levels of drugs and their metabolites.

Lack of Objective Markers of Drug Toxicity. Some products have well-established, valid biomarkers that can be measured to track certain safety concerns. For example, a dose-response association with proteinuria, creatine phosphokinase, and urine myoglobin levels can be monitored to assess the safety of HMG-CoA reductase inhibitors (Figure 27.1). However, there are often no specific markers (or pathognomonic clinical findings) of toxicity for many drugs. For most drugs under investigation—and most marketed drugs—practical tests to measure toxic drug or metabolite levels are not widely available [2]. Additionally, relying on product labeling of a drug in a similar class as a clue to investigate the toxicity of a drug is faulty, as labeling can be influenced by a number of factors including litigation and publicity.

The Overwhelming Volume of Data to be Analyzed. Any given drug safety researcher—whether a statistician, clinician, epidemiologist, or safety evaluator—can only analyze so much nonstandardized data in a given time period. Premarketing databases contain very detailed data on thousands or perhaps tens of thousands of subjects. In some cases, premarketing data may have been collected over several decades for a wide array of indications. Postmarketing drug safety databases may contain millions of adverse event reports. The Composite Health Care System II database maintained by the U.S. Department of Defense contains over 9 million medical records. The FDA's AERS database contains over 2.5 million adverse event reports collected since 1968. As mentioned above, AERS utilizes the MedDRA classification system for its adverse event coding system. For these reports, approximately 10,000 MedDRA-preferred terms have been coded for 4000 generic drugs in the database. Thus over 40 million drug-event combinations are theoretically possible. This situation, compled with the fact that the FDA currently receives over 1000 new reports of adverse events each day, exemplifies the daunting task that safety evaluators face when analyzing postmarketing adverse event data. With such a large volume of reports to review each day, exploring signals based on clinical judgment in combination with threshold reporting frequencies may not always be optimal or even practical. Such an approach makes it difficult to contextualize information regarding adverse events. How do we systematically access such huge databases to select appropriate variables for analyses? Without adequate drug exposure data and baseline rates of disease processes (which may be erroneously attributed to "adverse drug events") in specific populations at risk, how do we determine whether 20 cases of a specific drug-event combination is disproportionately frequent to merit further investigation?

Subjective Analysis Strategies. There are also too many *subjective* analysis strategies in place. What is convincing to one analyst is not convincing to another. For example, what should be done when there are outliers in the data, that is, measured values of findings (such as laboratory values) or events that deviate substantially from the reference range? If outliers are ignored, important safety findings may not be identified; on other hand, outliers may represent errors in data collection. This was the case for one patient in an NDA submission. The patient had a serum creatinine value of 13 mg/ml (over 10 times the normal value, by any reference!) but a normal serum BUN value.

Limited Knowledge of Exposure and Reporting Rates in Postmarketing Data. Unlike clinical trials and electronic medical records in clinical practice, postmarketing voluntarily reported data contain limited information about the total number of patients exposed and the duration of exposure. This problem is compounded by the fact that adverse events are often underreported [2,9].

27.4.5 Reproducibility

Traditional analytical methods make extensive use of computers, but typically these methods still require constant restructuring of the data and multiple analytical tools. This endless restructuring wastes time and productivity and also makes the analytical processes difficult to document, audit, and reproduce in real time. This situation also makes it difficult to reconstruct and update analyses in real time when *new* adverse event data become available or when *new* questions need to be asked. The application of comprehensive data standards allows the use of integrated, reusable software for analyzing adverse event data. This integration facilitates the reproducibility of the results.

27.4.6 Maintenance

Any computer database system will require maintenance. This maintenance includes such things as actively identifying and correcting data errors, ensuring that data can still be used with upgraded software and that this software can be used with upgraded hardware and data. Maintenance also includes actively testing and identifying computer bugs and adding new features and enhanced functions to the software.

27.5 EXAMPLES OF PRACTICAL COMPUTER-INTENSIVE TOOLS FOR SYSTEMATICALLY ASSESSING DRUG SAFETY DATA

27.5.1 Background

Although 500,000 individuals were enrolled in clinical trials that were submitted to the FDA during 1990–1995 [10], the lack of a repository of clinical trial data, standardized data, and interoperable systems precludes us from efficiently tapping and reanalyzing these data. This missed opportunity underscores the need for standardization and interoperable systems, as discussed above (see Section 27.4.1 on data standards and interoperable systems).

Drug safety reviewers spend a great amount of time learning the peculiarities of the data structure format and the variable names used with each NDA (and NDA supplement) submitted for marketing approval. As described above, for some NDAs the data from several studies must be incorporated into an integrated summary of safety data set and validated before performing a safety analysis; if every study uses a different data structure this is an arduous task. To rectify this situation, the FDA is using the Clinical Data Interchange Standards Consortium (CDISC) Submission Data Tabulation Model (SDTM) format adopted as a standard by the FDA in July 2004. The implementation of such data standards allows for development of standard and comprehensive analytical tools that can automatically generate standardized and comprehensive analyses that can be used across numerous NDAs.

27.5.2 Analysis of Premarketing Data with WebSDM™

An example of an analytical tool that utilizes CDISC data standards is WebSDM™ (Web Submission Data Manager) by Lincoln Technologies. The FDA has recently implemented WebSDM™ to analyze two NDAs in real time [11]. Although the original NDA data were submitted with nonstandard formats and the data had to be transformed into beforethe Study Data Tabulation Model format before being loaded into WebSDM™, the review process for these Z NDAs was more efficient than with standard methods. In this case the data was transformed to demonstrate the concept that the use of standardized data simplifies the analytical process. WebSDM™ saves time because it first ensures that the data submitted to the FDA complies with CDISC format and then uses standard methods that enable automation of the analytical processes. Typically, FDA reviewers receive different data formats for each NDA; however, WebSDM™ eliminates the need for reviewers and supervisors to learn where the variables for analyses for each NDA are located (Figure 27.3) and the different data formats for each NDA. For example, assessing potential liver injury by analyzing increases in serum alanine aminotransferase (ALT) and total serum bilirubin (TBILI) is done in one step instead of multiple cumbersome steps. It was also easier for the reviewers to fulfill the requirements of the NDA Review Template in a recent FDA guidance document for reviewers [12]. WebSDM™ also eliminates the need to reconfigure the data and the analytical tools for each new NDA analysis. WebSDM™ allows reviewers to use tailor-made, reusable tables and graphs of patient data in any NDA or supplement. The Sector Map graphical tool (with interactive drill-down capabilities) visualizes clinical trial data by highlighting higher-than-expected associations of adverse events compared to control groups. These features greatly simplify interpretation of the data. (See example with post-marketing data in Figure 27.4) These advanced graphical and analytical features are designed to simplify the interactive analysis of the clinical trial data.

27.5.3 Analysis of Postmarketing Data with MGPS and HBLR

For drugs already on the market, the FDA is utilizing the Multi-Item Gamma Poisson Shrinker (MGPS) statistical algorithm [9, 13] to systematically and simultaneously detect signals of higher-than-expected drug-adverse event associations in its postmarketing drug safety databases. To identify these signals, MGPS employs a disproportionality analysis of drugs and events, combined with Bayesian shrinkage. MGPS uses the independence model as the basis for computing the drug-event expected counts. MGPS includes a

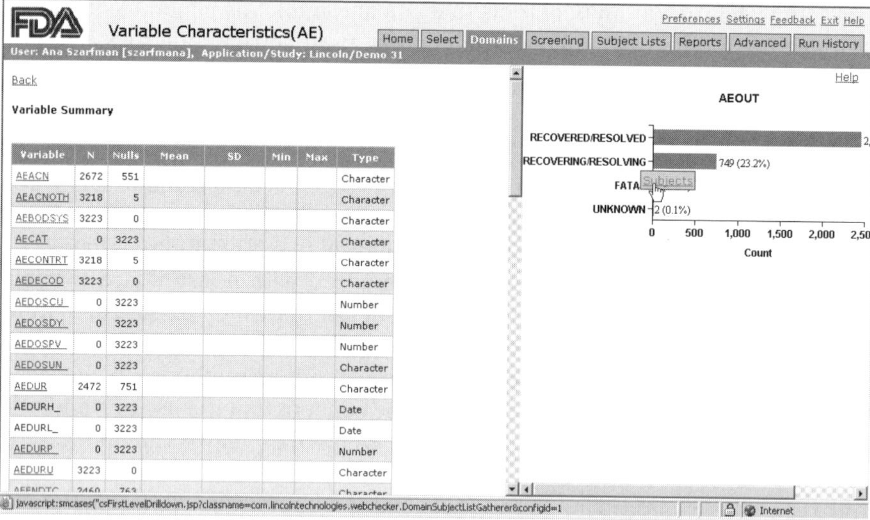

Figure 27.3 Once the data are transformed into CDISC standards and integrated with a drug safety analysis system, the data can be easily analyzed. In this figure we show a sample screen from WebSDM™ a drug safety analysis system being evaluated by the FDA. This screen allows the user to view different attributes of the variables in a user-specified data set. When a variable is selected, a graphical display of the data is produced on the right-hand side of the window. The user can then select to visualize a graphical display of the individual patient profiles under the variable in a different window.

Maentel–Haenszel style approach for adjusting the expected counts for potential strata heterogeneity. When applied to the FDA's AERS database, the MGPS program systematically stratifies the data by over 1000 categories (9 categories for age, 3 for sex, and 38 for year of report) to help adjust for background differences in relative reporting rates by these variables. The FDA thus far has focused its analytical efforts on the AERS database, but MGPS can be applied to any large drug safety database. The British Medicines and Healthcare Products Regulatory Agency (MHRA) has recently begun using MGPS as part of its pharmacovigilance program. MGPS also incorporates advanced graphical tools for analysis, including the Sector Map described previously (Figure 27.4).

The FDA is also exploring another statistical algorithm, the Hierarchical Bayesian Logistic Regression (HBLR), to study signals that may be influenced by polypharmacy. HBLR corrects for confounding induced by concomitant medications (each with its own potentially strong adverse event associations) throughout the database [14, 15]. HBLR uses a prior distribution (estimated from the data) to improve the modeling of the joint associations for up to hundreds of drugs with a logistic regression response variable.

HBLR adjusts for both "signal absorption" and "signal masking." Signal absorption is a phenomenon whereby an "innocent bystander" drug is falsely signaled as being associated with a particular adverse event simply because of its frequent coprescription with another drug that is associated with that same event. Signal masking occurs in a database when there is failure to detect a weak signal for a particular drug because of the presence of other strong signals for the same adverse event, usually because of the homogeneity of drugs in the database [16]. Our initial experience indicates that HBLR may be a useful adjunct to MGPS in postmarketing safety assessments, especially in polytherapy regimens [15]. Dr. William DuMouchel has presented an overview of future empirical Bayes methods for estimation of adverse event rates in clinical trials and active surveillance [17].

27.5.4 Other Data Resources

The number and size of databases containing drug safety information is growing rapidly, with some databases already containing millions of records [18, 19]. Analyzing several databases can help strengthen or refute a putative safety problem based on the results of the primary database analysis. Databases that can be analyzed include those maintained by various countries (e.g., the British General Practice Research Database or GPRD); various organizations (e.g., the World Health Organization and health maintenance organizations); various agencies (e.g., the U.S. Department of Defense, Department of Veterans Affairs, and Centers for Medicare and Medicaid ServicesAffairs), and others. Adapting new standard computer-intensive analytical tools to analyze data converted into standardized format will allow different experts to review each other's selection criteria and results so that conclusions can be more objectively studied and understood.

27.5.5 Validation of New Methods

Validation of new methods for analyzing drug safety data is challenging. There is no gold standard tool that can provide complete information about the whole spectrum of toxicity for a given drug and the magnitude and extent of this toxicity in specific subpopulations [9]. These facts, coupled with the discordant manner in which medical data are collected, make it very difficult to systematically analyze drug safety data in real time and to cross-reference multiple collections of medical data and results in a systematic way. The application of advanced computer methods offers a tremendous opportunity to analyze large databases in a timely and consistent manner and to learn about drug safety in a systematic way. These efforts will assist in creating gold-standard positive and negative signal definitions and methods given the data analyzed [20]. With these gold standards in place, we will be better able to further advance the art as well as the science of systematic drug safety assessment across databases.

Cerivastatin

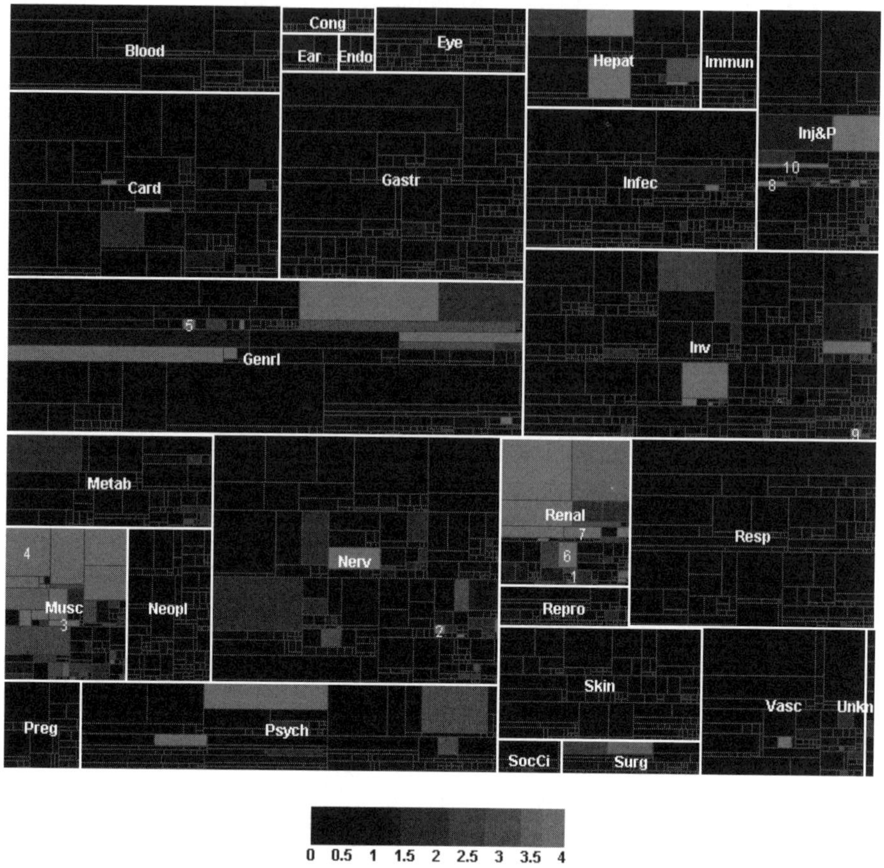

0 0.5 1 1.5 2 2.5 3 3.5 4

Rank	SOC	Term (PT)	EBGM	AERS cases
1	Renal	Myoglobinuria	15.416	104
2	Nerv	Myasthenic syndrome	12.449	1021
3	Musc	Myositis	12.198	2670
4	Musc	Rhabdomyolysis	11.501	12024
5	Genrl	Organ failure	10.121	685
6	Renal	Chromaturia	9.437	3034
7	Renal	Renal tubular necrosis	9.249	2547
8	Inj&P	Muscle injury	9.025	998
9	Inv	Myoglobin blood increased	8.807	527
10	Inj&P	Polytraumatism	8.497	1105

NOTES: Additional restrictions for graph:

Color controlled by: EBGM.
Size controlled by: relative importance.
Maximum intensity at signal score of 4.0.
Omit rare terms used fewer than 100.0 times
List 10 top scores
Show score indexes.
Group by HLT
Group by HLGT
Group by SOC
Lowest level displayed: PT

Print

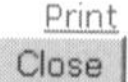

Figure 27.4 Sector map display of the MGPS data mining profile for a drug, using a dictionary of medical terms. This display shows the safety profile of cerivastatin, a drug withdrawn from the US market in August 2001 because of reports of fatal rhabdomyolysis, renal failure, and other organ failure [24]. The sector map shows strong signals for several serious muscle events including rhabdomyolysis and for renal failure (note the signals for "renal tubular necrosis" highlighted in the yellow pop-out note). The strong renal failure signals with this drug were unexpected. In addition, there were huge differences between cerivastatin and other statins regarding the magnitude of the renal failure signals. See color plate.

- *Color, size, position in space, grouping, and ranking of tiles* provide a "big picture" overview of the adverse event profile of a drug.
- *Color:* Red corresponds to stronger signals.
- *Size:* A large tile (with a white border) defines each SOC (System Organ Class) in the MedDRA dictionary.
- *Box size for each PT* (preferred adverse event term) is based on the number of serious cases of the term across all drugs in the AERS database. Thus, the box size of each PT is stable over different displays of different drugs.
- *Position in space:* SOCs and PTs are always represented in the same area of the sector map. The position of each SOC and PT is stable over displays of different drugs.
- *Grouping:* PTs are grouped by high level term (HLT), high level group (HLGT), and SOC.
- *Ranking:* PTs are ranked in descending order of EBGM values for each drug. EBGM: Signal Score. AERS cases: number of cases for the term in the AERS database. Note that the PT "renal failure acute" is ranked 43rd with cerivastatin and that "renal tubular necrosis" is ranked 12th with this drug. The PT "renal failure acute" has a larger box size than "renal tubular necrosis" because it has a much larger number of serious cases in the AERS database.

27.6 CONCLUSIONS

Even though great progress has been made since the passage of the Food, Drug, and Cosmetic Act in 1938, pharmaceutically related adverse events are still, unfortunately, responsible for a tremendous burden of pain and suffering in the United States [21] and old problems still persist across the world [22, 23]. Adverse events are also responsible for tremendous financial costs to taxpayers, insurance policyholders, insurance companies, and pharmaceutical companies. With such public health and economic costs in mind, we should carefully consider the strengths of new pharmacovigilance approaches while clearly acknowledging their limitations as well.

New tools that exploit the power of modern computer technology provide innovative approaches to help identify and investigate potential drug safety problems in a systematic way. These new computer methods can assist in pharmacovigilance efforts because the results of an analysis from a particular drug safety database can be compared to the results from other, independent databases (e.g., clinical trial, health maintenance organization, or military medical databases). With interoperable standards in place, statisticians, epidemiologists, and other analysts will be in a great position to improve drug safety and communication between all parties involved (consumers, clinicians, regulators, industry representatives, and legislators). By using the same software and data we can validate each other's selection criteria, results, and interpretation. As a result, researchers and policy makers will be better equipped to understand the limitations and biases of the data, leading to more objective decisions regarding drug safety.

REFERENCES

1. http://www.fda.gov/oc/history/elixir.html [accessed March 2006]
2. Szarfman A, Tonning JM, Doraiswamy PM. Pharmacovigilance in the 21st century: new systematic tools for an old problem. *Pharmacotherapy.* 2004; 24:1099–104.
3. http://www.genaissance.com/pharmacogenomics/glossary.asp#Informatics [accessed March 2006]
4. http://www.trains.com/Content/Dynamic/Articles/000/000/003/011gsqfq.asp [accessed on March 1, 2006]
5. 2005 FDA Science Forum: Advancing Public Health through Innovative Science. Washington, DC. April 27, 2005.
6. Video Clips. Workshop on statistical issues in drug safety monitoring. Schering-Plough Workshop June 2–3, 2005. Harvard School of Public Health. Section III: Pharmacovigilence and Datamining for Drug Safety Monitoring. Szarfman A, Levine JG, Tonning JM, "Use of Advanced Computer Methods to Simplify the Analysis of Complex Clinical Drug Safety Data." Available from URLs: http://biosunl.harvard.edu/events/schering-plough/oldagenda2004-05.html [accessed on March 2006] and http://webapps.sph.harvard.edu/content/Sch-Plo6205III_Unspecified_2005-06-02_04-03-PM.htm (3rd presentation in the video) [Accessed March 2006]
7. Barnett ST, James JA. Measuring the clinical development process. *Appl Clin Trials* 1995;4:44–52.
8. Szarfman A, Talarico L, Levine JG. Analysis and risk assessment of hematological data from clinical trials: toxicology of the hematopoietic system. In: Sipes IG, McQueen CA, Gandolfi AJ, editors, *Comprehensive toxicology.* Vol. 4. New York; Elsevier Science, 1997, p. 363–79.
9. Szarfman A, Machado SG, O'Neill RT. Use of screening algorithms and computer systems to efficiently signal higher-than-expected combinations of drugs and events in the U.S. FDA's spontaneous reports database. *Drug Saf* 2002;25:381–92
10. Evelyn B, Toigo T, Banks D, Pohl D, Gray K, Robins B, Ernat J. *Women's Participation in Clinical Trials and Gender-Related Labeling: A Review of New*

Molecular Entities Approved 1995–1999. June 2001. Office of Special Health Issues, Office of International and Constituent Relations, Office of the Commissioner, U.S. Food and Drug Administration. http://www.fda.gov/cder/reports/womens_health/women_clin_trials.htm [accessed October 2005].

11. Cooper CK, Levine JG, Tonning JM, Fram D, Millstein J, Rochester G, Szarfman A. Use of standards-based data and tools to improve the efficiency of the NDA Safety Review. 2005 FDA Science Forum. Abstract and Poster H-03. http://www.accessdata.fda.gov/scripts/oc/scienceforum/sf2005/Search/preview.cfm?abstract_id=339&backto=author [accessed March 2006].
12. Reviewer Guidance Conducting a Clinical Safety Review of a New Product Application and Preparing a Report on the Review. U.S. Department of Health 13a., and Human Services. Food and Drug Administration, Center for Drug Evaluation and Research (CDER) February 2005. http://www.fda.gov/cder/guidance/3580fnl.htm
13. DuMouchel W, Pregibon D. Empirical Bayes screening for multi-item associations. In: Seventh ACM SigKDD International Conference on Knowledge Discovery and Data Mining. San Francisco: ACM Press, 2001.
14. DuMouchel W. Manuscript in preparation.
15. Szarfman A, DuMouchel W, Fram D, Tonning J et al. Lactic acidosis: unraveling the individual toxicities of drugs used in HIV and diabetes polytherapy by hierarchical Bayesian logistic regression data mining (abstract). 11th Annual FDA Science Forum, April 27–28, 2005. http://www.accessdata.fda.gov/scripts/oc/scienceforum/sf2005/Search/preview.cfm?abstract_id=483&backto=author [accessed March 2006]
16. Gould L. *Pharmacoepidemiol Drug Safety* 2003;12:559–74.
17. Video Clips. Workshop on statistical issues in drug safety monitoring. Schering-Plough Workshop June 2–3, 2005. Harvard School of Public Health. Section III: Pharmacovigilence and Datamining for Drug Safety Monitoring. Szarfman A, Levine JG, Tonning JM, "Use of Advanced Computer Methods to Simplify the Analysis of Complex Clinical Drug Safety Data." Available from URLs: http://biosunl.harvard.edu/events/schering-plough/oldagenda2004-05.html [accessed on March 2006] and http://webapps.sph.harvard.edu/content/Sch-Plo6205III_Unspecified_2005-06-02_04-03-PM.htm (2nd presentation in the video) [Accessed March 2006]
18. http://www.gprd.com/home/ [accessed March 2006]
19. http://www.nttc.edu/resources/funding/dod/sbir2003/osd032.htm [accessed March 2006]
20. Levine JG, Tonning JM, Szarfman A. Reply: The evaluation of data mining methods for the simultaneous and systematic detection of safety signals in large databases: lessons to be learned. *Br J Clin Pharmacol.* 2006;61:105–13.
21. Lazarou J, Pomeranz BH, Corey PN. Incidence of adverse drug reactions in hospitalized patients: a meta-analysis of prospective studies. JAMA. 1998 Apr 15;279(15):1200–5.
22. Centers for Disease Control and Prevention (CDC). Fatalities associated with ingestion of diethylene glycol-contaminated glycerin used to manufacture acetaminophen syrup—Haiti, November 1995–June 1996 *MMWR Morb Mortal Wkly Rep* 1996;45:649–50.

23. Ferrari LA, Giannuzzi L. Clinical parameters, postmortem analysis and estimation of lethal dose in victims of a massive intoxication with diethylene glycol. *Forensic Sci Int* 2005;153:45–51.
24. FDA Talk Paper. Bayer Voluntarily Withdraws baycol. FDA talk paper no T01–34. 2001 Aug 8.

PART VIII

FURTHER APPLICATIONS AND FUTURE DEVELOPMENT

28

COMPUTERS IN PHARMACEUTICAL FORMULATION

Raymond C. Rowe and Elizabeth A. Colbourn

Contents

Computer Applications in Pharmaceutical Research and Development, Edited by Sean Ekins.
ISBN 0-471-73779-8

28.1 INTRODUCTION

Before a new drug can be released on the market, it must be formulated to produce a quality product that is acceptable to both regulatory bodies and patients and can be manufactured on a large scale. There are many formulation types depending on the route of administration of the active drug.

- *Capsules*—These are primarily intended for oral administration and are solid preparations with hard or soft shells comprised of gelatin or hydroxypropyl methyl cellulose and small amounts of other ingredients such as plasticizers, fillers, and coloring agents. Their contents may be powders, granules, pellets, liquids, or pastes.
- *Oral liquids*—These consist of solutions, suspensions, or emulsions of one or more active ingredients mixed with preservatives, antioxidants, dispersing agents, suspending agents, thickeners, emulsifiers, solubilizers, wetting agents, colors, and flavors in a suitable vehicle, generally water. They may be supplied ready for use or may be prepared before use from a concentrate or from granules or powders by the addition of water.
- *Tablets*—These are solid preparations each containing a single dose of one or more active drugs mixed with a filler/diluent, a disintegrant, a binder, a lubricant, and other ingredients such as colors. flavors, surfactants, and glidants. Tablets are prepared by compacting powders or granules in a punch and die and can exist in a variety of shapes and sizes. Tablets can also be formulated with a variety of polymers to provide a range of drug release profiles from rapid release over minutes to prolonged release over many hours. Tablets may also be coated either with sugar or with polymer films. The latter may be applied to enhance identification, in which case colored pigments may be added; to increase stability, in which case opacifying agents may be added; or to provide varying release profiles throughout the gastrointestinal tract.
- *Parenterals*—These are sterile preparations intended for administration by injection, infusion, or implantation. Injections are sterile solutions, emulsions, or suspensions comprising the active drug together with suitable pH adjusters, tonicity adjusters, solubilizers, antioxidants, chelating agents, and preservatives in an appropriate vehicle, water- or oil based. If there are stability issues, the formulation may be prepared as a freeze-dried sterile powder to which the appropriate sterile vehicle is added before administration. Infusions are sterile aqueous solutions or emulsions intended for administration in large volumes. Implants are sterile solid preparations designed to release their active drug over an extended period of time.
- *Topicals*—These are semisolid preparations such as creams, ointments, or gels intended to be applied to the skin or certain mucous membranes

for local action. They may be single- or multiphase comprising one or more active drugs mixed with emulsifiers, oils, soaps, gelling agents, or waxes with a continuous phase of either water or oil.

- *Eye preparations*—These are specifically intended for administration to the eye in the form of solutions, lotions, or ointments. All preparations must be sterile.
- *Suppositories and pessaries*—These are preparations intended for either rectal or vaginal administration of drugs. They are formulated with a suitable base that melts at body temperature.
- *Inhalation preparations*—These can be solutions, suspensions, or powders intended to be inhaled as aerosols for administration to the lung.

The process of formulation for any of the above is generically the same, beginning with some form of product specification and ending with one or more formulations that meet the requirements. Correct choice of additives or excipients is paramount in the provision of efficacy, stability, and safety. For instance, the excipients may be chemically or physically incompatible with the drug or they may exhibit batchwise variability to such an extent that at the extremes of their specification they may cause failure in achieving the desired drug release profile. In addition, some excipients, especially those that are hydroscopic, may be contraindicated if the formulation is to be manufactured in tropical countries. Hence formulators must work in a design space that is multidimensional in nature and virtually impossible to conceptualize.

Over the past decade a small number of visionary scientists have been experimenting with and developing advanced computing techniques. These include expert and knowledge-based systems for the generation of initial formulations and processing conditions ab initio; neural computing for modeling formulation and process data to explore relationships within the data set and optimize the formulation; and computer simulation for the development of mathematical models of the interaction between the formulation and the manufacturing process to predict outcomes. The idea behind this work is to assist the formulation of products with the added benefits of consistent decision making, decreased timelines, and cost savings. This chapter reviews the current situation.

28.2 EXPERT AND KNOWLEDGE-BASED SYSTEMS

There is a wide divergence as to what defines an expert system. Examples relevant to the formulation process are:

> "An expert system is a knowledge-based system that emulates expert thought to solve significant problems in a particular domain of expertise." [1]

"An expert system is a computer program that draws upon the knowledge of human experts captured in a knowledge base to solve problems that normally require human expertise." [2].

The first recorded reference to the use of expert systems in pharmaceutical product formulation was in the London *Financial Times* in the spring of 1989 [3], closely followed by an article in the autumn of the same year [4]. Both referred to the work then being undertaken by personnel at ICI Pharmaceuticals, UK (now AstraZeneca) to develop an expert system for formulating pharmaceuticals ab initio. Since that time several companies and academic institutions have reported their experiences.

28.2.1 Technology

In their simplest form expert systems comprise an interface allowing a two-way communication between the user and the system: a knowledge base where all the knowledge pertaining to the domain is stored and an inference engine where the knowledge is extracted and manipulated to solve the problem in hand. Inferencing strategies may be either forward chaining, which involves the system reasoning from the data and information gained by consultation with the user to form a hypothesis, or backward chaining, which involves the system starting with a hypothesis and then attempting to find data and information to prove or disprove the hypothesis. Both strategies are used in formulation expert systems.

Many potential sources of knowledge are necessary for the creation of an expert system. These range from the expertise often gathered over many years of work resident with the domain expert or, in the case of large complex domains, a number of experts; the data included in written documents (research reports, reference manuals, textbooks, operating procedures, and technical bulletins); and general information such as policy statements. It is the objective of the knowledge engineer to acquire or elicit this knowledge and structure it in a computer-usable format.

Knowledge acquisition is regarded as probably the most difficult task in the development of expert systems. It is both time consuming and tedious as well as being difficult to manage. The basic model is one of a team process whereby the knowledge engineer mediates between the expert or experts and the users of the system with face-to-face interviews. A technique that is often used in the acquisition process is the rapid prototyping approach whereby the knowledge engineer builds a small prototype system as early as possible. This is then shown to both the users and the experts, who can suggest modifications and additions. Hence the system grows incrementally as more knowledge is added. This methodology has been used successfully in the development of current formulation expert systems.

Once acquired, there are many ways of representing knowledge in the knowledge base. Probably the most common is the production rule, which expresses the relationship between several pieces of information by way of conditional statements that specify actions under certain sets of conditions—IF (condition 1) AND (condition 2) OR (condition 3) THEN (action) UNLESS (exception) BECAUSE (reason). Each rule is easy to understand, implements an autonomous piece of knowledge, and can be developed and modified independently of other rules. Unfortunately, a complex domain may require a large number of rules and other representation methodologies may be necessary. These include frames or templates for holding clusters of related knowledge; semantic networks for representing complex relationships between objects; and decision trees or tables for organizing knowledge in a tree or tabular format that is easy to understand and format. Generally, multiple methods are used to express formulation knowledge.

Expert Systems can be developed with conventional computer languages such as C or more recently JAVA, with specialized languages such as LISP and PROLOG, or with the assistance of development shells or toolkits. Conventional languages have the advantage of wide applicability and flexibility to create the strategies required but require considerable time and effort to create the basic facilities. Specialized languages have been used extensively in the development of expert systems because they retain the advantages of conventional languages but are faster to implement. Shells and toolkits are sets of programs written in either conventional or specialized languages that can form an expert system when loaded with knowledge. They compromise on applicability and flexibility but allow the rapid development of unique systems.

Shells differ in their secondary characteristics such as interfaces, knowledge representation, and associated algorithmic facilities. One such shell specially developed for product formulation is Logica's Formulogic (formerly Product Formulation Expert System, PFES). This is a reusable software kernel and associated methodology originally developed by a consortium of Shell Research Ltd., Schering Agrochemicals Ltd., and Logica UK Ltd under a UK GOVERNMENT-funded scheme in 1985–1987. Its generic capability of providing knowledge representation methods common to most product formulation tasks allows new applications to be developed rapidly and efficiently. It provides a decision support framework consisting of two levels: a task level that contains the problem solving steps involved in the formulation process and a physical level that contains specific knowledge about the properties of the ingredients [5, 6].

The technology referred to above is generally referred to as rule-based reasoning (RBR) because it relates to the structuring and use of knowledge in the form of rules abstracted during the acquisition process. Another technology used to develop expert systems is case-based reasoning (CBR). This can be explained in a single sentence: To solve a problem, remember a similar problem you have solved in the past and adapt the solution to solve the new problem [7]. CBR directly uses records of previous solutions both successful and unsuccessful as its principal knowledge base. The method of problem solving mimics that often used intuitively by many experts including formulators. Indeed, they often talk of their domain by giving examples rather than articulating their knowledge with logical rules. The CBR cycle can be described by the 4 Rs [8]: RETRIEVE the case(s) in the memory/case base that gives solutions to the problem similar to the current problem; REUSE the knowledge about that case to suggest a solution; REVISE and adapt the solution; and RETAIN the new solution in the memory/case base for future problem solving.

Case-based reasoning is very much dependent on the structure and content of its cases and their representation because case retrieval involves identifying those features in the problem that best match those in the case base. The dynamic addition of new cases means that CBR is intrinsically a learning methodology such that the performance of an expert system based on this approach will improve with time [9]. Systems may be developed with conventional computer languages or shells [7].

28.2.2 Applications

It is not surprising, considering the widespread use of tablets and capsules, that these domains have received most attention for the development of expert systems by both companies and academic institutions. However, it should be noted that other domains such as inhalation preparations, topicals, and parenterals have also been investigated. One system, the Galenical Development System developed at the University of Heidelberg, Germany, has been designed to provide assistance in the development of a range of formulations (aerosols, capsules, tablets, intravenous injections, pellets, and granules) starting from the chemical and physical properties of a drug. The project was initiated in 1990 [10] and has been extensively revised and enhanced in the interim [11, 12]. It should also be noted that many systems, especially those developed by companies, are rarely reported in the literature, and hence it is difficult to review all developments in the field.

Tablet Formulations. In this domain reported systems have been developed by personnel at Cadila Laboratories Ltd, in Ahmedabad, India, by ICI/Zeneca/AstraZeneca in the UK, by a consortium of pharmaceutical companies in Japan, and by Pfizer UK.

The Cadila system [13] has been designed to formulate tablets for drugs based on their physical (solubility, hydroscopicity, etc), chemical (functional groups), and biologically interrelated (dissolution rate) properties. The system first identifies the desirable properties for optimum compatibility with the drug, selects those excipients that have the required properties, and then recommends proportions based on the assumption that all tablet formulations comprise at least one binder, one disintegrant, and one lubricant. Other excipients such as fillers or glidants are then added as required. An example of a formulation proposed for acetaminophen (paracetamol) is shown in Table 28.1. The filler is unnamed, but it can be assumed that it will not be lactose because there is a rule embedded in the system that negates the use of lactose if the drug contains a secondary amine group, because it will promote a chemical interaction. Knowledge acquired through active collaborations with expert formulators over a period of 6–7 months is structured as decision tables with derived production rules. The system is written in PROLOG, is menu driven, and is interactive with the user. The prototype system when first implemented had 150 rules, but this rapidly expanded to over 300 rules to increase reliability. It is reported to have reduced by 35% the development time for a new tablet formulation and to be of benefit in planning the purchase and stocking of excipients.

The system developed at ICI/Zeneca/AstraZeneca has been widely reported [14–16]. The system was initiated in 1988 with enhancements and revisions taking place as a result of new knowledge and company changes. The system has been implemented with the Formulogic shell and knowledge acquisition by interview and structured with frames, objects, and production rules. The user is prompted to enter all the relevant physical, chemical, and mechanical properties (solubility, wettability, compatibility with excipients, and deformation behavior) of the drug together with the dose required. The system proposes a target tablet weight and then selects the excipients and calculates their concentrations to satisfy a series of predetermined constraints based on the manufacturability of the formulation. At all times the system may be overridden by the formulator if the recommendations are not to his/her satisfaction. The system also has a formulation optimization procedure implemented whereby the formulator enters the results from testing tablets prepared with the recommended formulation. These include disintegration time, tablet strength, tablet weight variation, and the presence of defects such as capping, lamination, etc. The system compares these with specifications and then alters the excipient concentrations. Help routines are embedded in the system, and explanations to recommendations can be accessed. It is now an integral part of the development strategy for tablet formulation. Recently, a prototype CBR system has also been developed and tested [17].

A computer-aided formulation system for tablets (Expert-Tab) has recently been developed by a consortium of 13 pharmaceutical companies coordinated

TABLE 28.1 An Example of a Tablet Formulation for Acetaminophen (Paracetamol) as Generated by the Cadila System

Drug	Acetaminophen (Paracetamol)	500.0 mg
Filler	Unnamed	20.0 mg
Binder	Pregelatinized starch	43.7 mg
Disintegrant	Sodium starch glycolate	5.0 mg
Lubricant	Stearic acid	2.5 mg

by Kyoto University in Japan [18–20]. Knowledge was acquired by questionnaires and discussions with experts, and the system was developed based on the majority decision. The system operates by using a relational database with decision trees to recommend excipients based on the flow, compression characteristics, disintegration, and solubility of the drug [19]. It is interesting to note that the formulation is based on it being able to be manufactured with fluidized bed granulation, the most commonly used method by 8 of the 13 companies. The system has been extensively evaluated [20] and is presently being enhanced.

A prototype system implemented with the Formulogic shell has recently been reported by Pfizer [21]. The system has been designed to use preformulation data on new drugs and recommend early development formulations, predict product properties, and select processing conditions suitable for scale-up.

Capsule Formulations. Expert systems for capsule formulation have been developed by personnel at the University of London in collaboration with Capsugel and Sanofi Research Division in Philadelphia.

The Capsugel system was originally developed as part of a Ph.D. program at the University of London [22]. The system is unique in that its knowledge base is broad, containing information on a large number of excipients, a frequently updated database of marketed formulations from Germany, Italy, Belgium, France, and the US, and a database of literature references associated with capsule formulation updated through monitoring of current literature. In addition, it contains the experience and nonproprietary knowledge of a number of international experts and the results from statistically designed experiments on capsule formulation. The system, implemented in C, uses decision trees and production rules for knowledge representation. Data on a new drug are collected by way of an input questionnaire, and the system uses a variety of methods to predict properties of the drug with various excipients before recommending a formulation with any necessary processing conditions. In addition, the system provides a statistical design to optimize the formulation. The system has a semiautomatic learning tool that monitors user habits and collects data on the use of excipients. This, together with the results from user questionnaires, provides the background to further enhancements. Field trials have proved that the system does provide reasonable formulations [23].

The system developed by personnel at Sanofi uses the Formulogic shell with specific preformulation data on the drug. The system recommends one first-pass clinical capsule formulation with as many subsequent formulations as desired to accommodate an experimental design [24]. An example of a formulation proposed for naproxen at a dose of 500 mg is shown in Table 28.2. In addition to the formulation the system provides advice on the milling of the drug, the process to be used for blending, and details of the capsule shell.

TABLE 28.2 An Example of a Capsule Formulation of Naproxen as Generated by the Sanofi System

Drug	Naproxen	100 mg
Filler	Lactose (hydrous)	224 mg
Disintegrant	Microcrystalline cellulose (PH105)	60 mg
Surfactant	Sodium lauryl sulfate	4 mg
Lubricant	Talc	12 mg

It also provides an explanation log listing the reasons for the decisions made.

Other Formulations. In addition to those described above, systems have been reported for parenterals [25], film coatings [26], and topicals [27]. All use the Formulogic shell, the last one winning a prize for the Boots Company in 1991. All contain elements of the features of systems discussed above.

28.2.3 Benefits and Issues

Although there is a great deal of interest in expert systems, there is still much uncertainty regarding tangible benefits. In a survey of 74 companies in the US in 1993 [28] the main benefits identified were improved productivity, more consistent decision making, increased accuracy, and improved competitiveness. However, it is more pertinent to discuss those benefits found by users of systems in pharmaceutical formulation. These include:

- Prompt availability of knowledge
- Existence of durable knowledge base not affected by staff turnover
- Generation of consistent, robust formulations
- Useful training system
- Reduction in duration of formulation process
- Cost savings in drug and excipients
- Freeing experts' time for innovation
- Improved communication and discussion

Of course, as with all new technology, there are still many issues surrounding the implementation of expert systems. Although reduced staffing has generally been seen to be one of the least important benefits, it can still be an issue with some individuals. Probably of more importance is the need for good project management as well as having an articulate, responsive, and collaborative expert. Within the domain of pharmaceutical product formulation, early skepticism among potential users has generally changed to a mood of enthusiastic participation.

28.3 NEURAL COMPUTING

The properties of a formulation are determined not only by the ratios in which the ingredients are combined but also by the processing conditions. Although relationships between ingredient levels, processing conditions, and product performance may be known anecdotally, rarely can they be quantified. Traditionally, formulators have tended to use statistical techniques such as a response surface methodology to investigate the design space, but optimization by such a method can be misleading, especially if the formulation is complex. Recent advances in mathematics and computer science have resulted in the development of three techniques that can be used to remedy the situation—neural networks (an attempt to mimic the processing of the human brain); genetic algorithms (an attempt to mimic the evolutionary process by which biological systems self-organize and adapt), and fuzzy logic (an attempt to mimic the ability of the human brain to draw conclusions and generate responses based on incomplete or imprecise information).

28.3.1 Technology

Like humans, neural networks learn directly from input data. The learning algorithms take two main forms. Unsupervised learning, where the network is presented with input data and learns to recognize patterns in the data, is useful for organizing amounts of data into a smaller number of clusters. For supervised learning, which is analogous to "teaching" the network, the network is presented with a series of matching input and output examples, and it learns the relationships connecting the inputs to the outputs. Supervised learning has proved most useful for formulation, where the goal is to determine cause-and-effect links between inputs (ingredients and processing conditions) and outputs (measured properties).

The basic component of the neural network is the neuron, a simple mathematical processing unit that takes one or more inputs and produces an output. For each neuron, every input has an associated weight that defines its relative importance, and the neuron simply computes the weighted sum of all the outputs and calculates an output. This is then modified by means of a transformation function (sometimes called a transfer or activation function) before being forwarded to another neuron. This simple processing unit is known as a perceptron, a feed-forward system in which the transfer of data is in the forward direction, from inputs to outputs, only.

A neural network consists of many neurons organized into a structure called the network architecture. Although there are many possible network architectures, one of the most popular and successful is the multilayer perceptron (MLP) network. This consists of identical neurons all interconnected and organized in layers, with those in one layer connected to those in the next layer so that the outputs in one layer become the inputs in the subsequent layer. Data flow into the network via the input layer, pass through one or more hidden layers, and finally exit via the output layer (Fig. 28.1). In theory, any number of hidden layers may be added, but in practice multiple layers are necessary only for those applications with extensive nonlinear behavior, and they result in extended computation time. It is generally accepted that the performance of a well-designed MLP model is comparable with that achieved by classic statistical techniques.

Unlike conventional computer programs, which are explicitly programmed, supervised neural networks are "trained" with previous examples. The network is presented with example data, and the weights of inputs feeding into each neuron are adjusted iteratively until the output for a specific network is close to the desired output. The method used to adjust the weights is generally called back propagation, because the size of the error is fed back into the calculation for the weight changes. There are a number of possible back propagation algorithms, most with adjustable parameters designed to increase the rate and degree of convergence between the calculated and the desired (actual) outputs. Although training can be a relatively slow process, especially if there are large amounts of data, once trained, neural networks are inherently fast in execution.

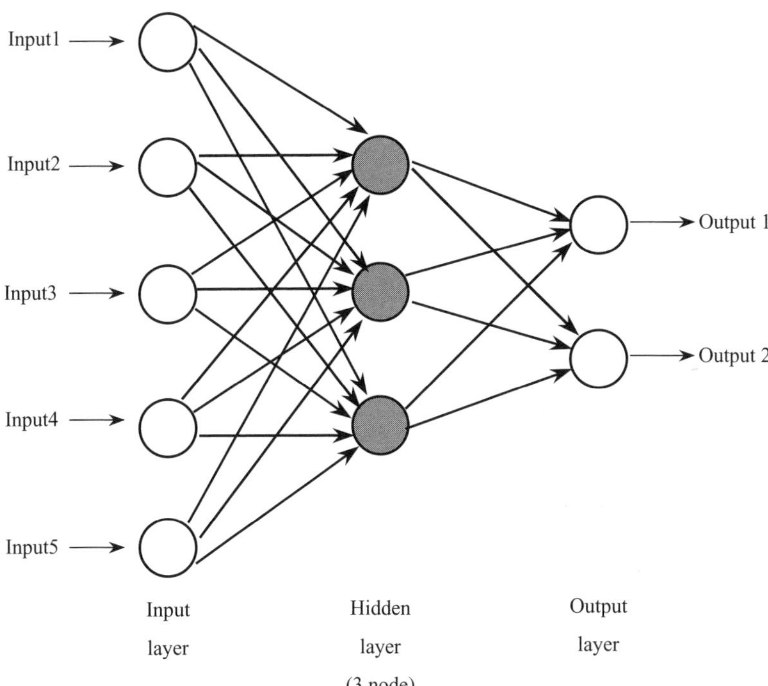

Figure 28.1 Diagram of a multilayer perceptron with one hidden layer.

Genetic algorithms are an optimization technique based on the concepts of biological evolution. Like the biological equivalent, genetic algorithms require a concept of "fitness," which is assessed according to how well the solution meets user-specified goals. Genetic algorithms work with a population of individuals, each of which is a candidate solution to the problem. Each individual's "fitness" is assessed, and if an optimum solution is not found, then a further generation of possible solutions is produced by combining large chunks of the fittest initial solutions by a crossover operation (mimicking mating and reproduction). As in biological evolution, the population will evolve slowly and only the fittest (i.e., best) solutions will survive and be carried forward. Ultimately, after many generations, an optimum solution will be found.

Genetic algorithms are especially useful for complex multidimensional problems with local minima as well as the global minimum. Unlike conventional more directed searches (like steepest descent and conjugate gradient methods), they are capable of finding the global minimum reliably. Effective use of genetic algorithms requires rapid feedback of the success or failure of the possible solutions, as judged by the fitness criteria. Hence, the combination of a genetic algorithm with a neural network is ideal. Such a combination (Fig. 28.2) is used in INForm, a software package available from Intelligensys Ltd., UK, in which formulations can be modeled with a neural network and then optimized with genetic algorithms.

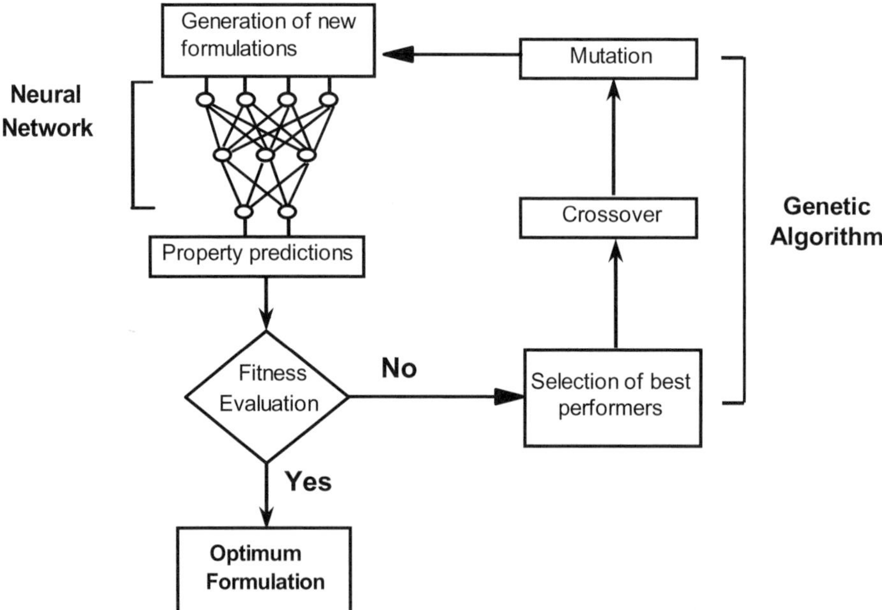

Figure 28.2 Diagram of a genetic algorithm linked to a neural network for modeling and optimization.

In defining the concept of "fitness," fuzzy logic provides a useful framework for describing complex formulation goals. Fuzzy logic, as the name implies, blurs the clear-cut "true" and "false" of conventional "crisp" logic, by assigning a noninteger number that describes the "membership" in a particular set as somewhere between 0 (false) and 1 (true). Therefore, in addition to the "black and white" of conventional logic, fuzzy logic allows "shades of gray" to be described intuitively and accurately. So, if the formulator is seeking a tablet with a disintegration time of less than 300 seconds, one with a disintegration time of (say) 310 seconds will not be rejected out of hand, but will be assigned a desirability of somewhat less than 100% (Fig. 28.3) according to its membership in the Low set.

More recently, coupling fuzzy logic with neural networks has led to the development of neurofuzzy computing, a novel technology that combines the ability of neural networks to learn directly from data with fuzzy logic's capacity to express the results clearly in linguistic form. Essentially the neurofuzzy architecture is a neural network with two additional layers for fuzzification and defuzzification. This has led to a powerful new modeling capability that not only develops models that express the key cause-and-effect relationships within a formulation data set but allows these to be expressed as simple actionable rules in the form IF (ingredient) . . . THEN (property), with an associated "confidence level." Neurofuzzy computing underpins FormRules, a software package from Intelligensys Ltd., UK that allows rules to be extracted directly from formulation data.

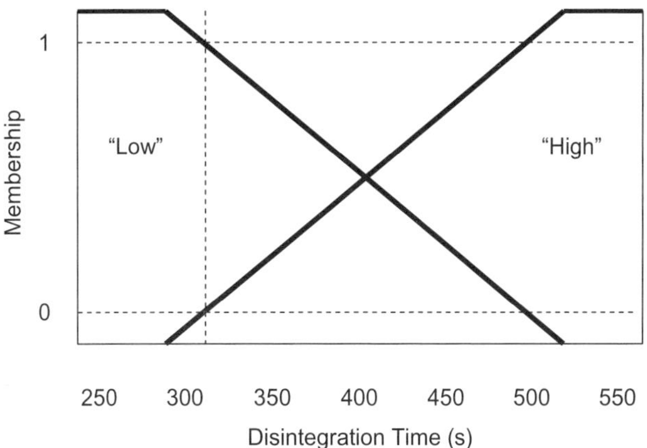

Figure 28.3 Fuzzy logic representation of the disintegration time of a tablet as Low or High.

28.3.2 Applications

The past decade has seen a dramatic increase in the number of reported applications of neural computing in pharmaceutical formulation [29–32]. Applications now cover a variety of formulations—for example, immediate and controlled release tablets, skin creams, hydrogel ointments, liposomes and emulsions, and film coatings. The following examples are by no means exhaustive, but they show where neural computing has been used successfully in modeling formulations.

Tablet Formulations (Immediate Release). Two papers in the mid-1990s reported the earliest studies on immediate release tablets. In the first, tablet formulations of hydrochlorothiazide [33] were modeled in an attempt to maximize tablet strength and select the best lubricant. In the other, a tablet formulation of caffeine was modeled [34] to relate both formulation and processing variables with granule and tablet properties.

Both of these studies were successful in demonstrating that neural networks performed better than conventional statistical methods. In a later paper [35], the data from the caffeine tablet formulation were subsequently reanalyzed with a combination of neural networks and genetic algorithms. This study showed that the optimum formulation depended on the relative importance placed on the output properties and on constraints applied both to the levels of the ingredients used in the formulation and to the processing variables. Many "optimum formulations" could be produced, depending on the trade-offs that could be accepted for different aspects of product performance. In a more recent paper [36], the same data have been studied with neurofuzzy computing. Useful rules relating the disintegration time to both formulation and processing variables were automatically generated.

In a series of papers, personnel from Novartis and the University of Basel in Switzerland have highlighted the pros and cons of neural networks for immediate release tablets [37–40]. In other studies neural networks have been found useful in modeling tablet formulations of antacids [41], plant extracts [42], theophylline [43], and diltiazem [44]. In a recent paper Lindberg and Colbourn [45] have used neural networks, genetic algorithms, and neurofuzzy to successfully analyze historical data from three different immediate-release tablet formulations.

Pigmented film coating formulations have recently been modeled and optimized to enhance opacity and reduce film cracking with neural networks combined with genetic algorithms [46, 47] as well as being studied with neurofuzzy [48]. In the latter study the rules discovered were consistent with known theory.

Tablet Formulations (Controlled Release). In this domain, the first studies were carried out in the early 1990s by Hussain and coworkers at the University of Cincinnati [49]. They modeled the in vitro release characteristics of a number of drugs from matrices consisting of a variety of hydrophilic polymers and found that in the majority of cases, neural networks with a single hidden layer had a reasonable performance in predicting drug release profiles. Later studies using similar formulations [50] have confirmed these findings, as have recent studies in Japan [51].

Neural networks have also been used in Slovenia, to model the release characteristics of diclofenac [52]; in China, to study release of nifedipine and nomodipine [53]; and in Yugoslavia to model the release of aspirin [54]. More recently, work in this area has been extended to model osmotic pumps in China [55] and enteric coated tablets in Ireland [56].

Topical Formulations. Topical formulations by their very nature are usually multicomponent, and it is not surprising that neural networks have been applied to deal with this complexity. The first work was performed on hydrogel formulations containing anti-inflammatory drugs in Japan in 1997 [57], followed up by further studies in 1999 [58] and in 2001 [59]. Lipophilic semisolid emulsion systems have been studied in Slovenia [60, 61] and transdermal delivery formulations of melatonin in Florida [62]. In all cases, the superiority of neural networks over conventional statistics has been reported.

Other Formulations. Neural networks have been applied to the modeling of pellet formulations to control the release of theophylline [63] and to control the rate of degradation of omeprazole [64]. They have also been applied to the preparation of acrylic microspheres [65] and to model the release of insulin from an implant [66]. In a recent study from Brazil, the release of hydrocortisone from a biodegradable matrix has been successfully modeled [67].

28.3.3 Benefits and Issues

Although there is a great deal of interest in neural computing, quantified information on the benefits has been harder to find. From the applications described above in this chapter, benefits that could be seen included

- Effective use of incomplete data sets
- Rapid analysis of data
- Ability to accommodate more data and retrain the network (refine the model)
- Effective exploration of the total design space, irrespective of complexity
- Ability to accommodate constraints and preferences
- Ability to generate understandable rules

In a survey [68] of the use of 93 neural computing applications in 75 UK companies covering all business sectors, the major benefits identified were improved quality, improved response times, and increased productivity. Eighty-four percent of users were satisfied or very satisfied with their systems, with only three percent expressing dissatisfaction. Business benefits specifically for the domain of product formulation (albeit for nonpharmaceuticals) have been given as [15]

- Enhancement of product quality and performance at low cost
- Shorter time to market
- Development of new products
- Improved customer response
- Improved confidence
- Improved competitive edge

As this new technology moves from the realm of academe into practical application, there are also issues regarding the implementation of neural computing. Users in the previously cited study were asked to identify where they had experienced problems. Thirty-nine percent had found problems related to software and lack of development skills; this will be reduced as commercial packages come into wider use and there is less need for bespoke in-house systems with their high programming and maintenance burden. However, even when commercial packages are used, there are a number of features that should be present before neural computing can be used to advantage. The problem must be numeric in nature, and reasonable quantities of data should be available to train an adequate model. The greatest benefits are achieved for multidimensional problems, where it is difficult to express any analytic model and difficult to abstract the rules by any other mechanism than neural computing. It helps if the problem is of practical importance, is part of the organization's essential activity, and meets a real business need. Pharmaceutical formulation meets these criteria well, and neural computing can be expected to provide significant benefits in industry in the future.

28.4 COMPUTER SIMULATION

Simulation is best described as the process of translating a real system into a working model in order to run experiments. A simulation does not duplicate a system; rather it is an abstraction of reality using mathematics to express cause-and-effect relationships that determine the behavior of the system. Hence the representation displayed on a computer may not always be pictorially similar to the real system, and, if it is, then it must be regarded as an added bonus. Software for computer simulation is often customized and based on that developed in academia. There are not many commercial packages available for pharmaceutical formulation.

28.4.1 Applications

In the domain of pharmaceutical formulation, computer simulation is a relatively new concept. This is not to say that it has not been attempted in the past. The mechanical modeling of the tablet compaction process with finite elements was first attempted in 1987 [69] and has been refined since [70, 71]. However, this methodology is based on the assumption that a tablet is a continuum, the properties of which can be defined by constitutive equations. It works well for tablet formulations comprising one ingredient but has little relevance to multicomponent formulations. Recently a combined finite-discrete element method for simulating multicomponent pharmaceutical powder tabletting has been proposed [72]. In this the irregular particle shapes and random sizes of powders are represented as a pseudoparticle assembly having a scaled-up geometry but based on the variations of real powder particles. The method is currently being evaluated and validated against experimental data, but initial results indicate that it does capture the characteristics of the pharmaceutical tableting process [73].

A prerequisite of tablet compaction is the initial filling of the tablet die with powder. Powder packing is one process that has received a great deal of attention, and commercial software for simulating this process is available (Macro Pac, Intelligensys Ltd., UK). This is software able to simulate the packing of multicomponent formulations of particles of any shape and size with a Monte Carlo technique. It is ideal for the simulation of the packing of pharmaceutical formulations into both tablet dies [72] and hard gelatin capsule shells [74]. A simulation of the packing of pellets into a hard gelatin capsule is shown in Figure 28.4.

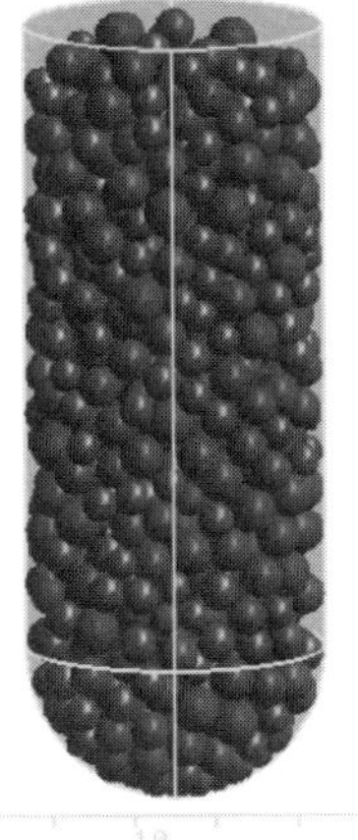

Figure 28.4 A computer simulation of a size 0 capsule filled with pellets with a size distribution of 0.8 and 1.2 mm.

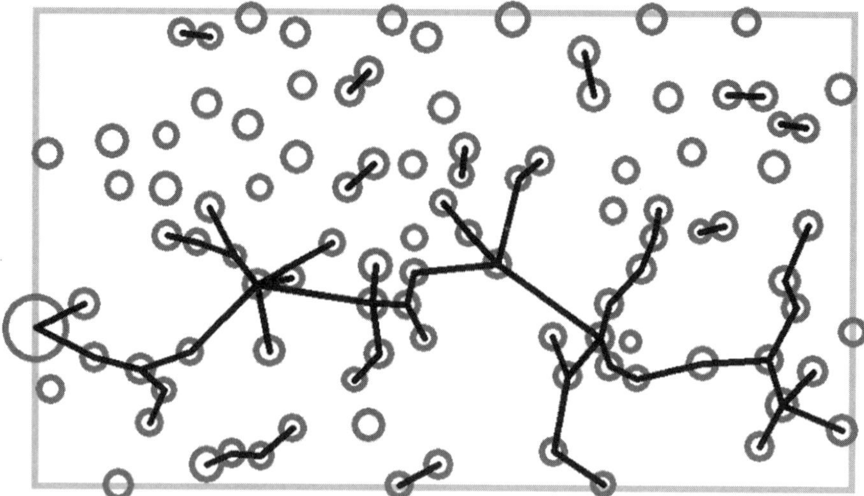

Figure 28.5 A computer simulation of crack propagation in a tablet film coating containing one population of an inclusion.

Solid inclusions in the form of pigments are often added to tablet film coatings to improve their color and/or their opacity. A potential problem is that of localized cracking around the individual particles or aggregates compromising the release control of the active drug. A simulation of crack propagation in such systems has been developed [75, 76], allowing the investigation of such effects of the addition of a second population of pigments, pigment particle size and size distribution, polymer molecular weight, addition of plasticizers, and many other factors affecting the film coating formulation. Recently this simulation has been made available as MacroCrack from Intelligensys Ltd., UK. A computer simulation of a crack (black line) propagating through a pigmented film coating is shown in Figure 28.5.

28.4.2 Benefits

There are many benefits of computer simulation:

- Many simulations performed with minimum effort
- Allows the investigation of the sensitivity of the system to small changes in parameters
- Assists in determining the accuracy to which the input parameters need to be controlled
- Allows the testing of the system in operating conditions that would be costly, dangerous, or time consuming to perform
- Excellent training tool

Recent work in this field has highlighted the potential in pharmaceutical formulation, and it is expected that there will be increasing activity in the future.

28.5 CONCLUSION

The next generation of formulators in the pharmaceutical industry are likely to find themselves using all of the above techniques routinely and to an increasing extent. Several pharmaceutical companies have already implemented some of them and made them available to formulators either as standalone programs or linked via an intranet. However, the largest benefit in the future will undoubtedly arise from the seamless integration of all of the techniques into a common decision support system allowing the *in silico* generation of formulated products ab initio with the added benefits of consistency, decreased timelines, and cost savings.

REFERENCES

1. Sell PS. *Expert systems—a practical introduction.* Basingstoke, UK: Camelot Press, 1985.
2. Partridge D, Hussain KM. *Knowledge—based information systems.* London: McGraw, 1994.
3. Bradshaw D. The computer learns from experts. *Financial Times London* 27 April 1989.
4. Walko JZ. Turning Dalton's theory into practice. *Innovation* 1989;18:24.
5. Turner J. Product formulation expert system. *Manufacturing Intelligence* 1991;14:13–15.
6. Bentley P. Product Formulation Expert System (PFES). In: Rowe RC, Roberts RJ, *Intelligent software for product formulation.* London: Taylor and Francis, 1998. pp. 27–41.
7. Goodall A. Preface. In: Althoff KD, *A review of industrial case-based reasoning tools.* Oxford: AI Intelligence, 1995.
8. Aamodt A, Plaza E. Case-based reasoning—foundational issues, methodological variations and system approaches. *AI Commun* 1994;7:39–59.
9. Watson I. *Applying case-based reasoning: techniques for enterprising systems.* San Francisco: Morgan Kaufmann, 1997.
10. Stricker H, Haux R, Wetter T, Mann G, Oberhammer L, Flister J, Fuchs S, SchmelmerV. Das Galenische Entwicklungs—System Heidelberg. *Pharm Ind* 1991;53:571–8.
11. Stricker H, Fuchs S, Haux R Rossler R, Rupprecht B, Schmelmer V, Wiegel S. Das Galenische Entwicklungs—System Heidelberg—Systematische Rezepturentwicklung. *Pharm Ind* 1994;56:641–7.

12. Frank J, Rupprecht B, Schmelmer V. Knowledge-based assistance for the development of drugs. *IEEE Expert* 1997;12:40–8.
13. Ramani KV, Patel MR, Patel SK. An expert system for drug preformulation in a pharmaceutical company. *Interfaces* 1992;22:101–8.
14. Rowe RC. Expert systems in solid dosage development. *Pharm Ind* 1993;55:1040–5.
15. Rowe RC, Roberts RJ. *Intelligent software for product formulation.* London: Taylor and Francis, 1998.
16. Rowe RC, Roberts RJ. Expert systems in pharmaceutical development. In Swarbrick J, Boylan JC, editors, *Encyclopedia of pharmaceutical technology* 2nd edition. New York: Marcel Dekker, 2002. pp. 1188–1210.
17. Rowe RC, Craw S, Wiratunga N. Case-based reasoning—a new approach to tablet formulation. *Pharm Tech Eur* 1999;11(2):36–40.
18. Kashihara T, Takahashi Y. Development of computer aided formulation system for tablet (Expert-Tab) 1. *Pharm Tech Japan* 2001;17:699–711.
19. Kashihara T, Development of computer aided formulation system for tablet (expert-Tab) 2. *Pharm Tech Japan* 2001;17:839–56.
20. Kusai A. Development of computer aided formulation system for tablet (expert-Tab) 3. *Pharm Tech Japan* 2001;17:1007–13.
21. Bentham C. Expert system in formulation design, In *Proceedings Computer Aided Formulation*, Coventry, UK 17th October 2001. Reading: Faraday Impact Partnership.
22. Lai S, Podczeck F, Newton JM, Daumesnil R. An expert system to aid the development of capsule formulations. *Pharm Tech Eur* 1996;12(9):60–8.
23. Kashihara T, Yoshioka M. Assessment in Japanese Focus Group. In Hashida M, editor, *Formulation design of oral dosage forms.* Yakagyo-Jiho, 1998. pp. 244–53.
24. Bateman SD, Verlin J, Russo M, Guillot M, Laughlin SM. The development and validation of a capsule formulation knowledge based system. *Pharm Tech* 1996;20(3):174–84.
25. Rowe RC, Wakerly MG, Roberts RJ, Grundy RU, Upjohn NG. Expert Systems for Parenteralo Development. *J Pharm Sci Technol* 1995;49:257–61.
26. Rowe RC, Hall J, Roberts RJ. Film coating formulation using an expert system *Pharm Tech Eur* 1998;10(10):72–82.
27. Wood M. Expert systems save formulation time. *Lab Equipment Digest* 1991 (December) 17–19.
28. Byrd TA. Expert systems in production and operations management; results of a survey. *Interfaces* 1993;23:118–29.
29. Achanta AS, Kowalsk JG, Rhodes CT. Artificial neural networks: implications for pharmaceutical sciences. *Drug Dev Ind Pharm* 1995;21:119–55.
30. Bourquin J, Schmidli H, van Hoogevest P, Leuenberger H. Basic concepts of artificial neural networks (ANN) modelling in the application to pharmaceutical development. *Pharm Dev Technol* 1997;2:95–109.
31. Takayama K, Fujikawa M, Nagai T. Artificial neural networks as a novel method to optimize pharmaceutical formulations. *Pharm Res* 1999;16:1–6.

32. Rowe RC, Colbourn EA. Applications of neural computing in formulation. *Pharmaceutical Visions* 2002. Spring Edition, 4–7.
33. Turkoglu J, Ozarslan R, Sakr A. Artificial neural network analysis of a direct compression tabletting study. *Eur J Pharm Biopharm* 1995;41:315–22.
34. Kesavan JG, Peck GE. Pharmaceutical granulation and tablet formulation using neural networks. *Pharm Dev Technol* 1996;1:391–404.
35. Colbourn EA, Rowe RC. Modelling and optimization of a tablet formulation using neural networks and genetic algorithms. *Pharm Tech Eur* 1996;8(9): 46–55.
36. Rowe RC, Colbourn EA. Generating rules for tablet formulations. *Pharm Tech Eur* 2000;12(1):24–7.
37. Bourquin J, Schmidli H, van Hoogevest P, Leuenberger H. Application of artificial neural networks (ANN) in the development of solid dosage forms. *Pharm Dev Technol* 1997;2:111–21.
38. Bourquin J, Schmidli H, van Hoogevest P, Leuenberger H. Comparison of artificial neural networks (ANN) with classical modelling technologies using different experimental designs and data from a galenical study on a solid dosage form. *Eur J Pharm Sci* 1998;6:287–300.
39. Bourquin J, Schmidli H, van Hoogevest P, Leuenberger H. Advantages of artificial neural networks (ANNs) as alternative modelling technique for data sets showing non-linear relationships using data from a galenical study on a solid dosage form. *Eur J Pharm Sci* 1998;7:5–16.
40. Bourquin J, Schmidli H, van Hoogevest P, Leuenberger H. Pitfalls of artificial neural networks (ANN) modelling technique for data sets containing outlier measurements using a study of mixture properties of a direct compressed tablet dosage form. *Eur J Pharm Sci* 1998;7:17–28.
41. Do Q M., Dang GV, Le NQ. Drawing up and optimizing the formulation of Malumix tablets by an artificial intelligence system (CAD/Chem). *Tap Chi Duoc Hoc* 2000;6:16–19.
42. Rocksloh K, Rapp F-R, Abu Abed S, Mueller W, Reher M, Gauglitz G, Schmidt PC. Optimization of crushing strength and disintegration time of a high dose plant extract tablet by neural networks. *Drug Dev Ind Pharm* 1999; 25:1015–25.
43. Chen U, Thosor SS, Forbess RA, Kemper MS, Rubinovitz RL, Shukla AJ. Prediction of drug content and hardness of intact tablets using artificial neural networks and near-infrared spectroscopy. *Drug Dev Ind Pharm* 2001;27:623–31.
44. Sathe PM, Venitz J. Comparison of neural networks and multiple linear regression as dissolution predictors. *Drug Dev Ind Pharm* 2003;29:349–55.
45. Lindberg N-O, Colbourn EA. Use of artificial neural networks and genetic algorithms—experiences from a tablet formulation. *Pharm Tech Eur* 2004;16(5): 35–9.
46. Plumb AP, Rowe RC, York P, Doherty C. The effect of experimental design in the modelling of a tablet coating formulation using artificial neural networks. *Eur J Pharm Sci* 2002;16:281–8.
47. Plumb AP, Rowe RC, York P, Doherty C. Effect of varying optimization parameters in optimization by guided evolutionary simulated annealing (GESA) using

a tablet film coat on an example formulation. *Eur J Pharm Sci* 2003;18:259–66.

48. Rowe RC, Woolgar CG. Neurofuzzy logic in tablet film coating formulation. *Pharmaceut Sci Technol Today* 1999;2:495–7.
49. Hussain AS, Yu X, Johnson RD. Application of neural computing in pharmaceutical product development. *Pharm Res* 1991;8:1248–52.
50. Hussain AS, Shivanand P, Johnson RD. Application of neural computing in pharmaceutical product development: computer aided formulation design. *Drug Dev Ind Pharm* 1996;20:1739–52.
51. Takahara J, Takayama K, Nagai T. Multi-objective simultaneous optimization technique based on an artificial neural network in sustained release formulations. *J Controlled Release* 1997;49:11–20.
52. Zupancic Bozic D, Vrecar F, Kozjek F. Optimization of diclofenac sodium dissolution from sustained release formulations using an artificial neural network. *Eur J Pharm Sci* 1997;5:163–9.
53. Sheng H, Wang P, Tu J.-S, Yuan L, Pin Q-N. Applications of artificial neural networks to the design of sustained release matrix tablets. *Chinese J Pharmaceut* 1998;29:352–4.
54. Ibric S, Jovanovic M, Djuric A, Parojcic J, Petrovic SD, Solomun L, Stupor B. Artificial neural networks in the modelling and optimization of aspirin extended release tablets with Eudragit L100 as matrix substance. *Pharm Sci Tech* 2003;4:62–70.
55. Wu T, Pao W, Chen J, Shang R. Formulation optimization technique based on artificial neural network in salbutamol sulfate osmotic pump tablets. *Drug Dev Ind Pharm* 2000;26:211–15.
56. Leane MM, Cumming I, Corrigan O. The use of artificial neural networks for the selection of the most appropriate formulation and processing variables in order to predict the in vitro dissolution of sustained release minitablets. *Pharm Sci Tech* 2003;4:218–29.
57. Takahara J, Takayama K, Isowa K, Nagai T. Multi-objective simultaneous optimization based on artificial neural network in a ketoprofen hydrogel formula containing σ-ethylmenthol as a percutaneous absorption enhancer. *Int J Pharm* 1997;158:203–10.
58. Takayama K, Takahara J, Fujikawa M, Ichikawa H, Nagai T. Formula optimization based on artificial neural networks in transdermal drug delivery. *J Controlled Release* 1999;62:161–70.
59. Wu P-C, Obata Y, Fijukawa M, Li CJ, Higashiyama K, Takayama K. Simultaneous optimization based on artificial neural networks in ketoprofen hydrogel formula containing σ-ethyl-3-burylcyclohexanol as a percutaneous absorption enhancer. *J Pharm Sci* 2001;90:1004–14.
60. Agatonovic-Kustrin S, Alany RG. Role of genetic algorithms and artificial neural networks in predicting phase behaviour of colloidal delivery systems. *Pharm Res* 2001;18:1049–55.
61. Agatonovic-Kustrin S, Glass BD, Wisch MH, Alany RG. Prediction of a stable microemulsion formulation for the oral delivery of a combination of antitubercular drugs using ANN technology. *Pharm Res* 2003;20:1760–5.

62. Kandimalla KK, Kanikkannon N, Singh M. Optimization of a vehicle mixture for the transdermal delivery of melatonin using artificial neural networks and response surface method. *J Controlled Release* 1999;61:71–82.
63. Peh KK, Lim CP, Qwek SS, Khoti KH. Use of artificial networks to predict drug dissolution profiles and evaluation of network performance using similarity profile. *Pharm Res* 2000;17:1386–98.
64. Turkoglu M, Varol H, Celikok M. Tableting and stability evaluation of enteric-coated omeprazole pellets. *Eur J Pharm Biopharm* 2004;57:277–86.
65. Yuksel N, Turkoglu M, Baykara T. Modelling of the solvent evaporation method for the preparation of controlled release acrylic microspheres using neural networks. *J Microencapsulation* 2000;17:541–51.
66. Surini S, Akiyama H, Morishita M, Nagai T, Takayama K. Release phenomena of insulin from an implantable device composed of a polyion complex of chitosan and sodium hyaluronate. *J Controlled Release* 2003;90:291–301.
67. Reis MAA, Sinisterra RO, Belchior JC. An alternative approach based on artificial neural networks to study controlled drug release. *J Pharm Sci* 2004; 93:418–28.
68. Rees C. *Neural Computing—Learning Solutions—User Survey.* Department of Trade and Industry, London, UK, 1996.
69. Al-Khattat IM, Al-Hassani STS. Towards a computer-aided analysis and design of tablet compaction. *Chem Eng Sci* 1987;44:707–12.
70. Michrafy A, Ringenbacher D, Tchoreloff P. Modelling the compaction behaviour of powders: Application to pharmaceutical powders. *Powder Technol.* 2002;127:257–66.
71. Wu C-Y, Ruddy OM, Bentham AC, Hancock BC, Best SM, Elliot JA. Modelling the mechanical behaviour of pharmaceutical powders during compaction. *Powder Technol* 2005;152:107–17.
72. Lewis RW, Gethin DT, Yang XS, Rowe RC. A combined finite-discrete element method for simulating pharmaceutical powder tableting. *Int J Num Meth Eng* 2005;62:853–69.
73. Yang XS, Lewis RW, Gethin DT, Rowe RC. Modelling of pharmaceutical powder compaction and tableting: effect of particle sizes and irregular shape. *Powder Technol.* 2005 in press.
74. Rowe RC, York P, Colbourn EA, Roskilly S. The influence of pellet shape, size and distribution on capsule filling-a preliminary evaluation of three dimensional computer simulation using a Monte Carlo technique. *Int J Pharm* 2005; 300:32–7.
75. Rowe RC, Roberts RJ. Simulation of crack propagation in tablet film coatings containing pigments. *Int J Pharm* 1992;78:49–57.
76. Rowe RC, Roberts RJ. The effect of some formulation variables on crack propagation in pigmented tablet film coatings using computer simulation. *Int J Pharm* 1992;86:49–58.

29

LEGAL PROTECTION OF INNOVATIVE USES OF COMPUTERS IN R&D

ROBERT HARRISON

Contents

29.1 INTRODUCTION

The days in which IP (intellectual property) strategists were separated into groups of pharmacologists (chemists or biologists) and other groups of computer scientists are slowly passing—in the same manner in which the tech-

Computer Applications in Pharmaceutical Research and Development, Edited by Sean Ekins.
ISBN 0-471-73779-8

nologies are increasingly overlapping in the scientific world. Pharmacology patent lawyers had typically spent their apprenticeship in the laboratory working with chemicals or using polymerase chain reaction (PCR) techniques; they understood how small molecular entities functioned and characterized sequences of RNA, DNA, and proteins. Their initial training was in drafting patents on gene sequences or on small chemical entities and methods of treating disease. Computer scientists, on the other hand, spent hours programming computers and later writing software and business method patents. Just as understanding the application of computers in pharmacology presents a challenge for researchers in both fields, it also means that the IP specialists also need to combine strategies from both fields to obtain the best possible legal protection for innovation.

A few years ago a study [1] carried out by the London-based consulting firm Silico Research reported that very few patent applications had been filed in bioinformatics. The reasons cited in the study for the scarcity of patents included the fact that many current bioinformatics products merely combined existing data sources into a single product and the difficulty of proving infringement of software patents. A further reason noted was that the industry was then so new that many patent applications might still be pending [2]. The United States Patent and Trademark Office (USPTO) recognized in 1999 that bioinformatics represented a special challenge and that same year created a special examination group—Art Unit 1631—to examine the increasing number of applications [3]. Since these studies were published, however, the growth in the number of bioinformatics patents seems to have stalled. This is probably a reflection of the state of the industry.

29.2 INTELLECTUAL PROPERTY RIGHTS

The term "intellectual property rights" is used to describe the legal instruments for protecting innovation. Although there are often differences in the laws governing these rights in different countries, almost all countries recognize the basic types of intellectual property that are summarized in Table 29.1 [4]. Member states of the World Trade Organisation have all committed to introducing these rights [5]. Of these rights, the most important in the application of computers to pharmaceutical research and development are patents, copyrights, and database rights.

29.2.1 Patents

Patents are the most important and strongest type of intellectual property. Patents protect inventions or technical innovations. Patents do not protect new designs (these are protected by copyright or registered designs), nor do

TABLE 29.1 Types of Intellectual Property Rights (IPR)

Type of IPR	Protects	Maximum Lifetime (generally—may vary from country to country)
Patent	Technical ideas	20 years from filing
Copyright	Literary works including computer programs	70 years from death of author or date of creation (in the case of joint works)
Database rights	Collection of data (only exists in the European Union and some other countries—the US is discussing the proposal)	70 years from the date of creation
Trade secrets	Secret nondisclosed information	Unlimited, as long as access is limited to a select group
Design	Aesthetic creation (generally not relevant in the pharmaceutical field)	Varies from country to country; 25 years in the European Union from application; 14 years in the United States from grant
Trademarks	Brand name or sign designating a product	Unlimited, as long as the trademark remains in use

they protect new brand names (trademark protection). Patents are granted for inventions that are novel (i.e., not known in the prior art) and are also not obvious—or have an inventive step—when compared to the prior art. In the application of computers to pharmaceutical applications, both hardware inventions and software inventions can be protected by patents. The hardware might consist of a microarray, a processor, memory and a display device. The software would consist of the set of instructions processed in the processor for processing data obtained from the microarray and stored in the memory. Hardware inventions are clearly patentable, and, despite misgivings in some quarters [6], it is now generally recognized that software can be protected by patents. In the United States, the decision of the Court of Appeal in the so-called "State Street" case [7] opened the way for much more far-reaching patent protection for computer-implemented inventions than had been previously granted. In that decision the Court stated that the sole test for determining whether an innovation is patentable is whether a "useful, concrete, or tangible" result was obtained.

The proposed European Directive (i.e., EU law) on the patenting of computer-implemented inventions [8] has led to a debate in Europe on the desirability of patents on software. The debate recently culminated in a vote by the European Parliament, which rejected the proposed legislation [9].

The European Patent Office (Munich, Germany) has issued a statement in which they stated that they would continue to grant patents in accordance with existing practice [10]. Under this practice the European Patent Office will grant patents on software or computer-implemented inventions when a technical effect is present [11], even if the European Patent Convention appears to state that patents cannot be granted for computer programs [12]. The European Patent Office realized fairly soon after its foundation in 1978 that this exclusion was illogical and, in one of the first decisions issued by the Boards of Appeal [13], pointed out that the wording of the European Patent Convention excluded only the patenting of computer programs *as such*. A general-purpose computer programmed for a special purpose is, however, not excluded from patentability as long as it produces a technical effect.

The initial decision—often called the VICOM decision after the applicant for the patent—was followed by further decisions of the Boards of Appeal that opened the way for the patenting of inventions implemented by means of computers. The reasoning behind these decisions has often been adopted by courts in other countries (not only in Europe, but elsewhere). The German Supreme Court, for example, has explicitly stated that the application of computers in chemistry or biology is acceptable patentable subject matter [14].

Patents on Algorithms. Whereas until recently much of the analysis of data in pharmaceutical research and development was carried out essentially by manual processes, the volume of data that is currently being generated means that increasingly sophisticated algorithms are being used to order, sort, and analyze the data.

No patent office will allow the patenting of an algorithm per se without reference to its practical application. The European Patent Convention clearly states that scientific theories and mathematical methods are not to be regarded as being inventions [15]. As discussed above, the USPTO (Washington, DC) and the US courts are looking for a concrete, useful, and tangible result to justify the grant of a patent. When an application of the algorithm is involved, patent protection can be secured. For example, the European Patent Office points out in its Guidelines for Examination that an electrical filter designed with a mathematical method would not be excluded from patentability [16].

This certainly suggests that any algorithm used in the analysis of data, such as DNA sequence or protein data, should be patentable as long as it is not couched in purely mathematical terms but is applied to achievement of a useful, concrete, and tangible result. Thus, for example, an algorithm such as the Smith–Waterman algorithm to identify homologies among proteins [17] would have been patentable because it offers a useful, concrete, and tangible result and is a means of obtaining information about the homologies. Similarly, an algorithm to mine data for potentially useful properties of a drug or for monitoring side effects of a drug is also protectable: An example would be an algorithm that efficiently searches annotations in databases for information about potential adverse side effects.

Patents on Human Interfaces. Most computer programs for use in pharmaceutical research and development must interact with a human researcher. Given the amount of data that can be potentially provided to the researcher, efficient means are needed to present the data in a readily understood manner. In Europe such methods of presenting information are excluded from patent protection [18]. However, several decisions from the European Patent Office indicate that patents might be granted if the information presented is more than just "mere" data. For example, the European Patent Office granted a patent on a method for displaying one of a set of predetermined messages indicating a specific event that may occur in an input/output device of a word processing system. The European Board of Appeal stated that giving visual indications automatically about conditions prevailing in an apparatus or system is basically a technical problem [19] and thus is not excluded from patentability. Applying the reasoning behind this decision to computer programs for use in pharmaceutical research and development, it is probable that the European Patent Office would have a generally favorable view of the patentability of an interface through which information is presented to a user about conditions prevailing in an apparatus or system, such as in a laboratory instrument. In the United States the Patent Office is likely to be less restrictive in issuing patents because the methods of presenting information are not excluded per se from patents. It is indeed possible that a patent granted in the United States would be refused in Europe for this reason.

Patents on Machine-Machine Interfaces. Unlike patents on machine-human interfaces, patents are regularly granted in both the United States and in Europe on the interfaces to a computer program. Such patents can be extremely valuable as they can allow the creator of the computer program to limit the access to the computer program only to others to whom a license to use the interface has been granted. During the course of the debate on patents for computer-implemented inventions in the European Parliament an amendment was proposed that would, in effect, have prevented the enforcement of patents on interfaces [20]. As mentioned above, this proposal has been dropped, and thus there is currently no restriction on patenting such interfaces. As discussed below, copyright protection on interfaces is, however, limited.

The use of patents on machine-machine interfaces can be illustrated by considering the example of a microarray. The data obtained by the microarray can be processed by any computer system running a suitable program. The data are transferred from the microarray to the computer system through an interface, and use of a patented interface can be restricted only to the patent holder and its licensees.

Patents on Data Structures. Much of the early interest in the application of computer programs to pharmaceutical research and development was focused on the construction of databases to record data generated by drug testing, high-throughput screening, or gene sequencing experiments. The experimental data in such early databases were often stored in a simple flat file structure. Subsequently, relational database structures were developed to allow the more efficient and significant analysis of the data stored therein. The structure of these databases can be protected by patents. It is unlikely, however, that a claim to a database structure per se without any reference to its application would be seen to be patentable because the structure by itself does not produce a useful, tangible, or concrete result. A patent application on the application of the database structure to a particular pharmaceutical problem would be more likely to be granted.

In the United States, this point was discussed in a decision that related to a computer memory with a novel hierarchical and relational data structure [21]. The patent was allowed in this case.

In a further case relating to the structure of data stored on or in a record carrier used in a picture retrieval system, the European Patent Office's Boards of Appeal have considered the issue of patentability of a data structure [22]. Initially the patent application had been rejected on the grounds that the presentation of data was excluded from patentability (see above). However, in accepting an appeal filed by the patent applicant, the Board pointed out that there was a difference between the functional data, which controlled the technical working of the system, and the cognitive information, which represented the picture that could be retrieved and displayed. The Board stated that functional data relates to data that control the technical operation of the system. These data do not relate to the presentation of information, and thus data structures containing this information should be patentable. On the other hand, the cognitive information relates to the picture that could be retrieved and displayed.

The reasoning behind the Board's decision can be applied not only to video or television systems but also to data structures used in computer programs in the pharmaceutical field. Consider, for example, genomic screening carried out with microarrays in which target cDNA sequences or oligonucleotides are placed at a number of sites on a chip and the material to be analyzed is washed over the chip. At some sites, some of the genetic material will become bound to the cDNA or oligonucleotides. The position of the sites is detected by fluorescence or another means. The sheer number of sites on a chip (Affymetrix, for example, has a chip with 400,000 sites) means that it is impossible for a human being to record all of the sites at which the genetic material is bound to the target. Instead the detection is carried out automatically, and the results are fed into a computer. The computer program processes the data and produce them in a form that can be understood and interpreted by a human.

Applying the Board's decision to the data generated in the use of microarrays would suggest that a data structure is patentable if the data relate to the control of a microarray experiment or to the display of information obtained from a microarray experiment. Furthermore, as data relating to the DNA sequences or protein structure are not merely "cognitive information," it is possible to argue that data structures containing the information on the DNA sequences or on the protein structure will be patentable.

In the microarray example described above, the information exchanged between the computer program that analyzed the microarray data and the microarray itself relates to conditions prevailing in the apparatus. Therefore, the interface between the processor implementing the computer program and the microarray should be patentable. Similarly, displays of DNA or protein sequence data on an output device give information about conditions prevailing in a microarray experiment, and a method for displaying this information should, consistent with the Board's reasoning, also be patentable.

29.2.2 Copyright

Copyright is traditionally used to protect literary works or works of art from copying or from the making of so-called derivative works, that is, new works based on a protected work. More recently, protection under the copyright laws has been extended to software. In the United States, software is protected as a literary work [23] and registration of the copyright is carried out at the US Copyright Office (www.copyright.gov). Until 1991, the situation in Europe was more complicated as protection was granted under national laws rather than on an EU-wide basis. Council Directive 91/250/EEC on the Legal Protection of Computer Programs of 14 May 2001 [24] introduced a common protection within the member states of the EU under which software was to be protected as a literary work. No requirements other than original authorship of the software were to be required before protection would be granted. The EU did not introduce a registration system for the protection of computer software under copyright law.

Most other major industrial countries have adopted similar rules, and in 2002 the World Intellectual Property Organisation (WIPO) Copyright Treaty of 1996 [25] entered into force for a number of countries, including Japan and the United States. Signatories to this treaty must ensure that computer programs are protected as literary works [26].

Compared to patent protection, copyright has a major disadvantage. Copyright only protects the so-called "expression" of the innovation, that is, the computer code, and protection does not extend to the innovation itself. In other words, the idea behind the program can be copied, as long as the code itself is not copied or adapted. Copyright protection can extend also to flow diagrams or pseudocode, and so these cannot be used to create a new (derived) program. Reverse engineering of computer code is also not allowed. However, in the European Union, use of reverse engineering is allowed if the intention is to obtain information about interfaces between computer programs [27].

29.2.3 Protection of Databases

In addition to the patenting of database structures (see 29.2.1), a database can be protected either by copyright protection or by so-called database rights. The extent to which information in the database can be protected by copyright varies widely depending on the country involved. In many countries, copyright protection is not available for information contained in databases. Other countries, such as Australia [28], consider that the arrangement and collection of the information may be so significant that copyright can be granted on the database. In contrast, the US Supreme Court in 1991 rejected the so-called "sweat of the brow" theory that previously had accorded copyright protection to informational compilations [29].

In 1996 the European Union adopted the European Database Rights Directive [30] to harmonize protection of the information contained within databases. The directive protects "a collection of independent works, data or other materials arranged in a systematic or methodical way and individually accessible by electronic or other means" [31]. Thus a developer of a database can prevent the extraction and/or reuse of all or a substantial part of the contents of the database [32]. This means that a party that creates, for example, a database comprising genome sequence data or protein structure data can stop others from using these data without permission. Unfortunately, protection under the European Database Rights Directive is limited only to persons or legal entities residing in the European Economic Area (the European Union, Norway, Iceland, and Liechtenstein) or in countries having similar protection schemes. It is only the database itself that is protected. The individual items of information contained within the database are not protected.

There have been several proposals to introduce a similar protection right in the United States, but these have not been successful to date.

29.2.4 Trade Secrets

Trade secret protection is probably the weakest of all intellectual property rights. The US Uniform Trade Secret Act defines a trade secret as information, including a formula, pattern, compilation, program device, method, technique, or process, that (1) derives independent economic value, actual or potential, from not being generally known to, and not being readily ascertainable by proper means by, other persons who can obtain economic value from its disclosure or use and (2) is the subject of efforts that are reasonable under the circumstances to maintain its secrecy [33].

Under this definition—which is similar to the definitions adopted by other countries—trade secret protection is available only for information that is known to a smallish group of persons and that is considered by that group to be confidential and economically valuable. Once the information becomes more widely known, it no longer qualifies for trade secret protection because its value has been lost. As a result, once the information has become generally known, it can be freely used by other companies for their own purposes.

Trade secrets (or "undisclosed information") are also protected under the TRIPS Agreement [34]. Despite this international agreement, there is a wide range of difference in the manner in which countries implement these provisions. Few countries, apart from the United States, have explicit provisions in their laws on the protection of trade secrets. In some countries, protection is only granted when a former employee takes confidential information to a new employer, whereas in other countries, protection is granted more widely. Unfortunately, once a trade secret is no longer a trade secret it can be freely used by anybody else who obtained the information fairly. The value of the trade secret is thus much more limited than, for example, patents or copyrights.

Trade secret protection can play a significant role in the protection of computer software. If the code is only released in object form and the source code is not readily available, then the source code—so long as it is only known to a limited group of programmers—remains covered by trade secret protection. As long as it is not published, any disclosure of the code would be considered to be an infringement of the creators' trade secrets. Data on the efficacy of new drugs, as long as their origination requires considerable effort, are also protected under the TRIPS Agreement [35]. The regulatory authorities are required to keep the information supplied confidential.

29.3 ENFORCEMENT OF RIGHTS

Obtaining IP protection is only the first step. The intellectual property rights obtained are only useful if they can be exploited and—ultimately—unauthorized users of the rights can be stopped from exploiting them.

This presents a fairly unique problem in the computer science field. IP rights are essentially national rights. They are only valid in the country in which they are granted or registered. A valid US patent is only valid in the United States, a Canadian copyright only valid in Canada. Even a so-called European patent is, in effect, a bundle of national patents valid in various European countries. This raises a problem in a situation in which, for example, the user of a computer program is in one country and the server is in another country.

Courts in both the United States and the United Kingdom have had to deal with this issue in patent infringements unrelated to pharmaceutical science.

In the United States, the dispute centered around the popular Blackberry e-mail devices [36]. A US company, NTP Inc., sued the makers of the Blackberry device, the Canadian company Research in Motion, for patent infringement. The Blackberry devices were being used in the United States and were connected to a US cell phone network. E-mails to the user were routed through Canada. Thus an e-mail sent from someone in the United States to another person in the United States would inevitably be routed through Canada. The court decided—citing an older decision—that because control of the delivery of the e-mail message to the Blackberry device was initiated through a US-based user, the use of the Blackberry device occurred within the United States, even though the messages might be transmitted outside the United States.

In the United Kingdom, a similar issue was decided with respect to a gaming system [37]. One of the UK's largest bookmakers, William Hill, had set up an Internet-based gaming system based on a computer system located in Antigua or Curacao. The UK Court of Appeal decided that even though the host computer on which the gaming system was located was outside of the UK, it had effect in the UK. Gamers could access the host computer from their (British based) home computers through the Internet. Thus the judge concluded that the there was infringement of the patent in the UK.

Both of these decisions are significant because they suggest that any scientist using unauthorized patented computer software in pharmaceutical research and development would be infringing the patent even if the computer (for example, a database server) was located in another country. Thus connecting to a database in another country or running the computer program on a remote server is unlikely to avoid—at least in the UK and in the US—patent infringement. No decisions are known from other countries on similar matters, but it is probable that the courts in other countries would be influenced in their own decisions by the British and US judges.

The two court decisions only relate to patent rights. The issue of whether a copyright infringement occurs when the user is located in one country and the copyrighted software is run on another computer in another country has, as far as the author is aware, not yet been the subject of litigation. However, because even running the copyrighted software remotely would lead to at least part of the software or the results of the program being displayed on the user's machine, it is probable that a court would consider that to be sufficient to be a copyright infringement.

29.4 CONCLUSION

The use of computers in developing new pharmaceutical products is nowadays commonplace, and a number of tools and databases have been developed to improve their use. Although intellectual property rights have to date rarely been the subject of court cases, protection is available and the courts are prepared to enforce these rights, even in an international context.

REFERENCES

1. Toner B. Bioinformatics patents remain a rarity in IP-heavy biopharmaceutical industry. *GenomeWeb*, 4 July 2001 (http://www.genomeweb.com)
2. Patent Applications generally remain unpublished for 18 months after their first filing.
3. Steinberg D. New PTO Unit examines Bioinformatics Application. *The Scientist* 27 November 2000;200:14(23);8.
4. Adapted from Robert Harrison, Protecting innovation in bioinformatics and in-silico biology. *Biodrugs* 2003:17(4):227–31.
5. TRIPS Agreement (Agreement on Trade Related Aspects of Intellectual Property). Available at URL http://www.wto.int/english/docs_e/legal_e/27-trips_01_e.htm.
6. Nichols R. The age of software patents. *Computer* April 1999:25–31.
7. *State Street Bank & Trust Co. Inc. v. Signature Financial Group* 149 F.3d 1368 (Fed Cir Jul 23, 1998).
8. Proposal for a Directive of the European Parliament and of the Council on the patentability of Computer-Implemented Inventions, COM (2002) 92 final. Available from URL http://europa.eu.int/comm/internal_market/en/indprop/comp/com02-92en.pdf.
9. Bodini S. EU software patent law is dead managing intellectual property. *Weekly News*, 11 July 2005. Accessible at http://www.managingip.com/?Page=9&PUBID=198&ISS=17456&SID=524170&SM=ALL&SearchStr=computer-implemented%20inventions
10. European Patent Office Press Release. European Patent Office continues to advocate harmonisation in the field of CII patents, 6 July 2005. Accessible at http://www.european-patent-office.org/news/pressrel/2005_07_06_e.htm
11. Programs for Computers in Guidelines for Examination in the European Patent Office, Part C, Chapter IV, Nr. 53, European Patent Office, October 2001. Available at URL http://www.european-patent office.org/legal/gui_lines/e/index.htm
12. European Patent Convention, Art 52 (2). Available from URL http://www.european-patent-office.org/legal/epc/e/ar52.html#A52
13. Decision T0208/84 of 15 July 1986 "Computer-related Invention/VICOM." *OJ EPO* 1987:14–23.
14. Decision X ZB 16/00 Suche Fehlerhafter Zeichenketten, 17 October 2001. Available from URL http://www.bundesgerichtshof.de
15. European Patent Convention, Art. 52 (2) (a). Available from URL http://www.european-patent-office.org/legal/epc/e/ar52.html#A52
16. See Ref. 10.
17. Smith TF, Waterman MS. Identification of common molecular subsequences. *J Mol Biol* 1981;147:195–7.
18. Art. 53 (2) (d) European Patent Convention. Available at URL http://www.european-patent-office.org/legal/epc/e/ar53.html#A53
19. T0115/85 "Computer-related Invention/IBM." *OJ EPO* 1990:30–4.
20. European Parliament Committee on Legal Affairs Recommendation for Second Reading on the Council common position for adopting a directive of the

European Parliament and of the Council on the patentability of computer-implemented inventions. Document Number 11979/1/2004—C6-0058/2005—2002/0047(COD).

21. *In re Lowry*, 31 USPQ 2d 1301 (Fed Circ 1994)
22. Decision T1194/97–3.5.2 of 15 March 2001. "Data Structure Product/PHILIPS" *OJ EPO* December 2000: 515–573.
23. 17 USC §102 (a) (1).
24. Copyright Directive EU Official Journal L 122, 17 May 1991 42–46
25. http://www.wipo.int/clea/docs/en/wo/wo033en.htm
26. Art. 4 WIPO Copyright Treaty. Available from URL http://www.wipo.int/treaties/en/ip/wct/trtdocs_wo033.html#P56_5626
27. Art. 6 of Copyright Directive (see Ref. 24).
28. *Telstra Corporation Limited v. Desktop Marketing Systems Pty Ltd* [2001] FXA 612 (15 May 2001).
29. *Feist Publications v. Rural Telephone Service Corp.*, 499 US 340 (1991)
30. OJ European Union No. L77, 27 March 1996, 20. (the "Database Directive")
31. Art. 1 Database Directive (see Ref. 30).
32. Art. 5 Database Directive (see Ref. 30).
33. §1 (4) Uniform Trade Secrets Act. Available at http://nsi.org/Library/Espionage/usta.htm
34. Art. 39 (2). Available at URL http://www.wto.int/english/docs_e/legal_e/27-trips_04d_e.htm#7
35. Art. 39 (3) (see Ref. 34.)
36. *NTP v Research in Motion*, US Court of Appeals for the Federal Circuit, 03-1615. Available at URL http://www.fedcir.gov/opinions/03-1615.pdf
37. *Menashe Business Mercantile v William Hill Organisation* 2002 EWCA Civ 1702. Available at URL http://www.hmcourts-service.gov.uk/judgmentsfiles/j1398/menashe_v_william_hill.htm

30

THE ETHICS OF COMPUTING IN PHARMACEUTICAL RESEARCH

MATTHEW K. MCGOWAN AND RICHARD J. MCGOWAN

Contents

30.1 INTRODUCTION

There is no doubt that computers, computing technology, and the consequent information systems have produced ethical challenges and conflicts. The challenges and conflicts have been presented not only to the practitioner facing new problems but also to the professional philosopher dealing with computer use at a conceptual level. As well, the challenges and conflicts are not only individual, often arising from practical experience, but also collective, involv-

Computer Applications in Pharmaceutical Research and Development, Edited by Sean Ekins.
ISBN 0-471-73779-8

ing judgments regarding policy and procedure. These broad observations are no less true for the use of computers generally as for the use of computers in pharmaceutical research.

We propose to examine the ethics of computing in pharmaceutical research and the challenges therein. We begin the examination with an overview of how philosophers regard computer ethics. The community of philosophers is uncertain that it is not facing, quite possibly, a whole new domain of inquiry with regard to computer ethics. After addressing the matter of how to regard computer ethics in terms of its philosophical classification, we identify the issues and areas in which philosophers have shown the most interest with regard to computer ethics, namely, the issues of privacy, liability, ownership, and power. As we address these areas, we note problems more specific to the computer user in pharmaceutical research and make suggestions about the place of ethics in pharmaceutical research. Finally, we look at some codes of conduct relevant to the use of computers.

30.2 PHILOSOPHY AND COMPUTER ETHICS

As a general observation, we can say that the philosophical community was slow to understand the ethical and conceptual challenges posed by the advent of computers. Although computers had existed for some time, the *Philosopher's Index*, which classifies and catalogs philosophical literature, had no entries under the heading of "computer ethics" until 1985. In the five years from 1985 to 1989, only three articles, monographs, or books were classified and listed under "computer ethics." There were only two such items listed between 1990 and 1994. However, 19 items were listed between 1995 and 1999 and 18 items were listed between 2000 and 2004.

Inasmuch as computers have been present in the workplace and at home since the late 1970s, the dearth of philosophical literature before 1995 suggests that interest in and awareness of the ethical challenges computers pose did not occupy much of the philosophical community's concern. A partial explanation for this situation may involve the manner in which the United States deals with privacy issues. Computer technology and computer use developed in America, but America deals with the issue of privacy on a piecemeal basis rather than as Europe deals with privacy, namely, with "comprehensive, overarching law" [1]. Therefore, the issue of privacy, one of the most important and early issues to arise with regard to computer use, was not a matter of debate on a national level. There was no demand for a "comprehensive, overarching law" or a comprehensive, overarching policy on the right to privacy. Little debate occurred on the issue of privacy until the problem of protecting privacy grew bigger.

Another reason philosophers were slow to provide ethical and conceptual analysis regarding computer use is that, more often than not, technology develops in a philosophical vacuum. That is, technology is developed by people with little training, formal or informal, in philosophy, including ethics. The ignorance of ethics on the part of technologists and computer gurus mirrors the ignorance (and subsequent disinterest) of philosophers about technology and technological development. Thus development occurs with unintended and unforeseen ethical consequences. It is not a question of technologists being "evil" or somehow malevolent—although that is possible for any group of people, philosophers included—but that the ignorance of the cognitive content in ethics and the initial lack of technological knowledge on the part of the philosophical community more easily permits problematic ethical results.

In making these observations, we may only be providing an echo of C. P. Snow's *The Two Cultures*, based on his Rede lecture for Cambridge University [2]. Snow's main point was that the lack of communication between the sciences and the humanities was a regrettable situation rife with negative consequences. *The Two Cultures* was meant to be both an admonition to thinkers and an invitation to have scientists and humanists work harder at understanding each other.

Snow followed that book with a modified version, *The Two Cultures: A Second Look* [3]. In this 1963 book, he suggested that a third culture would soon be upon us. As some have noted, for example, McGowan [4], that culture was fully upon us by the mid-1980s. But if we have three cultures, those of the scientist, the humanist, and the technologist, communication between the three could still improve along the lines Snow suggested.

If there had been better communication between humanists and technologists, philosophers might already have resolved the matter of how computer ethics should be viewed. Of the forty-two articles listed in the *Philosopher's Index* under the category "computer ethics," at least a dozen either focused on or touched upon the place of computer ethics in the pantheon of philosophy [see, e.g., 5–12]. The most basic question facing philosophers is the uniqueness of computer ethics.

Some have argued that computer ethics is a subdiscipline of applied ethics [5, 13]. As such, examining other subdisciplines of applied ethics would prove fruitful to resolving issues that arise in computer ethics. For instance, Wong and Steinke [13] argue that computer ethics shares many similarities with medical ethics and business ethics. They suggest that the fields of medical ethics and business ethics can be useful as models for computer ethics.

Others suggest that computer ethics is a type of professional ethics [14]. If this is the case, then computer ethics is not such a brand new thing and considered judgments already in the common body of knowledge suffice to resolve challenges posed by computers. In other words, the area of computer ethics is not so unique.

Proponents of the two positions just mentioned, that computer ethics is a subdiscipline of applied ethics and that computer ethics is a type of professional ethics, severely understate the case of computer ethics, according to others. Gorniak-Kocikowska [11], stating partial agreement with an earlier work by Moor, suggests that the "computer revolution" is not as similar to the Industrial Revolution—Moor's analogy—as it is to the printing press revolution. Gorniak believes a new ethical theory will be consequent upon the computer revolution.

For a book such as this one, that is, a book dealing primarily with scientific and technological questions, the history of computer ethics as a field of inquiry might be thought of as being beside the point. However, as Johnson [15] states, "this intimate connection between technology and human action is also important for understanding the uniqueness issue in computer ethics." In other words, how the question of the uniqueness of computer ethics is resolved bears upon the resolutions to questions arising from computer use, a point Floridi and Sanders [16] intimate as well. The situation for the pharmaceutical researcher is whether ethics and argumentation thereof applies generally or to the use of computers in pharmaceutical research specifically.

Inasmuch as philosophers have not resolved what they refer to as "the uniqueness question," we caution that the field of computer ethics is still very dynamic, malleable, and young. There will be a lot of rethinking of the issues related to computer use in the years ahead. Nonetheless, dealing with computers and their use is not a free-for-all where "anything goes," a viewpoint specifically attacked by Gottarbarn [14]. A considerable body of knowledge, in the form of considered opinions and judgments, exists.

30.3 ETHICAL ISSUES: PRIVACY, LIABILITY, OWNERSHIP, AND POWER

The single best source for quick and reasonably thorough access to the body of knowledge associated with computer ethics is Deborah Johnson's *Computer Ethics* (3rd edition, 2001). The first edition of that work [17], the first book listed under "computer ethics" in the *Philosopher's Index*, provides a conceptual framework for the issues of privacy, liability, ownership, and power. Despite its very early appearance in the short history of computer ethics, much of the analysis retains its value.

For one thing, the first part of the book presents a modest introduction to the basic considerations that applied ethics most often employs, namely, rights, justice, and utility. The concept of rights, which are an individual's entitlements to those liberties, choices, opportunities, and items having serious consequence for human life, is precisely what privacy depends on for protection. As well, the concept of rights significantly bears upon questions of ownership, that is, the right to property.

The concept of justice, that is, the matter of giving each person what is due that person, is necessarily connected to the distribution of benefits and burdens, whatever they might be and however they are conceived. The relationship between computer use and power will turn on the moral concept of justice, especially distributive justice. As many business ethics textbooks claim, for example, Velasquez [18], the formal rule of justice is that "equals should be treated equally and unequals treated unequally." Although this formal rule is silent about what features make individuals equal or unequal, the rule does incorporate basic notions of ethics into justice, namely, consistency and impartiality. We normally think that *ceteris paribus, omnes res pares esse debunt*—all things being equal, all things should be equal. The formal rule encapsulates that intuition. With regard to the issues related to computer ethics, matters pertaining to liability and power will rely heavily on the concept of justice.

However, all the issues enumerated may be dealt with using a consequentialist approach to moral decision making. The consequentialist approach looks, as the name suggests, at the consequences of an action or policy. The morally correct decision, a consequentialist maintains, is the decision that produces the act or policy, among all available acts or policies, that maximizes the net benefit for all parties concerned, taking into account all foreseeable consequences. The rule regarding consequences, known as the utilitarian principle, may come into conflict with the moral considerations of rights and of justice.

Suppose, for example, that a person has a highly contagious and highly fatal disease. The people who come into contact with the person stand a good chance of getting the disease themselves, and thus their lives would be in jeopardy. The greatest net benefit by way of action may be to make public the sick person's medical condition. However, there is a right to privacy that protects the sick individual's medical record from public release. Does the utilitarian gain override the individual's right to privacy and, even if so, are there certain conditions under which such information should not be made public?

30.3.1 Privacy

The previous sort of question is relevant to the matter of computer use and the issue of privacy. In fact, computer use may have altered the way we think and should think of privacy. Before the advent and prevalence of computers, intrusions into an individual's privacy were largely time- and place dependent. The intrusion could be done but only on a small scale. As Johnson [15] notes, however, computers have changed the nature of intrusion into privacy as well as the scale of intrusion into privacy. The result is a demand to rethink privacy and rethink the framework of applied ethics, especially because the scale of intrusion may change the qualitative nature of the offense.

Nonetheless, the rethinking would not alter the basic notion of the right to privacy. Philosophers have normally thought of the right to privacy as Justice Brandeis did over a century ago, namely, as "the right to be let alone" [19]. More narrowly defined, the right to privacy is thought of as the right of individuals to determine the nature, scope, and manner of information revealed about themselves [20]. The right to privacy is essentially a matter of an individual's controlling the information about himself or herself. And, as has been pointed out, the supplier normally controls that which he or she supplies [21]. Supplying information about an individual should be in the hands of the individual. It takes little effort to see that computer use in pharmaceutical research could produce violations of the right to privacy, construed broadly or narrowly.

But as philosophers have remarked and courts have ruled, the right to privacy is not absolute. In fact, the place and importance of the right to privacy are still being explored, as the Supreme Court decisions in *Roe v. Wade* (1973) and *Planned Parenthood v. Casey* (1992) demonstrate. As a result, decisions regarding the right to privacy are very often driven by context. Such may be the case with situations involving computer use, the right to privacy, and pharmaceutical research.

Philosophers have identified three general aspects with regard to the right to privacy. For any intrusion into the right to privacy, the elements of relevance, consent, and method must be considered. The element of relevance involves the necessity of the intrusion into privacy as bearing a direct relationship to the matter at hand. For instance, in employer-employee relationships, the employer may, at times, investigate work-related problems by encroaching upon the employee's private life. Such "encroachments" must be relevant to the job the employee does. For matters relating to pharmaceutical research, the most likely problem with regard to privacy is the possibility of learning more about an individual than the scope of the research permits. Generally speaking, such information must be disregarded and destroyed.

Assuming that standard codes of conduct, for example, the Nuremburg Code (1947) and the World Medical Association's Declaration of Helsinki, are followed by researchers, the element of consent will already have been satisfied. In fact, as far as the element of consent to the intrusion into privacy goes, the medical community's doctrine of "informed consent" is a very strict application of the element of consent. We may note that the specific "informed consent" of an individual human subject of research may not be adequate to the decisions surrounding data mining.

The third element involved with possible intrusions into the right to privacy specifies that the method of inquiring into the private life of an individual be ordinary and reasonable. This is an area in which technological development has had significant impact: What was extraordinary and unreasonable in the 1970s has now become standard practice. For instance, routine preemployment drug-testing of individuals was an unheard-of practice thirty or forty years ago. Now, preemployment drug-testing is accepted. The evolution of technology marks, again, an aspect of privacy that suggests a context-dependent right. The right to privacy protects physical and psychological privacy inasmuch as those aspects of privacy are "culturally recognized as private" (Velasquez [18]). The right to privacy stretches or contracts with cultural notions, and it is a simple fact that culture changes.

In fact, as Ware [1] points out, the threats to the right to privacy were viewed in the 1970s as originating primarily from the government. The phrase "Big Brother is watching" meant that government officials had control over information on citizens. Now, however, a huge information industry has evolved and the biggest threats derive from private parties. Pharmaceutical researchers need not and ought not contribute to the supply of information available about an individual. Furthermore, given the advent and techniques of data mining, researchers should take precautions and build prohibitors into research that would prevent identification of any individual subject of the research.

30.3.2 Liability

Johnson [17] identifies several topics related to liability, and she offers an important distinction as well. Among the topics related to liability and computer use in general are legal liability, the duty of honesty, the nature of contracts, misrepresentation, express and implied warranties, and negligence [17]. The relevant distinction concerns the nature of software as either a product or a service. Many of these topics hold little interest for the ethicist investigating computer ethics. For instance, legal liability is less important to philosophy than to jurisprudence.

On the other hand, a topic such as the duty of honesty, although generally stated, holds a lot of interest for the philosopher for the particular manner in which the duty of honesty might appear in research using human subjects. The duty of honesty governs informed consent with regard to health risks, but it could also serve as a springboard to inform human subjects of the potential risks to privacy as well, even if those risks are not well understood.

The distinction between software as a product and software as a service seems more relevant to research. As Prince [22] suggests, the fact that software is sold and used as a prepackaged item means that strict liability obtains. Should there be a defect in the software, the manufacturer is held liable. However, and especially with research, software is often written with a specific purpose in mind. As such, the programmer is providing a service rather than a product. In the case of software written specifically for a certain research purpose, the liability may not fall exclusively on the software provider. In those situations, it behooves the researcher to be very clear in knowing and stating his or her purposes to the programmer.

In addition to the increased precision in the communication between the researcher and the programmer, there will be an increase in the accuracy of the data involved in the research. As Mason [23] pointed out early on in the history of computer use, authenticity and correctness are necessary for accuracy. One current controversy in the pharmaceutical industry, in fact, depends on accuracy, which in turn affects liability. People in and out of the industry are discussing how best to make research visible to potential users of drugs.

Several companies, for example, Eli Lilly and Company, have said that their research will be made public so people may view the work and come to their own judgments about the efficacy of a drug. And, of course, scientific research is designed from the start so that results can be shared with other scientists and replicated.

The upshot of this trend toward visibility of research should reduce liability on the part of drug manufacturers and researchers, increase the likelihood that accuracy is enhanced, and produce more informed drug users. The question of accuracy undergirds the topic of liability, and if trends toward pharmacogenetics and individualized drug therapy hold, the importance of accuracy and subsequent liability will only increase.

With the increased importance of accuracy, though, comes an increase in knowledge about an individual. If the right to privacy demands protection, then there may need to be strict limits on who has access to programs, especially programs involving research. So, not only is there a need for technological "blockers" to protect against intrusions into programs, policy and procedure must strictly limit access to programs. Should no clear procedure be spelled out or no clear policy implemented, intrusions into programs and stored data largely become the liability of those most immediately connected to the program and the institution they are part of.

30.3.3 Ownership

One of the more philosophically interesting questions surrounding computers is the question of how to regard software. We lack clear analogs for programs. Whereas paintings, poetry, music, and prose have a lot of similarities, computer software does not consistently share similarities. The courts have struggled with this question as the question of applicable law has proved difficult to answer. So far, various devices have been used to encapsulate and resolve the question of ownership of software. And, of course, the question of ownership is circumscribed by the right to property.

But if the property is unlike any the world has yet seen, then it is not clear how such property should be regarded, let alone protected. In other words, the question of just what sort of property software is has not been satisfactorily answered, which contributes to the debate on the "uniqueness question." Nonetheless, devices such as copyrights, patents, encryption, trade secrets, and oaths of confidentiality and standard virtues like trustworthiness and loyalty have been tried to protect ownership and the right to property [17, 23].

Further complicating the matter of software as property and its place in pharmaceutical research is consideration of the very place of property in health care. The value of health, most philosophers agree, is intrinsic. It exists for itself and for no other reason. As such, health, like life and liberty, is an important and powerful end or goal. Ownership of property is a lesser end or goal.

Conflict can occur: Do property rights protect medical breakthroughs although great utilitarian gain might be realized by making the medical knowledge public? The phrasing of this question pits the right to property against utility. However, others [24] have cast the conflict in terms of competing notions of justice, namely, the notions of Rawls and of Nozick. In short, it may be that ownership of spectacularly useful medical knowledge of the sort sometimes contained in software may have to yield to utility or to a right to health care.

Although the matter of ownership seems to turn on an overwhelmingly broad conceptual question, the concrete reality is that programmers who provide a service may have some ownership rights over the research and its results. In short, not only is there a need to communicate between the researcher and the programmer for the sake of accuracy and liability, there is a need to resolve the issue of property rights, too. It is worth noting that questions pertaining to liability for malfunctioning programs also depend on the resolution of ownership.

30.3.4 Power

Johnson [17] identified the issue of power as a crucial matter for the development of computer ethics. Mason [23] made the same point when he identified accessibility as a concern for people investigating computer ethics. The issue of power may be important as never before, if Moor [10] is correct. He has suggested that the computer revolution has now gone through two distinct stages, namely, the introduction stage and the permeation stage. He believes the computer revolution is now entering a third stage, the power stage. This stage will necessarily deal with the impact of computers on human life especially in the areas of politics, socialization, and law.

While Moor asks for investigation, others have already made judgments. For instance, Joy [25] argues that limits must be placed on technology and its development. Others, for example, Weckert [26] do not share his rather pessimistic and alarmist view about how technology, especially the technology of computers, will affect human life. That there is debate surrounding computers as they affect society and its members is evidence that attention needs to be paid to this area. How do and will computers affect social relations?

This question is, for the purposes of this book, beyond any hope of being answered satisfactorily, involving as it does very broad issues related to the importance of property rights, to concepts of distributive justice, and to critical analysis of "power." After stating that "power" may broadly be construed as any capacity, Johnson [17] analyzes computer use in terms of several topics, including the matter of centralization or decentralization of power, computer use as favoring the status quo, the embedded values in computer use and programming, the impact on those who have and those who do not have access to computers, the effect computers may have on alienating people from what is rightfully theirs, and the place of the computer professional in resolving these matters. Of special concern to the computer user doing pharmaceutical research are the matters of computer use as favoring the status quo and the way computers might exclude groups or have embedded biases.

However, these sorts of concerns, we repeat, depend on resolution of other sorts of larger questions involving an adequate understanding of justice and fair distribution of resources. For instance, the answer to the empirical question of how the permeation of computers affects the status quo or whether computers contribute to the centralization or decentralization of power will not resolve the questions of whether the status quo should be maintained and whether centralization or decentralization of power is the better arrangement.

As is well-known in philosophy, certain feminist critics of science and technology, for example, Keller [27] and Harding [28], have argued that the scientific community has maintained the status quo in its exclusion of women and women's concerns. To the extent that a person believes that the scientific community has or has not excluded women, and to the extent that a person believes exclusion is unjust, that person may address the question of computer use favoring the status quo and excluding women. Although there are good reasons to think that the scientific community has not been the disaster that certain feminists think it is [29], any researcher should be well aware of the possibility of exclusion not only for the effect on scientific validity but also for the moral questions exclusion raises.

If this last claim is correct, then doing good research depends not only on scientific knowledge but also on moral knowledge. And, as the authors of this chapter have noted [30], the latter sort of knowledge is not always or meaningfully present in the curricula of graduate schools in science. Therefore, we agree that "ideally, research . . . is a cooperative venture between computer scientists, social scientists, and philosopher," [31] but also, if the research is in a scientific discipline, between the area scientist.

In short, we return to C. P. Snow's recommendation that the scientist and humanist converse more. The conversations, analysis, and discussion should include the third culture, the technologist. Therefore, although we have not provided specific and detailed analysis of issues related to computer use in the pharmaceutical industry, believing as we do that that sort of analysis is for the specialized philosopher doing conceptual analysis in computers ethics, we do urge that applied philosophers be part of the research team. Also, in the dynamic and flexible world of technology, applied philosophers—not just the people in the field of computers—should help draft policy statements and codes of conduct.

30.4 CODES OF CONDUCT RELEVANT TO THE USE OF COMPUTERS

A professional code of conduct serves several purposes: to allow a profession to regulate itself; to state the agreed-upon values of a profession; to make members aware of issues to which they might not otherwise be sensitized; and to provide guidelines for ethical behavior [17]. Pharmaceutical researchers have certain responsibilities and obligations in the pursuit of their profession. A recent study identified the ten most important behaviors that are sanctionable offences in scientific research, and subsequently used this list to survey scientists about whether they committed any of these offences [32]. As research scientists, pharmaceutical researchers should not exhibit these behaviors. We provide a list of the offences here (see Table 30.1) because the study found that over 30 percent of respondents had engaged in one or more of these offences in the three-year period before the survey.

By applying computers to pharmaceutical research, researchers introduce new ethical issues in the execution of their research. The Association for Computing Machinery (ACM), the United States' largest organization of computer professionals, was aware of such potential when it adopted its first Code of Professional Conduct in 1972. Other organizations of computer professionals have also developed codes of conduct to help guide the behaviors of their members. Table 30.2 provides a list of organizations of computer professionals that have codes of conduct, along with their respective web

TABLE 30.1 Top Ten Offenses in Scientific Research

1. Falsifying or "cooking" research data
2. Ignoring major aspects of human-subject requirements
3. Not properly disclosing involvement in firms whose products are based on one's own research
4. Relationships with students, research subjects, or clients that may be interpreted as questionable
5. Using another's ideas without obtaining permission or giving due credit
6. Unauthorized use of confidential information in connection with one's own research
7. Failing to present data that contradict one's own previous research
8. Circumventing certain minor aspects of human-subject requirements
9. Overlooking others' use of flawed data or questionable interpretation of data
10. Changing the design, methodology, or results of a study in response to pressure from a funding source

TABLE 30.2 Computing Organizations with Codes of Conduct

Professional Organization	Web Address
Association of Computing Machinery	www.acm.org
Association of Information Technology Professionals	www.aitp.org
The Australian Computer Society	www.acs.org.au
The British Computer Society	www.bcs.org/bcs
Canadian Information Processing Society	www.cips.ca
The Institute for the Management of Information Systems	www.imis.org.uk

addresses. The full versions of the current codes of conduct are available from the web sites. Even people who are not computer professionals themselves can use these guidelines to help ensure that they are following ethical computing practices.

We identify several principles here that are most salient to the application of computers to pharmaceutical research. Pharmaceutical researchers can apply the following principles to help guide their behavior in using computers for pharmaceutical research. ACM principle 2.01 states that one should "provide service in their areas of competence, being honest and forthright about any limitations of their experience and education." Thus researchers who do not have the appropriate expertise in developing computer applications should involve someone who does. Even for those who are appropriately qualified, ACM principle 3.10 says one should "ensure adequate testing, debugging, and review of software and related documents on which they work." For example, most spreadsheet applications contain errors.

Principle 3.13, "Be careful to use only accurate data derived by ethical and lawful means, and use it only in ways properly authorized," is important because computer technology makes it very easy to combine data from multiple sources, or even to collect data in the first place. Privacy and confidentiality are also important in data management (ACM principle 2.05 addresses this issue.) Principle 3.14 instructs one to "maintain the integrity of the data, being sensitive to outdated or flawed occurrences." A recent study found that pharmaceutical industry data disclosure practices is one of the three issues most frequently reported on in a negative manner by the press [33]. GlaxoSmithKline was recently sued by the state of New York for concealing the results of clinical trials of paroxetine [34]. Clinicians, health care institutions, and patients making decisions about the use of drugs or treatments can make more informed choices with access to all relevant data [34].

30.5 SUMMARY

The applications of computing technology have created new situations involving ethical challenges and conflicts. The community of philosophers is uncertain as to whether computer ethics represents a new area of study or simply new situations for ethical applications. However, there are four common issues in computer ethics: privacy, liability, ownership, and power. One can consider three ethical frameworks in examining ethical conflicts: rights (of individuals), justice (fairness), and consequentialism (utility). Researchers who use computer technology in pharmaceutical research must be aware of the issues of computer ethics in addition to other issues of conducting pharmaceutical research. Codes of conduct such as the one developed by ACM can help provide guidelines for ethical computing in pharmaceutical research.

REFERENCES

1. Ware WH. Contemporary privacy issues. In: Bynum TW, Maner W, John L. Fisher JL, editors, *Computing and privacy*. New Haven: Southern Connecticut State University Press, 1992:4–19.
2. Snow CP. *The two cultures*. London: Cambridge University Press. 1959.
3. Snow CP. *The two cultures: a second look*. London: Cambridge University Press. 1964.
4. McGowan R. The three cultures and children's T.V. *The Lion and the Unicorn* 1987;11.2:87–95.
5. Himma KE. The relationship between the uniqueness of compute ethics and its independence as a discipline in applied ethics. *Ethics Inform Technol* 2003;5.4:225–37.
6. Floridi L, Sanders JW. Mapping the foundationalist debate in computer ethics. *Ethics Inform Technol* 2002;4.1:1–9.
7. Marturano A. The role of metaethics and the future of computer ethics. *Ethics Inform Technol* 2002;4.1:71–1.
8. Tavani HT. The uniqueness debate in computer ethics: what exactly is at issue and why does it matter? *Ethics Inform Technol* 2002;4.1:37–54.
9. Bynum TW. Computer ethics: its birth and its future. *Ethics Inform Technol* 2001;3.2:109–12.
10. Moor JH. The future of computer ethics: you ain't seen nothing yet. *Ethics Inform Technol* 2001;3.2:89–91.
11. Gorniak-Kocikowska K. The computer revolution and the problem of global ethics. *Sci Eng Ethics* 1996;2.2:177–90.
12. Maner W. Unique ethical problems in information technology. *Sci Eng Ethics* 1996; 2.2:137–54.
13. Wong K, Steinke, G, The development of computer ethics: contributions from business ethics and medical ethics. *Ethics Inform Technol* 2000;6.2:245–53.
14. Gotterbarn D. Computer ethics: responsibility regained. *Natl Forum* 1991 (Summer): 26–31.
15. Johnson DG. Computer ethics. In: Frey RG, editor, *A companion to applied ethics*. Malden, MA: Blackwell Publishing Ltd, 2003:608–19.
16. Floridi L, Sanders JW. Artificial evil and the foundation of computer ethics. *Ethics Inform Technol* 2001;3.1:1–9.
17. Johnson DG. *Computer ethics*, third edition. Englewood Cliff, N.J.: Prentice-Hall, 2001.
18. Velasquez MG. *Business ethics—concepts and cases*, 5th ed. Upper Saddle River, NJ: Prentice Hall. 2002.
19. Brandeis LD, Warren SD. The right to privacy. *Harvard Law Rev* 1890;4,5:193–220.
20. Freid C. *An anatomy of values: problems of personal and social choice*. Cambridge: Harvard University Press, 1970.
21. Wright RA. Information as a commodity. In: Bynum TW, Maner W, John L. Fisher JL, editors, *Computing and privacy*. New Haven: Southern Connecticut State University Press, 1992;20–30.

22. Prince J. Negligence: Liability for defective software. *Oklahoma Law Rev* 1980;33:848–55.
23. Mason RO. Four ethical issues of the information age. *MIS Quarterly* 1986; 10 (March):4–12.
24. Gewertz NM, Amado R. intellectual property and the pharmaceutical industry: a moral crossroads between health and property. *J Business Ethics* 2004;55:295–308.
25. Joy B. Why the future does not need us. *Wired* 2000 8.04.
26. Weckert J. Lilliputian computer ethics. *Metaphilosophy* 2002;33.3:366–75.
27. Keller EF. *Reflections on gender and science.* New Haven, CT.: Yale University Press, 1985.
28. Harding S. *Whose science? Whose knowledge?* Ithaca, NY: Cornell University Press, 1991.
29. McGowan G, McGowan R. Attribution, cooperation, science, and girls. *Bull Sci Technol Religious Values* 1997;19.6:547–52.
30. McGowan MK, McGowan R. Ethics in an MIS education. *Philos Contemporary World* 1998;3(3):12–17.
31. Brey P. Method in computer ethics: toward a multi-level interdisciplinary approach. *Ethics Inform Technol* 2000;2.2:125–9.
32. Martinson BC, Anderson MS, de Vries R. Scientists behaving badly. *Nature* 2005;435(9):737–8.
33. Porth SJ, Sillup GP. Good news bad news. *Pharmaceut Executive* 2005 (April):106–110.
34. Anonymous. Open access to industry's clinically relevant data. *BMJ* 2004 (10 July); 329: 64–5.

31

THE ULTRALINK: AN EXPERT SYSTEM FOR CONTEXTUAL HYPERLINKING IN KNOWLEDGE MANAGEMENT

Martin Romacker, Nicolas Grandjean, Pierre Parisot, Olivier Kreim, Daniel Cronenberger, Thérèse Vachon, and Manuel C. Peitsch

Contents

Computer Applications in Pharmaceutical Research and Development, Edited by Sean Ekins.
ISBN 0-471-73779-8

31.1 INTRODUCTION

Drug discovery is an experimental process that relies on an increasingly diverse and complex set of platform technologies such as genomics, proteomics, metabolomics, high-throughput screening, and combinatorial chemistry. These technology developments are driving the diversity, complexity, and amount of experimental data to unprecedented levels. In addition, experimental data are supplemented with contextual information such as the detailed experimental plan, descriptions of the involved substances, and other relevant "metadata." Furthermore, data are interpreted in the scientific context in which they were captured. This leads to a wealth of scientific publications building on previous knowledge gained by the scientific community. This community is thus faced with an increasingly insurmountable amount of data and knowledge, stored in a growing collection of databases, information sources, and knowledge bases, each following its own distinct information management processes and serving often disconnected communities of users.

A major consequence of this data and knowledge explosion in drug discovery is the increasing need for effective information integration and federation capabilities bridging scientific domains such as biology, chemistry, and medicine. These capabilities allow scientists to rapidly and efficiently search, retrieve, and analyze key elements of information in a context-sensitive manner. The scientists can then apply their findings to the advancement of science and thereby accelerate the discovery of novel medicines. It is therefore becoming apparent that knowledge management systems allowing seamless information navigation across scientific domains are key enablers of drug discovery. Given the complexity and diversity of the relevant information sources, new adaptive and intelligent information navigation capabilities are required and are under development.

Scientific information—the contextual interpretation of experimental data—is published as "free text." The same applies to the annotation of experimental results, genes, proteins, and compounds and the description of medical conditions. This clearly indicates that scientific information is not structured, which creates a major challenge for its reuse, management, and statistical analysis. This fact has largely been recognized, and much research effort is focused on intelligent technologies that help to unlock the information captured in "free text."

In this chapter, we describe an expert system for knowledge management in drug discovery that uses a broad range of methods and knowledge sources (dictionaries and thesauri). This application is used to federate very diverse information sources and provide a Web-based environment for information extraction, navigation, and analysis. We then describe the underlying knowledge sources and models (ontologies and description of metadata) and the technologies for information extraction (text mining and parsing). Finally, an introduction to the Web-based user interface serves to illustrate the application.

31.2 THE VISION

We are all confronted daily with the complexity of finding and retrieving information relevant to our profession. Although Internet search tools (such as Google) have greatly contributed to the simplification of this process, there is still a long way to go before such tasks become really efficient. Indeed, a typical session using such search engines yields a number of hits, generally ranked by relevance. The users can then follow the hyperlinks and explore the top hits returned for their query. Although in simple cases the first few hits are relevant to the query, more refined searches are needed to disambiguate terms that have several meanings or are used in different contexts. The final assessment of the relevance of any link can only be done by reading the content of the target page. The users must therefore often follow several links and iteratively refine their query before the relevant answer is found. Furthermore, any new concept found within these pages will trigger a new and similar "search and explore" session. This is clearly not a satisfactory approach to information navigation, and far more refined query and information navigation methods must be developed to cope with the ever-increasing amount of available information.

To support the needs of drug discovery, we envision an expert system that would "understand" enough about biology, medicinal chemistry, and medicine to automatically identify and extract the key basic concepts and entities from free text and databases. These basic concepts would then be associated with meaningful rules leading to contextually relevant actions and tasks. This would lead to a markedly improved search engine and provide a context-sensitive information navigation environment with two main types of features: (1) The content of each result page would be read and categorized by the expert system—at loading time—enabling the selection of pertinent pages based on a treelike representation of the extracted concepts and entities, and (2) a new type of hyperlink, termed UltraLink, that associates each extracted entity with a set of meaningful links to other databases and applications.

31.3 FROM VISION TO IMPLEMENTATION

The UltraLink has been implemented on our Knowledge Space Portal (KSP), which is a Web-based application deployed at the Novartis Institutes for Biomedical Research (NIBR). The KSP is an information integration environment that enables scientists to search a diverse collection of internal and external sources, including the Internet (through Google). The system allows for the integration of diverse sources and applications and provides new ways to navigate information in a seamless manner. Databases are organized in clusters that are defined by the information domain (chemistry, biology, medicine, etc.) to which they belong. Individual databases or whole clusters can be combined and searched with a natural language query. A query interpreter enriches and transforms the queries to match the syntax of the corresponding search engines and normalizes and transforms the queries to our representation standards. The resulting list of documents is ranked by relevance. In contrast to standard search engines, the KSP not only displays the retrieved documents but also analyzes them for the concepts they contain. We now describe the technologies, methods, and knowledge resources needed to implement this vision.

31.3.1 Text Mining

Text mining is a relatively new technology for the life sciences that enables the retrieval and extraction of information contained in unstructured texts. The basic tasks of text mining can be defined as the identification of the entities in the universe of discourse and the detection of their relationships. A particular example of such identified entities is protein names, their function, and interactions with other molecules [1–4]. Identification means that we assign semantic values to the retrieved entities and relationships, in contrast to common search engines, which only match strings or sequences of strings in a given text. In our case the domains under consideration include medicine, biology, chemistry, and their related documents and databases.

To extract this knowledge from the various heterogeneous data sources made accessible to the KSP and the UltraLink, we combine several steps of normalization and analysis. These procedures are applied at loading time whenever the documents are displayed in the browser.

The first step applied to the text documents or database records is zoning. This process uses our (meta)knowledge about information structure and tags the relevant contexts of the documents or database records. This process also allows us to reduce (sometimes drastically) the search space to be covered by the entity recognition process. For example, within the life sciences the use of acronyms is widespread. However, acronyms are highly ambiguous and have to be interpreted according to the context in which they are encountered. For example "MS" has more than twenty different meanings and refers to diverse concepts such as (1) a well-known software company, (2) multiple sclerosis, and (3) Mississippi. This means that when a field in a record or document labeled as "disease" (through the zoning process) contains the entity "MS," the latter can be identified and disambiguated to "multiple sclerosis". Thus zoning allows us to correctly identify an entity in a given context and to extract even more information according to the metaknowledge related to the data source (such as attributes). This metaknowledge is part of a data structure, the Metastore, which we explain below.

The next steps consist of the extraction and normalization of terms from the zoned input document. To this end, we apply standard natural language processing techniques and normalize the extracted terms to their canonical form with string manipulations and morphological analysis. The former refers to the treatment of symbols (e.g., dashes), and the latter refers to variations of words due to inflection (e.g., plurals). These steps of information extraction rely on, and make extensive use of, our terminologies and ontologies.

31.3.2 Terminology Hub, Thesaurus, and Ontologies

Building and maintaining large-scale terminologies and ontologies is a time-consuming yet necessary activity without which we could not operate the Knowledge Space and the UltraLink. Many activities in this area are driven by community projects focused on specific domains such as the Gene Ontology [5] and the Foundational Model of Anatomy [6]. To build our terminology and ontology environment, we acquired and integrated such established resources. However, they do not cover our needed proprietary terminology, which we must construct and maintain internally. To this end, we regularly extract the new terms from our databases and use them to complement our established internal terminologies.

The integration of our distributed and very diverse knowledge sources in a single framework for retrieval (KSP) and navigation (UltraLink) leads to a huge naming and word space. The external terminologies that are widely used are not coherent (use of terms across data sources is impossible) and are only partially overlapping. This means that we need a unique and unified terminology that is able to adequately reference the different databases. To address this need we designed a terminology hub that enables coherent navigation between different terminologies, thus ensuring semantic interoperability when creating an UltraLink.

To create our terminology containing both internal terms and external terms we semiautomatically extract terms from available external resources (e.g., MeSH, EMTREE, UniProt). Then we fit the extracted terms to our data structure and preserve the reference to the source system because sometimes terms are very specific to certain databases. We refer to the terms specific to a database as *local terms*. These local terms are stored in a dedicated data structure, the Metastore. It must be noted that we refer to accession codes and identifiers used in databases such as UniProt, RefSeq, and GO as local terms (see Tables 31.1 and 31.2).

TABLE 31.1 Knowledge on Granulocyte-Macrophage Colony-Stimulating Factor as a PRODUCT

Term to UltraLink: *granulocyte- macrophage colony-stimulating factor*
Concept type: *PRODUCT*
Normalized term: Granulocyte-macrophage colony-stimulating factor—Cangene
Synonyms:
60154-12-3
83869-56-1
GM-CSF Cangene
Granulocyte-macrophage colony-stimulating factor
Granulocyte-macrophage colony-stimulating factor—Cangene
LEUCOTROPIN
Leucotropin
rhGM-CSF
Local terms:
Adis 8046
IDDB: DR7383

TABLE 31.2 Knowledge on Granulocyte-Macrophage Colony-Stimulating Factor as a TARGET

Term to UltraLink: *granulocyte-macrophage colony-stimulating factor*
Concept Type: *TARGET*
Normalized term: *Granulocyte-macrophage colony-stimulating factor*
Synonyms:
colony stimulating factor 2
colony stimulating factor 2 precursor
Colony-stimulating factor
CSF
GCSF
GM-CSF
Granulocyte macrophage colony stimulating factor
Granulocyte-macrophage colony-stimulating factor
Granulocyte-macrophage colony-stimulating factor—precursor
Molgramostin
Sargramostim
Local terms (nonexhaustive list of examples):
EMBL, e.g., *AC004511, AF373868,...*
Medline, e.g., *84245825, 85218749,...*
NCBI, e.g., *10090, 10116, 9606*
GO, e.g., *GO:000512, GO:0019221,...*
UniProt, e.g., *P01587,...*
PubMed, e.g., *1569568, 1737041,...*
Refseq, e.g., *NM_000758,...*
Species variants in Uniprot, e.g., *CSF2_HUMAN, CSF2_MOUSE, CSF2_RAT*

Besides the flat set of terms we also use and extract thesaurus relations such as "*synonymy*", "*broader_term*" and "*narrower_term*". By introducing these relationships we create a thesaurus from our terminology. The semantic knowledge encoded in the thesaurus is used for expansion of queries within the KSP and also for enriching the UltraLink.

Furthermore, we relate a canonical form of a term to a concept with a corresponding concept type. By convention, the identifier for a concept definition is the canonical form of its term; for example, the term "gene" is represented by a concept named "gene." The relationships inside the thesaurus guarantee that we can access a concept type for each term in our terminology by reference to the canonical form. Between the concepts, we introduce taxonomic relationships defining an ontology. Currently, our ontology contains a number of top-level concepts:

- Authors
- Companies and institutions
- Targets, comprising gene and protein names
- Compound nomenclature, compound codes, IUPAC names, SMILES strings
- Product names and generic drug names
- Modes of action
- Diseases and indications

31.3.3 Typed Concepts and Rules

Each concept has an interpretation specific to the scientific domain that defines the context in which a concept is located. A scientific domain can be described by various dimensions: a collection of standard practices, databases and information sources, tools, and computational approaches. Therefore, we can define a set of methods and rules for each concept that reflect the domain specific interpretation. For instance, a term denoting a concept with *TARGET* as concept type (gene or protein name) can be used to search genomic, proteomic, literature, as well as disease databases. Consequently, it is relatively straightforward to describe a set of methods for a concept (e.g., a subconcept of a *TARGET*) in a given scientific context and define them as rules. As we will see below, the UltraLink uses a database (the Metastore) describing these rules associated with each concept and corresponding references to context and scientific dimensions. Furthermore, this database contains such items as hyperlinks (URL), optional parameters, and other elements necessary to apply a specific rule.

31.3.4 Identifying Typed Entities

To identify entities in a portion of text and type them, we use the knowledge sources (terminology, thesaurus, and ontology) introduced in Section 31.3.2. The three levels are used by the following procedures:

- *Term Identification*: Identify the lexical items in a text, relate them to a term, and retrieve the corresponding reference term via thesaurus relations.
- *Concept Identification*: Identify the concept related to the reference term(s).
- *Type Assignment*: Assign the concept type related to a concept identifier.

The example below illustrates the identification of a term, how this identified term is associated with one or more concepts, and how a type is associated with the identified concepts creating the *typed entities*. The example also shows how the normalized term and local terms are used to drive the UltraLink.

The term "granulocyte-macrophage colony-stimulating factor" was identified in a document or record by our text mining tools. In our environment "granulocyte-macrophage colony-stimulating factor" is ambiguous because it is a synonym for two entries (normalized terms) in our thesaurus, namely for *Granulocyte-macrophage colony-stimulating factor—Cangene*, and for *Granulocyte-macrophage colony-stimulating factor* that are related to the concept types *PRODUCT* and *TARGET*, respectively.

Tables 31.1 and 31.2 show the corresponding knowledge that we extracted from our thesaurus and ontology to feed the UltraLink.

For the first interpretation (the *PRODUCT* reading), *Granulocyte-macrophage colony-stimulating factor—Cangene* is associated with a list of synonyms extracted from various sources of products and is referenced in two competitive intelligence databases: ADIS R&D Insight from Adis International Ltd and IDdb (Investigational Drugs database) from Current Drugs Ltd. The local terms in ADIS and IDDB are used to point to the original records in ADIS and IDDB and are only valid in the database they are pointing to.

The *TARGET* reading of *Granulocyte-macrophage colony-stimulating factor* is associated with a list of synonyms extracted from various sources of target names (protein and gene names) and is referenced in a large number of bioinformatics databases. The local terms are used to point to the original records, or for further searching purposes.

31.4 CREATING THE ULTRALINK

The UltraLink results from the identification of typed entities and the creation of contextual actions based on the type and context of the tagged entities.

As set forth above, terms are identified from free text and database records by text mining. The terms are then associated with relevant concepts, which in turn are associated with their associated concept types. This leads to the typed entities. As each concept type is associated with a number of properties, methods, and rules, the UltraLink provides a simple mechanism for associating these typed entities with contextual actions—as defined by a set of rules—that can be performed on these entities (Fig. 31.1).

The process to build UltraLinks follows these five steps:

1. Extraction and tagging using text mining techniques
2. Service invocation
3. Retrieving information from the Metastore
4. Filtering
5. Generating the UltraLinks

31.4.1 Extraction and Tagging

Briefly, the process normally involves the following procedures, applied sequentially. The first two (zoning and parsing) are dependent on the source

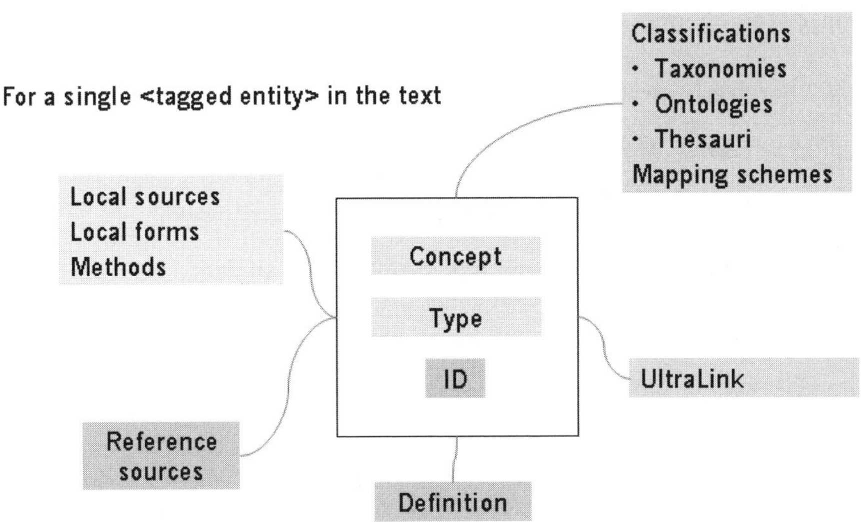

1. Get list of concepts for a given term to UltraLink
2. Get list of sources per concept type associated to the term to UltraLink
3. Get for each concept type which is associated to the term to UltraLink
   - the normalized form, the list of synonyms, the local terms in the various sources
4. Get the list of links for a specific source and the associated rules for launching the links

Figure 31.1 How an UltraLink is created.

being processed, whereas the others are independent of the source and can be applied to any textual information source.

- *Zoning*: tagging relevant contexts in a document. These "contexts" might be bibliographic or scientific and are identified either by the presence of tags in the documents or by the identification of some scientifically meaningful strings in the text.
- *Parsing*: extracting strings of characters based on pattern recognition and document layout.
- *Normalizing*: mapping strings of characters extracted by parsing to a set of normalized terms, either by applying a set of rules or by substituting typographical or morphological variants by a preferred term.
- *Lexical extraction*: extracting concepts from the text, using extensive lexicons referencing the various lexical forms a concept may take (e.g., synonyms, quasi-synonyms), each dictionary being triggered, controlled, or suppressed by contexts.
- *Classification*: assigning extracted variables to one or more nodes in a taxonomy.

The result is the assignment of a set of normalized properties (attribute and value) to each record, describing the content and context of the records. These properties are represented as a set of tags attached to each record.

31.4.2 Service Invocation

When a user clicks on a "typed entity" in the Web interface the UltraLink Web Service is called, a connection to the Web Service is established, and the component is accessed. A method named GetLinks is then called together with the following parameters: the type of the concept, the normalized form, and the raw text as encountered in the source document (the so-called lemma).

31.4.3 Retrieving Information from the Metastore

The Metastore is the data structure where we store different levels of meta knowledge underlying the UltraLink:

- The list of available data sources associated with a specific concept type (source, concept type, flag security, position in the list of displayed UltraLinks for that source)
- The list of normalized terms, synonyms and local terms for each concept type (e.g., DISEASES—COMPANIES—TARGETS—PRODUCTS—MODES OF ACTION) in each source, as deemed relevant for the creation of the UltraLink

The UltraLink component, called by the GetLinks method, queries the Metastore in the following ways:

- First with the specific concept type to obtain the list of sources relevant for that type
- Then with each source in that list to get the local term(s) related to the concept type that is bound to the normalized term.

The UltraLink component then generates a list of value pairs with the form (SOURCE, LOCAL_TERM) using the information extracted from the Metastore. It should be noted that an UltraLink is only generated if the data source contains information about the term under consideration.

31.4.4 Filtering

At this stage we can apply specific filters to customize the UltraLink for any application from which it was called. Because the UltraLink is a Web service that can be called by any application, we have rules defining its behavior based on the calling application. This means that certain value pairs described above can be removed based on explicit rules when the UltraLink is called from an application that should provide only a restricted navigation capability.

31.4.5 Generation of the UltraLinks

For each of the generated value pairs (SOURCE, LOCAL_TERM) an UltraLink can now be created and the substitution rules can be applied. To construct the contextual menu, the UltraLink component will fetch the title to display in the Web Interface as well as the URL to link to from the Metastore. It will then apply a set of substitution rules such as, for example:

- Replace the value of the entity to UltraLink by the local term.
- Replace the value of the entity to UltraLink by the normalized term.
- Or make any specific character substitution to ensure that the syntax expected by any given query engine is respected.

As a result, each term in a text that has been identified receives a set of associated UltraLinks.

Below we illustrate the processes leading to the UltraLink through a couple of examples. These examples will be reused in Section 31.5 describing the Web Interface:

- Psoriasis
- Tumor necrosis factor alpha
- Myeloblastic leukemia

Example on Psoriasis. The term *psoriasis* was identified by our text mining tools in a document or record. Table 31.3 depicts the corresponding knowledge that we extracted from our thesaurus and ontology to feed the UltraLink.

The disease *psoriasis* is associated with a list of synonyms extracted from various sources of disease names. Several methods as well as a set of rules

TABLE 31.3 Knowledge on Psoriasis

Term to UltraLink: *psoriasis*
Concept Type: *DISEASE*
Normalized term: *psoriasis*
Synonyms:
Psoriasis
psoriatic epidermis
psoriatic skin
willan lepra

TABLE 31.4 Contextual Menu generated for a Concept Type DISEASE

SOURCE	TITLE	CONCEPT TYPE	N0
CIAP	Portfolio Analysis	DISEASES	0
HON	Knowledge Map	DISEASES	4
KMAP	Search in HON	DISEASES	5
OMIMSRC	Search in OMIM	DISEASES	6
HARRISON	Search in Harrison	DISEASES	3
DEV_PRODUCTS	Products in Development	DISEASES	1
MARKET_PRODUCTS	Launched Products	DISEASES	2

are associated to the concept type "DISEASES" for display, search, and navigation purposes: The contextual menu, which will be generated just in time by extracting the relevant information from the Metastore, is based on the elements and their corresponding values listed in Table 31.4. SOURCE identifies the database under consideration, and TITLE shows the string displayed by the UltraLink. Finally, the CONCEPT TYPE and the position in the menu of the UltraLink are indicated (NO).

Example on Tumor Necrosis Factor Alpha. The term *tumor necrosis factor alpha* can be readily identified from text. The GetLinks method fetches the local terms associated with the normalized term for the various sources from the Metastore. The local terms are then used for pointing to the original records and linking to specific applications (Table 31.5).

Example on Myeloblastic Leukemia. The term *myeloblastic leukemia* can be easily identified in a document or record by text mining.

Table 31.6 lists the corresponding knowledge that we extracted from our thesaurus and ontology to feed the UltraLink. The large number of synonyms

TABLE 31.5 Knowledge on TNF Alpha

Term to UltraLink: *tumor necrosis factor alpha*
Concept Type: *TARGET*
Normalized term: *TNF alpha*
Synonyms:
Cachectin
TNF alpha
TNF-a
TNF-alpha
tumor necrosis factor alpha
Tumor necrosis factor ligand superfamily member 2
Tumor necrosis factor precursor
Local terms (nonexhaustive list of examples):
EMBL, e.g., *AB039224*
Flybase, e.g., *BC028148*
Medline, e.g., *22388257*
OMIM, e.g., *191160*
NCBI Taxonomy, e.g., *10090*
GO, e.g., *GO:0005164*
UniProt, e.g., *P01375, P06804*
Pubmed, e.g., *10089307*
Refseq, e.g., *NM_000594*
Species variants in Uniprot, e.g., *TNFA_HUMAN, TNFA_MOUSE*

TABLE 31.6 Knowledge on Myeloblastic Leukemia

Term to UltraLink: *myeloblastic leukemia*
Concept Type: *DISEASE*
Normalized term: *myeloid leukemia*
Synonyms:
myelocytic leukaemia
myeloid leukaemia
granulocytic leukaemia
granulocytic leukemia
myeloblastic leukaemia
myeloblastic leukemia
myelocytic leukaemia
myelocytic leukemia
myelocytomatosis
myelogenic leukemia
myelogenous leukaemia
myelogenous leukemia
myeloid leukaemia
myeloid leukemia
myeloid leukemoid reaction
myeloleukemia
myelomonoblastic leukemia
myelosis
neutrophil leukemia
promyeloblastic leukemia

indicates which terms are mapped to the normalized term and, therefore, are retrieved by a query in the KSP.

31.5 THE WEB INTERFACE

In Section 31.4, we explained the data structure that we use to represent and build an UltraLink. Now, we outline how the Web interface of the KSP assembles the information to user-friendly dialogs.

Figure 31.2A shows the results of a simple query sent to the KSP (list of ranked documents/records) and how the extracted concepts are displayed. The concepts are grouped into color-coded types (Figure 31.2B, keywords). The recognized entities are presented as a set of clickable concepts highlighted by the color corresponding to their type. For example, in the third hit "Tumor necrosis factor alpha," "myeloblastic leukemia," and "granulocyte/macrophage colony-stimulating factor" are highlighted. "Tumor necrosis factor alpha" is identified as being a "target." The collection of entities under concept types as shown in Figure 31.2B allows immediate navigation within and across these types.

When the user clicks on an identified concept the UltraLink creation process is called and displays a menu of possible links. Figure 31.2C shows the list of links that are generated at run time when the user clicks on "Psoriasis" (second document in the hit list in Fig. 31.2A), which has been classified as a disease. It can clearly be seen how the internal logical structures from the previous section are exposed to the user when calling the UltraLink (Fig. 31.2, B and C).

When a term is ambiguous, for example, when it can be associated with more than one concept type, these multiple readings are recognized automatically and displayed in tabular format. In Figure 31.3A granulocyte-macrophage colony-stimulating factor was categorized as a *PRODUCT* and as a *TARGET*. When the user clicks on the Products Tab, links to databases for products in development are shown. In this case the product cited exists in the competitive intelligence databases ADIS R&D Insight and IDdb (Investigational Drugs database). It should be noted that these databases are searched and accessed with their internal reference code (local term).

When the user clicks "View Granulocyte-macrophage colony-stimulating factor—Cangene in IDdb," the UltraLink jumps to the associated entry in IDDB (Fig. 31.3B).

Under the Target tab, another contextual menu, organized into submenus reflecting the nature of the links (search, display, blast, etc.) is displayed (Fig. 31.3C).

UltraLinks are not limited to "unzoned" text. They can be generated specifically on titles, abstract, full text publications, graphs, and chemical structures. Figure 31.3D shows a record from Medline-Embase where the abstract

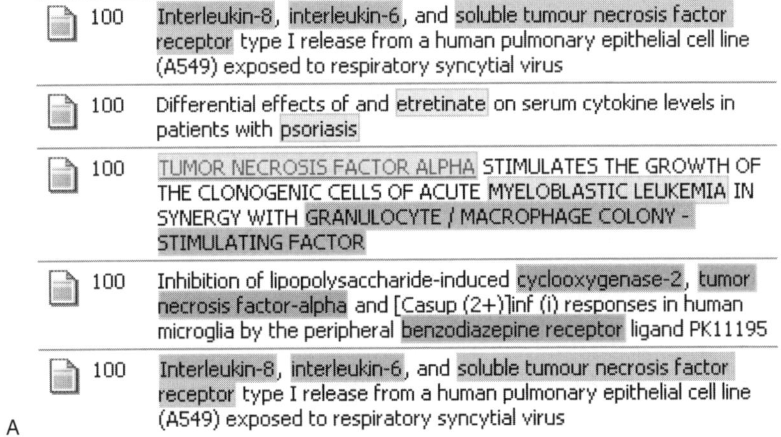

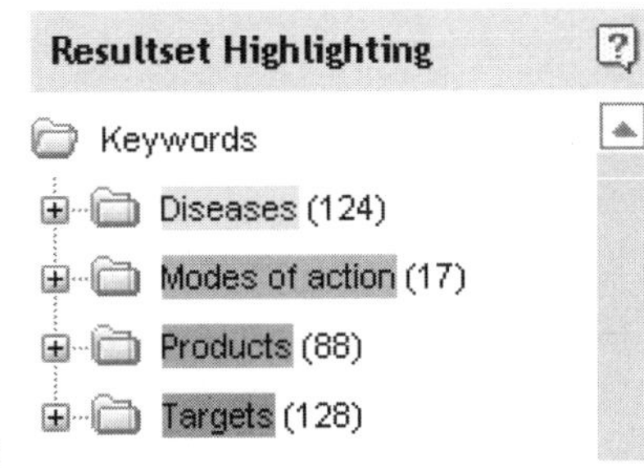

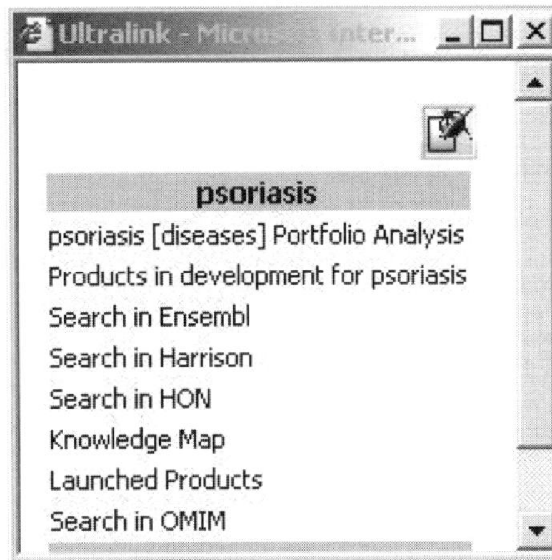

Figure 31.2 From search to UltraLink. A. results of a simple query. B. list of extracted entity types. C. list of links for “psoriasis”.

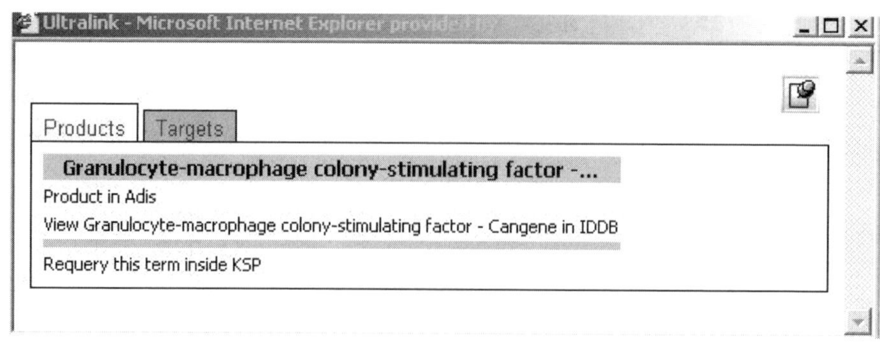

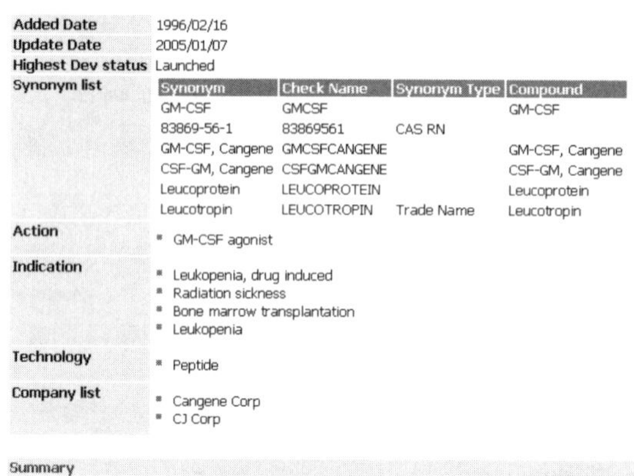

Added Date	1996/02/16
Update Date	2005/01/07
Highest Dev status	Launched

Synonym list

Synonym	Check Name	Synonym Type	Compound
GM-CSF	GMCSF		GM-CSF
83869-56-1	83869561	CAS RN	
GM-CSF, Cangene	GMCSFCANGENE		GM-CSF, Cangene
CSF-GM, Cangene	CSFGMCANGENE		CSF-GM, Cangene
Leucoprotein	LEUCOPROTEIN		Leucoprotein
Leucotropin	LEUCOTROPIN	Trade Name	Leucotropin

Action
- GM-CSF agonist

Indication
- Leukopenia, drug induced
- Radiation sickness
- Bone marrow transplantation
- Leukopenia

Technology
- Peptide

Company list
- Cangene Corp
- CJ Corp

Summary

Cheil Jedang (now CJ Corp), under license from Cangene, launched Leucotropin, a granulocyte-macrophage colony stimulating factor (GM-CSF) in Korea in 1998 [425841]. By December 1997, Cangene had completed phase I/II trials, in Canada, of Leucotropin for the treatment of leukopenia following therapy for CMV infection in AIDS patients [271809]. In October 2001, Cangene planned to complete a submission to the FDA during 2002 [442425]. In October 2003, Cangene filed for approval in Canada for the treatment of leukopenia in Hodgkin's disease and non-Hodgkin's lymphoma following stem cell transplantation [507934]. In September 2002, as part of an initiative aimed at improving Canada's readiness in the event of chemical, biological, radiological or nuclear incidents, Cangene planned to demonstrate the utility of Leucotropin as a treatment for white-blood cell damage resulting from radiation exposure [463946].

B

Ultralink - Microsoft Internet Explorer provided by Novartis

Products | Targets

Granulocyte macrophage colony stimulating factor

▶GeneBank
▶Blast
▶Search
Display Granulocyte macrophage colony stimulating factor (IPR000773)
Display Granulocyte macrophage colony stimulating factor (138960)
Display 3D Structure for Granulocyte macrophage colony stimulating factor
Display Source for Granulocyte macrophage colony stimulating factor
Display Granulocyte macrophage colony stimulating factor (PF01109)
▶PIR
Display Granulocyte macrophage colony stimulating factor (PR00693)
Display Granulocyte macrophage colony stimulating factor (PD007349)
Display Granulocyte macrophage colony stimulating factor (PS00702)
▶PubMed
▶UniProt
▶MISC
▶Avalon
View Granulocyte macrophage colony stimulating factor in Novartis LocusLink

C

Figure 31.3 Sample UltraLinks. A. UltraLinks for granulocyte-macrophage colony-stimulating factor *PRODUCT.* B. Granulocyte-macrophage colony-stimulating factor—Cangene in IDDB. C. UltraLinks for granulocyte-macrophage colony-stimulating factor *TARGET.*

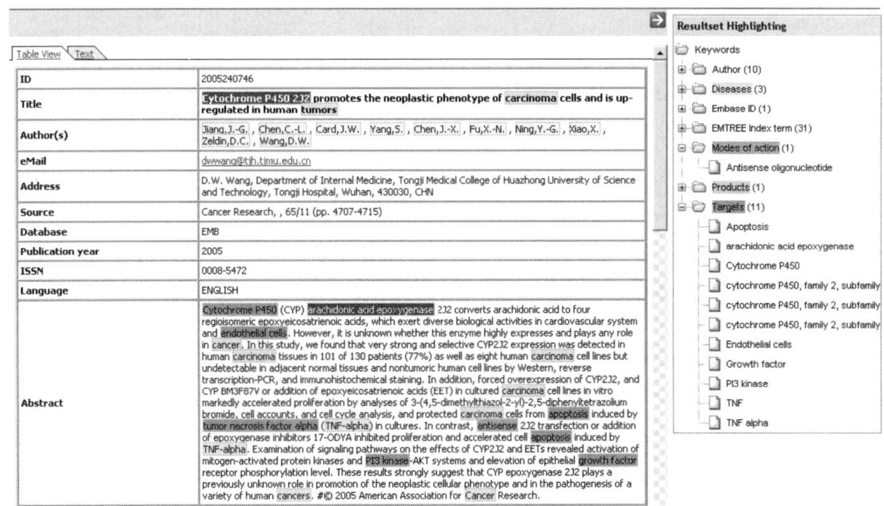

Figure 31.3 D. Annotated record from Medline-Embase.

has been annotated. The number of extracted concepts is of course larger on a full record than on a title only. The concept type of the extracted terms is defined for each source.

In the examples described above, the UltraLink is associated with the extracted concepts. To augment its flexibility and applicability, we allow for a dynamic UltraLink construction from a portion of text selected by the user. When the user selects a section of a document with the mouse, a list of UltraLinks is generated on the fly on release of the mouse button as shown in Figure 31.4A. Furthermore, the Web Interface allows for several UltraLink windows to be opened simultaneously as shown in Figure 31.4B.

31.5.1 Beyond the UltraLink

The purpose of the UltraLink is not only to comfortably navigate across distributed knowledge sources but also to access a variety of analysis tools. In this section, we illustrate this functionality through a few of the implemented tools, building on the previous "psoriasis" example.

Let's follow the UltraLink provided for "psoriasis" in Figure 31.2C:

- "psoriasis" [disease] Portfolio Analysis: It links to a proprietary strategic analysis platform that uses the normalized term for performing a portfolio analysis on published information (display of the number of products per phase of development for that disease in Fig. 31.5A).

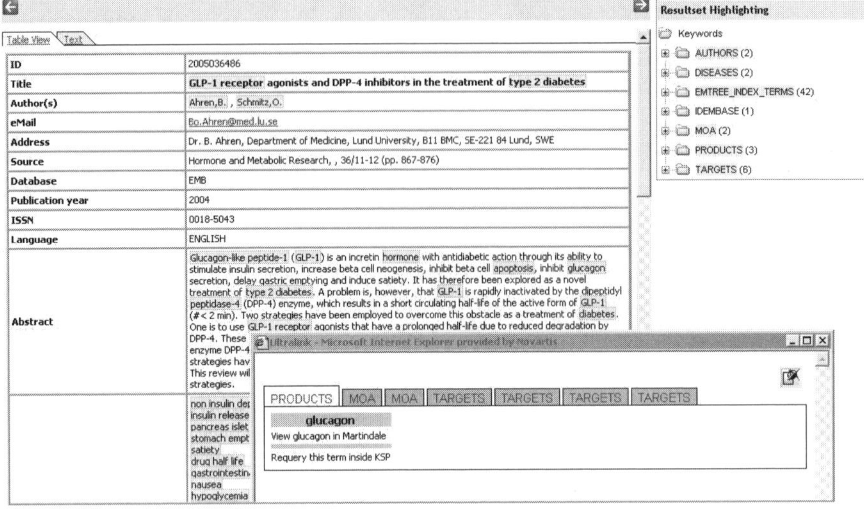

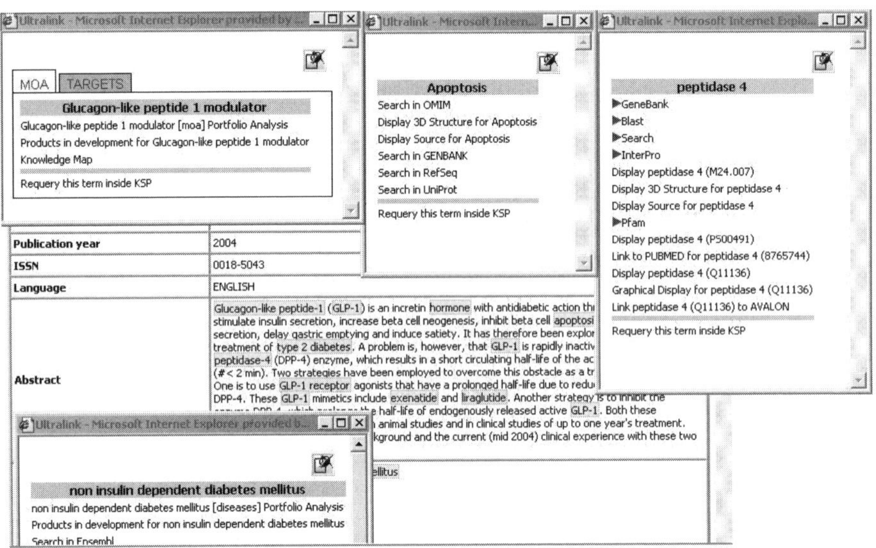

Figure 31.4 Further features of the UltraLink. A. UltraLinks can be generated for any section of text, by simply selecting a portion thereof with the mouse and releasing the mouse button. B. Multiple UltraLink windows can be kept when the pin icon is clicked.

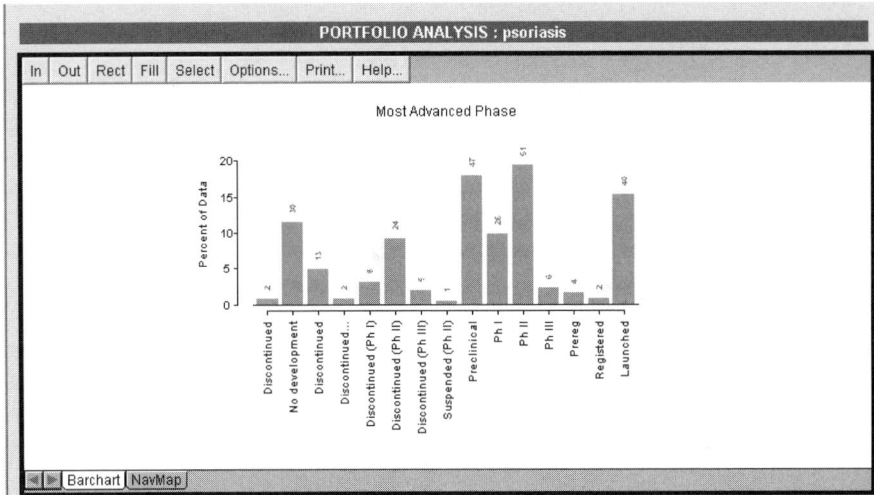

A

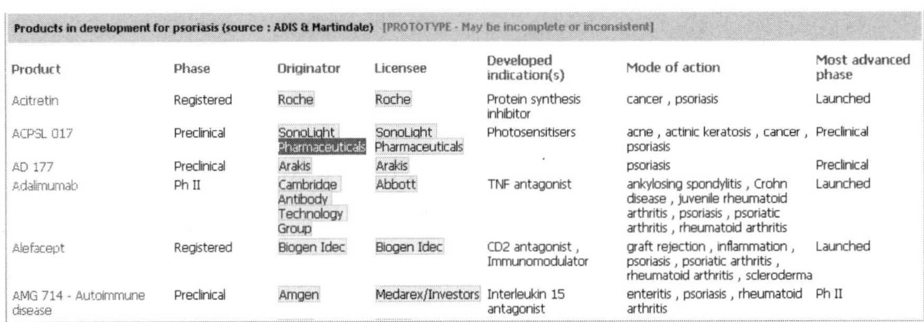

Products in development for psoriasis (source : ADIS & Martindale) [PROTOTYPE - May be incomplete or inconsistent]

Product	Phase	Originator	Licensee	Developed indication(s)	Mode of action	Most advanced phase
Acitretin	Registered	Roche	Roche	Protein synthesis inhibitor	cancer , psoriasis	Launched
ACPSL 017	Preclinical	SonoLight Pharmaceuticals	SonoLight Pharmaceuticals	Photosensitisers	acne , actinic keratosis , cancer , psoriasis	Preclinical
AD 177	Preclinical	Arakis	Arakis		psoriasis	Preclinical
Adalimumab	Ph II	Cambridge Antibody Technology Group	Abbott	TNF antagonist	ankylosing spondylitis , Crohn disease , juvenile rheumatoid arthritis , psoriasis , psoriatic arthritis , rheumatoid arthritis	Launched
Alefacept	Registered	Biogen Idec	Biogen Idec	CD2 antagonist , Immunomodulator	graft rejection , inflammation , psoriasis , psoriatic arthritis , rheumatoid arthritis , scleroderma	Launched
AMG 714 - Autoimmune disease	Preclinical	Amgen	Medarex/Investors	Interleukin 15 antagonist	enteritis , psoriasis , rheumatoid arthritis	Ph II

B

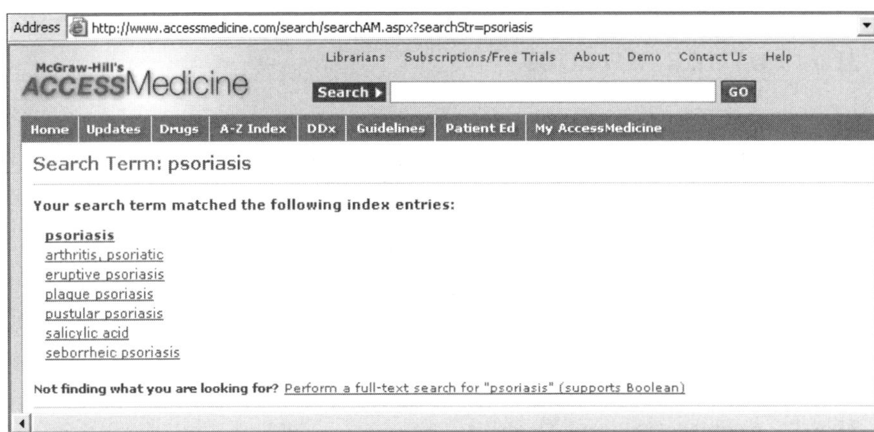

C

Figure 31.5 Sample of analysis tools offered by the UltraLink. A. Link to the Competitive Intelligence Analysis Platform. B. Extract of products in development for "psoriasis"—Source (ADIS, Martindale). C. Link to Harrison Online for "psoriasis". D. Knowledge Map for "psoriasis".

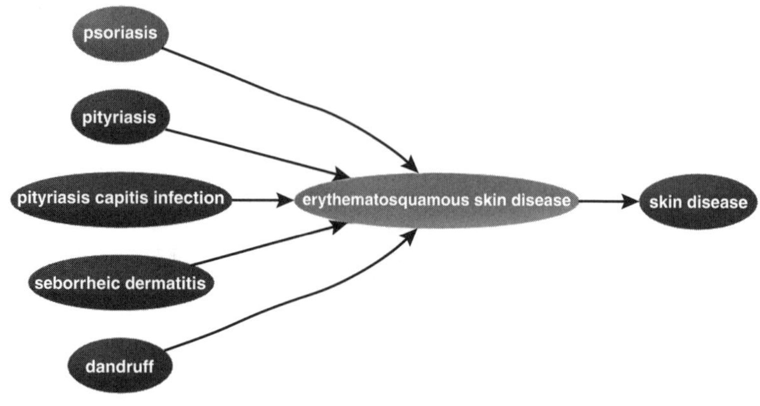

Figure 31.5 *Continued*

- Products in development for "psoriasis": It links to the strategic analysis platform using the normalized term and returns the list of products in development for that disease (Fig. 31.5B).
- Search in Harrison for "psoriasis": It links to the online version of Harrison's Principles of Internal Medicine using "psoriasis" as search term (Fig. 31.5C).
- Knowledge Map for psoriasis: It shows a graph of concepts linked to "psoriasis." The Knowledge Map is generated on the fly and uses the terminology that we maintain (Fig. 31.5D).

31.6 FUTURE OUTLOOK

The methods and technologies integrated in the UltraLink expert system are the subject of ongoing research activities in the scientific community. One of our primary objectives is to keep pace with scientific progress and continuously improve the reasoning and information extraction capabilities of our system. Our research focuses on architecture and usability, terminologies and knowledge representation, text mining and information extraction, and data analysis. In this section, we provide an overview of only a few of our activities and planned improvements to the UltraLink.

31.6.1 Architecture and Usability

We are developing a new version of the UltraLink, based on a federated service concept. The "federator UltraLink" will be responsible for connecting to "satellite UltraLinks" that in turn will access data and connect to applications in a domain-specific manner (e.g., bioinformatics, chemoinformatics, medical informatics). The federator will distribute the requests to a list of selected candidate satellites in parallel, and the resulting lists will be returned to the federator, which will consolidate them before sending them back to the user interface. This will increase the flexibility of the expert system at run time as modifications of rules and pointers and the addition of new UltraLinks can be done without interrupting the applications. Furthermore, the maintenance and updates of the "satellite UltraLinks" can be done by communities of domain experts independently.

The current implementation of the UltraLink uses a centralized set of terminologies, concepts, and rules, which may not correspond to the needs of every user. To further increase the flexibility of the expert system, we will implement a "personalized" version of the UltraLink. This should allow users to personalize the terminology, concepts, relationships, and rules used to identify typed entities and thereby create the UltraLinks best suited for their daily work. This will also enable us to design precustomized UltraLinks specifically tuned for chemists, biologists, and physicians.

31.6.2 Terminology and Knowledge Representation

The Semantic Web aims to simplify and provide a structure to the exponentially growing content of the Web, by using knowledge representations for searching and information retrieval [7]. Consequently, large-scale terminologies, formal ontologies, and knowledge representation are gaining importance. A recent trend in this field is the definition of syntactic and semantic information encoding standards by the Web consortium. Furthermore, efforts to build terminologies and ontologies are converging to a limited set of tools, languages, and reasoning devices, in particular Protégé (http://protege.stanford.edu), OWL (http://w3.org/TR/owl-ref/), and the corresponding classifiers (e.g., RACER) [8]. In this context, our research interests are threefold:

1. The ontology that underlies the information extraction and annotation process is solely based on taxonomic relationships. We intend to enrich our ontology with typed relationships. We are currently evaluating how typed relationships can extend the functionality of the UltraLink and how the expressivity for our ontology impacts the computational complexity of formal reasoning [9].

2. The knowledge domains that we deal with are very large and diverse (e.g., biology, chemistry, medical information). Therefore, we will need to work with knowledge representation maintained externally. For instance, semantic interoperability and knowledge syndication are addressed by, for example, KIF [10] or OntoLingua [11]. The above-mentioned convergence of representation standards offers new possibilities to automatically incorporate external knowledge sources into our terminologies and ontologies, and

thereby we can ensure a sufficient coverage of the knowledge-based methods within the UltraLink.

3. Ontological engineering is gaining in importance for the modeling of business processes and business objects. In this chapter, we have already exposed the metamodel that drives the UltraLink. However, we are continuously enlarging the ontology that feeds our business logic. It is also important to increase the expressive power of the modeling language and to integrate the rule system into a single formal framework.

31.6.3 Text Mining and Information Extraction

Large terminologies and amplified ontologies directly enable text mining and information extraction. We will extract more concepts from our texts and databases during the analysis process as broader knowledge repositories become available despite the fact that we will get more ambiguities during the identification step—because the entity recognition task covers many more concept classes that may interfere. Furthermore, our intention is to go beyond simple concept recognition by applying transformation algorithms that convert information such as chemical entities into other representations such as connection tables and SMILES strings. Thus the search space will encompass heterogeneous representation formats (text, graphical, IUPAC, SMILES, etc.) and queries will lead to increased precision and recall rates on queries. In addition, the introduction of typed relationships at the ontological level will be reflected in our ability to extract both entities (concepts) and the relationships between these entities through text mining [12]. Indeed, scientific publications contain relationships such as protein-protein or protein-compound interactions that are highly relevant to drug discovery. Mining these relationships and integrating them into the UltraLink will clearly add a new level of functionality to our expert system.

31.6.4 Data Analysis

Exploring documents for novel scientific knowledge is human-driven activity and is based on an iterative application of information extraction and analysis processes. This process generally leads progressively from the wider context to a narrower and relevant subset of documents containing the relevant information. As we cannot cope with huge amounts of information in a reasonable time frame, we need computerized tools to support these processes. These tools should provide data analysis capabilities such as data visualization, statistics, knowledge inference, and reasoning that can be applied to the concepts and data extracted from heterogeneous sources through text mining. The future UltraLink should execute a set of sophisticated actions, which themselves are based on a set of rules enabling knowledge inference and reasoning at each step. Machine learning, data mining, and computational intelligence methods provide approaches that can be used to implement such an environment. One can envisage three kinds of approaches: (1) descriptive methods that highlight useful features of the data set to ease exploration; (2) exploratory methods that guide the search by revealing potentially useful patterns; and (3) knowledge discovery methods that exploit many search paths and result sets to discover unanticipated or unknown facts (e.g., trends, relationships). Hereafter we describe three examples of complex ultra-actions applied to a set of documents resulting from a query designed to further analyze the result of queries:

1. Identify and extract chemical compounds from the text, transform them into structures and ask an external application to compute their chemical properties and toxicology alerts, and annotate the documents with these results. The added information might then be used for further analysis of the data set.
2. Identify and extract gene/proteins names and their interactions. Filter for specific interactions and query other information sources.
3. Extract concepts from a set of publications, identify experts for each concept, and then build an expert location system dynamically. This system would be based on extracted concepts, authors, institution, and cited authors.

31.7 CONCLUSION

Easy and effective access to relevant knowledge spread across disjoined and exponentially growing sources is becoming a crucial success factor for biomedical research. We have shown that we have developed and can provide a Web-based knowledge space (KSP) with search capabilities reaching beyond those of common search engines. Indeed, once documents are found and retrieved from a large set of diverse databases we analyze their content with text mining methods. During this analysis relevant terms are identified and concept types are assigned to them. A context-sensitive UltraLink is then associated with each identified entity providing concept-driven links to (1) navigate across a variety of available databases and (2) launch specific scientific applications. Our aim is that every query leads to relevant documents and applications with only three or at most four mouse clicks, independent of how complex the query may look. Our expert system enables a user to navigate across a knowledge space by using concepts like products, targets, and modes of action as starting points. The required knowledge is encoded in terminologies, thesauri, and ontologies and in descriptive metadata that provide the coordinates for navigation.

The KSP and, therefore, also the UltraLink are deployed within Novartis and are in daily use. We intend to further extend the abilities of the UltraLink. To achieve this objective we will concentrate our activities on text mining, ontological engineering, formal reasoning, enhancement of metaknowledge, and, finally, machine learning approaches.

REFERENCES

1. Blaschke K, Valencia A. Can bibliographical pointers for known biological data be found automatically? Protein interactions as a case study. *Comp Funct Genom* 2001;2:196–206.
2. Chaussabel D. Biomedical literature mining: challenges and solutions in the "omics" era. *Am J Pharmacogenet* 2004;4:383–93.
3. Chen H, Sharp BM. Content-rich biological network constructed by mining. *BMC Bioinformatics* 2004;5:147.
4. Daraselia N, Yuryev A, Egorov S, Novichkova S, Nikitin A, Mazo I. Extracting human protein interactions from MEDLINE using a full-sentence parser. *Bioinformatics* 2004;20(5):604–11.
5. Bada M, Stevens R, Goble C, Gil Y, Ashburner M, Blake JA, Cherry JM, Harris M, Lewis S. A short study on the success of the GeneOntology. *J. Web Semantics* 2004;I:235–40.
6. Rosse C, Mejino JLV Jr. A reference ontology for bioinformatics: the Foundational Model of Anatomy. *J Biomed Inform* 2003;36:478–500.
7. Berners-Lee T, Hendler J, Lassila O. The Semantic Web. *Sci Am* May 2001:35–43.
8. Haarslev R, Möller V. Description of the RACER system and its application. In *Proceedings of the International Workshop on Description Logics,* pages 1–3, DL 2001, Stanford, CA.
9. Baader F. A formal definition for expressive power of knowledge representation languages. In *Proceedings of the 9th European Conference on Artificial Intelligence, ECAI-90*, Stockholm, Sweden, 1990, p. 53–58.
10. Genesereth MR. Knowledge interchange format. In: *Proceedings of the 2nd International Conference on the Principles of Knowledge Representation and Reasoning*, Allen, 1991, p. 238–249.
11. Chaudhri VK, Farquhar A, Fikes R, Karp PD, Rice JP. Open Knowledge Base Connectivity 2.0. In: *Knowledge Systems, AI Laboratory*. 1998. (http://www.ai.sri.com/~okbc/spec/okbc2/okbc2.html)
12. Pyysalo S, Ginter F, Pahikkala T, Koivula J, Boberg J, Järvinen J, Salakoski T. Analysis of link grammar on biomedical dependency corpus targeted at protein-protein interactions. In: *Proceedings of the International Joint Workshop on NLP in Biomedicine and Its Applications.* Geneva, Switzerland, 2004, p. 15–21.

32

POWERFUL, PREDICTIVE, AND PERVASIVE: THE FUTURE OF COMPUTERS IN THE PHARMACEUTICAL INDUSTRY

NICHOLAS DAVIES, HEATHER AHLBORN, AND STUART HENDERSON

Contents

Computer Applications in Pharmaceutical Research and Development, Edited by Sean Ekins.
ISBN 0-471-73779-8

32.1 INTRODUCTION—ALL CHANGE

Despite enormous investment, the recent fall in Pharma's productivity has caused discomfort to investors and CEOs alike (summarized in numerous other chapters of this volume). To succeed, over the next 15 years the Pharma industry will not only make white powders; instead, it will sell a variety of products and therapeutic health packages that will include diagnostic tests, drugs, and monitoring devices and mechanisms, as well as a wide range of services to support patients. Companies that wish to deliver the highest standard of care to patients while delivering the sort of growth and shareholder returns seen in the early 1990s will need to move toward this product model as fast as their organizations will allow them. We believe that in the future, advances in molecular sciences and the integration of rapidly advancing information technologies will enable the industry to produce health care packages for specific disease pathologies, or targeted treatment solutions [1]. But although targeted treatment solutions (see Figure 32.1) represent the most promising source of future revenues, discovering and developing them poses problems with which pharmaceutical companies have never had to contend before.

Making such treatments involves the simultaneous development of drugs, diagnostics, and biomarkers, so it will substantially expand the scope of the discovery process. It will also blur the traditional boundaries between biology and chemistry, and between discovery and development, and accelerate the speed with which new products can be tested in humans. The data that are used will thus span a wider range of disciplines and be more complicated than those required to support conventional drugs. Similarly, the decisions that are made on the basis of the data—both scientific decisions about whether to push a molecule further down the pipeline and practical decisions such as how to micromanufacture biologics for preliminary clinical studies—will need to be made at a much earlier stage in the process.

The bottom line, then, is that targeted treatment solutions will demand much more of the R&D functions. The requirement for data integration and analysis will become even greater, as will the need to share data among a wider group of people—including regulators, research, development, and manufacturing partners, and in-house sales and marketing staff—much more rapidly than before.

The consequence of moving consciously toward this model will be the provision of a robust and scalable IT infrastructure and systems able to cope with exponentially growing data mountains that will need to be integrated and shared, accessed and mined in the most effective way. It will also require formidable computing power and sophisticated algorithms to be able to simulate both organs and whole body systems to reduce expensive failures in the clinic and predict much earlier the pharmacokinetic and pharmacodynamic properties and toxicological and efficacy profiles of molecules in pharmaceutical development. Finally, as computers pervade most of our working and domestic lives, they will increasingly become integrated into a health care network that will provide the infrastructure to deliver the pharmaceutical products of the future.

32.2 LIFTING THE DATA FOG

Pharmaceutical research is fundamentally about generating high-quality data and making sense of them to obtain new insights into disease and its treatment. But despite huge advances in information technology (IT), that task is steadily getting harder, particularly for R&D scientists and clinicians [2]. Mergers and acquisitions have left many large pharmaceutical companies struggling with legacy systems that cannot speak to each other, and the sheer volume of data is growing exponentially, as the new molecular sciences (genomics, genetics, proteomics, metabonomics, phosphonomics, glyconomics, etc.) come on stream. The nature of the research the industry performs is also becoming ever more complex, as are the data it uses to make decisions and the speed with which it must make decisions.

In fact, most pharmaceutical companies invest heavily in IT; according to META Group, the technology research firm, they spend between 4% and 5% of their annual gross revenues on hardware, software, and related services [3]. Forrester estimate that pharmaceutical companies spent $10 billion on IT in 2005 [4]. However, they often focus on technologies that will enable them to do more things rather than technologies that will help them to make sense of the data they possess—and this is what discovery scientists and clinicians most need. Mergers are a continuing confounding factor, and research from PricewaterhouseCoopers shows that between 1998 and 2002 (the latest year for which figures are available), there were 1584 mergers and acquisitions in the pharmaceutical industry [5]. The vast majority of these deals left the companies concerned struggling to reconcile totally different IT systems. Many of them have now harmonized the technologies supporting back-office activities like human resources and accounting, but integrating their R&D data is a far bigger challenge.

Although commonly used, the metaphor of drowning in data is a poor one because it fails to accurately describe the situation. When a person drowns he attempts to stay afloat and survive; most scientists and clinicians have given up, and many never even tried. A better metaphor is that a heavy fog has come down on the mountain they are navigating and that finding their next navigation point is going to take longer. Only those who are expert map readers are able to move quickly through the fog, and unfortunately, the number of people in R&D who are this capable is far too small. Capabilities that enable more scientists and clinicians to navigate this fog are essential to the reuse of existing information assets.

The volume and variety of data are also growing rapidly. As a compelling illustration, the University of California at Berkeley conducted a study that estimated that the volume of data created and stored in 2002 was five exabytes (10^{18}), essentially 800 MB for every person on Earth [6]. In fact, pharmaceutical industry analysts estimate that it now only takes six to nine months to generate a volume of new information that is comparable to what is already stored in all drug industry libraries and computers worldwide [7]. Combinatorial chemistry, high-throughput screening, genotyping and proteomic technologies, X-ray crystallography, clinical imaging, audio and video, electronic data capture from clinical trials, and other such tools have already generated numerous petabytes of data, but this is nothing compared to what is just around the corner. Where previously, for example, a company might generate 500 hits from high-throughput screening and conduct assays on the most promising compounds, with high-throughput profiling it can now conduct multiple secondary assays on all 500 hits, generating as many as 100,000 assays for one project alone. High-throughput biology—genomics, proteomics, metabonomics, and the like—will produce even more data. The genetic profile of a single person generates about two terabytes [8], and the number of different proteins in the human body is at least an order of magnitude greater than the number of genes. Furthermore, the industry convergence of health care and pharmaceuticals will mean there are more data coming from sources such as in-life trials and services associated with targeted treatment solutions. This will only increase exponentially the thickness of the data fog.

What is becoming increasingly clear is that this growth poses a very real management challenge for pharmaceutical IT. This is forcing the data maturation scale beyond storage and integration, instead focusing it on the ability of the end user to utilize the data for actionable decision making. After all, the purpose of generating data is to solve business problems.

32.3 KNOWING WHAT WE KNOW

When the volume of data exceeds the capabilities of individuals they must rely on intelligent agents to look for the patterns they are interested in. Again the vast majority of scientists and clinicians are not capable of expressing their information needs in a language such as SQL (structured query language). The ability to process natural language is critical to the success of these intelligent agents. Although it has been said time and again, it bears repeating here. Too often, pharmaceutical companies don't know what they know. That is to say, the focus in recent years has been primarily on creating data and new technological sources of data. Data utilization and knowledge creation has not kept pace with data creation. We have failed to move up the data hierarchy and derive full business value from the data that currently exist. To derive full business value from in-house data, it is necessary for those data to be accessible and integrated with other relevant data, to enable the end user to turn those data into useful information and scientific knowledge. Most, if not all, pharmaceutical companies have ongoing data integration projects. The historic approach of creating direct point-to-point interfaces between data stores has left many enterprise architects with a frightening and expensive tangle to unwind. It is critical that more strategic data integration approaches bring together their many silos of data creation in an attempt to provide scientists with the ability to make cross-discipline connections and insights.

Today, much of the utilization of computerized data is still predicated upon the paper paradigm. Desktop applications rely on the file/folder construct of a graphical user interface for storing documents and email. This was a step up in sophistication from the 1980s model of file system storage, in which users needed to know the exact location within directories and subdirectories (i.e., the full path name) to access and manipulate files. But with the typical end user now sitting in front of a computer with 40–100 GB of disk space (it is predicted that by 2010 most computers could have a terabyte of local storage), maintaining an efficient file system can be challenging and time consuming. Retrieving misplaced files is difficult at best, as the typical search functions of most operating systems perform a perfunctory search, querying files individually, looking for matches. In many instances, it is actually easier and faster to query the Internet for the needed information, rather than to locate a specific document on your personal computer. The advent of more sophisticated search engines will revolutionize the power of advance search capabilities for users. These search engines will enable the simultaneous searching of both structured and unstructured information. The business intelligence market (e.g., Business Objects; http://www.businessobjects.com/) and the content management market (e.g., Documentum; http://www.documentum.com/) are converging to build tools for the emerging information intelligence market. This is further supported by new players such as the ontology vendors (e.g., Biowisdom; http://www.biowisdom.com/).

A significant requirement of better searching is improvement of the semantic capabilities of search. The project to bring that meaning to the web is the Semantic Web project. The Semantic Web is a project that intends to create a universal medium for information exchange by giving meaning (semantics), in a manner understandable by machines, to the content of documents on the Web. Currently under the direction of the Web's creator, Tim Berners-Lee of the World Wide Web Consortium, the Semantic Web extends the World Wide Web through the use of standards, markup languages and related processing tools. Many pharmaceutical companies are working toward their own use of the semantic web technologies. The semantic web technologies such as RDF, OWL, and the datacentric customizable markup language XML will enable more efficient information gathering for scientists and clinicians but ultimately automated information gathering and research by computers.

An early pharmaceutical application of the Semantic Web is BioDASH (http://www.w3.org/2005/04/swls/BioDash/Demo/). This is a Semantic Web prototype of a Drug Development Dashboard that associates disease, compounds, drug progression stages, molecular biology, and pathway knowledge. It is based on the concept of a therapeutic topic model, something that exists in one form or another within the pharmaceutical industry. Normally this information resides across many internal databases and different groups in the R&D function; the tool achieves the challenge of using the information that already exists in a semantic approach rather than making new data models.

The Semantic Web Initiative supports two key needs in pharmaceuticals, first, the need to collect and represent complex forms of information in an intelligent, flexible form so that it is usable by computer tools and by scientists and clinicians and second, the need to gain insights or make decisions based on an aggregation of information that may share common entities, such as molecules, diseases, and intellectual property.

The ultimate in search engine technology and data maturation is the creation of personal computerized avatars. An avatar, from the Sanskrit *Avatara* meaning "embodiment," is a humanlike computer rendering of a search engine on steroids that facilitates information/knowledge retrieval. A trusted, intelligent agent, the avatar functions as a personal assistant, utilizing natural language search capabilities and knowledge repositories to draw upon the cumulative experience of others with similar needs, wants, and values to guide information retrieval, synthesis, and decision making. It is important to emphasize that the avatar will not only retrieve data but will also process those data, moving up the data hierarchy, creating information and knowledge. Interaction with your personalized avatar could occur via several interfaces: keyboards, speech, graphics and video displays that respond to touch, perhaps even via neural implants. The avatar, a "HAL"-like figure can currently be represented as a high-resolution graphical display, but it is not too far-fetched to imagine interaction with a hologram.

Data integration and more powerful search technologies are the IT backbone for deriving business value from the plethora of data fogging the pharmaceutical industry today. Fortunately, this is not a problem for this industry alone, and the best and brightest of IT minds and companies are focused squarely on this problem. In addition, further advances in how humans process data and information will also come to bear.

32.4 POWER AND PREDICTIVE BIOSIMULATION

32.4.1 Petaflop and Grid Computing

The simulation of events as complicated as the interaction of biological systems such as protein folding, cells, organs, and whole organisms requires both elegant algorithms and enormous computer power [9]. This chapter will not describe the intricacies of grid and supercomputing except to say that a new generation of petaflop computers will enable Pharma to begin large-scale biomolecular simulations. To give an example, the computational effort required to study protein folding is enormous. Proteins fold very rapidly, some as fast as a millionth of a second (microsecond). Although this is quick in human terms, it is a very long time for a computer to simulate. Even with a petaflop machine, it would take about three years to simulate 100 microseconds. Petaflop computing involves bringing different processes together in one huge machine (such as IBM's Bluegene; http://www.research.ibm.com/bluegene/). Grid computing works the opposite way; it splits a computing task into discrete packages, which are distributed to numerous computers. The answers are then posted back to a controlling hub. This approach harnesses the idle computing power locked in a company's many desktops and servers or in computers linked to the Internet. Therefore, it is a very economical means of solving problems that can be broken up into millions of tiny parts. It also provides a cost-effective base infrastructure for connecting research scientists working at different sites and enabling them to share data.

Pharma is tapping into the potential of grid computing to analyze sales and marketing data in real time, perform protein-folding predictions, screen for DNA sequence matches, and run sequence comparison algorithms. So, for example, Find-a-Drug (http://www.find-a-drug.org.uk/) is working on treatments for cancer, HIV, and severe acute respiratory syndrome (SARS); Drug Design and Optimization Lab (http://www.d2ol.com/) is screening target proteins for anthrax, Ebola virus, and other infectious diseases; Compute against Cancer (http://www.computeagainstcancer.org/) is studying the structure and behavior of cancer cells; and the Smallpox Research Grid (http://www.grid.org/projects/smallpox/) is seeking a cure for smallpox. IBM is also in the process of building the World Community Grid (http://www.worldcommunitygrid.org/index.jsp), which will be open to scientists around the world.

32.4.2 Predictive Biosimulation

Predictive biosimulation is the use of computer modeling to put all the pieces of the biological puzzle together in a dynamic model that shows how they interact and work as a whole (see Chapters 6 and 22). It goes hand in hand with high-performance computing because it requires enormous computing resources.

Genomics, genetics, proteomics, metabonomics, etc. have generated vast amounts of data, but it is not yet possible to integrate this material in comprehensive models of human organs or bodies. Scientists can correlate changes in gene expression and protein synthesis with a particular disease state, but they cannot distinguish changes that *cause* a disease from those that are *caused by* the disease [9]. Nor can they predict how those changes will affect the system as a whole. In short, they lack the biological context in which to interpret the data. Predictive biosimulation addresses this problem by using *in silico*—literally, "in computer"—modeling to integrate all the relevant data, reproduce the control principles of a biological system, and simulate how it will respond. Such models enable researchers to test hypotheses by "playing" with numerous permutations. Then researchers can identify potential molecular targets and compounds as candidates for treating disease. A number of organizations (described below) are currently building biological models of cells or organs. In addition, the development of industry-wide standards—like Bio Sequence Markup Language (BSML), Micro Array and Gene Expression Markup Language (MAGE-ML), and Health Level Seven Clinical Document Architecture (HL7 CDA)—will make the integration of data from a wide variety of sources much easier [9].

32.4.3 *In Silico* Biosimulation

In silico modeling is becoming a valuable and accurate prediction tool, despite its early spotty reputation. The increase in information from metabolomics, proteomics, and genomics projects, plus clinical data, and better integration between bioinformatics and cheminformatics, are helping researchers build more complete and more complex models that are beginning to produce lab-proven results. *In silico* modeling helps design better laboratory experiments and clinical trial protocols to define what should be measured; it doesn't remove the need for experimental research and clinical trials. Once the question is well-focused, a model can be used to explore how heterogeneity in the patient population or changes in trial design will affect response. It gives researchers a faster way to run "what if" scenarios [10].

32.4.4 Mathematical Modeling

Entelos (www.entolos.com) is developing mechanistic mathematical models of human disease that have been used across the pipeline from early target identification through Phase IV clinical trial design. They are just beginning stage II of a collaboration with the American Diabetes Association to develop a model of type 1 diabetes based on the nonobese diabetic (NOD) mouse. For this project, the key question is: Why have therapies that have looked so promising in preclinical animal models failed in humans? There are qualitative and quantitative differences between mouse and human physiology that significantly impact response to therapy, and very small differences mean a lot. By identifying and understanding those differences, researchers can better predict whether a therapy will be efficacious, and design more focused and effective drug trials.

In addition to the NOD mouse, Entelos has models for several human metabolic diseases (diabetes, obesity, and metabolic syndrome), inflammatory diseases (rheumatoid arthritis), and respiratory diseases (asthma and COPD).

32.4.5 Focusing on Metabolism

Genomatica (http://www.genomatica.com/index.shtml) focuses on metabolism because of its critical role in the majority of diseases and has developed a number of organism-specific cellular metabolism models that model certain types of metabolic problems, such as production and manipulation of small molecules by microbial cells and the effects of compounds on cellular metabolism under varying conditions. The SimPheny (simulated phenotype) computational platform helps users create predictive metabolic models of organisms ranging from bacteria to humans by integrating organism-specific metabolic models with experimental data and then simulate and analyze the metabolic capabilities within the context of the model. It provides a comprehensive description of the metabolic process so researchers can manipulate genes or biochemical parameters, or alter the environment or their own hypotheses *in silico*. It may have particular value in such difficult products as amino acids and antimicrobial compounds, and in producing the base chemicals for polymers. The next few years may see the development of a handful of models for microbial organisms and multicellular systems, followed eventually by models for human and other mammalian cells.

32.4.6 Biological Interactions

Compugen (www.cgen.com) is built around mathematical modeling, based on the experimental and clinical data provided by its partners and its internal labs, and Novartis (www.novartis.com) is using their models to study certain biological interaction networks. Although there are many companies addressing the need for network modeling (see Chapter 6), the goal of this particular collaboration is to demonstrate that they can incorporate data from diverse sources, analyze it, and predict new information regarding the relationship and timing events involved in specific types of biological networks. If successful, the model will be able to predict relationships between proteins that would have been extremely difficult to discover experimentally on an individual basis. The integration of data from diverse sources is important because any single source, for instance, microarray data, is often very noisy and difficult to reproduce. Such modeling projects are lending validity to *in silico* modeling techniques. They are also developing qualitative models for specific pathways related to well-known drugs, with the hope of gaining insights into diversity in patient response to treatment.

32.4.7 Predicting Pharmacological Properties

There have been considerable efforts toward modeling ADME/Tox properties and the biophysical properties of molecules (see chapters 18–20, 22, 28), including numerous commercial software solutions. Simulations Plus (http://www.simulations-plus.com/) have developed GastroPlus, a product that predicts dissolution/precipitation, transit, degradation, and absorption of drugs in the gastrointestinal tract, including the effects of transporter proteins like PepT1 and PGP. Simulation Plus ADMET Predictor allows researchers to predict some 50 different properties from molecular structure. It is used for very high-throughput *in silico* screening of large compound libraries and for estimates of key properties for single compounds. By using groups of artificial neural networks and averaging their outputs, it predicts properties critical to oral absorption as well as several pharmacokinetic properties and types of toxicity. It allows researchers to build structure-property models from their own data on their own servers and add them to ADMET Predictor models, thus keeping the information inhouse. Simulations Plus also recently released DDDPlus simulation software for in vitro dose disintegration and dissolution studies for formulation scientists. Formulations for new active ingredients require only one calibration experiment before the software will predict how formulation changes affect the dissolution rate. The value of this application occurs when you have such formulation changes as variations in amounts of active ingredients, excipients, and particle sizes. The program helps researchers simulate such changes and get results literally in seconds. MembranePlus, a similar product, will simulate and interpret Caco-2 and PAMPA in vitro membrane permeability.

32.4.8 Building the Predictive Infrastructure

To build such models, data must be structured in a way that enables these tools to work effectively across global organizations. Accelrys (www.accelerys.com) is an example of a company that blurs the line between modeling and bioinformatics. It doesn't build models, per se, but builds the bioinformatic databases needed to make the models. It also has virtual screening applications and products like Ligand Fit that are able to visualize how (components) interact at the atomic level and thereby help researchers prioritize what they do in the lab. Biogen Idec (www.biogenidec.com) and Eli Lilly (www.lilly.com) proved the point, each taking a separate approach to the same challenge and detailing their results in a joint paper [11]. Biogen Idec used Accelrys products to develop a pharmacophore *in silico*. Eli Lilly worked on the same target, but in a wet laboratory. Both developed a very similar lead compound, but the *in silico* lead was identified in two months, whereas identifying the lead in the wet laboratory took 18 months.

Despite such success, a lot more mapping of the complexity in the human body is required. Mapping the human genome was relatively straightforward compared to mapping the complexity and interactions of the human body.

32.5 PERVASIVE COMPUTING

Mark Weiser, a leading light at the Xerox PARC computer science laboratory, first defined the concept of ubiquitous or pervasive computing. In an article published in *Scientific American* in 1991 [12], he wrote: "The most profound technologies are those that disappear. They weave themselves into the fabric of everyday life until they are indistinguishable from it."

Weiser argues that what matters most is not technology itself but its relationship to humans. Over the past 50 years that relationship has undergone two major metamorphoses: We began with the mainframe, where many people share a computer, and migrated to the personal computer, where one person has one computer. We have subsequently moved onto the Internet, which provides widespread interconnection. But this, says Weiser, is simply a stepping stone to a third stage—an era of pervasive computing, where many computers share each of us.

Some of those computers will be the thousands we access in the course of browsing the Internet. Others will be embedded in walls, chairs, light switches, cars, and even the human body. In short, pervasive computing is the antithesis of virtual reality. Instead of creating an artificial world inside the computer, it invisibly enhances the world that already exists.

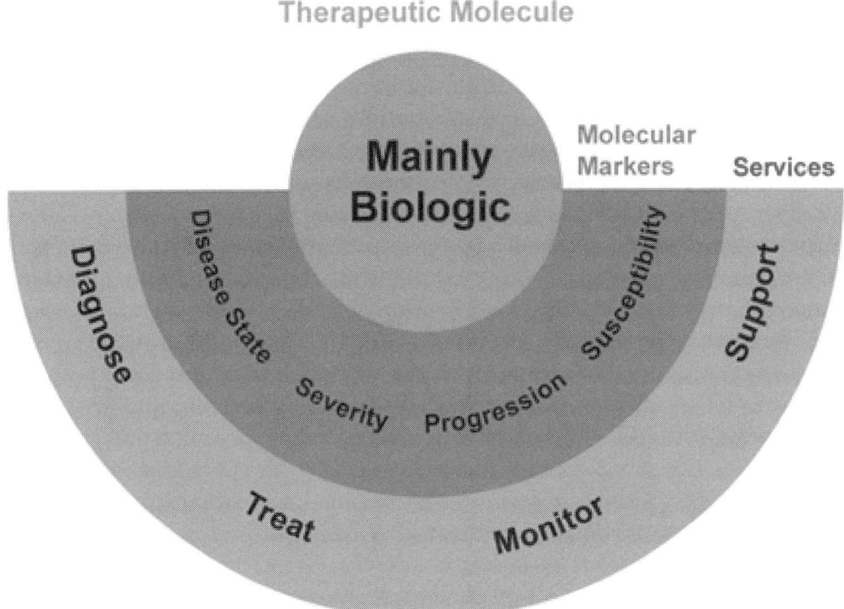

Figure 32.1 Targeted treatment solutions. Reproduced with permission from "Threshold of Innovation" (2005). IBM Business Consulting Services [1]. See color plate.

32.5.1 Pervasive Health Care

Pervasive computing has numerous applications, but it offers particular potential to the pharmaceutical and health care industries by facilitating the transmission and collection of biological data on a real-time basis outside a clinical setting. That, in turn, means it can be used to monitor patients and manage their health; to test new drugs in totally different ways; and to deliver health care anywhere, anytime [13].

In addition to such direct advantages, pervasive computing has a big social contribution to make. It can be used, for example, to enable patients and their relatives to keep in touch, and to help people with cognitive disabilities function on a daily basis. One illness that lends itself to such treatment is senile dementia, which is likely to be a growing trend in the graying populations of the Western World.

But although "pervasive healthcare," as it is sometimes called, promises to deliver huge benefits, there are still numerous challenges to be resolved. For a start, information about the health of patients is very sensitive, so any system that handles such data must be completely secure. It must also be unobtrusive and easy to use, because the vast majority of patients will not be technophiles eager to adopt the latest technology.

Finally, and for obvious reasons, any system that is used to provide pervasive health care must be completely robust, and this is currently the single biggest problem. Pervasive computing is still in its infancy and largely reliant on the methods of experimental computer science, where researchers design, develop, program, and assess prototypes. In other words, it is still at the "proof of concept" stage. But modern information-based medicine is rooted in statistical significance—repeated iterations of a test to prove that a treatment really works and does so without causing intolerable side effects. Moreover, the clinical trials that yield such evidence typically involve thousands of patients over a period of several months or years.

At present, most pervasive computing technologies are not sufficiently reliable to be used in such a context—and while there is any doubt about their robustness, the regulators will rightly refuse to accept data collected in this fashion. That said, some of the key components are already beginning to emerge, and although it is difficult to predict the precise crossover point, the moment at which they make the transition from prototype to practical reality is getting much closer (Fig. 32.2).

32.5.2 Wearable Devices and Wireless Networks

Thanks to advances in miniaturization and developments in sensors and measurement technologies, it is already possible to collect a considerable amount of health-related information from wearable or embedded devices, and numerous new devices are also in the pipeline (Table 32.1). Some of these devices function on a constant basis, whereas others take intermittent mea-

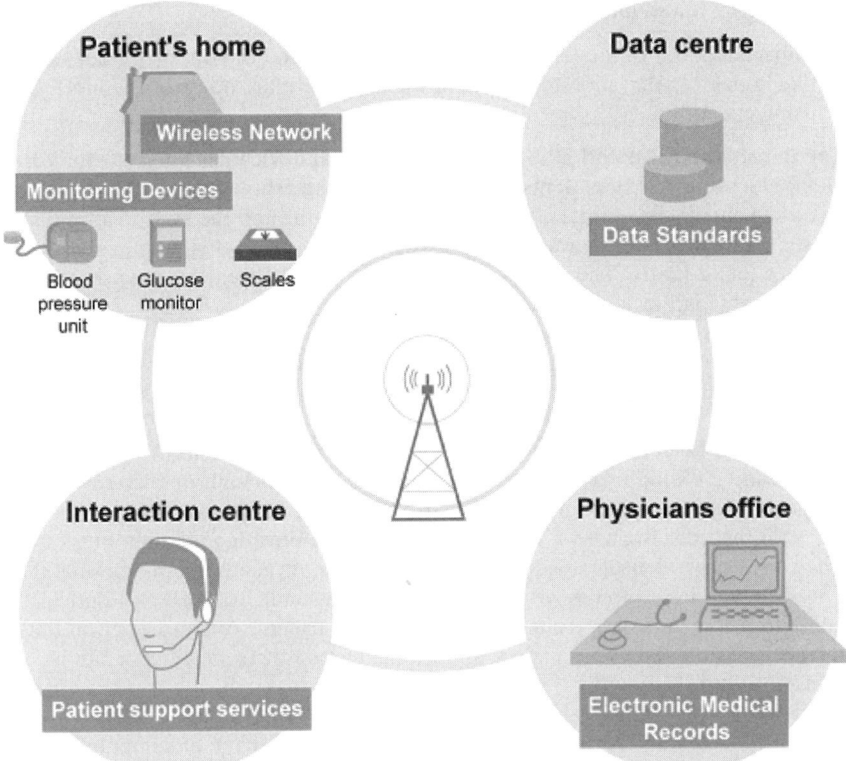

Figure 32.2 Infrastructure required for integrated health care. Reproduced with permission from "Threshold of Innovation" (2005). IBM Business Consulting Services [1]. See color plate.

surements. The surrogate markers they track determine which mode is most suitable; a device that monitors the heart rate in a patient with a history of cardiac events must be constant, for example, whereas a device that monitors lipid levels in the bloodstream of a patient who has high cholesterol need only be intermittent.

But reliable, portable monitoring devices are only one element in the equation. The second is the network across which the data they collect can be sent—and here two new technologies are particularly relevant: third-generation (3G) mobile telephony and a wireless network protocol known formally as 802.11 and colloquially as Wi-Fi.

The 3G networks using the Universal Mobile Telecommunications Systems standard have been in operation for a few years now. They offer an enormous increase in bandwidth and can theoretically transmit data at speeds of as much as two megabits per second (Mbps). They are also relatively easy to use.

TABLE 32.1 Small and Beautiful

Miniaturization and new fabrics have massively increased the opportunities for developing devices that monitor a patient's health. Here are a few of the most promising examples.

- ***The GlucoWatch:*** In mid-2001, the first wristwatch device designed to monitor blood glucose levels in patients with diabetes reached the market. It uses a small electrical current to extract a tiny amount of fluid through the skin. A thin plastic sensor on the back of the watch measures glucose levels in this fluid every 20 minutes for 12 hours. The device sounds an alarm if the wearer's glucose reaches dangerously high or low levels.
- ***The clip-on pedometer:*** Titan Industries is developing a clip-on device that tracks various parameters, including the number of calories the wearer has burned while walking around. The company is also exploring the potential for a similar device that monitors blood pressure.
- ***PC in a pill:*** Scientists in Israel have developed a wireless digital camera so small that it can be sealed in a capsule and swallowed. It takes high-quality color images while passing through the digestive tract. The images are transmitted to a portable recorder worn on a special belt and can be downloaded on a PC.
- ***The smart shirt:*** Sensatex, a New York-based company, is developing a shirt that is used to monitor patients' vital signs. The shirt is made of an electro-optical fabric that transfers data from the wearer to the garment. A transceiver on the shirt records the data and sends it to a wireless gateway, from which it can be transmitted to the doctor.
- ***Smart dust:*** Researchers at the University of California, Berkeley, have developed smart dust—tiny, intelligent wireless sensors that can communicate with each other, form autonomous networks, reprogram themselves, and monitor almost anything. They have already been tested for various military and nonmilitary applications, but their potential in providing pervasive health care is equally huge [15].

Wi-Fi runs at even faster speeds; the most common standard can now transmit data at a blistering 54 Mbps, although access is limited, except in large urban areas, and the technology has suffered from criticisms of being less secure. However, both these problems are being resolved. In the US, for example, IBM, Intel, and AT&T have formed a consortium to develop a nationwide wireless data network. Companies such as T-Mobile have developed global Wi-Fi networks and have even offered cell phone subscribers the ability to add Wi-Fi hotspot access to their cell phone plans. Airports, major hotel chains, and retailers such as Starbucks have created large networks of Wi-Fi hotspots that enable high-speed network connectivity. Indeed, vendors of enterprise software such as Siebel have taken advantage of this development in Wi-Fi availability. Siebel provides a feature known as TrickleSync. This automatically synchronizes data from the laptops of mobile professionals whenever the software detects a network connection. The time when such approaches are applied to synchronizing wearable medical devices is not far away. The new and much more secure encryption standards, Wi-Fi Protected Access—WPA—and more recently WPA2, are fast replacing the Wired Equivalent Privacy (WEP), which was less secure.

The third element required for pervasive health care is a hub at the relevant hospital or doctor's office, to which the data can be sent. The frequency of collection and transmission determines whether the data are electronically filtered and programmed to trigger an alert only when they fall outside certain preset parameters or are checked by a human agent. This hub will subscribe to the stream of data coming over as HL7 messages. It will be able to retrieve the messages it has permissions for. Using this publish and subscribe approach could also enable pharmaceutical companies to receive data during in-life trials. The data recorded through the devices or diagnostics, laboratory tests, and dispensary records and the information captured by the physician in the EMR will produce a stream of HL7 messages that can have permissions defined to enable the trial sponsor to subscribe during the conduct of the study. Although this messaging approach may sound somewhat futuristic, the reality is that examples of this exist today. A project known as the Healthcare Collaborative Network (http://www-03.ibm.com/industries/healthcare/doc/content/landing/972420105.html?g_type=pspot) aimed at improving patient care uses this publish and subscribe messaging approach. The project was launched in 2003 with the aim of improving patient care. The initial project participants are New York Presbyterian Hospitals, Vanderbilt University Medical Center and Wishard Memorial Hospital, as well as the Centers for Disease Control and Prevention, the Centers for Medicare and Medicaid Services, and the Food and Drug Administration.

Another example is the Canadian government, which has purchased the same technology to run a pilot for an early warning and response system for biological agent threats. Initially limited to Winnipeg, the system's goal is to create a readiness network for front-line health care workers.

With all the technology found in the modern hospital today, the lack of coordination between other parts of health care, the pharmaceutical industry, and the agencies is outdated. A network that connects these parts together will improve patient safety, improve care, speed the development of new treatments, and support new medical breakthroughs.

32.5.3 Tools for Pervasive Health Care

The tools for pervasive healthcare are evolving quite rapidly, then. But how will they work in practice? Here we outline some of the implications [12]. Most of the drugs currently on the market come in a one-size-fits-all format and are aimed at a mass population. But complex biomolecular and genetic variations in individuals, as well as the different environmental influences to which they are exposed, mean that many drugs do not work for a significant percentage of the patient population. Worse still, some drugs cause serious side effects in some people. Research conducted at University College,

London, shows, for example, that every year more than 800,000 patients using the UK National Health Service experience adverse drug reactions [13 and references therein].

As described above, targeted treatment solutions will include diagnostics for evaluating a patient's susceptibility to a particular disease; biomarkers for identifying the specific subtype from which he or she suffers, and for measuring its severity and progression; drugs for treating that disease subtype; and monitoring mechanisms to check the efficacy of the treatment and help the patient comply with his or her individual medical regimen.

Pervasive computing is one of the vital parts of this transition. In future, any company that wants to produce a new drug will develop relevant biomarkers as an intrinsic part of the target validation process. These biomarkers will be used to assess the toxicity and efficacy of the drug during the preclinical phase. They will also be used, in conjunction with remote monitoring devices, to determine how patients respond during clinical trials, both in terms of adverse effects such as hepatic toxicity (one of the biggest risks with any drug) and in terms of how effectively the drug impedes the progress of the disease subtype for which it is designed.

Forrester estimates that the market for personal medical monitoring will be $34 billion by 2015, rising from $5 billion in 2010. In 2003 they surveyed 12,000 US households in which 84% said they would, if they were ill, pay for services or equipment to help them stay in their home as long as possible. The question of who pays for such services remains a problem, as the same survey identified that only 9% of the consumers sought medical care not covered by their insurance.

Pharmaceutical companies may well end up footing some of the initial bill. The continuing publicized safety issues and the reaction of press, public, and lawyers drives home the issue that the concept of relative risk will never be understood. The fact that all drugs have side effects, especially when taken in large doses over long periods of time, is not seen in the context of the benefits they bring. As a result, pharmaceutical companies are already extending their pharmacovigilance efforts. Examples include the aim of connecting to data feeds in hospitals to support more detailed safety monitoring. Projects such as these will be the initial foray in connecting health care, the pharmaceutical industry, agencies, and ultimately the pervasive health care tools to create the collaborative network discussed above in this chapter.

32.5.4 In-Life Testing

However, pervasive computing will ultimately do much more; it will change the very way in which new drugs are tested. At present, all drugs go through three clinical phases, but the process is both very costly and very inefficient. Clinical trials cannot detect rare side effects and drug interactions, or sometimes even fairly common reactions. In fact, one recent study conducted by Harvard Medical School and Public Citizen, the US consumer advocacy group, estimates that 20% of all new drugs are eventually found to have serious side effects that are unknown or undisclosed at the time of their approval.

Pervasive computing will help to overcome these problems, by providing the means with which to conduct "in-life testing" [1]. Promising new drugs will first be tested in humans during late-stage discovery to prove their safety and efficacy. They will be tested still further in Phase II trials and submitted to regulators for conditional approval. They will then be launched on the market and subjected to extensive additional in-life testing, with a wide range of remote monitoring devices and networks.

In-life testing has various practical and economic advantages. It will dispense with the need to expose patients to placebos or dosing levels that are pharmacologically ineffective. It will be better able to pick up rare side effects and drug interactions, thus making the move from the laboratory to real life much safer. It will also reduce the frequency of the visits patients need to make to their doctor or hospital. Travel was one of the two biggest obstacles cited in a recent survey of potential trial patients. Similarly, it will reduce the amount of time that health care professionals need to spend in consultation with individual patients, enabling them to look after more patients more effectively.

32.5.5 Round-the-Clock Health Management

The same technologies that support in-life testing will enable health care professionals to monitor the rest of their patients from a distance. Pervasive computing is particularly suitable for monitoring people with chronic illnesses such as diabetes and coronary heart disease, by measuring their blood sugar levels, blood pressure, lipid levels, and other such biomarkers. It can also be used to track the constant elements of acute diseases, like the white blood cell count in patients with cancer, or to detect the danger signs suggesting an acute incident such as a heart attack or stroke.

32.5.6 Electronic Personalized Health Records

These data can then be fed into electronic medical records (EMR) such as those the NHS plans to introduce throughout the UK over the next 2 years. This represents a process that will ultimately both reduce the frequency with which patients have to visit their doctor and improve health care delivery. EMR or electronic personal health records (as they are also known) have already been established, or are being established, in many European nations, such as Denmark. The United States, with its decentralized health care industry, is behind the curve in these efforts. However, in early fall of 2005, IBM and eight other IT companies that form the Technology CEO Council (TCC), including Intel, HP, Dell, Motorola, EMC, Applied Materials, NCR, and Unisys committed to adopt electronic health records based on open standards. In addition to these private sector efforts, the US Department of

Veterans Affairs will also begin rolling out an on-line system for personal health records.

Beginning in 2006, IBM's active workforce, as part of their health benefits, will have access to a personal health record (PHR) application. With the new benefit, participating IBM employees in the United States will be able to input and manage information about their medications, allergies, medical histories, test results, and more. In addition, they may also create PHRs for eligible family members. The personal health record is protected by federal HIPAA privacy and security regulations. The new PHR feature is envisioned as one building block of a larger on-line health information resource that offers content tailored to personal needs and is designed to help participants actively manage their health. The long-term goal for such an electronic health record sytem is to make patient data securely available to health care providers such as hospitals and emergency personnel when and where the information is needed.

A complex national network will take several years to take shape, but this eventual integrated system will do more than just enable people to share their health records with doctors and hospitals. Such a global, information-rich, real-time system of health data can serve as an aid in identifying health trends, providing an early-warning indication of drug complications arising from concomitant medications or perhaps signaling the advent of pandemics (such as avian flu) or bioterrorism. In a TCC-commissioned study, 86% percent of US physicians surveyed said that a health care system that adopted information technology such as electronic health records would improve the overall quality of health care received by patients.

32.5.7 Trial Registries

In addition to the electronic personalized health record, another database that has the potential to revolutionize the pharmaceutical industry is the establishment of trial registries. One example of such a registry is www.clinicaltrials.gov, a NIH-sponsored voluntary registry. The International Committee of Medical Journal Editors (ICMJE) has stated that for clinical trial results to be considered for publication in journals that adhere to ICMJE standards, all clinical trials that started recruiting on or after July 1, 2005 must be registered with a public registry before the enrollment of their first patient. Ongoing trials not registered at inception will be considered by the ICMJE for publication if they were registered before September 13, 2005.

The impetus for the registration process is that by requiring registration at the start of a trial, the public will know the number of trials and their key milestones and end points. Unpublished trials would raise a potential flag to physicians. In addition, by knowing commitment to key milestones and end points up front, there is less chance of sugar coating results.

But the power of pervasive computing is not simply its ability to monitor the health of individual patients and trigger remedial action; it will also encourage compliance and persistence. Many patients do not stick to their treatment regimen, even when they risk becoming seriously ill. In one recent study of compliance levels in patients with high cholesterol, for example, only 33% of patients were still using a statin at the end of 12 months, and only 13% were still doing so at the end of five years [11 and references therein]. A number of factors contribute to such low levels of compliance, but a patient who knows that a drug is doing him/her good because there is visible proof of its efficacy is far more likely to keep taking it than one who has to rely on infrequent visits to the doctor.

However, it is important to identify where pervasive computing cannot add value, and to distinguish between what it can and cannot do. There is no point, for example, in using it for one-off tests to identify whether a patient has a particular disease subtype, such as breast cancer arising from overexpression of the Her-2 gene. It is only useful for measuring changes in an existing condition on an iterative basis. There is probably little point, either, in trying to monitor side effects that are better measured qualitatively, such as dizziness, rashes, headaches, and nausea; although these are common adverse reactions, they are essentially subjective.

Similarly, pervasive computing can only be used to monitor the *known* risks associated with a particular disease or drug, or those associated with a common drug combination (such as the cocktail of drugs for high blood pressure, angina, and high cholesterol that many elderly patients require). It cannot be used to measure unknown risks or unusual drug combinations.

But although pervasive computing may not be a universal panacea, it will certainly have a profound impact on drug development and health care delivery [14]. Moreover, one of the areas in which it promises to yield greatest fruit is in the treatment of the diseases that are now the world's biggest killers. According to a report published by the World Health Organization in 2002: "Non-communicable conditions, including cardiovascular diseases, diabetes, obesity, cancer, and respiratory diseases, now account for 59% of the 56.5 million deaths annually and 45.9% of the global burden of disease."

Pervasive computing will be one of the most powerful tools in combating this burden, in developing effective new drugs for patients with different disease subtypes; helping health care professionals and patients alike to monitor their condition; and enabling patients who might otherwise require hospitalization to enjoy an active, independent life for as long as possible.

32.6 SUMMARY

During the course of this chapter we have described the changing environment that will eventually see the pharmaceutical industry producing a range of products and services far removed from the blockbusters of today. This poses significant challenges to these corporate behemoths. The avalanche of data from new technologies and high-throughput biology will need to be accommodated, integrated, and shared effectively across these large, global organizations. Sophisticated search methods will be required to enable the mining of these huge data resources in order to facilitate faster, earlier, and informed decision-making. Powerful computers combined with more sophisticated algorithms will enable the *in silico* biosimulation of a range of experiments currently only possible in the laboratory, animals, or human subjects. The implications for predicting the physical properties, toxicology profiles, and efficacy of molecules in early stages of development would realize enormous time and cost savings, as well as ensure that as few human subjects as possible are exposed to adverse events and nonefficacious medicines.

We have also shown that the increasing integration of computers into our everyday life will include IT as a component of diagnosing, monitoring, and treating the diseases we are susceptible to and will eventually develop. There will need to be an extensive partnership between Pharma, regulators, payers, physicians, and patients for this to become a reality, but pervasive computing will play a central enabling role.

Although, as stated at the beginning of this chapter, novel IT strategies cannot transform the pharmaceutical industry; the discovery, development, and delivery to the patient of innovative new medicines meeting a variety of unmet medical needs is entirely dependent on the successful implementation and integration of powerful, predictive, and pervasive computing.

REFERENCES

1. Arlington S, Davies N, Barnett S, Palo J. IBM Business Consulting Services, *Pharma 2010: The Threshold of Innovation*. 2005. Copies available at http://www1.ibm.com/industries/healthcare/doccontent/resource/thought/390030105.html
2. Davies N, Peakman, T. Making the most of your discovery data. *Drug Discovery World*, 2004; Spring Edition.
3. META Group, *Worldwide IT Benchmark Report 2004*, Vol. 1 2004 IT Spending & Staffing Analysis: Pharmaceuticals & Medical Equipment. 2003; p.2.
4. Ramos, L. *Smart Spending Plans For Pharma IT. Six Winning Technology Opportunities For Life Sciences*, 2005; Forrester Research.
5. PricewaterhouseCoopers. Pharmaceutical Sector Insights: Annual Report 2002. 2003; p.4.
6. Mullin R. Dealing with data overload. *Chem Eng News* 2004; 22 March; 19–24.
7. How Much Information? at http://www.sims.berkeley.edu/research/projects/how-much-info-2003/execsum.htm#summary.
8. Cobbs C. Machines and genes: superfast computers aid today's genetic advances. *Orlando Sentinel* 2002; July 15, p.G1.
9. Silicon Reality. IBM Business Computing Services. 2004; Download at http://www1.ibm.com/businesscenter/smb/gb/en/gcllifescience/gcl_xmlid/17341/nav_id/lifesciences

10. *Genetic Engineering News* 2004.
11. Singh J, Ling LE, Sawyer JS, Lee W-C, Zhang F, Yingling JM. Transforming the TGFβ pathway: convergence of distinct lead generation strategies on a novel kinase pharmacophore for TGFβRI (ALK5). *Curr Opin Drug Discov Dev* 2004;7:437–45.
12. Weiser M. The computer for the 21st century. *Sci Am* 1991;265:66–75.
13. Davies N, Henderson S. Drugs, devices and the promise of pervasive computing. *Curr Drug Discov* 2003; October: 25–28.
14. Stanford V. Using pervasive computing to deliver elder care. *IEEE Pervasive Comput Mobile Ubiquitous Syst* 2002;1:10–13.
15. Ananthaswamy A. March of the motes. *New Scientist* 2003; 23 August 2003: 26–31.

INDEX

Computer Applications in Pharmaceutical Research and Development, Edited by Sean Ekins.
ISBN 0-471-73779-8